W9-AMM-505

Springer Series on Rehabilitation

Editor: Myron G. Eisenberg, PhD
Veterans Affairs Medical Center, Hampton, VA

Consulting Editor: Thomas E. Backer, PhD
Human Interaction Research Institute, Los Angeles, CA

1981 The Psychology of Disability
Carolyn L. Vash, PhD

1982 Disabled People as Second-Class Citizens
Myron G. Eisenberg, PhD, et al.

1982 Behavioral Approaches to Rehabilitation
Elaine Greif, PhD, and Ruth G. Matarazzo, PhD

1984 Chronic Illness and Disabilities Through the Life Span: Effects on Self and Family
Myron G. Eisenberg, PhD, et al.

1985 Handbook of Private Sector Rehabilitation
Lewis J. Taylor, PhD, CRC, et al.

1986 Applied Rehabilitation Counseling
T. F. Riggar, EdD, et al.

1988 Family Interventions Throughout Chronic Illness and Disability
P. Power, SdD, CRC, NCC, et al.

1991 Disability in the United States: A Portrait From National Data
Susan Thompson-Hoffman, MA, and Inez Fitzgerald Storck, MA, Editors

1991 Treating Families of Brain-Injury Survivors
Paul R. Sachs, PhD

1994 Personality and Adversity: Psychospiritual Aspects of Rehabilitation
Carolyn L. Vash, PhD

1997 Rehabilitation Counseling: Profession and Practice
Dennis Maki, PhD, and Ted Riggar, EdD

1998 Medical Aspects of Disability: A Handbook for the Rehabilitation Professional, second edition
Myron G. Eisenberg, PhD, et al.

Myron G. Eisenberg, PhD, is Director of Psychological Services, and Director of Research Services, at the Department of Veterans Affairs Medical Center in Hampton, VA, and is Associate Professor of both Physical Medicine and Rehabilitation and of Psychiatry and Behavioral Sciences at Eastern Virginia Medical School, Norfolk. He obtained his PhD from Northwestern University and received postdoctoral training at the University of Toronto's Clarke Institute. Dr. Eisenberg has published extensively in the area of rehabilitation, holds editorial board positions on several journals, is the immediate past-Editor of *Rehabilitation Psychology*, and is a member of several national task forces charged with investigating various quality-of-life issues of importance to persons with chronic disabling conditions. Dr. Eisenberg has received recognition at the local, regional, and national level for contributions he has made to the rehabilitation of persons with physical impairments. A Fellow and Past President of the American Psychological Association's Division of Rehabilitation Psychology, he is actively involved in heightening the public's awareness of the importance of rehabilitation through the promotion of research. In addition, he is interested in the development of standards that will establish a more effective and consistent basis for evaluating the performance of individual rehabilitation service providers.

Robert L. Glueckauf, PhD, is Professor and Director of the Center for Research on Telehealth and Health Care Communications in the Department of Clinical and Health Psychology at the University of Florida. He obtained his MS and PhD degrees in clinical psychology at Florida State University. Dr. Glueckauf is a Past President of the American Psychological Association's Division of Rehabilitation Psychology and currently serves as Associate Editor for Special Issues for *Rehabilitation Psychology*. Dr. Glueckauf has authored over 50 empirical and theoretical articles, books, and chapters in the field of health care and rehabilitation. As an advocate and scientist, he is committed to improving the quality of life of persons with disabilities through the promotion of community-based interventions and effective health care legislation. His current research activities include evaluation of the effectiveness of behavioral telehealth interventions for rural teens with disabilities and their families, process studies on the quality of interactions between telehealth providers and clients, and analysis of health care policy and its impact on psychological practice, education, and research.

Herbert H. Zaretsky, PhD, is currently Administrator, Department of Rehabilitation Medicine at the Rusk Institute, New York University Medical Center, and a faculty member of New York University's School of Medicine and College of Dentistry. He received his PhD from Adelphi University. Dr. Zaretsky has published extensively in the field of rehabilitation in such areas as psychological aspects of disability, geriatric rehabilitation, learning and conditioning with the neurologically impaired and spinal-cord injured, rehabilitation psychology and long-term care of the chronically ill, chronic pain management, and behavioral medicine applications to rehabilitation. In addition, he has participated in numerous symposia and panels on topics of current interest to rehabilitation, sponsored by the American Psychological Association. Dr. Zaretsky is a Fellow of the American Psychological Association and Past President of APA's Division of Rehabilitation Psychology. He is also a Consulting Editor for *Rehabilitation Psychology* and the *Archives of Physical Medicine and Rehabilitation* and the 1992 recipient of the Division's Distinguished Contribution to Rehabilitation Psychology Award. His present interests focus on the development of innovative multidisciplinary rehabilitation programs and the enhancement of the interdisciplinary team approach in the delivery of quality rehabilitation services.

Second Edition

MEDICAL ASPECTS OF DISABILITY

A Handbook for the Rehabilitation Professional

Myron G. Eisenberg
Robert L. Glueckauf
Herbert H. Zaretsky
Editors

Springer Publishing Company

Contents

services are being delivered. We are pleased that the book is being widely used and confident that information contained in it will prepare its readers for the challenges that await them in the world of clinical practice.

M.G.E.
November 1998

Preface

Medical Aspects of Disability: A Handbook for the Rehabilitation Professional responds to the need for a text that provides concise and current yet comprehensive and authoritative coverage of medical aspects of disabling conditions, including discussions of their functional presentation, prognosis, psychological and vocational sequelae, and other background information critical to the study of disability. It is a text designed to assist the student preparing for a career in the field of rehabilitation and the practitioner in need of a reference guide. Comprehensiveness of coverage in a single volume on a topic of this dimension has realistic limits, however. Therefore, readers looking for exhaustive coverage of specific conditions can turn to other sources, many of which are identified in this text's extensive reference lists.

People with disabilities are one of the largest minorities in the United States. The 1991 report of the National Institutes of Health's Institute of Medicine, *Disability in America*, recognized disability as the "Nation's largest public health problem." It identifies about 35 million Americans—one person in seven—as having a physical or mental disability that interferes with daily living.

The *Disability in America* report provides new information on the extent of disability in this country:

- More than 9 million people have physical or mental conditions that keep them from being able to work, attend school, or maintain a household.
- Disabilities are disproportionately higher among minorities, older people, and lower socioeconomic groups.
- Developmental disabilities (e.g., cerebral palsy, seizure disorders, mental retardation, hearing and vision impairments, spina bifida) are diagnosed in 80,000 children each year. There are as many as 4 million people of all ages with developmental disabilities.
- Between 10,000 and 20,000 people sustain spinal-cord injuries each year, resulting in quadriplegia in half the cases.

- The U.S. government spends about $60 billion annually to assist people with disabilities through medical and income support.
- People with disabilities, on average, are older and have lower incomes than others.

Additional information, obtained from the National Institutes of Health's *1990 Report of the Task Force on Medical Rehabilitation Research*, sheds further light on the magnitude of this issue by citing the following statistics:

- Almost 4% of the U.S. population has disabilities so severe they are unable to carry out the major activity of their age group (playing, attending school, working, or attending to self-care).
- An additional 6% of the population are restricted in their major activity.
- Disability imposes an economic cost estimated at 6.5% of the gross national product.
- The average American spends nearly 12 years in a state of limited functioning because of acute and chronic conditions.

Most recently, Congress has been applying a new focus to both the medical and socioeconomic issues affecting the 35 million Americans with disabilities. The Americans with Disabilities Act (ADA) of 1990, which went into effect on July 26, 1992, is the first major federal civil rights legislation in 26 years. It prohibits employment discrimination against people with disabilities, who are otherwise qualified. The ADA provides people with disabilities access to public places such as doctor's offices, restaurants, and businesses and to public transportation and telecommunications. The ADA has the potential of providing more employment opportunities for America's over 13 million working-age people with disabilities.

It is hoped that *Medical Aspects of Disability: A Handbook for the Rehabilitation Professional* will help equip the practitioner and the student alike with information necessary to make a critical difference in the quality of life and independence of persons with disabilities. This text's ultimate goal, however, is to add to the knowledge base needed for clinicians to effect the meaningful integration of persons with disabilities into this nation's social and vocational fabric.

Introduction to the First Edition

Over the past decade we have witnessed a rapid expansion in the development and utilization of rehabilitation services. The number of medical rehabilitation inpatient units, for example, has more than doubled since the early 1980s. As of 1989, there were 849 free-standing rehabilitation hospitals and medical rehabilitation units in acute care facilities (National Association of Rehabilitation Facilities, 1991); this statistic is undoubtedly an underestimate of the current number of inpatient facilities. The number of outpatient rehabilitation programs also has greatly increased. In 1980, 27% of U.S. hospitals offered outpatient rehabilitation treatment; as of 1987, almost 40% had rehabilitation programs (American Hospital Association, 1989).

Ironically, as a consequence of this growth, the field of clinical rehabilitation faces a number of challenging problems. There is a critical shortage of qualified rehabilitation specialists, particularly in psychology, physical therapy, occupational therapy, and nursing (e.g., McNett, 1980). Compounding this problem, graduate training programs responsible for educating rehabilitation professionals continue to be understaffed and have persistent difficulties attracting well-qualified faculty.

One of the most pressing concerns of rehabilitation educators is the predominance of the medical model in academic textbooks that address issues of functional performance and rehabilitation intervention (cf. Halter, Bond, & DeGraaf-Kaser, 1992; Wright, 1959, 1972). Most clinical rehabilitation texts (e.g., Kottke, Stillwell, & Lehman, 1982) have emphasized the importance of physiological and neuropsychological processes in shaping the daily activities of persons with disabilities. In contrast, only limited attention has been paid to the role of social-psychological factors (e.g., compliance with treatments, barriers to employment, family support) in predicting rehabilitation outcome (Wright & Fletcher, 1982).

One common assumption of the medical model is that severity of disability is highly predictive of psychosocial functioning. Put simply, the more severe the disability, the poorer the anticipated psychosocial and vocational prognosis. An unfortunate consequence of this form of reasoning is that health care professionals may be less likely to prescribe psychosocial interventions to those who most need it (i.e., the most severely disabled). It is enlightening to note that this widespread medical-model assumption has little scientific merit. Across several studies with different rehabilitation populations (see Eisenberg & Glueckauf, 1991), psychosocial factors have been found to exert a stronger influence on the quality of life of persons with disabilities than severity of illness. The same argument can be applied to the widely held belief that certain personality traits are routinely associated with certain medical disorders (see Pincus, Callahan, Bradley, Vaughn, & Wolfe, 1986). The editors of the current text have made a serious attempt to ensure that contemporary theory and research on adjustment to disability have been taken into account in discussing the implications of medical disabilities.

A troubling observation from both our graduate students and practitioners in the field also instigated the creation of this book. We have frequently heard that it is difficult to locate reading materials that adequately integrate current information on the medical characteristics, psychological assessment, and treatment of individuals with chronic disabilities. Rehabilitation faculties have also told us that they are hard pressed to find current textbooks providing broad coverage of the medical aspects of disabilities and their social and vocational consequences. We hope that the current text will meet the need for a state-of-the-art reference linking medical factors, assessment, and vocational intervention for persons with chronic disabilities.

We have organized the text into three major sections: (1) an introduction to key topics and issues that are directly relevant to acquiring a global understanding of the theoretical underpinnings of medical aspects of disability; (2) a series of review chapters covering the functional presentation, treatment, prognosis, and psychological and vocational implications of specific disabling medical conditions; and (3) a collection of chapters that address trends and emerging developments in the area. The primary function of the first section is to provide an overreaching framework for examining the major objectives and outcome expectations of rehabilitation intervention approaches. It also presents an overview of major body systems to facilitate understanding of the medical complications associated with specific complications associated with specific chronic disabilities. The second section of the text shifts to a description of the functional presentation, treatment, prognosis, and quality-of-life implications of a variety of physical and mental disabilities. We have given special emphasis to the potential psychological and vocational concerns associated with each medical condition. The third section considers a series of emerging trends and seminal developments, which are enlarging the scope of treatment options and shaping patterns of practice and service delivery.

The editors hope that the current text will encourage students and practitioners in health care disciplines and vocational rehabilitation to examine critically their assumptions about the relationships between medical disability and psychosocial and vocational functioning. If we have successfully met our objectives, the current text should sensitize the professional and student to the need to consider both medical and situational factors in assessing the impact of disability.

Finally, we have designed the current textbook for use in medical aspects of disability courses across the broad spectrum of rehabilitation disciplines, including nursing, vocational rehabilitation, psychology, and recreation, speech, occupational, and physical therapy. The material covered in each chapter can be easily assimilated by both advanced undergraduates and graduate students who are preparing for fieldwork or full-time employment in clinical rehabilitation. Classroom presentations and group discussions can be used to further enrich students' appreciation of the reciprocal relationships between physical and psychological functioning in chronic disabilities.

REFERENCES

American Hospital Association. (1989). *Survey of medical rehabilitation hospitals and programs—1988*. Chicago: American Hospital Association.

Eisenberg, M. G., & Glueckauf, R. L. (Eds.). (1991). *Empirical approaches to the psychosocial aspects of disability*. New York: Springer Publishing Co.

Halter, C. A., Bond, G. R., & DeGraff-Kaser, R. (1992). How treatment of persons with mental illness is portrayed in undergraduate psychology textbooks. *Community Mental Health Journal, 28*, 29–42.

Kottke, F. J., Stillwell, G. K., & Lehmann, J. F. (Eds.). (1982). *Krusen's handbook of physical medicine and rehabilitation* (3rd ed.). Philadelphia: W. B. Saunders.

McNett, I. (1980). Mental health services for handicapped fall between the cracks. *APA Monitor, 11*(4), 15.

National Association of Rehabilitation Facilities. (1991, November). *Medical rehabilitation: What it is and where it is: A discussion* (NARF Monograph Series). Washington, DC: Author.

Pincus, T., Callahan, L., Bradley, L. A., Vaughn, W., & Wolfe, F. (1986). Elevated MMPI scores for hypochondriasis, depression and hysteria in patients with rheumatoid arthritis reflect disease rather than psychological status. *Arthritis and Rheumatism, 29*, 1456–1466.

Wright, B. (1959). *Psychology and rehabilitation*. Washington, DC: American Psychological Association.

Wright, B. (1972). Value-laden beliefs and principles for rehabilitation psychology. *Rehabilitation Psychology, 19*, 38–45.

Wright, B., & Fletcher, B. (1982). Uncovering hidden resources: A challenge in assessment. *Professional Psychology, 13*, 229–235.

PART I

An Introduction to Key Topics and Issues

Chapter 1

Comprehensive Rehabilitation: Themes, Models, and Issues

Robert Allen Keith

Long-term demographic and epidemiological trends in industrial societies, including the United States, have changed the focus of health care. Communicable diseases such as smallpox and measles no longer exact a toll on life. Modern medicine, better hygiene and living conditions, and improved nutrition have had a profound effect on health. Since 1900, U.S. mortality rates have declined 50% (Rothenberg & Koplan, 1990). Not only are more people staying alive, they are living longer. Projections show the proportion of the population over age 65 increasing from about 11% in 1980 to over 18% by 2030 (Rice & Feldman, 1983).

These two trends, more individuals staying alive and more living longer, have greatly increased chronic disease rates. A major share of health care is now devoted to treating the consequences of coronary heart disease, strokes, cancer, and arthritis, to name the most prominent chronic diseases. Individuals with catastrophic injuries, such as brain injury or spinal cord injury, now survive more frequently. Chronic diseases and injuries result in large numbers who require specialized services to regain lost functions: the role of comprehensive rehabilitation.

Although there are many kinds of rehabilitation services, the focus here is on physical disability. The service area is medical rehabilitation with the array of professionals usually found on the comprehensive team: physiatrists (physical medicine specialists), other medical specialties, nurses, physical therapists, occupational therapists, psychologists, speech and language specialists, social workers, recreation therapists, and orthotists (individuals who design and make assistive devices, such as leg braces). The population they serve are individuals with strokes, brain injuries, spinal cord injuries, orthopedic disorders, neuromuscular diseases, and numerous other conditions. The scope of medical rehabilitation is wide, because programs begin with the remediation of basic self-care skills and often progress through improving cognitive functions (such as memory and attention) and social skills. To accomplish such an ambitious mission, the comprehensive team is needed.

Although medical rehabilitation is a relatively small part of health care, during the 1980s and early 1990s, it experienced considerable growth. According to the American Rehabilitation Association, which monitors statistics from the Health Care Financing Administration, there were 68 freestanding rehabilitation hospitals in 1985; by 1996 there were 195, a nearly threefold increase (American Rehabilitation Association, personal communication, 1997). In 1985 there were 386 rehabilitation units in acute care hospitals, and by 1996 the number had gone up to 841. The tally of comprehensive outpatient programs is more difficult to determine. Facilities choosing to participate in the Medicare Health Insurance Program rose from 86 in 1985 to 386 in 1996. Many outpatient providers choose not to participate in Medicare, however, so these numbers do not reflect the total outpatient count very accurately. They do illustrate the rapid growth of outpatient rehabilitation care.

The provision of rehabilitation in skilled nursing facilities is one of the fastest-growing rehabilitation services if anecdotal evidence from providers and payers can be believed. Because there is still no accepted definition or certification of such care, reasonable estimates of numbers are not available. Costs are considerably lower than for comprehensive hospital rehabilitation, although research on outcome comparisons is not well established. A study of stroke rehabilitation found costs and treatment intensity in a skilled nursing rehabilitation unit to be half of that in a hospital rehabilitation program with reasonably comparable outcomes (Keith, Wilson, & Gutierrez, 1995).

In spite of the vigorous growth, rehabilitation faces some uncertain times. All of health care is undergoing radical restructuring from managed care and an increasingly competitive marketplace. Treatment decisions, once the province of professionals, is now a responsibility shared with managers and payers. The philosophy of comprehensive rehabilitation is under heavy pressure as an expense no longer affordable. Despite the uncertainties in health care, medical rehabilitation has an important role in alleviating the increasing incidence of disability. The failure to meet this challenge will have heavy personal, social, and economic consequences (Pope & Tarlov, 1991).

THE ORIGINS OF REHABILITATION

The road to legitimacy has not been an easy one for rehabilitation medicine, for either physicians in this specialty or other health professionals in the field. An acquaintance with its origins helps to understand its current status and its response to changes in health care. The history of medical rehabilitation is scattered through various journals and presentations to professional societies. The best source of early beginnings is in Gritzer and Arluke's (1985) volume *The Making of Rehabilitation*. Most of this account is taken from that work. The focus is on physiatry, physical therapy, and occupational therapy. Although other professions have made important contributions to medical rehabilitation, these three have had the most prominent role in shaping the origins of the field.

Physiatry

The term *physiatry* is a confusing one for those unacquainted with the physical medicine and rehabilitation specialty designation because it is close to *psychiatry*, a more widely known term. It was chosen from a combination of the Greek *physis* (meaning nature) and *iatreia* (healing).

The basis for specialization began before World War I, when a group of physicians began using electrical stimulation and eventually added the modalities of hydrotherapy, heat, massage, and exercise. During the war these physicians, who called themselves physiotherapy physicians, joined other professionals in treating the consequences of injuries. After the conflict they returned to acute medicine.

World War II and the immediate postwar period brought significant changes to most health care professions, including physical medicine. Even though there were heavy demands for services, physical therapy physicians (yet another name) did not initially establish a claim for special competence. It remained for Howard Rusk, an internist outside physical medicine, to lay the groundwork for the modern field of physical medicine. He built a program on the use of convalescent time at an air force hospital that began to feature physician training in rehabilitation methods.

With status as a medical specialty in 1946 came a more explicit recognition of the commitment to rehabilitation. The emphasis was an important one because it marked a departure from the use of rest as the prescribed treatment during convalescence in favor of reconditioning. That emphasis has remained and, if anything, has become stronger in recent years with the general recognition of the importance of fitness.

Physical medicine and rehabilitation remains one of the smallest specialties in medicine, although the expansion of rehabilitation facilities has strengthened its position. The small number of physiatrists engaged in research is a matter of concern. The aggressive push by physical and occupational therapy for greater autonomy, particularly in independent practice, is a challenge to physician control, although the physiatrist is still acknowledged as the leader of the comprehensive treatment team.

Physical Therapy

The origins of physical therapy were also heavily tied to wartime needs. During World War I those individuals who had been orthopedic assistants were designated as reconstruction physiotherapy aides, and they began to work with physical therapy physicians.

In 1921 former military aides and a few physicians formed what was soon called the American Physiotherapy Association. There then followed a period of several years in which physiotherapy aides had to battle to establish their legitimacy and independence. Relations with medicine waxed and waned, with physicians insisting that aides call themselves physiotherapy technicians to differentiate themselves from physiotherapy physicians. By 1936 the American Medical Association was accrediting physiotherapy schools. Doctors also controlled the American Registry of Physical Therapy, which restricted the opening of private offices by technicians. According to Gritzer and Arluke (1985), even though there was lack of autonomy, the field of physiotherapy benefited from this association with medicine by establishing education and training standards that excluded those with poor preparation.

World War II did much to establish the status of modern physical therapy. When physicians acquired the title of physical medicine specialists instead of physical therapy physicians, those individuals who had been called aides or technicians were able to discard these terms for the designation of physical therapist.

The later history of physical therapy shows this field to be in a very strong position on the rehabilitation scene. In the early 1980s it broke the domination of the American Medical Association in the accreditation of physical therapists and set up its own accrediting organization. The close relationship with physiatry no longer remains because most referrals to physical therapists now come from other medical specialties (Institute of Medicine, 1989). A significant number have chosen independent practice rather than an institutional setting. The perception of the importance of physical reconditioning and the expansion of rehabilitation services has made physical therapy job growth greater than that of any other allied health occupation (Institute of Medicine, 1989).

Occupational Therapy

Gritzer and Arluke (1985) observe that the origins of occupational therapy can be traced to the belief that activity and work can be therapeutic, a connection first used for treating those with mental illness. Just prior to World War I, the first professional society for occupational therapy was formed. Early on, its members established the working principle that therapeutic activity should be physician-prescribed.

In the 1920s occupational therapy began to expand its base from mental institutions to include tuberculosis sanatoriums. The treatment of industrial accident injuries was also added to its domain. In the early years of World War II, occupational therapy still had to fight the view of its mission as diversional rather than therapeutic. Physical therapy physicians became interested in the potential of occupational therapy to bridge the gap between physical and vocational rehabilitation.

The postwar years have been marked by the push for greater autonomy and also by the continuing struggle to convey to other professionals and to the public just what it is that an occupational therapist does. The decision to opt for certification rather than licensure contributed to some ambiguity of status. It was only in 1987, for example, that occupational therapy was able to bill separately under Medicare. The inclusion of occupational therapy with physical therapy (later to include speech and language pathology) in the Medicare regulation mandating 3 hours a day of therapy has helped to consolidate occupational therapy's position in rehabilitation. Occupational therapists' unique expertise in sensory and cognitive retraining ensures that they will remain important members of the treatment team.

COMPREHENSIVE REHABILITATION OPERATIONS

Medical rehabilitation programs come in many forms, and they serve a variety of clients. In spite of this diversity, there has been a common philosophy of treatment that holds that the complex problems of individuals with severe disability require the services of a team of specialists; no one treater has the knowledge to cope with the complications involved. As already mentioned, there are serious challenges to the team concept. Using a full spectrum of specialists is admittedly expensive, particularly for an inpatient program. The prevailing philosophy among professionals is still for team care, although its form may be attenuated into lower intensity and skill levels, such as with skilled nursing facility rehabilitation.

Understanding rehabilitation operations requires a description of the kinds of facilities and programs, the caseloads that they serve, and some idea of how this group of professionals divides up the labor and goes about its usual routines. The rapidly changing health care scene means that some of the traditional forms of rehabilitation are being altered.

Types of Facilities

For many years there was no defining mechanism for determining the number of rehabilitation programs in the United States. Consequently, there were no reasonable estimates of the number and kinds of facilities in operation or of the populations they served. This uncertain identity obviously did not help the field's quest for greater visibility. It also meant that rehabilitation was often not included in health care planning or policy-making.

With the advent of a prospective payment system and the use of diagnosis related groups (DRGs) for Medicare in 1983, the situation changed. DRGs are based on the prediction of costs in groups of patients with similar problems, but some specialty hospitals had populations that were quite different from those of acute care hospitals. These facilities were designated as exempt from the use of DRGs and included rehabilitation hospitals.

To gain exemption, however, it was necessary to define what each of these facilities was, a task taken on by the Health Care Financing Administration (HCFA), the agency that makes policy for Medicare and Medicaid. In collaboration with professionals from rehabilitation, HCFA established a definition for inpatient medical rehabilitation that included, among other provisions, a case mix with at least 75% of patients in eight impairment groups and a coordinated multidisciplinary team (HCFA, 1983).

In the 1980s the American Hospital Association, as part of its annual survey of hospitals, began to include rehabilitation hospitals and units (Mullner, Nazum, & Matthews, 1983). The freestanding hospital is a self-contained facility devoted entirely to rehabilitation, without some services found in acute care, such as operating rooms and emergency rooms. The rehabilitation unit is a part of a larger acute care hospital.

Inpatient programs receive most patients from acute care hospitals. Because inpatients are still medically fragile and are severely impaired, close medical supervision and 24-hour nursing care are needed. All of the skills of the interdisciplinary team are required to assess the patient's skills, set up a treatment plan, and provide treatment. Treatment programs are usually intensive, that is, with a full schedule of therapy, because hospitalization is expensive.

Comprehensive outpatient rehabilitation facilities treat patients who do not require 24-hour nursing and who can remain home at night. These ambulatory services take a variety of forms, with a full range of disciplines and a treatment intensity that can vary from one session a month to several hours a week. The National Association of Rehabilitation Facilities (1988) (now the American Rehabilitation Association) recognizes several different outpatient programs. Day rehabilitation programs are for individuals who still require considerable medical monitoring and a full program but who are able to go home at night. Comprehensive outpatient programs have a full range of services but may use only portions of them for any one patient. Outpatient rehabilitation services, in distinction to programs, provide single or multiple therapies of a less coordinated nature. They may occur in either rehabilitation or acute care hospitals.

Residential rehabilitation focuses on community reentry and training for independent living in transitional living centers, community reentry programs, and independent living centers (National Association of Rehabilitation Facilities, 1988). The extent to which they are comprehensive in scope of service varies. Some programs may concentrate on a specific disability, such as head injury, spinal cord injury, or pain. Whereas transitional living centers (TLCs) commonly have a full therapy group, independent living centers operate with the goal of its members becoming autonomous of professional supervision.

Skilled nursing facilities with rehabilitation are a relatively new development in recuperative programs. Although nursing homes have traditionally admitted those with chronic long-term problems, often terminal, the skilled nursing facility (SNF) may have relatively short lengths of stay. Some of these facilities are able to offer many of the same services as the acute inpatient rehabilitation program at a lower cost. Services are typically less intensive than inpatient programs.

Specialty units emphasize care devoted to a single condition. One of the earliest examples was the unit dedicated to the treatment of spinal cord injury, a practice begun in England. Because of the high degree of skill required and the uniqueness of this catastrophic injury, spinal cord injury is commonly treated in a specialized unit.

Patients with cerebrovascular accidents or strokes are among the most frequent admissions to rehabilitation. Although most patients with strokes are treated as part of general rehabilitation, there are a number of specialty units. There have also been several studies demonstrating the effectiveness of such units in relation to other kinds of care (Jorgensen et al., 1995; Keith, 1996).

The 1980s was a period of rapid expansion of programs devoted to rehabilitation of those with brain injury, from only a dozen or so programs in 1980 to more than 600 in 1988 (Perry, 1989). For many years brain injury was not given much attention in rehabilitation, partially because methods of treatment and knowledge regarding this condition were not very good. An additional factor was the difficulty of doing therapy with individuals for whom behavior control is a problem. The advent of neuropsychology and of behavioral methods of treatment has helped considerably. Advances in imaging and other diagnostic techniques have greatly assisted understanding of brain-behavior linkages.

One of the most ubiquitous chronic disease problems, one with enormous economic consequences, is low back pain (Institute of Medicine, 1987). Individuals with this condition do not fit the usual rehabilitation regimen. Most can be seen on an outpatient basis, but the combination of relaxation and biofeedback, exercise, assertion training, and education about back mechanics requires a specialized program. There is still considerable controversy about the effectiveness of such programs, however (Deyo, Cherkin, Conrad, & Volinn, 1991).

Populations Served

Just as the lack of information about the number of facilities has hampered the development of medical rehabilitation, so too has the sparsity of caseload information been a hindrance. In recent years, however, a number of databases have been developed. The most extensive is that of the Uniform Data System (UDS) for Medical Rehabilitation (Hamilton, Granger, Sherwin, Zielezny, & Tashman, 1987). The assessment measure used in this system, the Functional Independence Measure (FIM) has rapidly become the most frequently used instrument for clinical and outcome uses. The UDS report for 1995, its most recent published account (Fiedler & Granger, 1997), was based on nearly 200,000 cases from 472 medical rehabilitation hospitals and units. According to this report, the most frequent groups seen in inpatient hospitals are patients with orthopedic conditions (34%) and with strokes (30%). Other important diagnoses include brain injury, spinal cord injury, amputations, and other neurological disorders.

Age is an important consideration in rehabilitation caseloads. In the UDS report mentioned above (Fiedler & Granger, 1997), the average age of all inpatients was 68 years, indicating the necessity of considering geriatric factors in treatment. Disabilities resulting from trauma, such as brain injury or spinal cord injury, have significantly lower ages, so many facilities have a split in age distributions.

Typical Program Operations

Although rehabilitation units do not all conduct their operations in the same way, programs have many common features because of the nature of the tasks involved.

Screening

The determination of the appropriateness of the individual for the services occurs before admission (in preadmission screening), after admission (in assessment), and during treatment (in monitoring progress). This continuing process is called utilization review and is one of the mechanisms to contain costs to ensure the proper fit between patient and services.

The admission criteria used in screening are a set of guidelines that presumably are predictive of rehabilitation success. The task is to select candidates with a middle band of severity. Those with continuing medical problems or those in a confused state would not be apt to take advantage of treatment. Likewise, individuals who easily walked about on their own might not need hospitalization and could use an outpatient program.

Diagnosis and Assessment

The distinction between these two terms is one that highlights the differences between acute care and rehabilitation. Diagnosis commonly refers to the process of determining the status of disease or other complaint and applying a remedy. In some cases, the cause is not identified, but the symptoms are still treated. Assessment, on the other hand, is concerned with the functional capacity of the patient and of his or her ability to profit from treatment.

The assessment process is a demanding test of the team's ability to coordinate the scheduling of time for various team members and to communicate their findings to each other. It is usually at the initial team conference that information about the patient is exchanged and evaluated, culminating in a treatment plan that anticipates the patient's progress through the various treatment stages.

Treatment

The treatment phase continues the intricate scheduling necessary to allow team members to have time with the patient. Because the time in program is costly, particularly for inpatient stays, it is mandatory that the patient's day be tightly scheduled. Many patients, particularly those older or frailer, may not be able to take advantage of a full schedule. With the current emphasis on shorter stays, patient endurance becomes a problem.

The division of labor requires that each team member be responsible for some area of functioning, with the patient passed from one discipline or department to another. Just transporting the patient from one treatment area to another takes time, of course, unless there is a unit in which all activities are concentrated. It has been found, for example, that stroke patients treated on a dedicated unit spent more time in treatment during the day than in units where patients went from one department to another (Keith & Cowell, 1987). In inpatient units, nurses see patients every day; physical and occupational therapy have sessions every working day (i.e., 5 or maybe 6 days a week). In 1983, HCFA published regulations for Medicare patients requiring that patients receive at least 3 hours a day of a combination of physical and occupational therapy (HCFA, 1983). Later, speech and language specialists were added to these two. Other disciplines, such as social work or psychology, usually see the patient less frequently. A study of traumatic brain and spinal cord injuries in eight rehabilitation hospitals found an average of 3.06 hours per day of billed therapy for brain injury and 2.64 hours per day for spinal cord injury (Heinemann, Hamilton, Linacre, Wright, & Granger, 1995). These figures do not include nursing or physician time.

Documentation and Progress Monitoring

Therapists spend an increasing amount of time writing notes in the medical record about the patient's progress and documenting what they did during a treatment session. Some of this is necessary for clinical management and judging patient gains in relation to the treatment plan, but much of it is for the benefit of third-party payers, who require detailed justification.

Although much information is exchanged informally among team members as they go about day-to-day duties, the team conference is the place where communication is the highest. Here reports from members are heard and information integrated and evaluated, with conclusions about progress and the direction of therapy. Many teams include the patient and family members in such deliberations at some point because they are as much a part of rehabilitation as are the professionals.

Discharge Planning

When the patient nears the goals set in the treatment plan, the focus shifts more toward the environment in which the patient is to live. Home visits by a team member is one way to evaluate home facilities, although payers are increasingly reluctant to pay for them. The extrapolation from one setting to another requires clinical experience and as much information as can be gained about family support and living arrangements. Patients usually leave with a discharge plan that includes medications, exercises or other routines, and referral back to a community doctor and frequently to the next phase of rehabilitation if appropriate. Follow-up arrangements for a clinic visit or a telephone call to determine the patient's status at some point postdischarge are frequently added.

THE TREATMENT TEAM AS REHABILITATION MODEL

Every human service has a practice ideology—the set of rules that govern its procedures. These guidelines are not arbitrary but have been built up by the experience of its practitioners over many years. An important contribution, particularly for well-established fields such as medicine, comes from empirical research, which helps to validate existing procedures and to suggest new ones.

A model helps also to establish the identity of a field and to aid in the differentiation between it and other fields and between experts and the laity. The comprehensive treatment team has become the centerpiece of modern rehabilitation medicine. Its model of treatment delivery distinguishes it from the rest of health care. The twin focus, on stabilizing and managing the medical effects of illness and injury and on the restoration of function, requires a unique configuration of professional skills. Although the comprehensive team philosophy is being challenged on economic grounds, it has not been replaced by any alternative.

Origins

The origins of the treatment team are a part of the history of rehabilitation medicine, although there are different explanations about why we have the current configuration of disciplines. The perception that there is a logical fit between the skills of the treaters and the problems of the patients they serve has been called the natural growth model by Gritzer and Arluke (1985). In this view, specialties were added to deal with increasingly complicated patient deficits and to get a better match between clinicians and the populations they served. Advances in technology and knowledge also require greater specialization.

A second view suggests that the current team arose from the attempts of each profession to make a place for itself in the marketplace, the political economy model. In this version, the establishing of professional territory, economic demand, and environmental factors, such as wars and government regulations, all play a role in solidifying who will be a member of the team.

A combination of both models is a reasonable explanation for the present comprehensive team. Certainly, there are rational reasons for the match between the technical skills of team members and the conditions they treat. Likewise, professional societies do maneuver to increase the power and economic advantage of their constituencies. However, the composition of the team is not fixed forever but may vary with changes in the health care climate.

Effectiveness of the Team

Even though the comprehensive team has been the treatment model in rehabilitation from the early days of the field, the amount of research on team functioning and effectiveness has been very modest. Reviews of research have concluded that coordinated interdisciplinary team care is superior to general medical care or uncoordinated rehabilitation (Keith, 1991; Ottenbacher & Jannell, 1993; Strasser & Falconer, 1997). Much of this work has concentrated on the use of specialty units or programs in the treatment of individuals with strokes. In a meta-analysis of clinical trials in stroke rehabilitation, Ottenbacher and Jannell (1993) found that programs of focused treatment across a variety of interventions were superior to standard medical care. One of the most convincing studies was community-based research in which all patients with strokes in two areas went either to a hospital with a stroke unit or one using general medical care (Jorgensen et al., 1995). Treatment on the dedicated stroke unit reduced the relative risk of death by 50%, reduced the risk of discharge to a nursing home by 40%, and nearly doubled the rate of home discharge.

The dynamics of the treatment team have begun to receive attention (Strasser & Falconer, 1997), with work on interprofessional relations, team building, involvement and participation, communication, and problem solving. The research is in an early phase of investigating what organizational and personal factors contribute to effective teams. A special 1997 issue of *Topics in Stroke Rehabilitation* is devoted to the topic of linking team processes to treatment effectiveness.

Just what it is that contributes to the superiority of comprehensive or specialty teams over alternatives is still a matter of conjecture. Early intervention appears to be one factor (Ottenbacher & Jannell, 1993). The amount or intensity of treatment might be expected to be higher in specialty teams, but such is not the case. Patients with strokes, for example, may receive more physical and occupational therapy under general medical care than with stroke units (Jorgensen et al., 1995). The effects of higher treatment intensity on outcomes, whether or not delivered by a specialty unit, have thus far been ambiguous (Keith, 1997b). Presumably better communication and relations among team members, better coordination of services, and greater expertise should result in more efficient and effective treatment. Until there is research linking organizational processes to outcomes, answers about what contributes to treatment effectiveness will remain speculative.

RESEARCH AND EVALUATION ISSUES

Research is essential to health care because it tests current clinical procedures and points to potentially new directions. The most vigorously applied areas are those with a solid foundation of basic research. Rehabilitation has an added dimension in its research repertoire in the form of program evaluation. It is one of the few human services that requires program evaluation for accreditation. Concern with program objectives, measures, outcomes, and accountability has had a beneficial long-term effect on the field. Programs have been able to present their results to both professional and lay audiences in much more specific form. Whereas the rest of health care has begun to focus on outcomes as a way to judge quality of care, rehabilitation has had this orientation for many years.

Theoretical and Conceptual Issues

Theories are the blueprints to help understand what goes on in rehabilitation and to chart research directions for the field. For many years there was little interest in theory-building, but that has begun to change.

Disablement Theory

One of the earliest theories in rehabilitation and one that continues to be the most prominent, concerns the consequences of disease and injury, that is, disablement. The World Health Organization (WHO) model (1980) is most frequently mentioned:

Disease → Impairment → Disability → Handicap

In it disease or injury leads to impairment, which involves deficits at the organ level. For example, paralysis results in loss of hand function and can be measured in physical terms. To understand the consequences of this loss, however, it is necessary to examine how meaningful tasks are affected, for example, the inability to write a letter or dial a telephone—a disability. Finally, there is the stage of handicap in which the disability results in deficiencies in social role functioning. Paralysis of the hand, to continue this example, might mean the individual could no longer be employed in a former job—the loss of work role.

The WHO model is useful in conceptualizing the links between physical states, the ability to perform tasks, and the social consequences of various levels of task performance. It implies greater linearity of causation between elements than exists, however. The concept of handicap is the least well elaborated, with disagreement about what the term means, although there are measurement scales with promise (Willer, Button, & Corrigan, 1997). Whiteneck, Fougeyrollas, and Gerhart (1997) reviewed the utility of WHO disablement concepts, particularly in relation to treatment outcomes, and added two factors. The subjective perceptions of individuals with disabilities is frequently included in outcomes, often in the form of satisfaction with service and with treatment results, and should be a part of the model. Environmental factors influence all of the stages of the WHO model and, according to these authors, should also be included.

Treatment Theory

The drive to identify the most cost-effective treatment methods has brought the realization that there must be a better understanding of the rationale of treatment. Most outcome research has not included detailed description of what treatment was given, so there has been little empirical basis on which to identify the elements of intervention that have the greatest effects.

An obvious place to begin formulation about treatment theory is to inventory the various factors that are the inputs, processes, and outcomes of rehabilitation. Keith and Lipsey (1993) described the determinants of rehabilitation outcomes as patient characteristics, internal facility factors (including staff qualifications and organization), external factors (family support, health care funding), and treatment (frequency, duration, type, and philosophy). Duncan, Hoenig, Samsa, and Hamilton (1997) divided their model into micro and macro elements. The micro side included patient factors, disablement status, the structure of the intervention, and the intervention method, including duration, frequency, intensity, and specificity. Macro elements spanned the expected outcomes, characteristics of providers, setting and system of care, and how services were provided. In their model of treatment effectiveness, Strasser and Falconer (1997) included hospital characteristics, treatment (dosage, timing, specificity, and efficacy), participants, team factors (social climate, interprofessional relations, and managerial practices), the environment, and patient outcomes.

Strategies for building treatment theory have emphasized the importance of detailed specification of assessment and treatment (Duncan et al., 1997; Keith, 1997a). Treatment strength has been advanced as a key concept in understanding how the various components of treatment interact with patient characteristics (Keith, 1997b), including purity, specificity, dose (intensity and duration), timing, and treatment characteristics. One implicit assumption about treatment is that greater exposure, in terms of duration and intensity, results in greater benefit. Keith (1997b) found that research on length of stay tends to confirm this assumption, although the uneven work on intensity is ambiguous. The greatest amount of research on specificity has been done on stroke rehabilitation units, with results that generally show greater benefit than with nonspecialized treatment. The various models that authors have constructed are useful for providing a conceptual framework for investigation, although it is apparent that research on treatment processes is in a beginning stage.

Learning Theory

Although learning plays a prominent role in physical and cognitive restoration, there has never been much interest in applying learning theory principles in rehabilitation. Operant conditioning and social learning theory have been used with considerable success in programs for pain management and traumatic brain injury, but wider use of these orientations has not occurred. To encourage learning theory applications in medical rehabilitation, the National Center for Medical Rehabilitation Research initiated a conference held at the National Institutes of Health in August 1997. There were overviews of traditional learning theories as well as those relating to motor learning and control, cognitive learning, and self-management theory. Discussion of key research issues included papers on the nature of recovery in relation to learning and on generalization and transfer of training. Applications of learning principles for various clinical populations were considered, as well as recommendations for research. The publications resulting from this conference may encourage the study of the effects of learning on restoration of function.

Measurement Issues

Uniform Data System

The greatest influence on patient assessment and data collection in the field has been the UDS. The system was designed with recognition of the importance of having data elements and a functional status measure that would be used uniformly throughout a large number of facilities. Under the initial leadership of Carl Granger and Byron Hamilton of the State University of New York at Buffalo, UDS now collects inpatient information from nearly 500 hospitals and units in 48 states (Fiedler & Granger, 1997). The FIM, which was developed for the system, has become the most widely used functional status instrument in rehabilitation and the object of dozens of research investigations. UDS annual reports of patient statistics furnish norms for inpatient hospitals for lengths of stay, characteristics of impairment groups, and other vital data for the industry (Fiedler & Granger, 1997).

Rasch Analysis

Most of the scales used to rate patient performance are constructed by assigning numbers to a series of attributes. For example, 1—fully independent, 2—requires minimal assistance, and so on. In terms of measurement theory, these are ordinal scales; that is, each step is greater or lesser than the next, but there is no set interval between steps. The difference between minimal and moderate assistance may not be the same as that between moderate and maximum assistance. Arithmetic operations, such as adding numbers for a total score, then become problematic. A statistical procedure devised by the Danish mathematician, Georg Rasch (1960), was designed to produce scales from ordinal data that have equal intervals and are unidimensional; that is, they measure one dimension of performance. Rasch analysis, then, is a method used to produce scales that have more powerful psychometric properties.

Benjamin Wright and J. M. Linacre of the University of Chicago have collaborated with several investigators to introduce Rasch analysis methods into the refinement of functional assessment methods (Wright, Linacre, & Heinemann, 1993). Rasch analysis has been used extensively with the FIM, confirming that its motor and cognitive scales are separate factors (Heinemann, Linacre, Wright, Hamilton, & Granger, 1993). Similar statistical methods have been used with the Patient Evaluation and Conference System (PECS) (Silverstein, Fisher, Kilgore, Harley, & Harvey, 1992) and for the measurement of handicap with the Craig Handicap Assessment and Reporting Technique (CHART) (Whiteneck, Charlifue, Gerhart, Overholser, & Richardson, 1992). The *Journal of Outcome Measurement*, a new publication devoted to outcome measurement in health, education, and the social sciences, has devoted much of its space to research using Rasch analysis.

Several new publications concerned with measurement have been forthcoming. McDowell and Newell have a second edition of their book *Measuring Health* (1996), a useful volume of evaluations of health status measures. A text more specifically focused on rehabilitation is *Functional Assessment and Outcome*

Measures for the Rehabilitation Health Professional by Dittmar and Gresham (1997). In addition to examining functional status scales, it also provides discussion of the rationale for such instruments. The *Journal of Rehabilitation Outcomes Measurement*, new in 1997, features work on the development of outcome measures and applications of outcome information.

Prominent Research Issues

Uncertainties regarding funding have not only affected the service delivery side of health care, they have also had an impact on research. Although government sources of research money are still available, at a modest level, rehabilitation providers are hard-pressed to find time and resources to conduct research. To reduce expenses, many programs have had to cut staff, leaving little time for research. Despite fiscal restrictions, however, there is still a significant amount of research being carried out.

Outcomes Research

Determining what strategies will improve health while adhering to cost restraints has become a major preoccupation of health care. *Outcomes research* is the term used to describe the search for cost-effective interventions. As a way to further this search, Congress, in 1989, created the Agency for Health Care Policy and Research (AHCPR). One of its missions is to identify the most effective treatment for illnesses affecting large numbers of the population. Toward that end, it has funded several patient outcomes research teams that search the research and clinical literature and conduct research on the most effective treatment for a particular condition, for example, benign prostate enlargement. This has resulted in an intensive scrutiny of the world's medical literature. Although most of these teams have been concerned with acute conditions, there are some illnesses relevant to rehabilitation. For example, a group has developed guidelines for poststroke rehabilitation (Gresham et al., 1995).

Outcomes have been of long-standing interest in rehabilitation. There is fairly good consensus about the general nature of treatment goals: improvement in functional performance, discharge to the least restrictive environment, reduction in the use of personal and health care services, and improvement in productive activity. There is less agreement about how to measure such outcomes. The underlying assumptions of measures, that is, their conceptual bases, have had relatively little examination (Keith, 1994). Independence is an underlying theme, involving social norms for what is desirable behavior.

A 1994 conference on evaluating the effectiveness of rehabilitation practices, sponsored by the National Center for Medical Rehabilitation Research, resulted in a volume devoted to issues of theory, measurement, and research in outcomes (Fuhrer, 1997). In that publication, Johnston, Stineman, and Velozo (1997) reviewed the status of outcomes research in medical rehabilitation and the direction that future work is apt to take. They concluded that a number of conditions had to be met before there would be much outcomes research of a sufficiently definitive nature to influence practices in the field. A system of uniform data and measures is necessary, as is the case for inpatient hospitals using the UDS (Fiedler & Granger, 1997). Similar systems need to be developed for other forms of care, such as outpatient facilities and for home rehabilitation. To establish the critical factors in treatment that are essential to patient progress, robust research designs are necessary, a condition not easily met without substantial funding. There are many able investigators in medical rehabilitation, so there is reason to be optimistic about the future of outcomes research.

Case-Mix Adjustment

According to Stineman (1995), "Case-mix measures are patient classification systems that relate each type of patient to the usual amount of resources consumed as approximated by episode length (length of stay [LOS]), episode cost, or costs of daily services (intensity)." They are a way to group patients with similar degrees of severity and complexity so that predictions can be made about how much treatment will be required. In acute care hospitals, DRGs comprise a patient classification system that is used to calculate levels of reimbursement for prospective payment. In this system, a facility receives a fixed amount of money, depending on the patient group. The ability to predict accurately is important if costs are to be managed. Rehabilitation hospitals have been exempt from using this payment system because case-mixes are different from those in acute care hospitals.

The HCFA has the responsibility for seeking a case-mix system that can be used by Medicare for reimbursement in medical rehabilitation. Stineman (1995) has reviewed the options available for case-mix adjustment in rehabilitation. There is, first, the function related groups (FRGs) derived from a sample of facilities studied by Rand (Harada, Kominski, & Sofaer, 1993). A system based on UDS data and the FIM, called the FIM-FRGs, uses four predictor variables: diagnosis leading to disability, admission scores for motor and cognitive FIM subscales, and patient age (Stineman et al., 1994). A third potential case-mix classification is that of the Resource Utilization Group (RUG), which was devised for use in nursing homes (Fries et al., 1994). Thus far there has been no decision on which system HCFA will adopt. The implications for rehabilitation hospitals are far-reaching, however, because Medicare funds a high proportion of admissions.

Practice Guidelines

A third area of research with potentially far-reaching consequences for rehabilitation is that of practice guidelines. Pioneering studies of the way treatment is administered, by Wennberg and Gittelsohn (1973, 1982), established that there are often wide variations in procedures across geographic areas and practitioners. Presumably, such deviations from established methods of treatment can be costly because patients receive less than optimal care. One way to supply potentially useful information about costs, service use, and quality of care is by monitoring the practice patterns of physicians and other professionals (Shapiro, Lasker, Bindman, & Lee, 1993). Such profiling of practice patterns can result in the identification of practices of a series of providers, called practice-based norms, or in adherence to an accepted practice guideline, a standards-based norm. Managed care organizations are interested in such guidelines because greater uniformity of procedures means greater predictability of costs. If well-established procedures are followed, it should also result in better quality of care.

Thus far, in rehabilitation, there have been no formal surveys of practitioner methods, although there have been guidelines based on experts' assessment of research and clinical literature. Those advanced for poststroke rehabilitation, already mentioned, are the most prominent example. As guidelines from various sources are promulgated, pressures for greater uniformity in treatment procedures will continue to mount.

COMPREHENSIVE REHABILITATION: PRESENT AND FUTURE

The end of the 20th century is the most tumultuous period in the short history of medical rehabilitation. Although reliable statistics on the status of the field are difficult to come by, it is obvious to even the casual observer that restructuring of rehabilitation organizations is proceeding at a fast pace. Acquisitions, mergers, and coalition formation for the purposes of both vertical and horizontal integration are responses to an increasingly competitive marketplace. Rehabilitation facilities have commonly been small agencies without affiliations other than those with local community hospitals. With larger health care groups, including for-profit chains, acquiring inpatient units, outpatient clinics, subacute facilities, and private offices of physical therapists and occupational therapists, there has been significant consolidation.

Because it has been the most costly, inpatient rehabilitation has had the most radical changes. Length of stays for stroke, for example, have dropped dramatically, from an average of 32 days in 1990 to 23 days in 1995 (Granger, Ottenbacher, & Fiedler, 1995; Fiedler & Granger, 1997). In markets with high managed care penetration, such as California, many patients formerly referred to inpatient rehabilitation hospitals are now being seen in subacute care in nursing homes. Some patients formerly viewed as inpatient candidates are being seen in outpatient clinics or for home rehabilitation. Comprehensive care, the treatment philosophy that has guided the field since its early days, is increasingly questioned as the essential foundation for professional practice. Economics, in addition to traditional clinical methods, is shaping treatment delivery. The news is not all bad, however. Many facilities are now more efficient than in the past. There are also more alternative forms of care. Home rehabilitation, for example, allows an individual to remain in familiar surroundings and to try out skills of immediate relevance to a particular home setting.

The Future

Although these are times of instability throughout health care, the changes have brought new ideas and methods that may prove, in the long run, to be of benefit to those with disabilities as well to the providers of care.

Managed care. The predominant force that will continue to shape the future of rehabilitation is the way services will be funded. Managed care plans, now unevenly spread across the country, will become the principal source of payment. It is estimated that, by the year 2000, 80% of Medicare beneficiaries will be enrolled in some form of managed care (Wheatley, DeJong, & Sutton, 1997). A survey of rehabilitation facilities in areas with high penetration by managed care organizations provides a view of the future (Wheatley et al., 1997). Reimbursement for acute inpatient rehabilitation has been slashed drastically; many patients are being sent to lower levels of treatment intensity. The number of programs that specialize in the treatment of one diagnosis are being reduced. Therapists are being stretched to care for a variety of patients, although, as already indicated, agencies are being forced to become more efficient.

Quality of life. The shift in health care, from treating infections and injuries to dealing with the effects of chronic disease, has produced an interest in the wider ramifications of recovery to the quality of life of those treated. This broader perspective has been part of rehabilitation, although quality of life has generally not been included in its vernacular. Quality-of-life formulations include not only the objective status and circumstances of the individual but also his or her subjective views about life quality and life satisfaction. Dijkers (1997) has reviewed the concept and its measures, noting that quality of life is still poorly defined, with little research involving rehabilitation services. There is an obvious tension between concerns for quality-of-life issues and reductions in services through cost-cutting. The emphasis on consumer-oriented health care requires, however, that there be continued discussion about the implications of outcomes on the lives of treatment recipients.

Fitness. Keeping fit has become a national preoccupation, although the continuing increase in obesity shows that the preoccupation is not always translated into action. Nevertheless, health club membership and participation in running, cycling, and other vigorous sports attests to the interest in fitness. The distinction between exercise for fitness and for recovery during rehabilitation has become blurred, as it should. Regular exercise is a cornerstone of physical medicine and is a key to the success of restorative treatment (Sullivan, 1996). There have been significant barriers to vigorous exercise by those with disabilities. Professionals have sometimes been fearful of pushing patients too hard. Although exercise regimens are often recommended for discharged patients, it has usually been as a way to maintain gains during treatment and not as an avenue of fitness.

Community hospitals have begun to recognize the connection between maintaining fitness and maintaining health and are opening fitness centers. Some rehabilitation hospitals have formed partnerships with existing commercial health clubs to offer rehabilitation services within such clubs (Smith, 1996). Sports medicine, yet another manifestation of interest in fitness, is a specialty with modalities very close to those of rehabilitation medicine. The experience of rehabilitation specialists is highly relevant to the pursuit of fitness.

A Final Note

Times of instability are disquieting for everyone associated with health care—patients, professionals, managers, and payers—but there is also opportunity. Altering traditional rehabilitation has produced a diversity of services whose ramifications are as yet poorly understood. In this process professionals have had to adapt to methods that are not in keeping with their previous training and experience. The emphases on outcomes and the patient's perspective are commendable, but it is not clear yet how this has benefited patients. There are concerns about quality of care amid the rampant commercialism. It will take time to sort out the good features of these changes from the bad. Meanwhile, therapists will continue to treat those in need of restoration, with the hope that the system will provide sufficient resources to do a decent job. Regardless of restructuring, the population will continue to age, the incidence of disability will continue to climb, and rehabilitation services will still be needed.

REFERENCES

Deyo, R. A., Cherkin, D., Conrad, D., & Volinn, E. (1991). Cost, controversy, crisis: Low back pain and the health of the public. *Annual Review of Public Health, 12*, 141–156.

Dijkers, M. (1997). Measuring quality of life. In M. J. Fuhrer (Ed.), *Assessing rehabilitation practices: The promise of outcomes research* (pp. 153–179). Baltimore: Paul H. Brookes.

Dittmar, S. S., & Gresham, G. E. (Eds.). (1997). *Functional assessment and outcome measures for the rehabilitation health professional.* Gaithersburg, MD: Aspen.

Duncan, P. W., Hoenig, H., Samsa, G., & Hamilton, B. (1997). Characterizing rehabilitation interventions. In M. J. Fuhrer (Ed.), *Assessing medical rehabilitation practices: The promise of outcomes research* (pp. 307–317). Baltimore: Paul H. Brookes.

Fiedler, R. C., & Granger, C. V. (1997). Uniform Data System for Medical Rehabilitation[SM]: Report of first admissions for 1995. *American Journal of Physical Medicine and Rehabilitation, 76*, 76–81.

Fries, B. E., Schneider, D. P., Foley, W. J., Gavazzi, M., Burke, R., & Cornelius, E. (1994). Refining a case-mix measure for nursing homes: Resource utilizations groups (RUG-III). *Medical Care, 23*, 668–685.

Fuhrer, M. J. (Ed.). (1997). *Assessing medical rehabilitation practices: The promise of outcomes research.* Baltimore: Paul H. Brookes.

Granger, C. V., Ottenbacher, K. J., & Fiedler, R. C. (1995). The Uniform Data System for Medical Rehabilitation: Report of first admissions for 1993. *American Journal of Physical Medicine and Rehabilitation, 74*, 62–66.

Gresham, G. E., Duncan, P. W., Stason, W. B., Adams, H. P., Jr., Adelman, A. M., Alexander, D. N., Bishop, D. S., Diller, L., Donaldson, N. E., Granger, C. V., Holland, A. L., Kelly-Hays, M., McDowell, F. H., Myers, L., Phipps, M. A., Roth, E. J., Siebens, H. C., Tarvin, G. A., & Trombly, C. A. (1995). *Post-stroke rehabilitation guideline technical support.* Rockville, MD: U.S. Department of Health and Human Services, Public Health Service, Agency for Health Care Policy and Research.

Gritzer, G., & Arluke, A. (1985). *The making of rehabilitation.* Berkeley: University of California Press.

Hamilton, B. B., Granger, C. V., Sherwin, F. S., Zielezny, M., & Tashman, J. S. (1987). A uniform national data system for medical rehabilitation. In M. J. Fuhrer (Ed.), *Rehabilitation outcomes* (pp. 137–147). Baltimore: Paul H. Brookes.

Harada, N., Kominski, G., & Sofaer, S. (1993). Development of a resource-based classification scheme for rehabilitation. *Inquiry, 30*, 54–63.

Health Care Financing Administration. (1983). *Medicare provider reimbursement manual: Part 1.* Washington, DC: U.S. Department of Health and Human Services.

Heinemann, A. W., Hamilton, B., Linacre, J. M., Wright, B. D., & Granger, C. (1995). Functional status and therapeutic intensity during inpatient rehabilitation. *American Journal of Physical Medicine and Rehabilitation, 74*, 315–326.

Heinemann, A. W., Linacre, J. M., Wright, B. D., Hamilton, B. B., & Granger, C. (1993). Relationships between impairment and physical disability as measured by the functional independence measure. *Archives of Physical Medicine and Rehabilitation, 74*, 566–573.

Institute of Medicine. (1987). *Pain and disability.* Washington, DC: National Academy Press.

Institute of Medicine. (1989). *Allied health services: Avoiding crises.* Washington, DC: National Academy Press.

Johnston, M. V., Stineman, M., & Velozo, C. A. (1997). Outcomes research in medical rehabilitation: Foundations from the past and directions for the future. In M. J. Fuhrer (Ed.), *Assessing medical rehabilitation practices: The promise of outcomes research.* Baltimore: Paul H. Brookes.

Jorgensen, H. S., Nakayama, H., Raaschou, H. O., Larsen, K., Hubbe, P., & Olsen, T. S. (1995). The effect of a stroke unit: Reductions in mortality, discharge rate to nursing home, length of hospital stay, and cost: A community-based study. *Stroke, 26,* 1178–1182.

Keith, R. A. (1991). The comprehensive treatment team in rehabilitation. *Archives of Physical Medicine and Rehabilitation, 72,* 269–274.

Keith, R. A. (1994). Conceptual basis of outcome measures. *American Journal of Physical Medicine and Rehabilitation, 74,* 73–80.

Keith, R. A. (1996). Rehabilitation after stroke: Cost-effectiveness analyses. *Journal of the Royal Society of Medicine, 89,* 631–633.

Keith, R. A. (1997a). The role of treatment theory. In M. J. Fuhrer (Ed.), *Assessing medical rehabilitation practices: The promise of outcomes research* (pp. 257–274). Baltimore: Paul H. Brookes.

Keith, R. A. (1997b). Treatment strength in rehabilitation. *Archives of Physical Medicine and Rehabilitation, 78,* 1298–1304.

Keith, R. A., & Cowell, K. S. (1987). Time use of stroke patients in three rehabilitation hospitals. *Social Science and Medicine, 24,* 529–533.

Keith, R. A., & Lipsey, M. W. (1993). The role of theory in rehabilitation assessment, treatment, and outcomes. In R. L. Glueckauf, L. B. Sechrest, G. R. Bond, & E. C. McDonel (Eds.), *Improving assessment in rehabilitation and health* (pp. 33–58). Newbury Park, CA: Sage.

Keith, R. A., Wilson, D. B., & Gutierrez, P. (1995). Acute and subacute rehabilitation for stroke: A comparison. *Archives of Physical Medicine and Rehabilitation, 76,* 495–500.

McDowell, I., & Newell, C. (1996). *Measuring health,* 2nd ed. New York: Oxford University Press.

Mullner, R., Nazum, F., & Matthews, D. (1983). Inpatient medical rehabilitation: Results of the 1981 survey of hospitals and units. *Archives of Physical Medicine and Rehabilitation, 64,* 354–358.

National Association of Rehabilitation Facilities. (1988). *Medical rehabilitation: What it is and where it is—a discussion.* (NARF Monograph Series). Washington, DC: Author.

Ottenbacher, K. J., & Jannell, S. (1993). The results of clinical trials in stroke rehabilitation research. *Archives of Neurology, 50,* 37–44.

Perry, L. (1989). Providers see potential in treating brain injury. *Modern Healthcare, 19,* 58.

Pope, A. M., & Tarlov, A. R. (Eds.). (1991). *Disability in America.* Washington, DC: National Academy Press.

Rasch, G. (1960). *Probabilistic models for some intelligence and attainment tests.* Copenhagen: Danmarks Paedogogiske Institute, and (1980). Chicago: University of Chicago Press.

Rice, D. P., & Feldman, J. J. (1983). Living longer in the United States: Demographic changes in health needs of the elderly. *Health and Society, 61,* 362–396.

Rothenberg, R. B., & Koplan, J. P. (1990). Chronic disease in the 1990s. *Annual Review of Public Health, 11*, 267–296.

Shapiro, D. W., Lasker, R. D., Bindman, A. B., & Lee, P. R. (1993). Containing costs while improving quality of care: The role of profiling and practice guidelines. *Annual Review of Public Health, 14*, 219–241.

Silverstein, B., Fisher, W. P., Kilgore, K. M., Harley, J. P., & Harvey, R. F. (1992). Applying psychometric criteria to functional assessment in medical rehabilitation: 2. Defining interval measures. *Archives of Physical Medicine and Rehabilitation, 73*, 507–518.

Smith, R. (1996, August/September). Fitness centers that offer therapy. *Rehab Management, 9*, 79–81.

Stineman, M. (1995). Case-mix measurement in medical rehabilitation. *Archives of Physical Medicine and Rehabilitation, 76*, 1163–1170.

Stineman, M. G., Escarce, J. J., Goin, J. E., Hamilton, B. B., Granger, C. V., & Williams, S. V. (1994). A case-mix classification system for medical rehabilitation. *Medical Care, 32*, 366–379.

Strasser, D. C., & Falconer, J. A. (1997). Linking treatment to outcomes through teams: Building a conceptual model of rehabilitation effectiveness. *Topics in Stroke Rehabilitation, 4*, 15–27.

Sullivan, T. (1996, August/September). Exercise for people with disabilities. *Rehab Management, 9*, 46, 48, 50–51.

Wennberg, J., & Gittelsohn, A. (1973). Small area variations in health care delivery. *Science, 142*, 1102–1108.

Wennberg, J., & Gittelsohn, A. (1982). Variations in medical care among small areas. *Scientific American, 246*, 120–134.

Wheatley, B., DeJong, G., & Sutton, J. P. (1997). Managed care and the transformation of the medical rehabilitation industry. *Health Care Management Review, 22*, 25–39.

Whiteneck, G. G., Charlifue, S. W., Gerhart, K. A., Overholser, J. D., & Richardson, G. N. (1992). Quantifying handicap: A new measure of long-term rehabilitation outcomes. *Archives of Physical Medicine and Rehabilitation, 73*, 519–526.

Whiteneck, G. G., Fougeyrollas, P., & Gerhart, K. A. (1997). Elaborating the model of disablement. In M. J. Fuhrer (Ed.), *Assessing medical rehabilitation practices: The promise of outcomes research* (pp. 91–102). Baltimore: Paul H. Brookes.

Willer, B., Button, J., & Corrigan, J. D. (1997). The concept of handicap in rehabilitation and research. In M. J. Fuhrer (Ed.), *Assessing medical rehabilitation practices: The promise of outcomes research* (pp. 127–151). Baltimore: Paul H. Brookes.

World Health Organization (WHO). (1980). *International classification of impairments, disabilities, and handicaps*. Geneva: Author.

Wright, B. D., Linacre, J. M., & Heinemann, A. W. (1993). Measuring functional status in rehabilitation. *Physical Medicine and Rehabilitation Clinics of North America, 4*, 475–491.

Chapter 2

Body Systems: An Overview

Jung H. Ahn

The human body consists of a complex combination of histoanatomical systems and biochemical materials (Clemente, 1985; DeLisa & Stolov, 1981; Ganong, 1991). In this chapter, however, the body is topographically divided for an adept understanding as follows: the skin, the musculoskeletal system, the nervous system, the respiratory system, the cardiovascular system, the hematopoietic system, the digestive system, the genitourinary system, the endocrine system, the visual system, and the auditory and vestibular systems.

SKIN

The most superficial system of the body is the skin, which consists of two parts: an epidermis and a dermis. The epidermis is an outer, keratinized layer of the skin. The bottom layer of the epidermis is called the basal cell layer. The dermis is an inner, connective tissue layer containing nerve endings, tactile corpuscles, and blood vessels. The sweat glands, sebaceous glands, and hair follicles are also contained in the dermis, and they pass upward through the epidermis. The skin is constantly exposed to external hazards, and therefore it is of utmost importance to protect it from any disabling trauma.

MUSCULOSKELETAL SYSTEM

The musculoskeletal system includes bones, cartilages, ligaments, tendons, and muscles. It serves to provide mechanical support for the body, protect vital internal organs, store minerals, and produce blood. The skeletal system also works as a lever system on which muscles act across joints to result in body movements. The skeletal muscle is made of contractile muscle fibers (myofibrils) surrounded by the sarcoplasmic reticulum and the T-system. The muscle fiber consists of protein chains of actin and myosin. During muscle contraction the strands of actin and myosin slide past each other (Figure 2.1) in the presence of Ca^{++} released from the sarcoplasmic reticulum via the T-system, thus shortening the fiber. The trigger to start this contraction comes from the motor nerve attached to each muscle fiber. The attachment occurs at the motor end plate, where acetylcholine (a neurotransmitter) is released at the moment an electrical impulse traveling in the motor nerve reaches the muscle fiber.

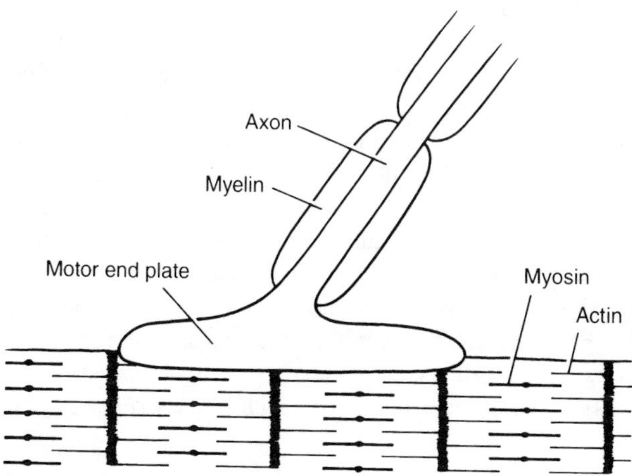

FIGURE 2.1 Very schematic representation of the terminal branch of a motor neuron attaching to a muscle fiber via the motor end plate. When the nerve's electrical impulse reaches the motor end plate, acetylcholine is released. The impulse then travels in both directions along the fiber. During contraction, the strands of actin and myosin slide past each other, thus shortening the fiber.

From DeLisa and Stolov: Significant Body Systems in *Handbook of Severe Disability* edited by Stolov and Clowers, U.S. Department of Education, Rehabilitation Service Administration, 1981.

Tendons attach the contracting part of the muscles to bones. They are composed largely of parallel collagenous fibers that are closely bound into fibrous bundles, forming tough cords. They include some elastic fibers.

Ligaments are also composed of collagenous fibers and some elastic fibers. They connect two or more bones and also stabilize joints. A ligamentous injury can be more problematic than a fracture and often requires prolonged immobilization. Congenital lax ligaments result in hypermobility of joints. Cartilage has a high content of collagen and proteoglycans combined with H_2O, giving it a gel-like consistency. It has essentially no blood supply but receives nourishment by diffusion from nearby capillaries. Three kinds of cartilages are recognized: fibro-, elastic, and hyaline. Fibrocartilage has a large concentration of less elastic collagen fibers and is dominant in intervertebral disks. Elastic cartilage has many elastic fibers, as is evident in the external ear. Hyaline cartilage contains few fibrils and is slightly elastic. It covers the opposing surfaces of movable joints such as the articular cartilage, which may wear out and become calcified with aging. Such changes are described as degenerative joint disease or osteoarthritis.

Joints are divided into the fibrous joint (immobile), the cartilaginous joint (slightly movable), and the synovial joint (movable). The fibrous joints are seen in the skull. Intervertebral disks are the cartilaginous joints. Limb joints are covered by the synovial membrane, which produces the viscous fluid in the joint space. The cartilaginous and synovial joints are susceptible to degenerative joint disease, and the synovial joint is prone to developing inflammation.

Bone is a hard, calcified connective tissue with 35% organic substance, 45% inorganic substance, and 20% water. Bone tissue consists of the matrix and the specialized cells of the bone, including osteoids (bone cells), osteoblasts (bone-forming cells), and osteoclasts (bone-destroying cells). The matrix contains mineral salts, mainly calcium phosphate. There are two major types of mature bone: sponge and compact. There are 206 bones in the adult human body; they can be divided into flat bones (e.g., skull), short bones (e.g., carpal bones), and long bones (e.g., humerus) or axial bones and appendicular bones (Figure 2.2, Table 2.1).

TABLE 2.1 Human Bones

Axial bones		Appendicular bones	
Spine	26	Upper extremities	64
Skull	28	Lower extremities	62
Hyeid bone	1		126
Ribs & sternum	25		
	80		

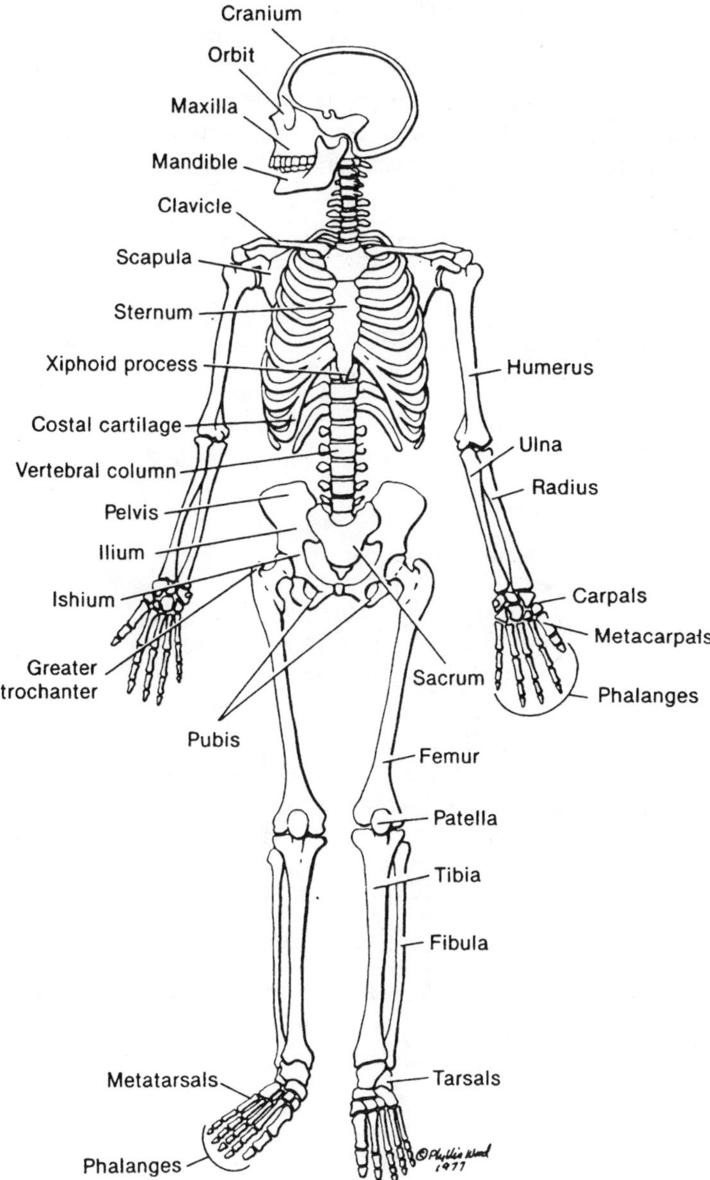

FIGURE 2.2 The gross structure of bones.

The gross structure of bones (Figure 2.3) is typically composed of the bone marrow, spongy bone, cortical bone, and periosteum. During growth, the red marrow, which manufactures the red blood cells, in most bones changes to the yellow marrow (fatty marrow) usually by about 6 years of age. The periosteum is a thick, fibrous membrane that covers the entire surface of a bone except its articular cartilage; it has two layers: an inner osteogenic layer and an outer connective tissue layer with blood vessels and nerve fibers.

NERVOUS SYSTEM

The nervous system is divided into the central nervous system (CNS) and the peripheral nervous system (PNS). The CNS includes the brain and the spinal cord. The PNS includes the cranial nerves, the spinal nerves, and the autonomic nervous system.

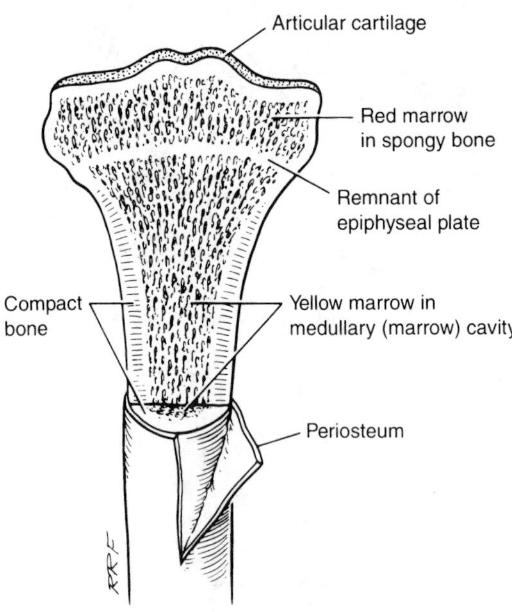

FIGURE 2.3 Cutaway section of an adult long bone showing the medullary cavity containing yellow marrow. In this section, only a residual line remains of the epiphyseal plate.

From DeLisa and Stolov: Significant Body Systems in *Handbook of Severe Disability* edited by Stolov and Clowers, U.S. Department of Education, Rehabilitation Service Administration, 1981.

The basic functional unit of the nervous system is the neuron, and there are about 1 trillion neurons in the human nervous system. The neuron consists of a cell body, dendrites, and an axon (Figure 2.4). The terms *axon* and *nerve fiber* are synonymous. Most axons are long and encased in a sheath called myelin, which acts as an insulator and aids the rapid transmission of conducting impulses away from the nerve cell body. The cell body is responsible for maintaining the functional and anatomical integrity of the axon. The length of the path traveled by afferent or efferent information is longer than any single axon. Therefore, chains of neurons are necessary to convey messages through the entire nervous system. The system for transfer from one neuron to the next is the synapse, in which a chemical neurotransmitter is released, triggering the next neuron into action.

Central Nervous System

The brain and spinal cord are covered by the meninges and surrounded by the cerebrospinal fluid (CSF). The brain is further protected by the skull, as the

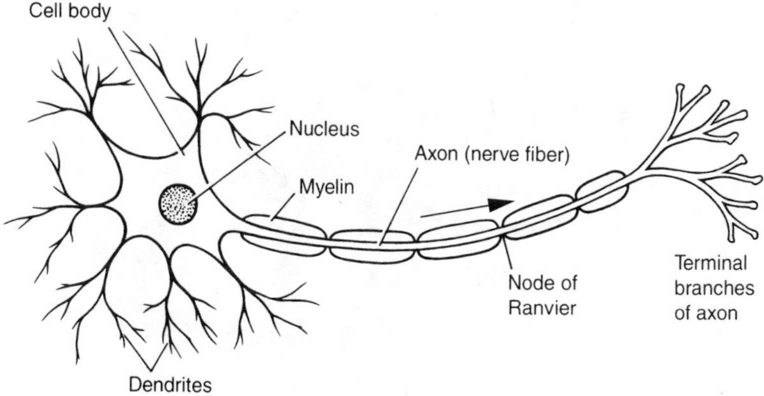

FIGURE 2.4 Basic myelinated nerve cell. Dendrites receive input from terminal branches of other axons. When sufficiently activated, the cell body transmits an electrical impulse down its axon. Myelin protects the axon and, together with the nodes of Ranvier, allows for very fast conduction. Nonmyelinated, slower-conduction axons also exist. Axon diameters range: 1–6 × 10^{-4} cm. Arrow indicates direction of impulse travel.

From DeLisa and Stolov: Significant Body Systems in *Handbook of Severe Disability* edited by Stolov and Clowers, U.S. Department of Education, Rehabilitation Service Administration, 1981.

spinal cord is protected by the vertebral column. The meninges include the pia mater, arachnoid mater, and dura mater. The CSF, formed in the choroid plexuses around the cerebral vessels and along the ventricular walls, fills the subarachnoid space and cerebral ventricles and is absorbed through the arachnoid villi into the cerebral venous sinuses. The fluid also serves as a medium through which nutrients and wastes can be exchanged between the blood and the CNS.

The brain is divided into the cerebrum, the cerebellum, and the brain stem (Figure 2.5). The cerebrum, consisting of left and right convoluted cerebral hemispheres, is the largest part of the brain. Its thin outer layer consists of gray matter (the cortex), and its interior portion consists of white matter. Each cerebral hemisphere is divided into the frontal, parietal, temporal, and occipital lobes.

The frontal lobe deals with emotions, abstract thinking, and judgment. The motor speech center (Broca's area) is also located in the frontal lobe. Essentially all right-handed individuals and about 85% of all left-handed individuals have

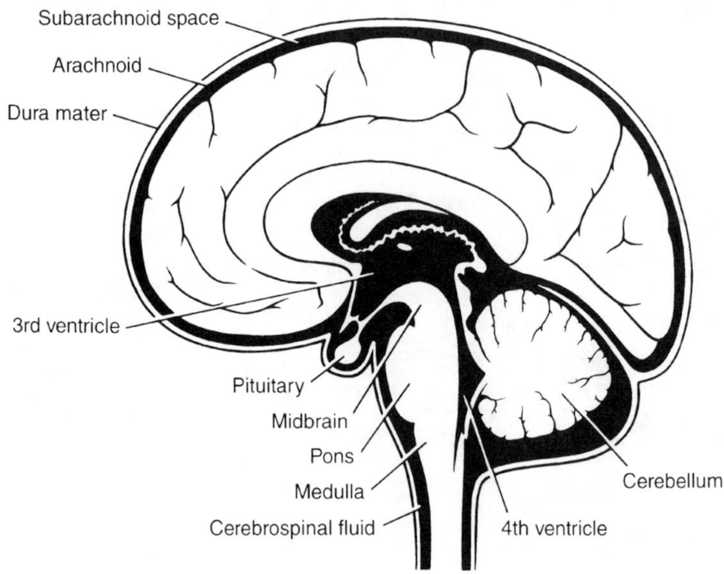

FIGURE 2.5 Midline section through the cerebrum, cerebellum, and brain stem. This section passes through the third and fourth ventricles, both of which are midline structures. Note cerebral spinal fluid bathing the brain.

From DeLisa and Stolov: Significant Body Systems in *Handbook of Severe Disability* edited by Stolov and Clowers, U.S. Department of Education, Rehabilitation Service Administration, 1981.

the speech center on the left side. The frontal lobe and the parietal lobe are demarcated by the central sulcus. The motor cortex is in the precentral gyrus of the frontal lobe and is responsible for voluntary movements on the opposite side of the body. It is important to be aware that most motor fibers of the corticospinal tract cross the midline in the medulla. The primary olfactory cortex is contained in the base of the frontal lobe.

The parietal lobe is concerned with integrating sensations. The postcentral gyrus is the major sensory receptive area (sensory cortex) for the highest integration and coordination of afferent information from the opposite side of the body, dealing with pain, temperature sense, proprioception, and fine touch. The sensory cortex is connected by the thalamic radiation from the thalamus, which is a sensory relay station. Nerve fibers mediating sensations via the spinal cord to the thalamus are the spinothalamic tracts and the dorsal columns.

The temporal lobe is located under the frontal and parietal lobes. Its cortex is the primary area where auditory stimuli are received. Wernicke's area for auditory comprehension is at the posterior end of the superior temporal gyrus. It is also one of the centers for dreams, memory, and emotions. The occipital lobe is located in the posterior part of each cerebral hemisphere, and its cortex is the primary area where visual stimuli are received.

The basal ganglia include the caudate nucleus, putamen, and globus pallidus. Close to the basal ganglia lies the internal capsule, which contains the important motor tracts (pyramidal tracts) descending from the motor cortex on their way to the spinal cord. The basal ganglia constitute part of the extrapyramidal system, which is made up of those areas in the CNS other than the pyramidal and cerebellar systems. They are concerned with the programming and initiation of movement and posture.

The hypothalamus is located below the thalamus and is intimately associated with the pituitary gland. It plays an important role in regulating the secretion of pituitary hormones. It also serves as a higher center for the autonomic nervous system and controls complex behavioral and emotional reactions, such as appetite, sexual behaviors, fear, and rage.

The limbic system consists of a rim of cortical tissue around the hilum of the cerebral hemisphere and a group of associated deep structures: the amygdala, the hippocampus, and the septal nuclei. It is directly concerned with smell and also with the control of feeding behavior, circadian rhythms, sexual behavior, rage, fear, and motivation.

The cerebellum can be found under the occipital lobe and is connected behind the brain stem. Like the cerebrum, it has right and left hemispheres, united by the vermis, and also has an outer layer of gray matter with numerous sulci and gyri. Almost all information to and from the cerebellum is transmitted by way of the midbrain. The cerebellum has three main functions: (1) maintenance of equilibrium and balance of the trunk, (2) regulation of muscle tension involved in the spinal nerve reflexes and posture and orientation of limbs, and (3) regulation of the coordination of fine limb movements.

The brain stem consists of the midbrain, the pons, and the medulla oblongata. Cranial nerves, except for the olfactory nerve and the optic nerve, originate in the brain stem. Cardiovascular and respiratory centers are located in the medulla. The reticular formation in the brain stem is generally associated with states of consciousness and alertness.

The spinal cord functions like a telephone cable between the brain and the PNS. Unlike the cerebrum and cerebellum, the spinal cord consists of gray matter centrally and white matter peripherally. The zone of gray matter resembles a butterfly in cross section. Anterior projections of gray matter, termed anterior horns, are the site of the final synapse for efferent motor impulses leaving the cord. Poliomyelitis is a viral disease that affects this area. Posterior projections of gray matter, termed dorsal horns, convey afferent sensory information entering the cord from sensory organs. The peripheral zone of the cord consists of white matter and contains various ascending and descending tracts. For example, the spinothalamic tract carries pain and temperature impulses up to the thalamus, the posterior columns carry propioceptive impulses up to the medulla, and the corticospinal tract delivers impulses downward from the motor cortex to initiate muscle activity.

The blood supply to the brain is derived from bilateral internal carotid and vertebral arteries, which are interconnected at the base of the brain at a vascular circuit known as the Circle of Willis. The middle cerebral artery supplies the lateral surface of most of the frontal lobe, nearly all of the parietal lobe, most of the temporal lobe, and part of the occipital lobe. The anterior cerebral artery supplies the medial surface of the frontal and parietal lobes. The precentral (motor) and postcentral (sensory) gyri representing the lower limbs lie within the distribution of this artery. The posterior cerebral artery supplies the upper pons, midbrain, much of the inferomedial aspect of the temporal lobe, and most of the occipital lobe. The blood supply to the brain stem and the cerebellum comes mostly from branches of the basilar artery, which is formed by bilateral vertebral arteries. The vertebral arteries also give rise to a single anterior spinal artery and two posterior spinal arteries, which run longitudinally along the spinal cord. This longitudinal arterial supply of the cord is further supplemented by radicular vessels at the cervicothoracic and thoracolumbar junctional areas.

Peripheral Nervous System

The cranial nerves (Table 2.2), with the exception of the olfactory and optic nerves, are defined as part of the PNS. At the spinal level, the PNS originates with the spinal nerves. Each spinal nerve has two roots: anterior (ventral) motor

TABLE 2.2 Human Cranial Nerves

Name	Number	Innervation		
		Motor	Sensory	Parasympathetic
Olfactory	I		Olfactory epithelium	
Optic	II		Retina	
Oculomotor	III	See Table 2.3 Levator palpebrae		Sphincter of iris Ciliary muscle
Trochlear	IV	See Table 2.3		
Trigeminal	V	Chewing muscles	Face	
Abducent	VI	See Table 2.3		
Facial	VII	Facial muscles orbicularis oculi	Ant. 2/3 of tongue	Salivary glands (submandibular and sublingual)
Vestibulo-cochlear	VIII		Inner ear	
Glosso-pharyngeal	IX	Swallowing muscle	Post. 1/3 of tongue Middle ear	Parotid gland
Vagus	X		Epiglottis External ear	Visceral organs Vocal cord
Accessory	XI	Sternocleidomastoid Trapezius		
Hypoglossal	XII	Tongue muscles		

root and posterior (dorsal) sensory root. The anterior root contains the axons of the cell bodies in the anterior horn of the spinal cord. The posterior root has its cell bodies located in the sensory nerve ganglion outside but close to the cord. There are 31 pairs of spinal nerves (8 cervical, 12 thoracic, 5 lumbar, 5 sacral, and 1 coccygeal).

The spinal cord ends at the upper level of the second lumbar vertebra. Because the spinal column is longer than the spinal cord itself, some of the spinal nerves, particularly at the lower levels, have to travel down a significant distance before actually leaving the bony canal. The very lower end of the cord is called the conus medullaris, and a bundle of spinal nerves passing downward within the aura mater below the first lumbar vertebra is referred to as the cauda equine. The phrenic nerve, which originates from the C3-5 spinal nerves, innervates the diaphragm.

All muscles in the upper extremities are controlled by the brachial plexus, which is a nerve complex formed by the C5-7-8-T1 spinal nerves. The main peripheral nerves of the brachial plexus include the axillary, musculocutaneous, median, ulnar, and radial nerves. These nerves contribute to both motor and sensation in the upper extremity.

The thoracic spinal nerves mainly innervate the thorax and abdomen, although the first and second thoracic nerves contribute partly to the upper extremities. All thoracic spinal and first and second lumbar spinal nerves contain sympathetic nerve fibers that innervate the viscera.

The lumbar and first and second sacral spinal nerves innervate the lower extremities in terms of motor control and sensory perception. The main peripheral nerves in the lower extremities include the femoral nerve, superior and inferior gluteal nerves, sciatic nerve, common peroneal nerve, and tibial nerve.

The pudendal nerve, originating from the S2-3-4, innervates the external genitalia, the perianal area, and the sphincter. The coccygeal nerve supplies the skin in the region of the coccyx. The autonomic nervous system (ANS) is divided into the sympathetic division and the parasympathetic division. The ANS regulates the activities of the viscera, such as the stomach and intestines, the heart, the smooth muscles of arteries, the sweat glands, the salivary glands, and the urinary bladder. The sympathetic preganglionic efferent nerve fibers, mostly myelinated, leave the spinal cord through the anterior roots of all of the thoracic spinal nerves and the upper lumbar spinal nerves. After exiting from the spinal canal, these nerve fibers branch off the spinal nerves to join a chain of ganglia that lies on either side of the spinal column, where they have their first synapse. The second sympathetic (postganglionic) fiber, mostly unmyelinated, then returns to the spinal nerves to be distributed to autonomic effectors in the areas supplied by these spinal nerves. Some postganglionic fibers may proceed directly to the viscera in the various sympathetic nerves rather than returning to the spinal nerve. Some preganglionic fibers pass through the paravertebral ganglion chain and end on the postganglionic neurons located in collateral ganglia close to the viscera.

The parasympathetic system is composed of cranial nerves III, VII, IX, and X, and the second, third, and fourth sacral spinal nerves. When the vagus (X) nerve is activated, the heart rate becomes slower, and the gastrointestinal tract becomes more active. The sacral parasympathetic nerves forming the pelvic nerve are important for contracting the detrusor muscle of the urinary bladder, for advancing the feces in the distal colon, and for erecting the penis.

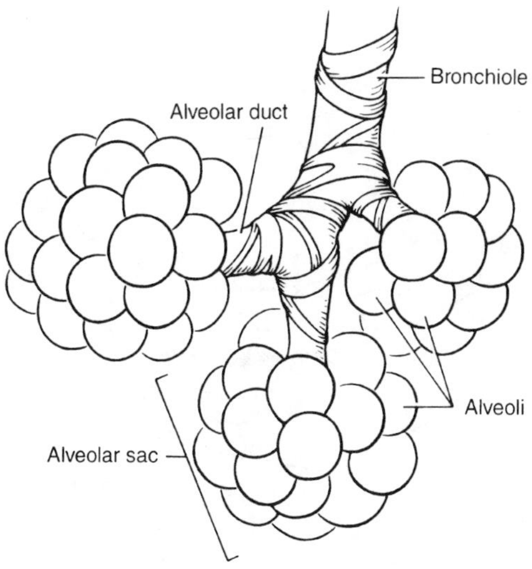

FIGURE 2.6 Schematic showing the structure of the alveolar ducts, alveolar sacs, and alveoli.

From DeLisa and Stolov: Significant Body Systems in *Handbook of Severe Disability* edited by Stolov and Clowers, U.S. Department of Education, Rehabilitation Service Administration, 1981.

RESPIRATORY SYSTEM

The respiratory system includes the nose, nasal passages, nasopharynx, larynx, trachea, bronchi, and lungs. Each lung is covered by the pulmonary pleura, and the inner surface of the chest wall is lined by the parietal pleura. The potential space between these two pleurae is known as the pleural cavity. The right lung is divided into a superior lobe, a middle lobe, and an inferior lobe. The left lung is divided into a superior lobe and an inferior lobe. Nutrition to the tissue of the lungs is provided by the bronchial arteries. While the pulmonary arteries are delivering the venous blood to the lungs, the inspired air keeps traveling down to the alveoli (Figure 2.6), which are surrounded by pulmonary capillaries. There are 300 million alveoli in the human body, and the total area of the alveolar walls making contact with capillaries (Figure 2.7) in both lungs, to exchange carbon dioxide for oxygen, is about 70 m^2. As oxygen diffuses into the blood, the hemoglobin molecule in the red blood cell immediately takes up oxygen, permitting more into the plasma.

Inspiration is an active process, primarily accomplished by contractions of the diaphragm, and expiration during quiet breathing results from the passive

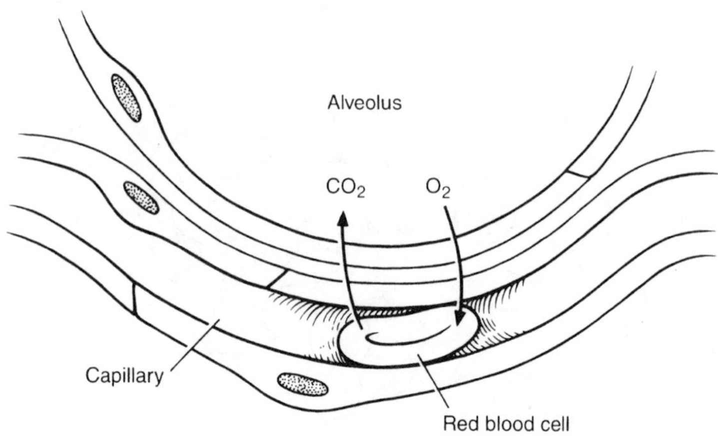

FIGURE 2.7 Schematic representation of the exchange of oxygen and carbon dioxide through the thin walls of the alveolus and a red blood cell of a capillary.

From DeLisa and Stolov: Significant Body Systems in *Handbook of Severe Disability* edited by Stolov and Clowers, U.S. Department of Education, Rehabilitation Service Administration, 1981.

recoiling of the lungs. Inspiration can be aided by using neck muscles and external intercostals. For forcible expiration, good strength of the abdominal muscles and the internal intercostals is necessary.

Besides gas exchange, the respiratory system secretes immunoglobulin to resist respiratory infections and has macrophages in the alveoli that serve to ingest inhaled bacteria and small particles. The hairs in the nostrils prevent large particles from entering the airway. Coughing and ciliary movements of the proximal airway with mucus are also capable of removing particles from the respiratory tract.

CARDIOVASCULAR SYSTEM

Blood circulation throughout the body is accomplished by means of the cardiovascular system. The driving force for moving the blood is provided by the pumping action of the heart. The pulmonary circulation, driven by the right heart, delivers venous blood to the lungs, where the carbon dioxide is effectively removed and the oxygen is replenished. The systemic circulation, driven by the left heart,

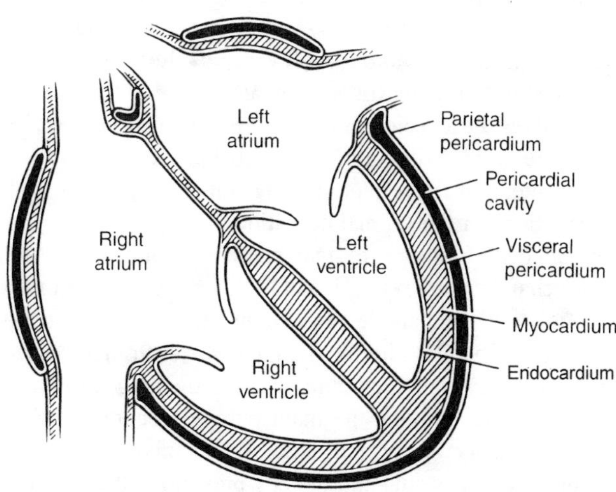

FIGURE 2.8 Schematic representation of the four chambers of the heart, the three layers of the heart wall, and the two layers of the pericardium.

From DeLisa and Stolov: Significant Body Systems in *Handbook of Severe Disability* edited by Stolov and Clowers, U.S. Department of Education, Rehabilitation Service Administration, 1981.

delivers oxygenated blood to active tissue of the body. The blood vessels leading from the heart are arteries, and the blood vessels returning the blood, containing increased carbon dioxide and decreased oxygen, to the heart are veins. The lymphatics take the extra fluid in the interstitial tissue and bring the fluid back into the blood, promoting turnover of tissue fluid.

The heart is about the size of a man's first. Two thirds of it lies to the left of the midline, within the chest cavity and between the lungs. The heart (Figure 2.8) is enclosed by a double-layered loose sac, the pericardium. A small amount of fluid between the two layers lubricates the surfaces to allow the heart to change its shape without much friction as it pumps. The wall of the heart has three distinct layers: the epicardium (outer thin membrane), the myocardium (thick middle layer of cardiac muscle), and the endocardium (inner layer). The pumping action is achieved by the myocardium, which is a special form of muscle, somewhat like skeletal muscle but not subject to the same type of voluntary control. The heart has four chambers: right atrium, right ventricle, left atrium, and left ventricle. Blood from the systemic circulation enters the right atrium through the inferior and superior vena cave. It passes through the tricuspid valve into the right ventricle. Right ventricular contraction propels the blood through the pulmonary semilunar valve into the pulmonary artery for pulmonary circulation. The blood from the lungs enters the left atrium through the pulmonary vein and passes through the mitral valve into the left ventricle. Left ventricular contraction propels the blood through the aortic semilunar valve into the aorta for systemic circulation. All valves—tricuspid, mitral, and semilunar—can pass blood in only one direction in the normal situation. The walls between the two ventricles and the two atria, the interventricular septum and the interatrial septum, block mixing of the two circulations in the normal condition.

Each cardiac cycle consists of two parts: diastolic and systolic. During diastole, all four chambers are relaxed, and both atria receive and fill with blood. Systole begins first with right and left atrial contraction, propelling blood through the tricuspid and mitral valves into the right and left ventricles, respectively. The myocardium of the atria is relatively thin, whereas the myocardium of the ventricles is thick. Ventricular systole, the main pumping action, forcefully propels blood into the pulmonary artery and aorta. When this contraction occurs, the tricuspid and mitral valves slam shut, thereby preventing the flow of blood back into the atria. The closures of these valves produce the first heart sound that can be heard with a stethoscope. The rush of blood out of the ventricles causes the pulse beat that can be felt at the wrist and other areas of the body where arteries are prominent. The rush of blood into the pulmonary artery and aorta distends the walls of these vessels. When ventricular contraction stops, the vessels recoil and the semilunar valves slam shut, thereby preventing the flow of blood back into the ventricles. The second heart sound is associated with the closure of the semilunar valves.

Cardiac murmurs are abnormal sounds heard over the heart and usually signify disease of the heart valves: stenosis or insufficiency. Abnormal sounds can also be heard outside the heart (i.e., carotid bruit when a carotid artery is partially occluded and thyroid bruit when a thyroid goiter is highly vascular).

Blood pressure recorded (usually in the arm) consists of two numbers that refer to the systolic pressure and the diastolic pressure. Pressures are recorded in millimeters of mercury (mmHg) and are written as systolic pressure over diastolic pressure (e.g., 120/80). The magnitudes of the pressures are dependent not only on the force produced by the thick myocardium of the ventricles but also by the resistance to flow produced by the progressively narrowing peripheral arterial vessels.

The heart has an inherent capacity to contract rhythmically. Each cycle originates in a special bundle of myocardial cells (sinoatrial node [SA node, or the pacemaker]) in the wall of the right atrium. These cells initiate electrical impulses at a regular interval without benefit of any external stimulation. The impulses travel in the walls of the atria, causing atrial contraction, and rapidly reach the atrioventricular (AV) node, which also lies in the right atrial wall near the interatrial septum. Impulses delay here slightly until atrial systole is completed.

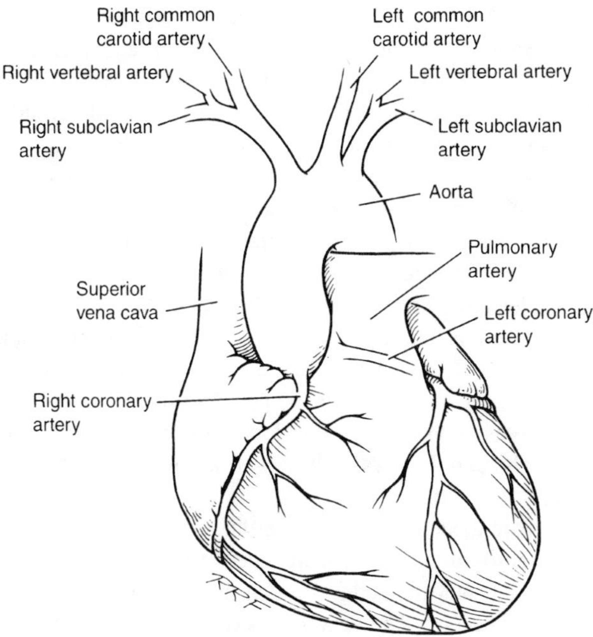

FIGURE 2.9 The two coronary arteries encircle the heart and supply blood to all portions of the myocardium. Each coronary artery can supply both atria and both ventricles, thus providing the heart with a safety factor in the event of disease in one of the coronary arteries. The vertebral and carotid arteries supply blood to the brain.

From DeLisa and Stolov: Significant Body Systems in *Handbook of Severe Disability* edited by Stolov and Clowers, U.S. Department of Education, Rehabilitation Service Administration, 1981.

From the AV node, impulses travel down two bundles of special muscle fibers (bundle of His) on the right and left side of the interventricular septum. The two bundles branch out as Purkinje fibers and spread over both ventricles, causing ventricular contraction. The parasympathetic fibers from the vagus nerve cause the SA node to slow down, and the sympathetic nerve fibers from the upper thoracic cord are responsible for speeding up the SA node. A number of chemicals and hormones, such as epinephrine and thyroxine, can accelerate the heart rate.

The major branches of the aorta distribute blood to the head, abdomen, and extremities. The right and left coronary arteries (Figure 2.9), which also originate from the aorta, supply the heart itself. Some branches of these two coronary arteries anastomize (interconnect). Arterial walls are composed of three layers: the intima (inner layer with endothelial cells), the media (middle layer with smooth muscle and elastic connective tissue fibers), and the adventitia (outer fibrous layer). As these arteries branch further, they become progressively thinner-walled and smaller in diameter. The smallest divisions of the arteries are the arterioles, whose main component is smooth muscle. The diameter of arterioles can be altered, even to the extent of closure, by sympathetic activation, hypertrophy of the arteriole smooth muscle, or arteriolosclerosis. The changes in the diameter of these vessels not only determine the quantity of blood delivered to capillaries but also influence the blood pressure.

The arteries lead into the microscopic capillaries that lie in close approximation to the fluid bathing the living cells (interstitial fluid). Capillary walls are very thin, consisting of only a thin lining of endothelial cells. This thin wall permits the passage of nutrients and oxygen into the interstitial fluid and also permits waste products and carbon dioxide from the cells to permeate into the venous system. The capillary walls, however, are relatively impermeable to the plasma proteins.

The venules are the smallest veins, yet larger than capillaries. They unite to form veins that return blood to the heart. The walls of veins have the same three layers as the arteries, but the media is much thinner. Many veins have valves to prevent the reflux of blood. The venous blood pressure is lower than the arterial blood pressure. The superior vena cava collects venous blood from the head, upper extremities, and thorax, and the inferior vena cava receives blood from the rest of the body. Although blood from all of the veins of the lower extremities is directly received by the inferior vena cava, visceral venous blood is first drained into the liver by the portal vein. In the liver the portal vein ends in sinusoids (capillary-like vessels in the liver) from which the blood is conveyed to the inferior vena cava. Both superior and inferior venae cavae open into the right atrium of the heart.

The lymphatic system is also an important vascular network, consisting of lymphatic capillaries, lymphatic collecting vessels, and lymph nodes through which the lymphatic fluid (lymph) recirculates from the tissue space of most organs into the venous system. Lymphatic capillaries allow the passage of extracellular fluids through their walls and reabsorb considerable amounts of proteins into the circulation. Unlike the capillary walls, the walls of the lymphatics are permeable to the macromolecules, and the proteins therefore are returned to the blood stream via the lymphatics. Two main lymphatic vessels are the thoracic duct, which ends in the left subclavian vein after draining the lymphatic fluid from most of the body, and the right lymphatic duct, which ends in the right subclavian vein after draining the fluid from the right side of the head and neck, the right upper extremity, the right side of the thorax, right lung, and right side of the heart. The lymph nodes manufacture lymphocytes, which have the ability to produce antibodies against many different foreign invaders (antigens). The main forces pushing lymph up toward the heart are skeletal muscle contractions, negative intrathoracic pressure during inspiration, the suction effect of high-velocity venous blood flow, and rhythmic contractions of the large lymphatic ducts.

HEMATOPOIETIC SYSTEM

Blood cells include white blood cells (leukocytes), red blood cells (erythrocytes), and platelets. During fetal life, blood cells are formed not only in the bone marrow but in the liver and spleen as well. In addition, the thymus is a lymphocyte-producing organ. Shortly after birth, however, most of the blood cells are formed in the bone marrow, specifically the red marrow.

The white blood cells include granulocytes (neutrophils, eosinophils, and basophils), lymphocytes, and monocytes. There are normally 4,000 to 11,000 white blood cells per microliter of human blood. These provide powerful defenses for the body against tumors and infections (viral, bacterial, and parasitic).

The red blood cells carry hemoglobin, binding oxygen during circulation. They survive an average of 120 days, and their normal count is 5.4 million per microliter of blood in men and 4.8 million per microliter in women. Old red blood cells are destroyed by macrophages, and the hemoglobin of those is eventually converted into bilirubin. The formation of red blood cells (erythropoiesis) is controlled by a circulating glycoprotein hormone (erythropoietin) that is secreted primarily by the kidneys. Erythropoiesis is also stimulated by anemia or hypoxia and is inhibited by a rise in the circulating red blood cell level to supernormal values.

Platelets are smaller than the red blood cells and contain granules. Between 60% and 75% of platelets that have been extruded from the bone marrow are in the circulating blood, and the remainder are mostly in the spleen. Platelets play a significant role in the blood-clotting mechanism. They have a half-life of about 4 days.

Bone marrow is soft fatty tissue found in the medullary cavity of bones and consists of two types: red and yellow. Red marrow is a hematopoietic tissue producing granulocytes, red blood cells, and platelets. Some lymphocytes are formed in the bone marrow, but most are formed in the lymph nodes, thymus, and spleen from precursor cells that originated from bone marrow. Yellow marrow consists of fat cells for the most part and a few primitive blood cells. Red marrow is found in the flat and short bones.

The spleen is a highly vascular organ and is situated principally in the left hypochondriac region of the abdomen. It contains many platelets and macrophages and removes abnormal red blood cells. Additionally, the spleen plays a significant role in the immune system.

The thymus is situated between the sternum and great vessels. Although prominent in the infant, it is hardly recognizable in the adult. The thymus forms lymphocytes and is also believed to enable the body to produce the antibodies and to reject foreign tissue and cells.

DIGESTIVE SYSTEM

The digestive system grossly consists of the mouth, teeth, tongue, salivary glands, throat, esophagus, stomach, duodenum, jejunum, ileum, cecum, colon, rectum, and anal sphincter, as well as the liver, gallbladder, and pancreas. The salivary glands are present in the parotid, submandibular, and sublingual regions, secreting saliva into the mouth. The stomach secretes gastric acid (HCl) and various digestive enzymes that make the chewed food creamy, enabling further digestion by the intestine. The liver is the largest gland in the body and is situated in the upper part of the abdomen, on the right side just under the diaphragm. It manufactures the plasma proteins concerned with blood clotting and detoxifies many drugs and toxins. It also converts sugars into glycogen, stores glycogen and blood, and secretes bile. The bile is concentrated in the gallbladder, a pear-shaped sac lodged on the liver. The bile is poured into the small intestine via the bile ducts. The pancreas is also a large gland, excreting the digestive pancreatic juice and secreting insulin; it is located transversely behind the stomach. The pancreatic duct opens into the duodenum.After chewing and swallowing of food, digestion and fluid absorption are major physiological events occurring in the gastrointestinal tract. Intestinal peristaltic movements then propel its contents down to the rectum, resulting in defecation.

GENITOURINARY SYSTEMS

The male reproductive organs include the testes, the epididymis, the vas deferens, the seminal vesicles, the ejaculatory duct, and the penis. The testes, consisting of convoluted seminiferous tubules, are suspended in the scrotum by the spermatic cords and produce the spermatozoa. The interstitial cells of the testes, which are nested between the tubules, secrete testosterone into the blood stream. Spermatozoa leaving the testes are not fully mobile but continue their maturation and acquire motility while they are passing through the epididymis. The vas deferens conveys spermatozoa to the ejaculatory duct. The seminal vesicles secrete a fluid that is added to the sperm. The ejaculatory duct begins at the base of the prostate, and the semen is propelled out of the urethra by contraction of the bulbocavernosus muscle. The penis is composed of the corpus spongiosum and the corpora cavernosa, with arterial, venous, and lymphatic vessels. Erection of the penis is basically due to engorgement of the elastic tissue when it is filled with blood.

The female genital organs include the ovaries, containing a number of immature ova, the uterine tubes, the uterus, and the vagina, along with the external genitalia. The uterus is composed of the endometrium (inner mucous membrane), the myometrium (middle muscular coat), and the perimetrium (external serous coat). After puberty, the uterine endometrium develops periodic changes, under hormonal influence, that manifest menstrual bleeding. The changes in the uterus are closely correlated with cyclic changes in the ovary. The length of the cycle is usually 28 days. During the menstrual cycle there are also cyclic changes in the breasts, with distension of the mammary ducts, hyperemia, and edema of the interstitial tissue affected by estrogen and progesterone. At about the 14th day of the menstrual cycle, only one matured ovum is extruded from the ovary into the abdominal cavity (ovulation). The ovum is taken up by the fimbriated end of the uterine tube and is conveyed to the uterus. Fertilization of the ovum by the sperm usually occurs in the midportion of the tube. When one sperm cell fuses to the ovum, embryonic development begins. The developing embryo then moves down the tube into the uterus. Without fertilization, the ovum is passed out through the vagina.

The urinary organs include the kidneys, the ureters, the urinary bladder, and the urethra. The kidney is grossly composed of the outer cortex, the inner medulla, and the renal pelvis. In the kidneys, the glomerular capillaries filter a fluid resembling the blood plasma into the renal tubules (glomerular filtration). The tubules then reabsorb glucose and some of the water and solutes (tubular reabsorption) and secrete some electrolytes (tubular secretion) to the tubular fluid. In this manner physiological levels of blood electrolytes are maintained. Finally, the urine is formed and is conveyed from the renal pelvis via the ureters down to the urinary bladder. The detrusor muscle of the bladder contracts to expel the urine out through the urethra and relaxes to act as a reservoir for the urine until the next voiding becomes necessary. In addition to their excretory function, the kidneys work as endocrine organs, secreting erythropoietin to enhance the formation of red blood cells in the bone marrow and renin to maintain the blood pressure.

ENDOCRINE SYSTEM

The major endocrine glands are the thyroid gland, the parathyroid glands, the pituitary gland, the adrenal glands, and the pancreas.

The thyroid gland is located in the anterior neck and secretes thyroxine (an oxygen-consumption-stimulating hormone) and calcitonin (a calcium-lowering hormone). The secretion of thyroxine is regulated by thyroid-stimulating hormone (TSH), which is one of the anterior pituitary hormones. The parathyroid glands are situated on the thyroid gland, two on each side, and produce parathormone for calcium metabolism.

The pituitary gland is seated in the sella turcica of the spheroid bone and is composed of anterior, intermediate (rudimentary), and posterior lobes. The anterior lobe, which is under hypothalamic control, secretes growth hormone (GH), TSH, adrenocorticotropic hormone (ACTH), follicle-stimulating hormone (FSH) luteinizing hormone (LH), and prolactin. FSH and LH act on the ovaries and control the function of the testes. Prolactin stimulates lactation. The posterior lobe secretes oxytocin, for uterine contractions at term and ejection of milk during lactation, and vasopressin (antidiuretic hormone [ADH]) for inhibition of renal diuresis.

The adrenal glands are situated at the upper pole of each kidney and are therefore sometimes referred to as the supradrenal glands. The adrenal gland is composed of the outer cortex and the inner medulla. The adrenal cortex elaborates steroid hormones, which are derivatives of cholesterol. The function of the adrenal cortex is regulated by pituitary ACTH. The adrenal medulla synthesizes the catecholamines, including epinephrine, norepinephrine, and dopamine.

As an endocrine organ, the pancreas secretes insulin and glucagon for the metabolism of carbohydrates, proteins, and fats.

VISUAL SYSTEM

The ocular system is situated peripherally in orbit. The eyeball (Figure 2.10) is composed anteriorly of the cornea, an avascular transparent structure, but mostly of the opaque posterior segment, which consists of an outer thick layer (sclera), a middle vascular layer (choroid), and an inner neural layer (retina). In addition, the anterior part of the sclera is covered by the conjunctival membrane. The iris, which is a circular, colored disk suspended in the aqueous humor, contains circular and radial muscle fibers that, respectively, constrict and dilate the pupil. A space between the cornea and the iris is called the anterior chamber. The crystalline lens is located immediately behind the iris. The lens is encircled by the ciliary processes, which produce the aqueous humor in the posterior chamber (a small space between the iris and the lens). The aqueous humor then flows into the anterior chamber via the pupil. Posterior to the lens there is a large cavity containing a transparent semigelatinous material that is known as the vitreous body. The vitreous body is surrounded posteriorly by the retina, which consists of an outer pigmented layer and an inner neural wall (retina proper). The retina proper is further microscopically divided into 10 layers, which contain visual receptors (rods and cones) and nerve cells. However, a small area in the

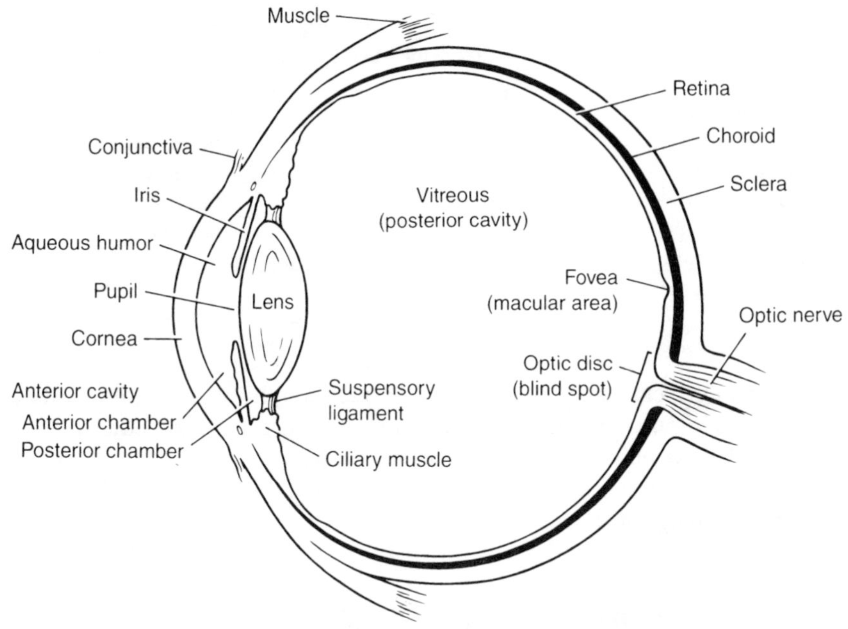

FIGURE 2.10 Schematic section of the human eye. The lens, the suspensory ligament, and the ciliary muscle divide the eye into anterior and posterior cavities. The iris further divides the anterior cavity into anterior and posterior chambers. Note the two extraocular muscles attached to the sclera.

From DeLisa and Stolov: Significant Body Systems in *Handbook of Severe Disability* edited by Stolov and Clowers, U.S. Department of Education, Rehabilitation Service Administration, 1981.

retina, where the optic nerve leaves the eye, has no visual receptors and is known as the blind spot. This region is also known as the optic disk.

Generally speaking, visual images are formed in the retina and conveyed to the occipital lobes of the brain via the optic nerves. For details, the visual field of each eye is divisible into the temporal field and the nasal field. Images from the temporal field are formed in the nasal portion of the retina, and images from the nasal field are formed in the temporal portion of the retina. The nerve fibers of the retina then convey visual impulses, which are transmitted by the optic nerve. However, the fibers from the nasal portion of the retina cross over in the optic chiasm, and the fibers from the temporal portion of the retina continue on the same side. These fibers combine (half from the nasal portion of retina and

TABLE 2.3 Extraocular Muscles

Name	Innervation cranial nerve	Eye movement
Superior rectus	III	Elevation/intorsion
Inferior rectus	III	Depression/extorsion
Medial rectus	III	Adduction
Lateral rectus	VI	Abduction
Superior oblique	IV	Intorsion/depression
Inferior oblique	III	Extorsion/elevation

half from the temporal portion of the other) to form the optic tract. Impulses are conveyed via the optic tract and end in the lateral geniculate body, where the fibers synapse on the cells, whose axons form the geniculocalcarine tract (the tract that finally conveys visual impulses to the occipital lobe of the cerebral cortex) (Figure 2.11).

AUDITORY AND VESTIBULAR SYSTEM

The receptors for hearing and equilibrium are located in the inner ears. The ear is divisible into the external ear, the middle ear (tympanic cavity), and the inner ear (labyrinth). The external ear includes the auricula, which collects sound, and the external auditory canal extending to the eardrum.

The middle ear is an air-filled space in the temporal bone that opens into the nasopharynx via the eustachian tube. This tube is usually closed, but it opens during chewing, swallowing, and yawning and thereby maintains the equality of air pressure on both sides of the eardrum. There are three movable auditory ossicles: the malleus, the incus, and the stapes, whose leverlike linkage serves to amplify the pressure of the sound. Sound waves passed through the external ear, eardrum, and ossicles are transformed into movements of the stapes, which set up fluid waves in the inner ear (Figure 2.12). There are also two small skeletal muscles: the tensor tympani and the stapedius. Their role is to reduce the oscillations of the ossicles to protect the inner ear from acoustic injury during a loud noise.

The inner ear is located in the petrous portion of the temporal bone and is divided into the bony labyrinth and the membranous labyrinth. The bony labyrinth consists of the cochlea, the vestibule, and the semicircular canals and contains a clear fluid, the perilymph. The perilymph surrounds most parts of the membranous labyrinth, which also contains a fluid, the endolymph. The cochlea, resembling

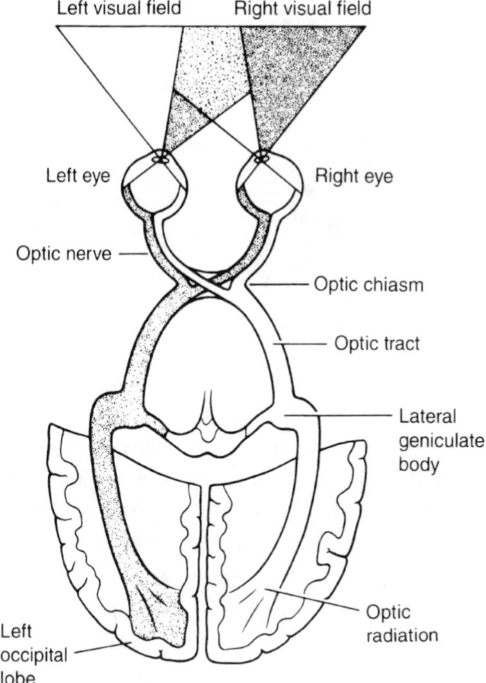

FIGURE 2.11 Note crossover of optic nerve fibers from both nasal retinas at the optic chiasma, with the result that the right visual field can project onto the left occipital cortex, and vice versa.

From DeLisa and Stolov: Significant Body Systems in *Handbook of Severe Disability* edited by Stolov and Clowers, U.S. Department of Education, Rehabilitation Service Administration, 1981.

a snail shell, contains the organ of Corti in its basal turn. This organ contains hair cells, innervated by the cochlear (auditory) division of the eighth cranial nerve, which function as auditory receptors. Auditory impulses then pass through the medial geniculate body in the thalamus and ultimately reach the auditory cortex of the temporal lobe.

In contrast, the vestibule and semicircular canals of the inner ear serve to maintain body equilibrium. There are two membranous sacs, called the utricle and the saccule, in the vestibular portion of the membranous labyrinth. These contain hair cells, as do the semicircular canals, that are innervated by the vestibular division of the eighth cranial nerve. Depending on body position, they

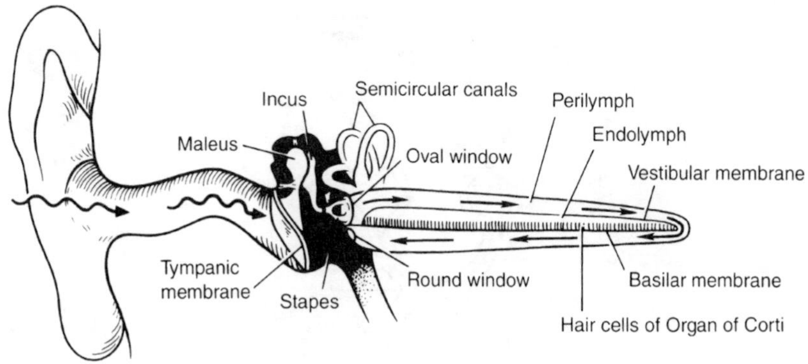

FIGURE 2.12 Schematic drawing of sound wave transmission. Sound wave vibrates the tympanic membrane, which in turn oscillates the malleus, incus, and stapes. Stapes vibrating in oval window agitates perilymph, which transmits vibration to vestibular membrane and then to endolymph to reach the hair cells of the organ of Corti. Wave dissipates at the round window. Note the two muscles anchoring the malleus and incus.

From DeLisa and Stolov: Significant Body Systems in *Handbook of Severe Disability* edited by Stolov and Clowers, U.S. Department of Education, Rehabilitation Service Administration, 1981.

are stimulated by otoliths in the maculae of the utricle and saccule and by the endolymph in the ampula of the semicircular canals. However, the anatomical pathways within the brain underlying vestibular function are yet to be clearly unveiled.

REFERENCES

Clemente, C. A. (1985). *Gray's anatomy* (American 30th ed.). Philadelphia: Lea and Febiger.

DeLisa, J., & Stolov, W. A. (1981). Significant body systems. In W. A. Stolov & M. R. Clowers (Eds.), *Handbook of severe disabilities* (pp. 19–54). Washington, DC: U.S. Department of Education, Rehabilitation Services Administration.

Ganong, W. A. (1991). *Review of medical physiology* (15th ed.). Los Altos, CA: Lange Medical Publications.

PART II

Disabling Conditions and Disorders

Chapter 3

Acquired Immune Deficiency Syndrome and Human Immunodeficiency Virus

Robert H. Remien, James Satriano, and Alan Berkman

Since the first case descriptions of what is now known as acquired immune deficiency syndrome (AIDS) appeared in the literature in the early 1980s (CDC, 1981), much has been learned about the disease. The causative agent of the disease, the human immune-deficiency virus (HIV), belongs to a family of viruses that have RNA as their core genetic material and are known as retroviruses. They are known as retroviruses because the process of converting RNA into DNA is the reverse of the normal cellular process.

For HIV to infect a host cell, the viral RNA must be converted into DNA, which can then be integrated into the host cell's DNA. Reverse transcriptase is the enzyme responsible for this conversion process. Once incorporated into the host cell, the viral genetic material causes the cell to produce more viral particles, which then bud from the host to infect other cells. Essentially, HIV converts healthy cells into virus factories.

HIV does not attack all the cells of the body but has a special affinity for cells known as lymphocytes and phagocytes. These are a class of white blood cells that circulate in the blood stream and are present in blood-forming organs of the body. These cells represent our major defense against foreign materials that have gained entry into the body.

IMMUNE FUNCTIONING

The functioning of an intact immune system is a well-orchestrated interplay of many factors (see Siegal, 1987, for a detailed explanation). Immune system cells are created in the bone marrow and consist of phagocytes (of which a macrophage is a special type) and two kinds of lymphocytes (T cells and B cells). When the body detects an invading organism, the phagocytes are the first line of defense. Macrophages will attack the invading virus and break off and display a piece of its surface protein, known as an antigen, so that other immune cells can identify the invader as a threat. The macrophages displaying the viral antigen muster the T cells into action. There are four different types of T cells (helper, killer, suppressor, and memory) created in the thymus. The antigen-carrying macrophage first activates helper T cells (also known as CD4+ lymphocytes) that are specific to the antigen being displayed. There are millions of types of helper T cells, each responsive to a different kind of antigen. The antigen fits the specific T-cell receptor like a key into a lock. The activated helper T cells travel to the spleen and lymph nodes, where they stimulate the production of killer T cells that are also specific to the antigen displayed by the macrophage. The killer T cells migrate to the site of the invading organism and, through a chemical process, kill the invader and any infected cells.

The antigen-displaying macrophage also activates the production of another type of immune system weapon, known as the B cell. The B cells are the immune system cells responsible for the production of antibodies. Antibodies are protein molecules made by the B cells and are, like the helper and killer T cells, specific to the antigen displayed by the macrophage. Antibodies can act against an invader in several ways. They destroy invading cells indirectly, by stimulating chemical reactions against them. They bind to the surface of the invaders, thereby causing them to clump together into aggregates and thus become more attractive targets for the phagocytes. Also, by binding to the surface of invading viruses, antibodies prevent the virus from binding with and thus infecting other cells.

When the battle is won and invading viral particles and infected cells have been destroyed, the suppressor T cells come into play. These cells, as their name implies, release a chemical that subdues the activated B and T cells and brings the production of new lymphatic cells to a halt. In the aftermath, memory B and T cells remain, giving the individual immunity to that specific strain of virus. However, very similar viruses can bear antigens with subtle differences, and immunity to one strain may not provide protection from another.

HIV VIROLOGY

HIV is a particularly insidious virus in that its major targets are the very cells of the immune system designed to protect against viral assault. HIV enters the body via blood or body fluids and is probably concealed in infected phagocytes or lymphocytes. The envelope protein of HIV (gpl20) has a high affinity for the

CD4 protein found on the surface of helper T cells and macrophages. However, several studies using both human and animal cells have demonstrated that the CD4 receptor alone is not sufficient for HIV to successfully infect a host cell. Macrophage-tropic strains of HIV, the type of HIV most commonly transmitted sexually, requires a coreceptor called CCR-5; T-cell tropic HIV uses a coreceptor called CXCR-4. Individuals can carry mutations of the CCR-5 coreceptor that may make them resistant to infection with macrophage-tropic strains when homozygous, and slow the progression of established HIV infection when heterozygous (Samson, Libert, & Doranz, 1996). It is believed that the envelope protein of HIV (gpl20) has a high affinity for the surface molecule of the CD4 protein found on the surface of helper T cell (CD4+ receptor). Once these molecules fuse, the viral RNA is released into the CD4+ cell. The viral enzyme reverse transcriptase converts the viral RNA into DNA, which is then integrated into the host cell's genome. The viral genetic components replicate within the host cell, and new viral particles are assembled and bud from the host cell to infect other cells (Shaw, Wong-Staal, & Gallo, 1988).

The reason that HIV damages the immune system is that it infects the very cells designed to fight off invading organisms, the macrophages and helper T cells. By infecting helper T cells and converting them into viral factories whose progeny can infect other cells, HIV slowly disables the immune system. As the number of healthy T cells drops, the immune system is made less effective in defending against other invading organisms, and the person becomes susceptible to opportunistic infections (Koenig & Fauci, 1988).

EPIDEMIOLOGY

The HIV infection in the United States was first noted among homosexual men in New York and California in 1981, as clusters of rare protozoal pneumonia (*pneumocystis carinii* pneumonia [PCP]) and rare skin cancer (Kaposi's sarcoma [KS]) began to be reported. At that time it was unclear how these diseases came about, and it was several years before a blood/body fluid-borne virus was discovered as the etiological agent. By that time, well-delineated disease clusters were established (Kaslow & Francis, 1989). Infection rates among homosexual men continued to rise. Also noted were escalating infection rates among intravenous drug users and blood transfusion recipients, especially hemophiliacs who received frequent transfusions of blood products. By the mid-1980s it was well established that HIV was transmitted through sexual contact, blood, and blood products, but at that time the disease was largely confined to males in this country. Soon reports of women infected by sexual partners began to emerge. These women were, by and large, the sexual partners of bisexual men or men who used intravenous drugs. As the rates of infected women began to rise, the virus was discovered to infect some of their children. It is believed that a percentage of infants become infected either in utero, during the birth process, or following birth through breast-feeding. Less frequent but news-making cases of transmission have occurred: from health care worker to patient, from patient to health care worker, and through organ or tissue transplantation.

Globally, the dominant mode of HIV transmission has been and remains heterosexual sex. Outside the U.S. and Europe, the ratio of infected men to women is 1:1. During the middle and latter part of the 1990s, the epidemiological pattern in large urban areas of the U.S. increasingly resembles that of Africa, Asia, and Latin America, with a growing proportion of new HIV infection occurring in young women with unprotected heterosexual sex as their primary risk factor (CDC, 1997).

- In the United States in 1996, approximately 70,000 new AIDS cases were reported to CDC.
- From 1981 through 1996, a total of 573,800 persons aged >13 years with AIDS were reported by state and local health departments.
- In 1996, non-Hispanic Blacks accounted for 41% of adults reported with AIDS, and women accounted for an all-time high of 20% of adults reported with AIDS.
- In 1996, the number of AIDS deaths declined in the United States for the first time since AIDS surveillance was initiated by the CDC.
- In 1997, it was estimated by UNAIDS that there are 30.6 million people with HIV/AIDS worldwide. That figure is expected to reach 40 million in the year 2000.
- Approximately 16,000 people, including 2,000 infants, become infected with HIV every day. More than 90% of those individuals live in developing countries with little or no access to antiretroviral treatment.

FUNCTIONAL PRESENTATION OF MEDICAL CONDITION/DISABILITY

Course of Illness

Infection with HIV can occur when contaminated blood or body fluids (especially sperm or vaginal fluids) come into contact with the bloodstream or mucosal tissue. The most common modes of transmission are sexual (unprotected anal, vaginal, or oral intercourse), blood-borne (transfusion or contaminated blood or blood products, needle-stick injuries, the use of "dirty" intravenous drug-injection equipment), or from mother to child (either perinatally or through breast-feeding). It should be noted that the course of illness described below does not hold for all individuals infected with HIV. Also, it should be stressed that the time of progression from HIV infection to AIDS may be considerable (more than 10 years), and it is still not clear if all HIV-infected individuals will develop AIDS.

Following contact with fluids contaminated with a sufficient number of viral particles, acute HIV infection may occur. The initial reaction to infection with

HIV may be a constellation of flu-like symptoms that can include fever, headache, and sore throat. These symptoms may last from a few days to a few weeks before dissipating (Yarchoan & Pluda, 1988). The immune system develops antibodies to HIV, indicating an immunological response, albeit an ineffective one. The development of antibodies to HIV usually occurs within 2 to 6 months after initial infection but in some cases may be delayed for up to 2 1/2 years (Imagawa et al., 1989; Ranki et al., 1987; Wolinsky et al., 1989). The currently licensed HIV tests (ELISA and Western blot) are tests for viral antibodies, not direct tests of the virus itself. There now exists an HIV RNA viral load assay that provides a direct measure of circulating virus per unit of blood (Ho, 1996). This measure can show the presence of HIV infection, even in the absence of a positive antibody test. Thus, one could be infected with HIV and be able to transmit it to others and still test HIV-negative by Western blot, if one had not yet developed viral antibodies. The Centers for Disease Control (CDC; 1992) adopted revised guidelines for the diagnostic classification of HIV-infected individuals as of 1993. This system has clinical categories with three CD4+ lymphocyte (helper T cell) ranges. The categories refer to HIV-related symptoms, and the levels refer to the absolute number of helper T cells per cubic millimeter of blood. The proposed CDC diagnostic classification system can be found in Table 3.1.

Following infection, patients generally enter a phase of asymptomatic HIV infection or persistent generalized lymphadenopathy (PGL; i.e., swollen lymph nodes) (Yarchoan & Pluda, 1988). During this phase of the illness patients may look and feel well. As noted above, this phase can last more than 10 years, and some HIV-infected individuals may never develop AIDS; we don't yet know. This phase corresponds to clinical category A in the CDC classification system.

The development of symptoms associated with moderate immune deficiency corresponds to CDC category B. The symptoms might include but are not limited to peripheral neuropathy, thrush, shingles, and pelvic inflammatory disease. The

TABLE 3.1 1993 Revised Classification System for HIV Infection and Expanded AIDS Surveillance Case Definition for Adolescents and Adults*

	Clinical categories		
CD4+ Cell counts	(A) Asymptomatic or PGL	(B) Symptomatic, not (A) or (C) conditions	(C) AIDS-indicator conditions
(1) > 500	A1	B1	C1
(2) 200–499	A2	B2	C2
(3) < 200 AIDS-indicator cell count	A3	B3	C3

*The shaded cells illustrate AIDS defining conditions.

development of these conditions is attributed to HIV, and their treatment is complicated by the virus.

Category C describes a list of conditions associated with severe immune deficiency. The list of AIDS-defining conditions can be found in Table 3.2. These are the conditions that result in a diagnosis of AIDS.

It should be noted that many AIDS activist groups object to the omission of many opportunistic infections developed by HIV-positive women from the list of AIDS-defining conditions. Women with conditions such as persistent or recurrent vaginal infections should consider the possibility of HIV infection. And for women with HIV infection, close gynecological follow-up is essential. Aggressive treatment of secondary infections at the earliest possible time is just as important in women as men.

TABLE 3.2 Conditions Included in the 1993 AIDS Surveillance Case Definition

Candidiasis of bronchi, trachea, or lungs
Candidiasis, esophageal
Cervical cancer, invasive
Coccidioidomycosis, disseminated or extrapulmonary
Cryptococcosis, extrapulmonary
Cryptosporidiosis, chronic intestinal (> 1 month duration)
Cytomegalovirus disease (other than liver, spleen, or nodes)
Cytomegalovirus retinitis (with loss of vision)
HIV encephalopathy
Herpes simplex: chronic ulcer(s) (> 1 month duration); or bronchitis, pneumonitis, or esophagitis
Histoplasmosis, disseminated or extrapulmonary
Isosporiasis, chronic intestinal (> 1 month duration)
Kaposi's sarcoma
Lymphoma, Berkitt's
Lymphoma, immunoblastic
Lymphoma, primary of brain
Mycobacterium avium complex or *M. Kansasii*, disseminated or extrapulmonary
Mycobacterium tuberculosis, any site (pulmonary or extrapulmonary)
Mycobacterium, other species or unidentified species, disseminated or extrapulmonary
Pneumocystis carintii pneumonia
Pneumonia, recurrent
Progressive multi focal leukoencephalopathy
Salmonella septicemia, recurrent
Toxoplasmosis of brain
Wasting syndrome due to HIV

Source: U.S. Centers for Disease Control and Prevention (1992).

As can be seen in Table 3.1, the current CDC classification system proposes that the diagnosis of AIDS be given to individuals in categories A and B who have CD4+ lymphocyte (helper T cell) counts of less than 200 per cubic millimeter of blood. Normal CD4+ counts are generally greater than 800. Although these individuals would not have developed an AIDS-defining infection, the blood counts are representative of severe immune deficiency.

When an individual is in a severe state of immune suppression, he or she is subject to repeated bouts of the illnesses listed in Table 3.2. Generally, the patient succumbs to one or a combination of opportunistic infections within a period of months to a few years of the onset of severe immune deficiency.

Functional Presentation of Disability

Prior to the development of severe immune deficiency, the HIV-infected individual may have no disabling condition at all. However, later in the course of the disease, many of the opportunistic infections described above can have a protracted course and may lead to prolonged periods of illness and hospitalization. Generally, the onset of the symptoms of AIDS is considered to be a disabling condition.

Aside from the physical disability due to opportunistic infection, HIV can directly infect the central nervous system (CNS) and result in a progressive dementing illness. Although the AIDS dementia complex (ADC) (Navia, Jordan, & Price, 1986) is estimated to affect over two thirds of patients prior to the terminal phase of the disease, it is rarely the first presenting symptom of the disease process (McArthur et al., 1989; Miller et al., 1990). Price and Brew (1988) developed a clinical staging system for the AIDS dementia complex that can be found in Table 3.3.

As can be seen from the characteristics of AIDS-associated dementia, cognitive, motor, and behavioral abilities are affected. It is important to note, however, that some opportunistic infections may result in altered mental states that mimic ADC but respond well to medical treatment. Therefore, all patients showing changes in mental status should be referred for a medical workup. Their symptoms may be as subtle as a slightly disturbed gait or very elusive memory complaints.

In patients with end-stage ADC, organic psychotic symptoms may be present; they most commonly involve hallucinations and/or delirium. It should be noted that as the dementia progresses, the patient will require increasing amounts of assistance in activities of daily living. For example, moderately demented patients may require supervision in taking medication and preparing food. End-stage patients typically require 24-hour nursing care and supervision in all activities.

TREATMENT AND PROGNOSIS

Survival rates for persons diagnosed with AIDS vary across studies in different geographical regions and research or clinical settings. Although some studies

TABLE 3.3 Clinical Staging of the AIDS Dementia Complex

Stage	Characteristics
Stage 0	Normal mental and motor function.
Stage 0.5 (equivocal/subclinical)	Absent, minimal, or equivocal symptoms without impairment of work or capacity to perform ADL. Mild signs may be present. Gait and strength are normal.
Stage 1 (mild)	Able to perform all but the most demanding aspects of work or ADL but with unequivocal evidence or functional intellectual or motor impairment. Can walk without assistance.
Stage 2 (moderate)	Able to perform basic activities of self-care but cannot work or maintain the more demanding aspects of daily life. Ambulatory, but may require a single prop.
Stage 3 (severe)	Major intellectual incapacity or motor disability.
Stage 4 (end stage)	Nearly vegetative. Intellectual and social comprehension and output are at rudimentary level. Nearly or absolutely mute. Paraplegic with or without incontinence.

Source: Price and Brew (1988).

showed a correlation of survival with gender, race, and mode of transmission, it appears that social and health care system factors explain these results. Undefined genetic factors, age, and comorbid infections, such as tuberculosis, do appear to influence survival. Until recently, low CD4+ cell count was thought to be the best predictor of disease progression and death (Stein, Korvick, & Vermund, 1992); it has now been demonstrated that the best single laboratory predictor of progression or death is the viral RNA level in the blood plasma (Mellors, Rinaldo, & Gupta, 1996). Clinically, those individuals whose only AIDS-defining condition is a low CD4+ count or Kaposi's sarcoma have the longest survival (i.e., range of 1 to 9+ years), whereas those with neurological disorders, whether due to opportunistic infections or neoplasms, have the shortest survival period (e.g., median survival of 4 months).

There have been improved survival rates for people diagnosed with AIDS since the start of the epidemic. As health care providers became more familiar with the manifestations of HIV infection, they were able to identify and treat potentially curable infections earlier and more accurately. In fact, more recent studies have shown that the experience of the health care provider is a significant predictor of prognosis in patients with HIV. By the late 1980s, prophylaxis against PCP had become widespread and significantly decreased the morbidity and mortality associated with that infection. At approximately the same time, antiretroviral treatment with a single nucleoside reverse transcriptase inhibitor (e.g., AZT, DDI, DDC) became available and did provide limited clinical benefit for those with advanced disease. Complementing these biomedical advances was better overall psychosocial management of HIV-infected and AIDS-diagnosed patients. Although some patients are receiving better all-around treatment that improves their survival and quality of life, many still do not have access to adequate care, and for others there exist psychological, cultural, and social barriers to receiving that care.

Starting in 1996, there has been a dramatic change in the clinical management of HIV in the United States. The introduction of a powerful new class of antiretroviral drugs, the protease inhibitors, have now made it possible for combinations of three or more drugs to suppress viral load below the limit of detection in many, if not most, HIV-infected individuals (Bartlett, 1996). There is growing clinical-trial data that significant treatment-induced decreases in viral load can translate into decreased morbidity and mortality in those with advanced disease; there is a biological rationale, but little data, to support that assumption among those with earlier and asymptomatic disease.

Readily available accurate viral load measurements has perhaps been as important as the development of combination HIV drug therapy to the new treatment paradigm. The optimal goal of therapy has now become the suppression of viral load to undetectable levels, and viral load now guides decisions on both initiation and changes in antiretroviral therapy (Carpenter, Fischl, & Hammer, 1997). Treatment guidelines developed in 1997 by both the International AIDS Society—U.S. branch and the Department of Health and Human Services strongly encourage the initiation of at least three drug-combination therapies in all persons symptomatic with HIV, in many who are asymptomatic, in individuals who develop primary HIV infection and in health care workers who have a significant occupational exposure to HIV. In addition, antiretroviral therapy, either monotherapy with AZT or combination therapy depending on individual circumstances, is strongly recommended for all HIV-infected women who become pregnant (Centers for Disease Control, 1994).

The decision to start medical treatment can be a difficult one, psychologically, for people with HIV infection because initiating treatment signifies the acceptance of a life-threatening illness. It also means starting treatment that will most likely need to be continued for the rest of the patient's life. Additionally, there is the legitimate concern about negative side effects and a theoretical risk of developing a resistance to antiviral properties of specific medications. It's reassuring to many patients to know that the treatment regimen that is started initially will not necessarily be the one that will be followed a few years down the road. The thinking is that additional treatments and new treatment combinations will be available as advances are made in the understanding and management of HIV illness.

It is hard for patients to know when to begin antiviral therapies. The new treatment guidelines recommend a "treat early, treat hard" approach that encourages people living with HIV to start three or four drug combination therapies early in the disease process when the immune system is still largely intact. There is some evidence that early treatment is more likely to result in suppression of viral replication and minimize the chance that drug-resistant viral mutations will emerge. However, the current treatment regimens are extremely complex, often involving 10 or more pills taken at four or five dosing intervals with varying relationships to meals. Further compounding the difficulty of adherence is the reality that side effects are common with powerful combination therapy, making patients who were asymptomatic from their HIV infection feel worse than before they started treatment. This combination of factors poses a considerable obstacle to high levels of adherence by almost all patients, and there is evidence that even minor problems with adherence can rapidly lead to clinically significant drug resistance. Therefore, the decision to begin therapy must be approached extremely carefully, and made only after full discussion of potential benefits and risks.

Patients with advanced HIV disease (AIDS) obviously must confront all the same difficulties concerning adherence discussed previously, but there is more compelling evidence that combination therapy can slow down the progression of their disease and improve the quality of their lives. Treatment guidelines recommend that all patients with CDC-defined AIDS and also those with symptomatic infection without AIDS be started on combination therapy that includes at least one protease inhibitor. Unlike asymptomatic patients, many persons with more advanced disease have a dramatic improvement in the overall quality of their lives and find that the problems posed by side-effects is compensated for by increased energy and a sense of well-being. However, AIDS patients often take several prophylactic drugs as well as complicated regimens for comorbid diseases, and the potential for drug–drug interactions and drug toxicity is significant. For example, psychotropic medications such as bupropion, midazolam, and triazolam are contraindicated in patients taking Ritonavir, one of the protease inhibitors. In addition, other manifestations of advanced disease, such as anorexia and wasting, may make it difficult for patients to adhere to the dietary requirements of the antiretroviral regimens and to absorb the drugs.

Although initiation of effective antiretroviral therapy often results in increased CD4+ counts and some recovery of immune function, the consensus among providers is that prophylaxis against opportunistic diseases such as PCP and Mycobacterium avium complex (MAI) should not be stopped. Many immunologists believe that HIV can cause irreversible damage to dedicated memory cells that makes it impossible for an individual to regain a full repertoire of immune responses even if the CD4+ count rises significantly. It will take years of clinical observation to determine if partially reconstituted immune systems can keep patients free of opportunistic infections and malignancies.

The medical management of HIV-positive and AIDS patients is complex and rapidly changing. Great strides have been made but much remains to be done. It is important that patients have access to physicians who are knowledgeable and experienced with HIV care and that patients themselves are informed about the disease and a range of treatment strategies. Management of this disease requires consistent updating and flexibility in approach on the part of both doctor and patient.

Without discussing specific treatments, here are some general guidelines for HIV-seropositive individuals based on the Health and Human Services guidelines and the advice of both patient advocacy and physician groups:

• All patients should work on remaining healthy by eating well, exercising, being careful about use of alcohol and recreational drugs and practicing safer sex. Patients should be reminded that sexually transmitted infections can both increase the risk of transmitting HIV to others and can raise an infected individual's viral load.

• Patients should attempt to find a physician experienced in the management of HIV who is willing to spend the necessary time to answer their questions fully. Decisions about when to initiate antiretroviral therapy, and which medications best fit the patient's lifestyle should normally take place over several visits.

• Guidelines strongly recommend that all patients who are symptomatic with HIV-related conditions, or who have AIDS, should be treated with combination antiretroviral therapy that includes one or more protease inhibitors.

• Guidelines recommend that asymptomatic patients with CD4+ T cells <500/mm or with viral load >20,000 (by RT-PCR) be offered combination therapy. The strength of this recommendation is based on the prognosis for disease-free survival as determined by viral load and CD4+ count and by willingness of the patient to accept therapy after being fully informed of potential risks and benefits.

• For those individuals infected with HIV who are asymptomatic and have >500 CD4+ T cells and <20,000 viral load, some experts would recommend treatment and some would delay treatment and observe. There is little clinical evidence that supports powerful combination therapy in this group.

• Once an individual starts on therapy, viral load and CD4+ measurements should be done approximately every three to four months. Changes in therapy will be dictated by clinical and virological response.

• Established guidelines for initiation of prophylaxis for various opportunistic infections should be followed based on a patient's lowest CD4+ count.

PSYCHOLOGICAL AND VOCATIONAL IMPLICATIONS

It has become increasingly clear that psychologists and other mental health workers can and do play a primary role in the overall management and care of HIV-infected people and people living with AIDS. Both research and clinical experience show us that adverse social and psychological consequences are associated with various stages of the HIV illness spectrum. Notable time points that often require mental health intervention include initial knowledge of one's antibody status, onset of physical symptoms, receiving an AIDS-defining diagnosis, and entering the terminal phase of the illness. Significant psychological reactions can occur during any and all of these phases of HIV illness. Such reactions include psychological distress—typically depression, despair, hopelessness, anxiety, and panic reactions—and psychiatric disorders, usually depressive, anxiety or adjustment disorders. Vegetative symptoms often include sleep and appetite disturbances, headaches, and fatigue. It is important to note that the stigma associated with this disease is an additional psychological burden to those infected and affected by this disease. Some studies have indicated significantly higher rates of suicide and suicidal ideation (e.g., Marzuk et al., 1988).

Conversely, some studies have shown that there can be remarkable psychological resilience in HIV-infected persons in both asymptomatic (Williams, Rabkin, Remien, Gorman, & Ehrhardt, 1991) and symptomatic stages. Research has consistently shown there to be an association between lower psychological distress and good social supports, active coping strategies, and an optimistic attitude in people living with chronic and life-threatening illnesses. The goals of psychological intervention include addressing these factors, namely, reducing isolation, facilitating good social supports, teaching and enhancing positive coping strategies, and helping to maintain hope. A psychological study of long-term survivors with AIDS found low rates of clinical depression and a positive quality of life, even in the context of profound illness (Remien, Rabkin, Katoff, & Williams, 1992). Participants in this study were all connected to a community-based service organization, and a majority of them had received individual psychotherapy since their AIDS diagnosis. Additionally, they were active in the medical management of their disease and worked hard to obtain what they felt was optimal medical care. As new treatment options are made available it becomes increasingly complicated for patients to make treatment decisions regarding when to initiate and/or change medication regimens and which combination therapies to use. It is equally challenging to initiate and maintain strict adherence to complicated dosing schedules. The counselor can play a role in facilitating the medical management of this disease and assisting in overcoming barriers to adherence.

Because persons with HIV infection and AIDS may experience a range of mental health needs, it is important that mental health services be available to them, including the following:

1. Crisis intervention. Interventions should be designed to enhance adaptive and integrative functioning through past and newly acquired coping skills. Whenever possible, having crisis services available in medical or community settings can provide early intervention and possibly prevent further crisis.

2. Individual therapy. A wide range of individual therapies can be helpful for the person with HIV infection and AIDS, including supportive, cognitive-behavioral, and insight-oriented approaches. It is important to address the patient's ability to manage distress and crises, deal with the ramifications of perceived loss, recognize and resolve grief, enhance support systems, maintain hopefulness, and maximize decision-making skills.

3. Family interventions. The overall goals of family intervention include enhancing the family's ability to support each other, focusing on the immediate crisis and environmental situation, facilitating the grieving process, and encouraging the use of community social supports and resources. Case management,

couples counseling, family therapy, home visits, and multiple family group interventions can be used to address these goals.

4. Support groups. Support groups can be extremely useful for people coping with HIV infection and AIDS because they allow for the enhancement of social support. A range of modalities may be useful, including cognitive-behavioral groups, therapy groups, and self-help groups. Both short-term and long-term closed groups can provide predictable consistency and ongoing social support. Drop-in groups can be especially useful for persons requiring immediate support.

5. Substance abuse treatment. Treatment of substance use problems associated with HIV infection is important for several reasons, including the prevention of further HIV transmission, health concerns for the infected individual, and the effect of psychoactive substance use on decision-making capability. Relapse in substance use is common following significant stressors, such as knowledge of a seropositive antibody status, the onset of medical symptoms, or receiving an AIDS-defining diagnosis.

There are also prevention issues that the counselor can address with HIV-infected persons. Once an individual knows the test result to be positive, he or she shoulders a significant responsibility for preventing further transmission. As many years of intervention research have shown, the initiation and, more important, the maintenance of safer sexual practices is not easily accomplished, even for the most committed. HIV-infected individuals also need psychological counseling to facilitate frank discussions of sex behavior and honest disclosure to sex partners. Some studies show that individuals who changed their sexual behavior to lessen the risk of transmission were more distressed than those who maintained high-risk behaviors. To forestall recidivism, the psychological cost of changing sexual behavior must be acknowledged, and mental health supportive services should be made available to assist individuals in making and maintaining behavior changes.

It is important for mental health workers to educate themselves about all aspects of HIV illness, including medical aspects and treatment strategies, which continue to evolve over time. It is also essential that counselors be familiar with information, medical, social, and legal resources available in the community to which they can refer patients and their significant others.

In review, psychologists and other mental health professionals can provide much needed services to HIV-infected and -affected people. These include helping patients, their friends, and families to deal with the initial trauma of an HIV or an AIDS-defining diagnosis; helping them to cope with the multiple psychological ramifications of the illness; assessing and monitoring the psychological and mental status of their patients; facilitating the medical management of this disease by encouraging patients to become active in their own medical care and helping them to access good medical (including psychiatric) intervention; helping to bring about positive behavior change; encouraging patients to access community resources and family support; facilitating the maintenance of hope while confronting this illness; and facilitating the optimal management of the dying process when that is the acknowledged outcome.

REFERENCES

Bartlett, J. (1996). Protease inhibitors for HIV infection. *Annals of Internal Medicine, 124,* 1086–1088.

Carpenter, C. C., Fischl, M. A., Hammer, S. M., Hirsch, M. S., Jacobsen, D. M., Katzenstein, D. A., Montaner, J. S. G., Richman, D. D., Saag, M. S., Schooley, R. T., Thompson, M. A., Vella, S., Yeni, P. G., & Volberding, P. A. (1997). Antiretroviral therapy for HIV infection in 1997. *Journal of the American Medical Association, 277,* 1962–1969.

Centers for Disease Control. (1981). *Pneumocystis* pneumonia—Los Angeles. *Morbidity and Mortality Weekly Report, 30,* 250.

Centers for Disease Control. (1992). 1993 revised classification system for HIV infection and expanded AIDS surveillance case definition for adolescents and adults. Atlanta: Author.

Centers for Disease Control. (1994). Zidovudine for the prevention of HIV transmission from mother to infant. *Morbidity and Mortality Weekly Report, 46,* 285–287.

Centers for Disease Control. (1997). Update: Trends in AIDS incidence, deaths, and prevalence—United States, 1996. *Morbidity and Mortality Weekly Report, 46*(8), 165–173.

Ho, D. D. (1996). Viral counts in HIV infection. *Science, 272,* 1123–1125.

Imagawa, D. T., Lee, M. H., Wolinsky, S. M. Sano, K., Morales, F., Kwok, S., Shinsky, J. J., Nishanian, R. U., Giorgi, J., Fahey, S. V., Dudley, J., Visscha, B. R., & Detels, R. (1989). Human immune-deficiency virus type I infection in homosexual men who remain seronegative for prolonged periods. *New England Journal of Medicine, 320,* 1458–1462.

Kaslow, R. A., & Francis, D. P. (1989). *The epidemiology of AIDS.* New York: Oxford University Press.

Koenig, S., & Fauci, A. (1988). AIDS: Immunopathogenesis and immune response to the human immune-deficiency virus. In V. DeVita, S. Hellman, & S. Rosenberg (Eds.), *AIDS etiology, diagnosis, treatment and prevention.* Philadelphia: J. B. Lippincott.

Marzuk, P., Tierney, H., Tardiff, K., Gross, E., Morgan, E., Hsu, M., & Mann, J. (1988). Increased risk of suicide in persons with AIDS. *Journal of the American Medical Association, 259,* 1333–1337.

McArthur, J. C., Cohen, B. A., Selnes, O. A., Kumer, A. J., Cooper, K., McArthur, J. H., Soucey, G., Connblath, D. R., Chmiel, J. S., Wang, M. C., Starkey, D. L., Ginsburg, H., Ostrow, D. G., Johnson, R. T., PhaiS J. R., & Polk, B. F. (1989). Low prevalence of neurological and neuropsychological abnormalities in otherwise healthy HIV-1-infected individuals: Results from the multicenter AIDS cohort study. *Annals of Neurology, 26,* 601–611.

Mellors, J. W., Rinaldo, C. R., Gupta, P., White, R. M., Todd, J. A., & Kingsley, L. A. (1996). Prognosis in HIV-1 infection predicted by the quantity of virus in plasma. *Science, 272,* 1167–1170.

Miller, E. N., Selnes, O. A., McArthur, J. C., Satz, P., Becker, J. T., Cohen, B. A., Sheridan, K., Machado, A. M., Van Gorp, W. G., & Visscher, B. (1990). Neuropsychological performance in HIV-1-infected homosexual men: The multicenter AIDS cohort study (MACS). *Neurology, 40,* 197–203.

Navia, B. A., Jordan, B. D., & Price, R. W. (1986). The AIDS dementia complex: 1. Clinical features. *Annals of Neurology, 19,* 517–524.

Piette, J., Mor, V., & Fleishman, J. (1991). Patterns of survival with AIDS in the United States. *Health Services Research, 26,* 75 95.

Price, R. W., & Brew, B. J. (1988). The AIDS dementia complex. *Journal of Infectious Diseases, 158,* 1079–1083.

Ranki, A., Valle, S. L., Krohn, M., Antonen, J., Allain, J. D., Leuther, M., Franchini, G., & Krohn, K. (1987). Long latency precedes overt seroconversion in sexually transmitted human immune-deficiency infection. *Lancet, 2,* 589–593.

Remien, R. H., Rabkin, J. G., Katoff, L., & Williams, J. B. W. (1992). Coping strategies and health beliefs of AIDS longterm survivors. *Psychology and Health, 6,* 335–345.

Samson, M., Libert, F., Doranz, B. J., Rucker, J., Liesnard, C., Farber, C. M., Saragosti, S., Lapoumeroulie, C., Cognaux, J., Forceille, O., Muyldermans, G., Verhofstede, C., Burtonboy, G., Georges, M., Imai, T., Rana, S., Yi, Y., Smyth, R. J., Collman, R. G., Doms, R. W., Vassart, G., & Parmentier, M. (1996). Resistance to HIV-1 infection in Caucasian individuals bearing mutant alleles of the CCR-5 chemokine receptor gene. *Nature, 382,* 722–725.

Shaw, G. M., Wong-Staal, F., & Gallo, R. C. (1988). Etiology of AIDS: Virology, molecular biology, and evolution of human immune-deficiency viruses. In V. DeVita, S. Hellman, & S. Rosenberg (Eds.), *AIDS etiology, diagnosis, treatment and prevention.* Philadelphia: J. B. Lippincott.

Siegal, F. P. (1987). The immune deficiency in AIDS. In G. Wormser, R. Stahl, & E. Bottone (Eds.), *AIDS and other manifestations of HIV infection.* Park Ridge, NJ: Noyes Publications.

Stein, D. S., Korvic, J. A., & Vermund, S. H. (1992). CD4+ lymphocyte cell enumeration for prediction of clinical course of human immunodeficiency virus disease: A review. *Journal of Infectious Diseases, 165,* 352–363.

Williams, J. B. W., Rabkin, J. G., Remien, R. H., Gorman, J. M., & Ehrhardt, A. A. (1991). Multidisciplinary baseline assessment of homosexual men with and without human immune-deficiency virus infection. *Archives of General Psychiatry, 48,* 124–130.

Wolinsky, S. M., Rinaldo, C. R., Kwok, S., Snisky, J. J., Gupta, P., Imagawa, D., Frazedegan, H., Jacobson, L. P., Grovit, K. S., Lee, M. H., Chmiel, J. S., Ginsburg, H., Kaslow, R. A., & Phair, J. R. (1989). Human immune-deficiency virus type I infection a median of 18 months before a diagnostic Western blot: Evidence from a cohort of homosexual men. *Annals of Internal Medicine, 111,* 961–972.

Yarchoan, R., & Pluda, J. M. (1988). Clinical aspects of infection with AIDS retrovirus: Acute HIV infection, persistent generalized lymphadenopathy, and AIDS-related complex. In V. DeVita, S. Hellman, & S. Rosenberg (Eds.), *AIDS etiology, diagnosis, treatment and prevention.* Philadelphia: J. B. Lippincott.

Chapter 4

Alzheimer's Disease

Barry Reisberg, Emile H. Franssen, Liduïn E. M. Souren, and Reuben R. Cespon

Presently, more than 34 million persons in the United States are age 65 or older, representing over 12% of the U.S. population. Similar demographic changes over the course of this century are evident in other developed nations. Current evidence suggests that approximately 10% to 15% of community-residing elderly persons may be afflicted with Alzheimer's disease (AD) or closely related dementing illnesses of late life (Evans et al., 1989; Katzman, 1986). Consequently, it is estimated that in the United States more than 4 million persons may have AD. AD is the fourth leading cause of death in the elderly, after heart disease, cancer, and stroke, and is the single major cause of institutionalization of aged people in the United States and in many other industrialized nations in the world. Current studies have indicated that a large majority of the more than 1.5 million residents in nursing homes in the United States manifest a dementia syndrome generally associated with AD (Chandler & Chandler, 1988; Rovner, Kafonek, Filipp, Lucas, & Folstein, 1986). The dimensions of the institutional burden associated with AD are even more striking when it is noted that well under 1 million persons are in U.S. hospitals at any particular time.

The course of AD has been described in increasing detail over the past several years. The cognitive, functional, and behavioral concomitants at each stage of the illness can now be described in detail. The clinically observable symptomatology of AD dramatically changes in form from the earliest manifest deficits to the most severe stage; therefore, recognition and differentiation of the stages of this illness is imperative for proper diagnosis, prognosis, management, and treatment. Progressive cognitive changes that occur are manifest in concentration, recent memory, past memory, orientation, functioning and self-care, language, praxis ability, and calculation, among other areas (Reisberg, London, et al., 1983; Reisberg, Schneck, Ferris, Schwartz, & de Leon, 1983). Characteristic behavioral symptoms are also a frequent component of AD (Kumar, Koss, Metzler, Moore, & Friedland, 1988; Reisberg, Franssen, Sclan, Kluger, & Ferris, 1989; Rubin, Morris, Storandt, & Berg, 1987). These behavioral symptoms peak in occurrence at various points in the course of AD and subsequently recede in magnitude and frequency with the progression of the disease. A comprehensive view of the nature and progression of these cognitive, functional, and behavioral changes is critical for the optimization of residual capacity and the identification and management of excess disability in these patients.

An outline of global cognitive, functional, and behavioral changes in normal aging and progressive AD is provided in the Global Deterioration Scale (Reisberg, Ferris, de Leon, & Crook, 1982), outlined in Table 4.1 and described in greater detail below.

GLOBAL DESCRIPTION OF NORMAL BRAIN AGING AND AD

Reisberg et al. (1982) described seven major clinically distinguishable global stages from normality to most severe AD. These stages and their implications are as follows:

Stage 1: No cognitive decline. Diagnosis: Normal. No objective or subjective evidence of cognitive decrement is seen. Only a minority of elderly persons fall within this category, perhaps 20% of persons over age 65. The prognosis is excellent for continued adequate cognitive functioning.

Stage 2: Very mild cognitive decline. Diagnosis: Normal aging. The majority of persons over age 65 have subjective complaints of cognitive decrement such as a subjective perception of forgetting names of people they know well or of forgetting where they placed particular objects such as keys or jewelry. These subjective complaints may be elicited by comparing the person's perceived abilities with their perceptions of their performance 5 to 10 years previously.

Complaints of cognitive impairment may also occur with other, much more serious conditions common in the elderly, notably dementia and depression. Persons with the generally benign complaints associated with this stage can usually recall the names of two or more primary school teachers, classmates, or friends and are oriented to the time of day, date, day of week, month, season, and year (although, of course, occasional minor errors may occur). Increasing

TABLE 4.1 Global Deterioration Scale (GDS) for Age-Associated Cognitive Decline and Alzheimer's Disease

GDS stage	Clinical characteristics	Diagnosis
1 No cognitive decline	No subjective complaints of memory deficit No memory deficit evident on clinical interview	Normal
2 Very mild cognitive decline	Subjective complaints of memory deficit, most frequently in following areas: (a) forgetting where one has placed familiar objects (b) forgetting names one formerly knew well No objective evidence of memory deficit on clinical interview No objective deficit in employment or social situations Appropriate concern with respect to symptomatology	Normal aging
3 Mild cognitive decline	Earliest clear-cut deficits Manifestations in more than one of the following areas: (a) patient may have gotten lost when traveling to an unfamiliar location (b) co-workers become aware of patient's relatively poor performance (c) word- and name-finding deficit become evident to intimates (d) patient may read a passage or book and retain relatively little material (e) patient may demonstrate decreased facility remembering names upon introduction to new people (f) patient may have lost or misplaced an object of value (g) concentration deficit may be evident on clinical testing Objective evidence of memory deficit obtained only with an intensive interview Decreased performance in demanding employment and social settings Denial begins to become manifest in patient Mild to moderate anxiety frequently accompanies symptoms	Mild neurocognitive disorder

TABLE 4.1 *(continued)*

GDS stage	Clinical characteristics	Diagnosis
4 Moderate cognitive decline	Clear-cut deficit on careful clinical interview Deficit manifest in following areas: (a) decreased knowledge of current and recent events (b) may exhibit some deficit in memory of one's personal history (c) concentration deficit elicited on serial subtractions (d) decreased ability to travel, handle finances, etc. Frequently no deficit in following areas: (a) orientation to time and place (b) recognition of familiar persons and faces (c) ability to travel to familiar locations Inability to perform complex tasks Denial is dominant defense mechanism Flattening of affect and withdrawal from challenging situations occur	Mild Alzheimer's disease
5 Moderately severe decline	Patient can no longer survive without some assistance Patient is unable during interview to recall a major relevant aspect of their current life, e.g., (a) address or telephone number of many years (b) the names of close members of their family (such as grandchildren) (c) the name of the high school or college from which they graduated Frequently some disorientation to time (date, day of the week, season, etc.) or to place An educated person may have difficulty counting back from 40 by 4s or from 20 by 2s Persons at this stage retain knowledge of many major facts regarding themselves and others They invariably know their own names and generally know their spouse's and children's names They require no assistance with toileting or eating, but may have difficulty choosing the proper clothing to wear	Moderate Alzheimer's disease

(continued)

TABLE 4.1 ***(continued)***

GDS stage	Clinical characteristics	Diagnosis
6 Severe cognitive decline	May occasionally forget the name of the spouse upon whom they are entirely dependent for survival Will be largely unaware of all recent events and experiences in their lives Retain some knowledge of their surroundings, the year, the season, etc. May have difficulty counting by 1s from 10 backward and sometimes forward Will require some assistance with activities of daily living: (a) may become incontinent (b) will require travel assistance but occasionally will be able to travel to familiar locations Diurnal rhythm frequently disturbed Almost always recall own name Frequently continue to be able to distinguish familiar from unfamiliar persons in their environment Personality and emotional changes occur; these are quite variable and include the following: (a) delusional behavior, e.g., patients may accuse spouse of being an imposter; may talk to imaginary figures in the environment, or to their own reflection in the mirror (b) obsessive symptoms, e.g., person may continually repeat simple cleaning activities (c) anxiety symptoms, agitation, and even previously non-existent violent behavior may occur (d) cognitive abulia, e.g., loss of willpower because an individual cannot carry a thought long enough to determine a purposeful course of action	Moderately severe Alzheimer's disease
7 Very severe cognitive decline	All verbal abilities are lost over the course of this stage Early in this stage words and phrases are spoken but speech is very circumscribed Later there is no speech at all, only grunting Incontinent of urine; requires assistance toileting and feeding Basic psychomotor skills (e.g. ability to walk) are lost with the progression of this stage The brain appears to no longer be able to tell the body what to do Generalized and cortical neurological signs and symptoms are frequently present	Severe Alzheimer's disease

From: Reisberg et al. (1982). Copyright 1983 by Barry Reisberg, MD.

evidence points to complaints of impaired cognition in a majority of elderly persons even in the absence of dementia and depression. The term *age-associated memory impairment* has been suggested for this condition (Crook et al., 1986). The American Psychiatric Association's *Diagnostic and Statistical Manual of Mental Disorders*, 4th edition, refers to this condition as "age-related cognitive decline." Clinical interview reveals no objective evidence of memory deficit, and there are no deficits in employment or social situations.

Present prognostic data do not indicate that these symptoms of subjectively impaired cognition and functioning are precursors of further decline in the majority of elderly with these common, age-associated complaints (Flicker, Ferris, & Reisberg, 1993). Although medications and nostrums are frequently taken for these perceived deficits, there remains no convincing evidence of their efficacy.

Stage 3: Mild cognitive decline. Diagnosis: Mild neurocognitive disorder compatible with incipient AD. Subtle evidence of objective decrement in complex occupational or social tasks may become evident in various ways. For example, the person may become confused or hopelessly lost when traveling to an unfamiliar location; relatively poorer performance may be noted by co-workers in a demanding occupation; persons may display overt word- and name-finding deficits; concentration deficits may be evident to family members and on clinical testing; relatively little material may be retained after reading a passage from a book or newspaper; and/or an overt tendency to forget what has just been said and to repeat oneself may be manifest. A teacher who had routinely recalled the names of all the students in his class by the end of a semester now may have difficulty recalling the names of any students. This same teacher may, for the first time, begin to miss important appointments. Similarly, a professional who had previously completed hundreds, perhaps thousands, of reports in the course of her lifetime may, for the first time, be unable to complete a single report. The person may lose or misplace objects of value, and concentration deficit may be evident on clinical testing. Mild to moderate anxiety is frequently observed and is an appropriate reaction to the awareness of impairment.

The prognosis associated with these subtle but objectively identifiable symptoms varies. In some cases, these symptoms are the result of brain insults, such as small strokes, which may not be evident from the clinical history, neurological examination, or neuroimaging findings. In other cases, symptoms are due to subtle and perhaps not clearly identifiable psychiatric, medical, and neurological disorders of diverse etiology. These symptoms are benign in many of the subjects who report them. However, in other cases, these symptoms do represent the earliest symptoms of AD and may last as long as 7 years before deficits associated with subsequent stages of AD become manifest. The diagnosis of AD in this stage, however, can be made with confidence only in retrospect.

Stage 4: Moderate cognitive decline. Diagnosis: Mild AD. Clinical interview reveals clearly manifest deficits in various areas, such as concentration, recent and past memory, orientation, calculation, and functional capacity. Concentration deficit may be of sufficient magnitude that patients may have difficulty subtracting serial 4s from 40. Recent memory may be affected to the degree that some major events of the previous week are not recalled, and there may be superficial or scanty knowledge of current events and activities. Detailed questioning may reveal that the spouse's knowledge of the patient's past is superior to the patient's own recall of his or her personal history, and the patient may confuse the chronology of past life events. The patient may mistake the date by 10 days or more but generally knows the year and the season. The patient may manifest decreased ability to handle such routine activities as marketing or managing personal and household finances.

Psychiatric features that may be prominent in this stage include decreased interest in personal and social activities, accompanied by a flattening of affect and emotional withdrawal. These behavioral changes are related to the person's decreased cognitive abilities rather than to depressed mood. However, they are frequently mistaken for depression. True depressive symptoms may also be noted but are generally mild, requiring no specific treatment. In cases where depressive symptoms are of sufficient severity to warrant treatment, a low dose of an antidepressant is frequently effective in reducing affective symptoms. At this stage patients are still capable of independent community survival if assistance is provided with complex but essential activities such as bill paying and managing the patient's bank account. Denial is the dominant defense mechanism protecting the patient from the devastating consequences of awareness of dementing illness.

The diagnosis of probable AD can be arrived at with confidence in this stage. It is possible to follow patients through the course of this stage, whose mean duration has been estimated to be approximately 2 years (Reisberg, 1986).

Stage 5: Moderately severe cognitive decline. Diagnosis: Moderate AD. Cognitive and functional deficits are of sufficient magnitude that patients can no longer survive without assistance.

Patients at this stage can no longer recall major relevant aspects of their lives. They may not recall the name of the current president, their correct current address or telephone number, or the names of schools they attended. Patients at this stage frequently do not recall the current year and may be unsure of the weather or season. Concentration and calculation deficits are generally of sufficient magnitude as to create difficulty in subtracting serial 4s from 40 and possibly even serial 2s from 20. Often the patient cannot recite the months of the year backward. Patients at this stage retain knowledge of many major facts regarding themselves and others and require no assistance with toileting or eating, but they may have difficulty choosing the appropriate clothing to wear for the season or the occasion and may begin to forget to bathe regularly unless reminded.

Psychiatric symptoms in Stage 5 are in many ways similar, although generally more overt, than those noted in Stage 4. The patient's denial and flattening of affect tend to be more evident. True depressive symptoms, with mild to moderate mood dysphoria, may occur. Anger and other more overt behavioral symptoms of AD, such as anxieties, paranoia, and sleep disturbances, are frequently evident. Paranoid and delusional ideation peak in occurrence at this stage, with almost 75% of patients exhibiting one or more delusions. Delusions such as people stealing their belongings or money, that one's house is not one's home, or that one's spouse is an impostor are common. Aggressivity may include verbal outbursts, physical threats and violence, or a general agitation. Depending on the nature and magnitude of the psychiatric symptomatology, treatment with an antidepressant or an antipsychotic medication may be indicated. When the latter is used, the dictum for the treatment of psychosis in the elderly applies: "Start low and go slow."

Patients who are living alone in the community at this stage require at least part-time assistance for continued community survival. When additional community assistance, such as day care or home health aides, is not feasible or available, institutionalization may be required. Patients who are residing with a spouse frequently resist additional assistance at this stage as an invasion of their home. The duration of this stage is approximately a year and a half (Reisberg, 1986; Reisberg, Ferris, et al., 1996).

Stage 6: Severe cognitive decline. Diagnosis: Moderately severe AD. Cognitive and functional deficits are of sufficient magnitude as to require assistance with basic activities of daily living.

Recent and remote memory are increasingly affected. Patients at this stage frequently have no idea of the date and may occasionally forget the name of the spouse upon whom they are dependent for survival but usually continue to be able to distinguish familiar from unfamiliar persons in their environments. Patients know their own names but frequently do not know their addresses, although they may be able to recall some important aspects of their domicile, such as the street or town. Patients have generally forgotten the schools they attended but recall some aspect of their early lives, such as their birthplace, their former occupation, and one or both of their parents' names. Concentration and calculation deficits are of such magnitude that patients in Stage 6 frequently have difficulty counting backward from 10 by 1s and may even begin to count forward during this task.

Agitation and even violence frequently occur in this stage. Language ability declines progressively so that, by the end of Stage 6, speaking is impaired in obvious ways. At this point in the late sixth stage, stuttering and word repetition are common; patients who learned a second language in adulthood sometimes revert to a varying degree to their childhood language; other patients may use neologisms, or nonsense words, interspersed to a varying degree in the course of their speech.

In this stage, emotional and behavioral problems generally become most manifest and disturbing, with 90% of patients exhibiting one or more behavioral symptoms (Reisberg, Franssen, et al., 1989). A fear of being left alone or abandoned is frequently exhibited. Agitation, anger, sleep disturbances, physical violence, and negativity are examples of symptoms that commonly require treatment at this point in the illness. Although low doses of antipsychotics may be useful, higher doses are frequently necessary for many patients, and a satisfactory response is sometimes difficult to obtain. Medication must continuously be monitored and adjusted, either upward or downward, as the disease advances.

The magnitude of cognitive and functional decline, combined with disturbed behavior and affect, make caregiving especially burdensome to spouses or other family members at this stage. They literally must devote their lives to helping patients who can no longer even recall their names, much less appreciate the kindness and care being provided. The caregivers' burden must be alleviated, for example, through regular participation in a dementia caregiver's support group, utilization of day care and respite centers for patients, or utilization of home health aides either part-time or full-time. Clinical experience suggests that if behavioral disturbances are not successfully managed, they become the primary reason for institutionalization, and successful management of the disturbances can postpone this need. The mean duration of this stage is approximately 2 1/2 years (Reisberg, 1986; Reisberg, Ferris, et al., 1996).

Stage 7: Very severe cognitive decline. Diagnosis: Severe AD. A succession of functional losses in this stage results in the need for continuous assistance in all aspects of daily living. Verbal abilities are severely limited early in this stage, to approximately a half dozen different intelligible words during the course of an average day, frequently interspersed with unintelligible babbling. Eventually, only a single word remains: commonly "yes," "no," or "OK." Subsequently, the ability to speak even this final single word is largely lost, although the patient may utter the seemingly forgotten word a year or more later. All vocalizations are eventually reduced to grunts or screams, which have been interpreted as signs of distress and muted with tranquilizers. Such a procedure, of course, may merely serve to dull remaining consciousness and thinking capacities of the patient (Auer, Sclan, Yaffae, & Reisberg, 1994). Although agitation can be a problem for some patients at this stage, psychotropic medication can frequently be discontinued successfully.

Nursing homes may be better equipped than spouses for the management of patients in this stage, but if family members maintain the patient at home, round-the-clock health care assistance may be necessary to manage incontinence and basic activities of daily living such as bathing and feeding. Human contact continues to make a great difference in the quality of life of a patient, whether in the home or in an institution. A loving voice, attention, and touch are important for the patient's emotional and physical well-being.

AD patients who survive until some point in the seventh stage generally die from pneumonia, traumatic or decubital ulceration, or a less specific failure in the central regulation of vital functions. Although approximately half of all patients who reach this stage are dead within 2 to 3 years, patients may potentially survive for 7 years or longer in this final stage.

FUNCTIONAL CHANGES IN AD

Understanding the progression of AD from the standpoint of change and deterioration in functional abilities is of great importance to both clinicians and families. In terms of a primary diagnosis, as well as differential diagnosis, it is useful to determine whether the nature of the dementia is consistent with uncomplicated senile dementia of the Alzheimer type, because dementing processes associated with other causes proceed differently from those of AD. Knowledge of the functional progression of AD can assist in this differential diagnostic process and, additionally, in identifying possible remediable complications of the illness. Furthermore, even the most severe AD patients can be assessed in terms of a functional level when all traditional mental status and psychometric assessment measures would produce uniform bottom (zero) scores (Reisberg, Franssen, et al., 1996). Functional assessment is presently capable of producing a detailed, meaningful map of the entire course of AD and, from the standpoint of physical rehabilitation, is extremely important in describing the AD patient's level of incapacity and areas of residual capacity.

Requirements for the management of AD fall into two categories: those relating to the patient and those relating to the primary caregiver. It is essential for the benefit of both that management advice be appropriate to each stage of the illness.

FUNCTIONAL DESCRIPTION OF AD

A practical diagnostic and assessment tool, the Functional Assessment Staging of Alzheimer's Disease (FAST) (Reisberg, 1988; Sclan & Reisberg, 1992) permits identification of the stages of characteristic decline in functional activities in AD and their estimated duration (outlined in Table 4.2). These stages of functional deterioration in AD correspond with the Global Deterioration Scale (GDS) stages described above. Table 4.2 indicates the corresponding mean Mini-Mental State Examination (MMSE) scores for each of the FAST stages and substages (Folstein, Folstein, & McHugh, 1975). Research has indicated strong relationships between progressive functional deterioration assessed on the FAST and progressive cognitive deterioration in AD (e.g., Pearson correlation coefficients of ~0.8 or greater between MMSE and FAST scores have been reported [Reisberg et al., 1984; Sclan & Reisberg, 1992]). Therefore, the relationships shown between FAST and MMSE scores are close approximations of likely findings in individual

TABLE 4.2 Functional Assessment Stages (FAST) and Time Course of Functional Loss in Normal Aging and Alzheimer's Disease

FAST stage	Clinical characteristics	Clinical diagnosis	Estimated duration in AD[a]	Mean MMSE[b]
1	No decrement	Normal adult		29–30
2	Subjective deficit in word finding or recalling location of objects	Age-associated memory impairment		27–28
3	Deficits noted in demanding employment settings	Mild neurocognitive disorder	7 years	24
4	Requires assistance in complex tasks, e.g., handling finances, planning dinner party	Mild AD	2 years	19–20
5	Requires assistance in choosing proper attire	Moderate AD	18 months	15
6a	Requires assistance in dressing	Moderately severe AD	5 months	9
b	Requires assistance in bathing properly		5 months	8
c	Requires assistance with mechanics of toileting (such as flushing, wiping)		5 months	5
d	Urinary incontinence		4 months	3
e	Fecal incontinence		10 months	1
7a	Speech ability limited to about a half-dozen words	Severe AD	12 months	0
b	Intelligible vocabulary limited to a single word		18 months	0
c	Ambulatory ability lost		12 months	0
d	Ability to sit up lost		12 months	0
e	Ability to smile lost		18 months	0
f	Ability to hold head up lost		12 months or longer	0

Adapted from Reisberg (1986). Copyright 1984 by Barry Reisberg, MD.

[a]In subjects without other complicating illnesses who survive and progress to the subsequent deterioration stage.

[b]MMSE = Mini-Mental State Examination score (Folstein et al. (1975)). Estimates based in part on published data summarized in Reisberg et al. (1989).

patients, although there is variability. Functionally, the late stages of AD can be subdivided into Stages 6a–e and Stages 7a–f. Consequently, a total of 16 functioning stages can be recognized that describe in detail the characteristic changes with the progression of AD. In uncomplicated dementia of the Alzheimer's type, progression through each of the functional stages described below occurs in a generally ordinal (sequential) pattern (Sclan & Reisberg, 1992).

Stage 1: No objective or subjective functional decrement. The aged subject's objective and subjective functional abilities in occupational, social, and other settings remain intact, compared with prior performance. The prognosis is excellent for continued adequate cognitive functioning.

Stage 2: Subjective functional decrement but no objective evidence of decreased performance in complex occupational or social activities. The most common age-related functional complaints are forgetting names and locations of objects or decreased ability to recall appointments. Subjective decrements are generally not noted by intimates or co-workers, and complex occupational and social functioning is not compromised.

When affective disorders, anxiety states, or other remediable conditions have been excluded, the elderly person with these symptoms can be reassured with respect to the relatively benign prognosis, which is excellent for continued adequate cognitive functioning. This reassurance may alleviate fears in the patient that these common symptoms presage a malignant deterioration, which, in the great majority of cases, they do not.

Stage 3: Objective functional decrement of sufficient severity to interfere with complex occupational and social tasks. This is the stage at which persons may begin to forget important appointments for the first time in their lives. Functional decrements may become manifest in complex psychomotor tasks, such as ability to travel to new locations. Persons at this stage have no difficulty with routine tasks such as shopping, handling finances, or traveling to familiar locations, but they may stop participating in demanding occupational and social settings. These symptoms, although subtle clinically, can considerably alter lifestyle. When psychiatric, neurological, and medical concomitants apart from AD have been excluded, the clinician may advise withdrawal from complex, anxiety-provoking situations. Because patients at this stage can still perform all basic activities of daily living satisfactorily, withdrawing from complex activities may result in complete symptom amelioration for a period of years.

Stage 4: Deficient performance in the complex tasks of daily life. Aspects of decreased functioning from former levels are apparent. At this stage, shopping for adequate or appropriate food and other items is noticeably impaired. The patient may return with incorrect items or inappropriate amounts of a certain item. The individual may have difficulty preparing meals for family dinners and may display similar deficits in the ability to manage complex occupational and social tasks. Family members may note that the patient no longer is able to balance the checkbook, no longer remembers to pay bills properly, and may make significant financial errors. Persons who are still able to travel independently to and from work may not recall names of clients or details of their employment duties. Because choosing clothing, dressing, bathing, and traveling to familiar locations can be adequately performed at this stage, patients may still function independently in the community although supervision is often useful.

Maximizing the patient's functioning at this stage is the goal of the family and health professionals. Financial supervision and structured or supervised travel should be arranged. Identification bracelets or clothing labels with a name, address, and telephone number may be useful.

Stage 5: Deficient performance in basic tasks of daily life. At this stage patients can no longer function independently in the community. The patient not only requires assistance in managing financial affairs and marketing but also begins to require help in choosing the appropriate clothing for the season and the occasion. The patient may wear obviously incongruous clothing combinations or wear the same clothing day after day unless supervision is provided.

At this stage, some patients develop anxieties and fears about bathing. Another functional deficit that frequently becomes manifest at this stage is difficulty in driving an automobile. The patient may slow down or speed up the vehicle inappropriately or may go through a stop sign or traffic light. Occasionally, the patient may have a collision with another vehicle for the first time in many years. The patient may be sufficiently alarmed by these deficits to voluntarily discontinue driving. Frequently, however, intervention and coercion are necessary from family members or even from the patient's physician or licensing authorities.

It is important that functional abilities be maximized. Patients are still capable of putting on their clothing with minimal guidance once it has been selected for them. They are also capable of bathing and washing themselves, even though they may have to be cajoled into it. A supportive environment that provides adequate stimulation, in addition to adequate protection, is desirable.

Stage 6: Decreased ability to dress, bathe, and toilet independently. Throughout the course of Stage 6, which lasts for approximately 2 1/2 years and encompasses five substages, increasing deficits in dressing and bathing occur. In addition to not being able to choose the proper clothing, early Stage 6 patients develop difficulties in putting on their clothing properly. Other dressing difficulties include putting on street clothing over night clothing, putting clothing on backward or inside out, and putting on multiple and inappropriate layers of clothing. The patient may also have difficulty zippering or buttoning their clothing or tying their shoelaces and may even put their shoes on the opposite feet. More overt dressing difficulties develop as this stage progresses and the patient requires increasing assistance in dressing.

A bathing difficulty that becomes apparent at this stage is a decreased ability to adjust the temperature of bath or shower water. Subsequently, taking a bath or shower without assistance becomes increasingly problematic, with difficulty getting into and out of the bath and washing properly. Fear of bathing may develop, combined with resistance or negativistic behavior. This fear of bathing sometimes precedes actual difficulties in handling the mechanics of bathing.

Later in the course of this stage, patients begin to have difficulties with the mechanics of toileting: initially, they may forget to flush the toilet, dispose of toilet tissue improperly, and clean themselves inadequately. Subsequently, urinary incontinence begins, followed by fecal incontinence by the end of Stage 6, both of which appear to be the result of decreased cognitive capacity to respond appropriately to urinary or fecal urgency. Assisting the patient to use the toilet often helps to forestall and remediate incontinence. Anxieties regarding toileting are frequently noted in the latter part of Stage 6. Patients may go to the toilet repeatedly even in the absence of a true need for elimination.

Motor capacity deficits also become notable during stage 6. Walking becomes more halting and steps generally become smaller and slower, but the ability to ambulate is still maintained. Because orientation in space is affected, patients may approach a chair and sit down with greater difficulty. Patients may also require assistance in walking up and down a staircase.

Full-time home health care is frequently useful at this time, and it may be appropriate or necessary to discuss nursing home placement with the caregiver and family members. Management strategies and supportive techniques must be developed to assist the patient in bathing, dressing, and toileting, as well as in minimizing the emotional stress of the caregiver.

Stage 7: Loss of speech and locomotion. This final stage of AD is marked by decreased vocabulary and speech abilities. Speech becomes increasingly limited, from a vocabulary of fewer than a half-dozen different words to a single distinguishable word that may be uttered repeatedly, and eventually speech becomes limited to only grunting and crying out.

Prior to the loss of ambulatory ability, patients may exhibit a twisted gait, take progressively smaller and slower steps, or lean forward, backward, or sideways while walking. Eventually, the ability to walk unassisted is lost with the progression of AD. Approximately a year after ambulatory ability is lost, the ability to sit up without assistance (such as lateral chair rests) is also lost. Subsequently, the ability to smile and to hold up the head independently is also lost. At this point, grunting and grasping may still be observed, and patients can still move their eyes, although familiar persons or objects are apparently no longer recognized. Approximately 2 to 3 years after the onset of Stage 7, generally after the loss of ambulatory ability, many patients die. However, some patients survive in this stage for 7 years or longer. Pneumonia, which is often associated with aspiration, is a frequent cause of death.

Full-time assistance at home or in an institution is a necessity at this stage, and as AD patients are increasingly well cared for, it is likely that more will survive to these final substages of the illness.

FEEDING CONCOMITANTS OF AD

Progressive changes in the ability to prepare meals and in feeding skills have been observed in AD patients and enumerated in accordance with the corresponding GDS and FAST stages (Reisberg et al., 1990). These feeding concomitants of Alzheimer's disease are outlined in Table 4.3. The progression of these distur-

TABLE 4.3 Feeding Concomitants of Alzheimer's Disease

GDS stage	Clinical characteristics
1–2	No objective or subjective decrement in the ability to adequately prepare meals, order food and beverages in a restaurant setting, or in table etiquette
4	Decreased facility in preparing and/or serving relatively complex meals, and/or decreased facility in ordering food and beverages in restaurant setting
5	Decreased ability in preparing simple foods or beverages (e.g., coffee or tea); may occasionally make mistakes in eating food (e.g., improper use of seasoning or condiments)
6	(a) Occasional difficulty with proper manipulation or choice of eating utensils (b) Meat and similar foods must be cut up for the patient (c) No longer trusted to use a knife; may also eat foods that would have formerly been refused (d) No longer trusted to properly use a knife and decreased ability to use a fork, but can still properly use a spoon; may also display occasional misrecognition of dietary substances (pica) (e) Capable of going to the refrigerator or cupboard but has difficulty discerning and choosing food, may have difficulty chewing hard food
7	(a) Capable of picking up spoon or fork; will occasionally drop food or misutilize silverware (e.g., may attempt to drink soup or other liquids with a fork); capable of reaching for a cup when desirous of fluid (b) Must be assisted in actual feeding; generally, patients are not permitted to handle a knife or fork; may not be able to properly lift a cup (c) Can reach for and pick up food with hands; cannot properly pick up a fork or a spoon but can grasp a spoon or other utensil; must be spoon-fed but can chew (d) Cannot distinguish foods from nondietary substances; will reach out for objects, including food

bances in meal preparation and self-feeding, as with the progression of deterioration in cognitive and functional abilities, appears to be characteristic of AD.

RIGIDITY AND CONTRACTURES

In the latter stages of AD, rigidity becomes increasingly manifest (Franssen, Kluger, Torossian, & Reisberg, 1993; Franssen, Reisberg, Kluger, Sinaiko, & Boja, 1991). Initially, this rigidity is of a paratonic type, that is, elicited in response to an irregular motion of an extremity, such as an irregular movement of an elbow. Later, the rigidity becomes increasingly evident. Figure 4.1 depicts the emergence of paratonic rigidity in AD. Although infrequently manifest in patients with mild AD (GDS Stage 4), approximately 50% of patients with moderate AD (GDS Stage 5), 75% of patients with moderately severe AD (GDS Stage 6), and virtually all patients with severe AD (GDS Stage 7) manifest at least a mildly detectable form of paratonic rigidity.

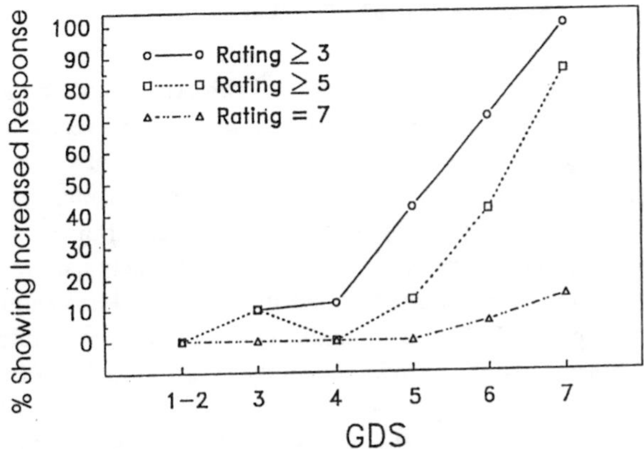

FIGURE 4.1 Percentage of subjects with increased paratonic rigidity in normal aging and AD of progressively increasing severity.

The graph depicts the percentages of subjects showing paratonia as a function of the Global Deterioration Scale (GDS) stage, using three different ratings of activity. Paratonic rigidity, defined as stiffening of a limb in response to contact with the examiner's hand and an involuntary resistance to passive changes in position and posture, was graded according to the amount of passive force necessary to elicit it. A rating of 1 denotes an absence of paratonic rigidity, whereas a rating of 7 indicates that minimal passive force is required for elicitation of the sequence.

Further details regarding the scoring procedure can be found in Franssen (1993). Data and figures are from Franssen et al. (1991). Reproduced with permission of the author.

One probable result of this increasing rigidity is the development of contractures. Contractures are irreversible deformities of joints, limiting range of motion. In a study by Souren et al. (Souren, Franssen, & Reisberg, 1995), a contracture was defined as a limitation of 50% or more of the passive range of motion of a joint, secondary to permanent muscle shortening, ankylosis, or both. Souren and associates found that contractures meeting this definition were present in 10% of moderately severe AD patients with incipient incontinence (i.e., FAST stages 6d and 6e AD patients) (Figure 4.2). In severe AD, contractures are very common. Forty percent of incipient averbal AD patients (FAST stages 7a and 7b), manifested contractures, and 50% of incipient nonambulatory AD patients (FAST Stage 7c) manifested these deformities. By late Stage 7 (in immobile patients, FAST stages 7d–f), 95% of AD patients manifested these deformities. Furthermore, at all stages, when contractures occurred, they tended to be present in more than one extremity. There is anecdotal evidence based on patient observations that contractures may be prevented until very late in the course of AD by maintenance of patient activities and movements.

TREATMENT IMPLICATIONS

Cognitive and functional deficits in patients with AD characteristically follow the progression outlined in the preceding sections. However, other disorders frequently associated with the presence of dementia do not necessarily follow this characteristic pattern. It has been observed that the characteristic pattern of functional loss in AD in particular is useful in differential diagnosis (Reisberg, 1986; Reisberg, Ferris, & Franssen, 1985). Common functional presentations of non-AD dementing disorders are outlined in Table 4.4. For example, normal-pressure hydrocephalus (NPH) commonly presents with gait disturbance as the earliest symptom, antedating any overt cognitive disturbance. In NPH this ambulatory disturbance is commonly followed by urinary incontinence. Only subsequently, after the advent of ambulatory disturbance and urinary incontinence in NPH, may cognitive disturbances become manifest. As summarized in Table 4.2, the sequence of functional loss in AD is different. In AD overt cognitive disturbance precedes urinary incontinence, which in turn precedes ambulatory loss.

Creutzfeldt-Jakob disease is a rare form of rapidly progressive dementia that presents with ambulatory disturbance as the earliest symptom in approximately one third of cases. In AD the ambulatory disturbance is a much later event. The two conditions also may be distinguished temporally. The course of AD extends over many years, as outlined in Table 4.2, and is frequently much slower than the relatively rapid course of the acute and subacute forms of Creutzfeldt-Jakob disease.

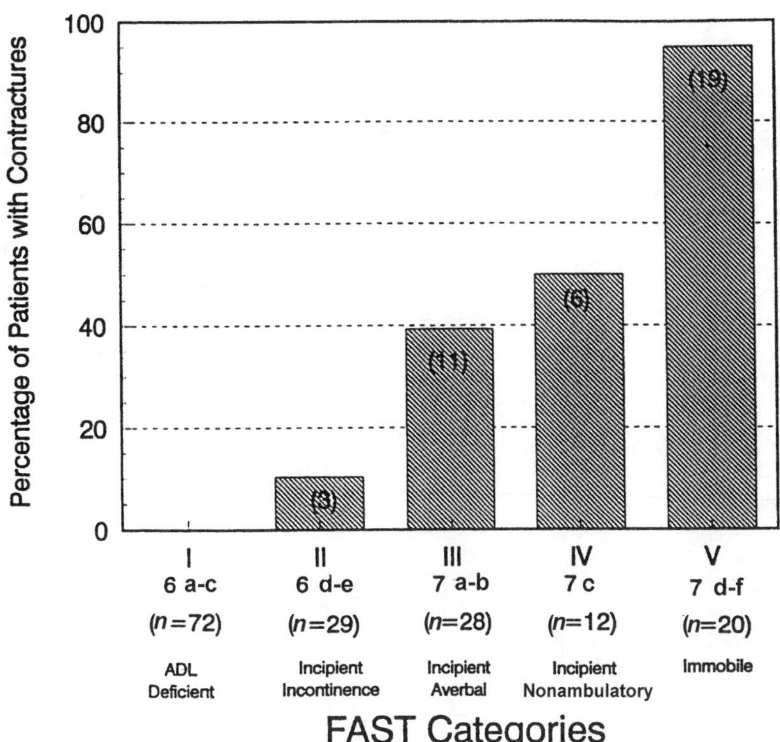

FIGURE 4.2 Percentages of patients with contractures in FAST Stage 6 and Stage 7 AD.

All subjects fulfilled criteria for probable AD. FAST (Functional Assessment Staging [Reisberg, 1988]) categories are as follows: *I*. ADL (activities of daily life) deficient, 6a, b, and c; *II*, incipient incontinence, 6d and e; *III*, incipient nonverbal, 7a and b; *IV*, incipient nonambulatory, 7c; and *V*, immobile, 7d, e, and f. The numbers in parentheses indicate the number of patients with contractures in the functional categories. The significance of change in the prevalence of contractures from the preceding functional categories is as follows: between functional categories I and II: $p < .01$; between functional categories II and III: $p < .05$; between functional categories III and IV: not significant; and between functional categories IV and V: $p < .01$.

Across the five functional categories, there are significant differences in the proportions of patients with contractures ($X^2 = 88.4$, $df = 4$, $p < .001$). The prevalence of contractures was highly correlated with FAST staging levels ($r = 0.70$, $p < .001$).

Data and figure are adapted from Souren et al. (1995).

TABLE 4.4 Functional Loss in Non-Alzheimer Disorders Associated with Progressive or Gradual Onset of Dementia and FAST Characteristics in AD

	Functional loss in non-Alzheimer disorders			FAST AD distinctions	
Disorder	Pathology or presumed etiology	Functional loss in non-AD disorder[a]	Equivalent FAST stage	Functional loss in AD per FAST	FAST stages in AD
Normal pressure hydrocephalus	Dilated cerebral ventricles	1. Gait disturbance	7c	1. Loss of ability to perform complex tasks	4
		2. Urinary incontinence	6d	2. Urinary incontinence	6d
		3. Loss of ability to perform complex tasks	4	3. Ambulatory (gait) disturbance	7c
Creutzfeldt-Jakob Disease	Prion	1. Gait disturbance	7c	1. Loss of ability to perform complex tasks	4
		2. Loss of ability to perform complex tasks	4	2. Gait (ambulatory) disturbance	7c
Multi-infarct Dementia	Multiple cerebral infarctions	1. Loss of speech	7a–7b	1. Loss of ability to perform complex tasks	4
		2. Loss of urinary continence	6d	2. Loss of ability to pick out clothing properly	5
		3. Loss of ability to put on clothing	6a	3. Loss of ability to put on clothing without assistance	6a
		4. Loss of ability to bathe without assistance	6b	4. Loss of ability to bathe without assistance	6b
		5. Loss of ambulatory capacity	7c	5. Loss of urinary continence	6c
		6. Loss of ability to perform complex tasks	4	6. Loss of fecal continence	6d
		7. Loss of ability to pick out clothing	5	7. Loss of speech	6e
		8. Fecal incontinence	6e	8. Loss of ambulatory capacity	7a–7b

TABLE 4.4 *(continued)*

Functional loss in non-Alzheimer disorders				FAST AD distinctions	
Disorder	Pathology or presumed etiology	Functional loss in non-AD disorder[a]	Equivalent FAST stage	Functional loss in AD per FAST	FAST stages in AD
Dementia Syndrome of Depression ("Pseudodementia")	Affective disorder associated with neurotransmitter imbalance	1. Loss of ability to perform complex tasks	4	1. Loss of ability to perform complex tasks	4
		2. Refusal to put on clothing (associated with negativity)	6a	2. Inability to pick out clothing properly	5
		3. Refusal to bathe (associated with negativity)	6b	3. Inability to put on clothing without assistance	6a
		4. Loss of ability to pick out clothing properly	5	4. Inability to bathe without assistance	6b
Dementia associated with hyponatremia	Electrolyte disturbance	1. Loss of ability to perform complex tasks	4	1. Loss of ability to perform complex tasks	4
		2. Loss of ability to pick out clothing properly	5	2. Loss of ability to pick out clothing properly	5
		3. Loss of ability to dress, bathe, and toilet independently	6a–6c	3. Loss of ability to dress, bathe, and toilet independently	6a–6c
		4. Loss of ambulation capacity	7c	4. Loss of urinary and fecal continence	6d–6e
		5. Loss of urinary and fecal continence	6d–6e	5. Loss of speech	7a–7b
		6. Loss of speech	7a–7b	6. Loss of ambulatory capacity	7c

(continued)

TABLE 4.4 *(continued)*

Functional loss in non-Alzheimer disorders				FAST AD distinctions	
Disorder	Pathology or presumed etiology	Functional loss in non-AD disorder[a]	Equivalent FAST stage	Functional loss in AD per FAST	FAST stages in AD
Dementia associated with diffuse CNS metastasis	Neoplastic diffuse cerebral trauma	1. Loss of ability to perform complex tasks	4	1. Loss of ability to perform complex tasks	4
		2. Loss of ability to dress, bathe, and toilet independently	6a–6c	2. Loss of ability to dress, bathe, and toilet independently	6a–6c
		3. Loss of ambulation capacity	7c	3. Loss of urinary and fecal continence	6d–6e
		4. Loss of urinary and fecal continence	6d–6e	4. Loss of speech	7a–7b
		5. Loss of speech	7a–7b	5. Loss of ambulatory capacity	7c

[a]The sequences of functional loss shown are typical for normal pressure hydrocephalus and Creutzfeldt-Jakob disease; the sequence for multiinfarct dementia is one of various common presentations; the sequences in the dementia syndrome of depression, dementia associated with hyponatremia, and dementia associated with diffuse CNS metastasis are previously observed examples of the presentation of these dementias. It should be noted that in some of the non-AD disorders, particularly multiinfarct dementia, the "sequence" described may appear abruptly, rather than over an extended time interval. From: Reisberg et al. (1990).

Multiinfarct dementia, or dementia associated with an overt, large infarction, may produce speech disturbance as the only symptom. Alternatively, the infarction may produce urinary incontinence as the major overt manifestation. Commonly, ambulatory loss may be the major sequela of a stroke. Clearly, the evolution of functional losses in AD follows a very different and much more stereotyped pattern (as outlined in Tables 4.2 and 4.3). As shown in Table 4.4, the evolution of functional disturbance in dementia associated with multiple infarctions may follow a very different course from that which is characteristic of AD.

Depression is a psychiatric disturbance associated with mood dysphoria and other symptoms. Among these other symptoms are negativity and subjective complaints of cognitive impairment. Occasionally, the depression produces a dementia-like syndrome that is potentially reversible when the underlying mood disturbance is treated. This potentially reversible dementia syndrome of depression, formerly called pseudodementia, does not necessarily follow the functional course outlined in Table 4.2. For example, as outlined in Table 4.4, depression may be accompanied by a refusal to dress and bathe as a result of the patient's negativity. However, the patient may be able to point to exactly the clothes he or she wishes to wear. In AD the loss of ability to pick out clothing properly precedes the loss of ability to put on one's clothing properly.

As outlined in Table 4.4, dementia associated with hyponatremia or other electrolyte disturbances, CNS metastases, and other conditions all may follow a course markedly at variance with the course of AD as outlined in the FAST.

In a patient with AD, a variety of coexisting conditions may result in functional disturbances that may occur prematurely or nonordinally (i.e., out of sequence) in terms of the FAST predictions. Examples of conditions that may be associated with premature (i.e., nonordinal) functional losses in an AD patient are outlined in Table 4.5. For example, if an AD patient is at GDS Stage 5 and FAST Stage 5 and develops urinary incontinence, this incontinence may, at this early point in AD, be a remediable complication, perhaps secondary to a urinary tract infection.

Similarly, if a patient with AD at GDS Stage 5 and FAST Stage 5 develops loss of independent ambulation, this may be the result of a stroke or possibly of a variety of potentially treatable conditions common in the elderly, such as medication-induced parkinsonian symptoms, arthritis, a fracture, and so on. Table 4.5 provides an extensive list of causes of premature functional losses in an AD patient, many of which are potentially remediable.

The relationship between the FAST and the GDS or the FAST and the MMSE also is useful in the identification of excess functional disability that may be remediable. Specifically, if an AD patient is notably more impaired functionally than cognitively (e.g., a GDS Stage 5 patient who is at Stage 6d on the FAST), this is an indication of the likely presence of excess functional disability. For

TABLE 4.5 Differential Diagnostic Considerations in Cases of Deviations from FAST

Stage	FAST characteristics	Differential diagnostic considerations (particularly if FAST stage occurs prematurely in the evolution of dementia)
1.	No functional decrement, either subjectively or objectively, manifest	
2.	Complains of forgetting location of objects; subjective work difficulties	2. Anxiety neurosis, depression
3.	Decreased functioning in demanding employment settings evident to co-workers, difficulty in traveling to new locations	3. Depression, subtle manifestations of medical pathology
4.	Decreased ability to perform complex tasks such as planning dinner for guests, handling finances, and marketing	4. Depression, psychosis, focal cerebral process (e g., Gerstmann's syndrome)
5.	Requires assistance in choosing proper clothing, may require coaxing to bathe properly	5. Depression
6.	(a) Difficulty putting on clothing properly	6. (a) Arthritis, sensory deficit, stroke, depression
	(b) Requires assistance in bathing, may develop fear of bathing	(b) Arthritis, sensory deficit, stroke, depression
	(c) Inability to handle mechanics of toileting	(c) Arthritis, sensory deficit, stroke, depression
	(d) Urinary incontinence	(d) Urinary tract infection, other causes of urinary incontinence
	(e) Fecal incontinence	(e) Infection, malabsorption syndrome, other causes of fecal incontinence
7.	(a) Ability to speak limited to one to five words	7. (a) Stroke, other dementing disorder (e.g., diffuse space-occupying lesions)
	(b) Intelligible vocabulary lost	(b) Stroke, other dementing disorder (e.g., diffuse space-occupying lesions)

TABLE 4.5 *(continued)*

Stage	FAST characteristics	Differential diagnostic considerations (particularly if FAST stage occurs prematurely in the evolution of dementia)
	(c) Ambulatory ability lost	(c) Parkinsonism, neuroleptic-induced or other secondary extrapyramidal syndrome, Creutzfeldt-Jakob disease, normal pressure hydrocephalus, hyponatremic dementia, stroke, hip fracture, arthritis, overmedication
	(d) Ability to sit up independently lost	(d) Arthritis, contractures
	(e) Ability to smile lost	(e) Stroke
	(f) Ability to hold up head lost	(f) Head trauma, metabolic abnormality, other medical abnormality, overmedication, encephalitis, other causes

From Reisberg (1986).

example, the patient may have coexisting arthritis and AD. As a result of the combination of arthritis and dementia, in addition to not being able to handle finances and to pick out clothing without assistance (deficits that occur only because of the patient's AD), the patient may be unable to dress, bathe, and toilet without assistance, the latter resulting in occasional urinary incontinence. The arthritis may or may not be remediable. Similarly, the excess functional disability may or may not be remediable. Interestingly, when excess functional disability occurs in AD patients, it tends to occur "along the lines of the FAST." It appears that AD predisposes to functional losses outlined on the FAST. When an insult occurs, the closer the AD patient is to the inevitable point of loss of a functional ability on the FAST, the more predisposed the AD patient is to the premature loss of that capacity on the FAST. Not only illnesses but psychological stressors may produce these premature losses. For example, if an AD patient at GDS Stage 6 and FAST Stage 6c is moved to an unfamiliar environment, the patient may develop urinary and fecal incontinence that remits when the patient is returned to familiar surroundings. Subsequently, these capacities will, tragically, be lost with the advance of AD.

Knowledge of the FAST progression of AD, in conjunction with the global concomitants, feeding concomitants, and other aspects, also provides invaluable information on the potential for treatment of disability, even in AD, that is uncomplicated by the presence of additional pathology. For example, strategies for forestalling incontinence can be contemplated in FAST Stage 6c. In FAST Stage 6d or 6e, treatment of incontinence requires different strategies, such as frequent toileting. With the advance of deficits in FAST Stage 7, strategies and goals for the management of incontinence must be modified.

Other symptoms in AD, notably symptoms associated with the behavioral syndrome as outlined in Table 4.6, also require treatment. These symptoms are commonly treated with neuroleptics or other psychotropic medications. It should be noted that treatment of these symptoms may also be related to the treatment of functional disabilities. For example, it has been observed that AD patients with excess functional disability in relation to the magnitude of their cognitive disturbances may frequently have particularly marked behavioral disturbances. Conversely, marked behavioral disturbances may be associated with excess functional disability. This excess functional disability may be remediated in part by successful treatment of the behavioral symptoms.

TABLE 4.6 Behavioral and Psychological Pathologic Symptomatology in Alzheimer's Disease

Paranoid and Delusional Ideation

The "people are stealing things" delusion. Alzheimer's patients can no longer recall the precise whereabouts of household objects. This is probably the psychological explanation for what apparently is the most common delusion of AD patients, that someone is hiding or stealing objects. More severe manifestations of this delusion include the belief that persons are actually coming into the home to hide or steal objects; the patient may actually speak with or listen to the intruders.

The "house is not one's home" delusion. AD patients, as a result of their cognitive deficits, may no longer recognize their home. This appears to account, in part, for the common conviction of the AD patients that the place in which they are residing is not their home. Consequently, while actually at home, AD patients commonly request that their caregiver "take me home." They may also pack their bags for their return home. More disturbing to the caregiver and of greater potential danger to the patient are actual attempts to leave their house to go "home." Occasionally, attempts to prevent the patient's departure may result in anger or even violence toward the caregiver on the part of the patient. Such violence is extremely upsetting to the spouse caregiver.

The "spouse (or other caregiver) is an impostor" delusion. With the evolution of cognitive deficit, AD patients no longer recognize their caregivers as well as previously. Perhaps for this reason, a frequent delusion in the AD patient is that persons are impostors. In some instances anger and even violence may result from this conviction.

The delusion of "abandonment." With the evolution of intellectual deficit in AD, a degree of insight into their condition remains relatively preserved. Although AD patients are largely aware of their cognitive deficits, denial protects them from this awareness.

TABLE 4.6 *(continued)*

Similarly, they may be aware of the burden they have become. These insights are probably related to the common delusion of abandonment, institutionalization, or of a conspiracy or plot to institutionalize the patient.

The delusion of "infidelity." The insecurities described above are also related to the AD patient's occasional conviction that a spouse is unfaithful to them, sexually or otherwise. This conviction of infidelity may also apply to other caregivers.

Other suspicions, paranoid ideation, or delusions. Although the above specific delusions are the most commonly observed in AD, others may also be present (e.g., phantom boarder [strangers are living in the home]; regarding activities in which one no longer participates [e.g., working, traveling]; regarding former family members or former status of family members [e.g., father is still alive; daughter is still a child]; delusion of doubles [e.g., there are two of the same person]). Suspicion and paranoid ideation may occur regarding strangers, people staring, people plotting to do harm, etc.

Hallucinations

Visual hallucinations. These can be vague or clearly defined. Commonly, AD patients will see intruders or dead relatives at home or have similar hallucinatory experiences.

Auditory hallucinations. Occasionally, in the presence or absence of visual hallucinations, AD patients may hear dead relatives, intruders, or others whispering or speaking to them. Sometimes the voices are only heard when caregivers are not present.

Other hallucinations. Less commonly, other forms of hallucinations may be observed in AD patients (e.g., smelling a fire).

Activity Disturbances

AD patients' decreased cognitive capacity renders them less capable of channeling their energies in socially productive ways. Since motor abilities are not severely compromised until the final stage of the illness, patients may develop various psychological/motoric solutions for their need to channel their energies. A few of the most common examples are the following:

Wandering. For a variety of reasons, including inability to channel energies, anxieties, and delusions such as those described above and decreased cognitive abilities per se, AD patients frequently wander away from the home or caregiver. Restraint may be necessary, and this, in turn, may provoke anger or violence in the patient.

Purposeless activity (cognitive abulia). AD patients may not be able to carry a thought long enough to complete a purposeful movement. This results in a variety of purposeless, frequently repetitive activities, including opening and closing a purse or pocketbook, packing and unpacking clothing, repeatedly putting on and removing clothing, opening and closing drawers, incessant repeating of demands or questions, or simply pacing. Among the most severe manifestations of this syndrome is repetitive self-abrading.

Inappropriate activities. These occur primarily as a result of decreased cognitive capacities, increased anxieties and suspiciousness, and excess physical energies. They

(continued)

TABLE 4.6 *(continued)*

include storing and hiding objects in inappropriate places, such as throwing clothing in the wastebasket, putting empty plates in the oven, etc. Attempts by the caregiver to prevent these inappropriate activities may be met by anger or even violence.

Aggressivity

Verbal outbursts. As already noted, these can occur in association with many of the behavioral symptoms already described. They can also occur as an isolated phenomenon. For example, an AD patient may begin to use unaccustomed foul or abusive language with intimates and/or with strangers.

Physical outbursts. This also can occur as part of the aforementioned syndromes or as an isolated manifestation. The AD patient may, in response to frustration or seemingly without cause, strike out at the spouse or caregiver.

Diurnal Rhythm Disturbance

Sleep problems are a frequent and significant part of the behavioral syndrome of AD. They may, in part, be the result of decreased cognition, which upsets habitual and other diurnal cues; the energy and motoric changes occurring in the illness; and the neurochemical processes predisposing to agitation and psychosis.

Day/night disturbance. The most common sleep problem in AD patients is multiple awakenings in the course of the evening. These can occur in the context of an overall decrease in sleep or in association with increased daytime napping.

Affective Disturbance

The depressive syndrome of AD is primarily reactive in nature. The syndrome tends to occur somewhat earlier in the course of AD than many of the other symptoms described above and appears to be related to the pattern of insight and denial in the patient.

Tearfulness. This predominant depressive manifestation generally occurs in brief periods. If queried as to the reason for their tearfulness, patients might respond that they are crying because of the person whom they once were or "because of what is happening to them"—they may say that they "forgot the reason." This tearfulness frequently may be a precursor of more severe behavioral symptomatology.

Other depressive manifestations. A depressive syndrome may coexist with AD, just as other illnesses may coexist with AD. A full discussion of this conjunction is beyond the scope of this chapter. However, thoughts of death, generally not accompanied by overt affective symptoms or dysphoria, do occur as part of the depressive behavioral syndrome of AD. In some instances, these thoughts can be accompanied by suicidal threats or gestures.

Anxieties and Phobias

These may be related to the previously described behavioral manifestations of AD. They also can occur independently.

Anxiety regarding upcoming events (Godot syndrome). This common syndrome appears to result from decreased cognitive and, more specifically, memory abilities in AD

TABLE 4.6 *(continued)*

patients and from their inability to channel their remaining thinking capacities productively. Consequently, the patient will repeatedly query with respect to an upcoming event. These queries may be so incessant and persistent as to be intolerable.

Fear of being left alone. This is the most commonly observed phobia in AD. As a phobic phenomenon it is entirely out of proportion to any real danger. For example, the anxieties may become manifest as soon as the spouse goes into another room.

Adapted from Reisberg et al. (1986).

CONCLUSIONS

AD is a very common condition in elderly persons, marked by a characteristic cognitive and functional course of disability. Knowledge of this characteristic course is essential for the identification and treatment of excess functional disability. This treatment can, in turn, alleviate suffering in the patient and burden in the caregivers of AD victims.

ACKNOWLEDGMENT

This work was supported in part by grants AG03051 and AG08051 from the National Institute on Aging of the U.S. National Institutes of Health and by the Zachary and Elizabeth M. Fisher Alzheimer's Disease Education and Resources Program at the New York University Medical Center.

REFERENCES

Auer, S. R., Sclan, S. G., Yaffee, R. A., & Reisberg, B. (1994). The neglected half of Alzheimer's disease: Cognitive and functional concomitants of severe dementia. *Journal of the American Geriatrics Society, 42,* 1266–1272.

Chandler, J. D., & Chandler, J. E. (1988). The prevalence of neuropsychiatric disorder in a nursing home population. *Journal of Geriatric Psychiatry and Neurology, 1,* 71–76.

Crook, T., Bartus, R. T., Ferris, S. H., Whitehouse, P., Cohen, G. D., & Gershon, S. (1986). Age-associated memory impairment: Proposed diagnostic criteria and measures of clinical change. Report of a NIMH work group. *Developmental Neuropsychology, 2,* 261–276.

Evans, V. A., Funkenstein, H., Albert, M. S., Soherr, P. A., Cook, N. R., Chown, M. J., Hebert, L. E., Hennekens, C. H., & Taylor, J. O. (1989). Prevalence of Alzheimer's disease in a community population of older persons. *Journal of the American Medical Association, 262,* 2551–2556.

Flicker, C., Ferris, S. H., & Reisberg, B. (1993). A longitudinal study of cognitive function in elderly persons with subjective memory complaints. *Journal of the American Geriatrics Society, 41,* 1029–1032.

Folstein, M. F., Folstein, S. E., & McHugh, P. R. (1975). Mini-mental state: A practical method for grading the cognitive state of patients for the clinician. *Journal of Psychiatry Research, 12,* 189–198.

Franssen, E. (1993). Neurologic signs in ageing and dementia. In A. Burns (Ed.), *Aging and dementia: A methodological approach* (pp. 144–174). London: Edward Arnold.

Franssen, E. H., Kluger, A., Torossian, C. L., & Reisberg, B. (1993). The neurologic syndrome of severe Alzheimer's disease: Relationship to functional decline. *Archives of Neurology, 50,* 1029–1039.

Franssen, E. H., Reisberg, B., Kluger, A., Sinaiko, E., & Boja, C. (1991) Cognition independent neurologic symptoms in normal aging and probable Alzheimer's disease. *Archives of Neurology, 48,* 148–154.

Katzman, R. (1986). Alzheimer's disease. *New England Journal of Medicine, 314,* 964–973.

Kumar, A., Koss, E., Metzler, D., Moore, A., & Friedland, R. (1988). Behavioral symptomatology in dementia of the Alzheimer's type. *Alzheimer Disease and Associated Disorders, 2,* 363–365.

Reisberg, B. (1986). Dementia: A systematic approach to identifying reversible causes. *Geriatrics, 41,* 30–46.

Reisberg, B. (1988). Functional assessment staging (FAST). *Psychopharmacology Bulletin, 24,* 653–659.

Reisberg, B., Borenstein, J., Franssen, E., Shulman, E., Steinberg, G., & Ferris, S. H. (1986). Remediable behavioral symptomatology in Alzheimer's disease. *Hospital and Community Psychiatry, 37,* 1199–1201.

Reisberg, B., Ferris, S. H., Anand, R., de Leon, M. J., Schneck, M. K., Buttinger, C., & Borenstein, J. (1984). Functional staging of dementia of the Alzheimer's type. *Annals of the New York Academy of Sciences, 435,* 481–483.

Reisberg, B., Ferris, S. H., de Leon, M. J., & Crook, T. (1982). The Global Deterioration Scale for the assessment of primary degenerative dementia. *American Journal of Psychiatry, 139,* 1136–1139.

Reisberg, B., Ferris, S. H., & Franssen, E. (1985). An ordinal functional assessment tool for Alzheimer's-type dementia. *Hospital and Community Psychiatry, 36,* 593–595.

Reisberg, B., Ferris, S. H., Franssen, E., Shulman, E., Monteiro, I., Sclan, S. G., Steinberg, G., Kluger, A., Torossian, C., de Leon, M. J., & Laska, E. (1996). Mortality and temporal course of probable Alzheimer's disease: A five-year prospective study. *International Psychogeriatrics, 8,* 291–311.

Reisberg, B., Ferris, S. H., Kluger, A., Franssen, E., de Leon, M. J., Mittelman, M., Borenstein, J., Rameshwar, K., & Alba, R. (1989). Symptomatic changes in CNS aging and dementia of the Alzheimer type: Cross-sectional, temporal, and remediable concomitants. In M. Bergener & B. Reisberg (Eds.), *Diagnosis and treatment of senile dementia* (pp. 193–223). Berlin: Springer-Verlag.

Reisberg, B., Franssen, E., Bobinski, M., Auer, S., Monteiro, I., Boksay, I., Wegiel, J., Shulman, E., Steinberg, G., Souren, L., Kluger, A., Torossian, C., Sinaiko, E., Wisniewski, H. M., & Ferris, S. H. (1996). Overview of methodologic issues for pharmacologic trials in mild, moderate, and severe Alzheimer's disease. *International Psychogeriatrics, 8,* 159–193.

Reisberg, B., Franssen, E., Sclan, S. G., Kluger, A., & Ferris, S. H. (1989). Stage specific incidence of potentially remediable behavioral symptoms in aging and Alzheimer's disease: A study of 120 patients using the BEHAVE-AD. *Bulletin of Clinical Neuroscience, 54,* 95–112.

Reisberg, B., London, E., Ferris, S. H., Borenstein, J., Scheier, L., & de Leon, M. J. (1983). The Brief Cognitive Rating Scale: Language, motoric, and mood concomitants in primary degenerative dementia. *Psychopharmacology Bulletin, 19,* 702–708.

Reisberg, B., Pattschull-Furlan, A., Franssen, E., Sclan, S. G., Kluger, A., Dingcong, L., & Ferris, S. H. (1990). Cognition related functional, praxis and feeding changes in CNS aging and Alzheimer's disease and their developmental analogies. In K. Beyreuther & G. Schettler (Eds.), *Molecular mechanisms of aging* (pp. 18–40). Berlin: Springer-Verlag.

Reisberg, B., Schneck, M. K., Ferris, S. H., Schwartz, G. E., & de Leon, M. J. (1983). The brief cognitive rating scale (BCRS): Findings in primary degenerative dementia (PDD). *Psychopharmacology Bulletin, 19,* 47–50.

Rovner, B. W., Kafonek, S., Filipp, L., Lucas, M. J., & Folstein, M. F. (1986). Prevalence of mental illness in a community nursing home. *American Journal of Psychiatry, 143,* 1446–1449.

Rubin, E., Morris, J., Storandt, M., & Berg, L. (1987). Behavioral changes in patients with mild senile dementia of the Alzheimer's type. *Psychiatry Research, 21,* 55–61.

Sclan, S. G., & Reisberg, B. (1992). Functional assessment staging (FAST) in Alzheimer's disease: Reliability, validity and ordinality. *International Psychogeriatrics, 4,* 55–69.

Souren, L. E. M., Franssen, E. M., & Reisberg, B. (1995). Contractures and loss of function in patients with Alzheimer's disease. *Journal of the American Geriatrics Society, 43,* 650–655.

Chapter 5

Traumatic Brain Injury

Thomas M. Dixon and Barry S. Layton

Brain injuries resulting from trauma constitute a major source of neurological disability throughout the world. Acquired damage to the brain affects the biological substrate that underlies fundamental functional capacities such as motor control, sensation, perception, cognition, memory, personality, and emotion. The physical and neurobehavioral sequelae of brain impairment often produce devastating consequences involving the ability to live independently, maintain competitive employment, sustain intimate relationships, and generally to establish a meaningful existence. Clearly then, the rehabilitation of brain injuries represents a vital challenge to survivors, families, and professionals.

For the purposes of this discussion, the term "traumatic brain injury" (TBI) refers to the disruption of brain structure and/or function from the sudden application of physical force, usually involving a blow to the head or penetration of the skull by a foreign object. Other descriptions applied to this phenomenon are head injury, concussion, craniocerebral trauma, and posttraumatic encephalopathy. The term TBI, rather than head injury, is preferred because it correctly indicates the focus of damage. The National Head Injury Foundation has recently acknowledged the importance of this nomenclature by renaming itself the Brain Injury Association.

DISTINCTIVE CHARACTERISTICS OF DISABILITY FROM TBI

TBI possesses at least three distinctive characteristics as a disability. First, in many other disabling conditions, the cognitive and emotional characteristics of the individual remain intact, permitting deployment of the full range of preinjury intellectual and affective resources in compensation for lost function. However, brain injury almost always disrupts intellect and emotion, limiting available resources for coping. Cognitive and emotional impairments, therefore, not only become a focus for painful feelings of loss but also interfere with psychological adaptation.

Second, the psychosocial impact of TBI is different from that of developmental cognitive disabilities. Intellectual difficulties beginning early in life (e.g., mental retardation) create limited expectations for productivity and social integration. TBI, on the other hand, often abruptly diminishes the social and vocational roles of individuals who have achieved a stable adaptation or who anticipate doing so at a level determined by irretrievable preinjury capacities.

A third distinguishing feature of TBI as a disability is that it frequently is invisible. Observers casually notice problems associated with physical losses such as paraplegia or limb amputation, but casual inspection often does not reveal the cognitive disorders that form the core of disability as a result of brain injury. TBI without accompanying physical deficits may evolve into a silent affliction conferring unique problems on the injured individual.

EPIDEMIOLOGY

The rate of survival from TBI has increased over the past 20 years due to advances in emergency medical procedures and neurosurgical techniques. As a result, the cumulative number of people with TBI currently is expanding; many individuals who formerly would have died as a result of accidents or assaults now are saved in the acute period following injury. The decrease in fatality in combination with the overrepresentation of TBI among young people creates a population with chronic disability because survival of acute hospitalization and emergence from coma often predicts a normal life span.

TBI outnumbers many other forms of neurological disability, including spinal cord injury, multiple sclerosis, Parkinson's disease, Guillain-Barre syndrome, motor neuron disease, and myasthenia gravis (Alexander, 1995). Table 5.1 shows

TABLE 5.1 Causes of Traumatic Brain Injury

Motor vehicle accidents	44%
Falls	21%
Assaults	12%
Sports accidents	10%
Gunshots	6%

From Kraus et al., 1984.

the major causes of TBI. According to recent reviews, population studies reveal an incidence rate of approximately 200 TBIs requiring hospitalization per 100,000 people in the United States (Kraus & Sorenson, 1994; Torner & Schootman, 1995). Estimates of incidence vary based on the region of the United States under survey as well as the means by which researchers define TBI.

Each year, roughly 500,000 TBIs occur, and 50,000 result in death. For injuries involving a visit to the emergency room or hospital admission, 80% are classified as mild TBI; 10%, moderate; and 10%, severe (Kraus & Sorenson, 1994). Incidence data may not reflect many cases of mild TBI that either are undiagnosed or treated outside hospitals.

Certain groups face increased risk of TBI. With respect to age, people between the ages of 15 and 24 have the highest rate of injury. Risk gradually declines through the middle-age years and then rises again after age 60. Older adults have increased TBI incidence and mortality, especially due to falls, with generally poorer neuropsychological recovery, compared to younger people. With respect to gender, TBI occurs 2 to 2.8 times more frequently in males than in females (Kraus & Sorenson, 1994). In addition, males are more likely to die as a result of TBI, presumably because of greater exposure to high-risk activities. Alcohol intoxication represents another major risk factor. Corrigan (1995) examined the available studies and found a 36% to 51% incidence of intoxication at time of injury. A significant number of people intoxicated at injury probably meet criteria for substance abuse, and some evidence indicates that these individuals may have less adequate recovery than those without a diagnosis of substance abuse.

The prevalence of persisting disability related to TBI is not precisely known. Certainly not everyone who suffers a TBI becomes disabled. Torner and Schootman (1995) suggest that determining the number of people who receive rehabilitation, extended care, or disability payments for TBI would offer a practical method of assessing prevalence, but such information has not yet been documented. Based on an algorithm of the available data, Kraus and Sorenson (1994) estimate that TBI causes 83,000 new disabilities per year.

TBI results in an enormous economic cost to society in the form of medical expenses, rehabilitation services, lost productivity, and disability payments. A recent multicenter study of TBI revealed that the average charge (adjusted to 1995 dollars) for acute care and inpatient rehabilitation of severe TBI equaled $164,238 (Harrison-Felix, Newton, Hall, & Kreutzer, 1996). Max, MacKenzie, and Rice (1991) estimated the total cost to society for head injuries in 1985 at $37.8 billion.

MECHANISMS OF INJURY AND PATHOPHYSIOLOGY

The type and magnitude of physical force to the brain determine the nature, location, and extent of trauma. Levin, Benton, and Grossman (1982) and Lishman

(1987) summarize the physical mechanisms of TBI in detail. Brain injuries are commonly classified as closed or open, depending on whether the skull remains intact or is penetrated by a bullet or other object. Closed head trauma occurs when the head undergoes a sudden change in momentum—either acceleration or deceleration. Consider the prototypical case of an automobile collision. The vehicle traveling at a high rate of speed collides with an immovable object, such as a telephone pole. The occupant suffers rapid deceleration as the head hits the dashboard or windshield, followed by acceleration as the head whips back in an arc. These blows cause the brain to move within the skull, thereby generating rotational forces—an abnormal twisting or swirling of the delicate gelatinous neural tissue. As a consequence of its movement, the brain also may come into forcible contact with bony prominences of the skull, such as the orbital ridges that form a shelf supporting the frontal lobes. The brain also may recoil from one side of the skull to the other, causing what is referred to as coup/contrecoup injury.

The physical mechanisms outlined above cause a variety of pathological changes in the nervous system. Rotational forces produce diffuse axonal injury (DAI)—that is, stretching, swelling, or shearing of axons throughout the brain. DAI includes damage to long axons (white matter) in the brain stem, initially producing a period of unconsciousness of variable duration and impairment of vital functions (Adams, Graham, & Gennarelli, 1985). Also, injury to connecting axons impairs communication between the two cerebral hemispheres and between cortical and subcortical structures. As a result of DAI, various areas of the brain function with less efficiency because they have been deprived of input from other cerebral regions or are less able to convey their output to control behavior.

Another primary form of damage resulting from TBI consists of laceration and focal cortical contusion, or bruising of brain tissue. The frontal and anterior temporal lobes are especially vulnerable to contusion because they sit within the skull's jagged inner surface. In injuries that do not entail high-speed acceleration/deceleration (e.g., falls, blunt blows to the head with an object, penetrating missile wounds), focal cerebral contusions may occur in the absence of underlying DAI.

Following the moment of injury, numerous secondary complications can develop that affect survival and ultimate outcome. For example, cerebral swelling or edema may increase tissue volume within the rigid cranial vault, creating an elevation in intracranial pressure and associated conditions of reduced blood flow (ischemia) and loss of oxygen (hypoxia). Leakage from ruptured blood vessels may produce space-occupying blood clots, known as hematomas, that compress the brain tissue and necessitate neurosurgery for evacuation.

In the past 10 years, scientific investigation of secondary mechanisms of brain injury has focused on the biochemical basis of neuronal death (Stein, Glasier, & Hoffman, 1994). Microvascular disruption and stretching of axons from the initial injury initiates a cascade of adverse events at the cellular level. Excessive release of neurotransmitters, overexcitation due to influx of calcium ions into cells, and degradation of membranes by oxidation gradually destroy neurons. Currently, pharmacological strategies to limit this destructive cascade are being investigated.

Medical complications in the early stages of TBI may contribute to nerve cell loss. Relatively common occurrences include posttraumatic epilepsy, infections, and pulmonary dysfunction (Miller, Pentland, & Berrol, 1990).

FUNCTIONAL PRESENTATION OF TBI

Brain injuries produce distinctive physical, cognitive, and behavioral syndromes corresponding to the nature and extent of neuroanatomical damage. Diffuse axonal injury produces areas of neuronal fallout throughout the brain and tends to result in generalized loss of cognitive efficiency and adaptive capacity. In addition, TBI often results in focal injury that affects circumscribed areas of the brain and produces specific symptoms according to location. Focal damage also may have nonspecific consequences because disparate regions of the brain operate together in functional systems; therefore, suppressing the activity in one area alters the operation of the whole system. Virtually any behavioral or neurocognitive syndrome can result from TBI, depending on the specific site(s) of injury. However, the prototypical acceleration/deceleration TBI comprises some degree of DAI, accompanied by frontotemporal cerebral contusions.

The manifestations of TBI vary not only in relation to lesion type but also as a function of unique attributes of the injured person. Considering the relationship between personality style and coping with TBI, one early observer (Symonds, 1937) concisely stated: "It is not only the kind of head injury that matters but the kind of head." Individual differences in age, premorbid education, intelligence, family support, social context, and psychological adjustment interact with neurological deficits, giving rise to heterogeneity in the functional impact of a given impairment. For example, a mild brain injury in a business executive or air traffic controller might have disastrous consequences, whereas, at least in some vocational situations, a more severe injury may not interfere with effective functioning.

Nature of Impairments After TBI

This section provides a brief, selective overview of neuropsychological syndromes following TBI. Common signs and symptoms of brain impairment include disturbances of motor and sensory abilities, language and communication, visual-perceptual skills, attention, memory, executive functions, personality, and awareness. The interested reader will wish to explore basic texts by Lezak (1995),

Lishman (1987), Prigatano et al. (1986), and Walsh (1994) to gain a greater appreciation of this complex topic.

Motor and Sensory Impairments

Damage to the precentral gyrus or motor strip of the cerebral cortex produces paralysis (hemiplegia) or weakness (hemiparesis) on the side of the body contralateral to the affected hemisphere. Thus, left-sided weakness of the upper and lower extremities usually signals right brain damage, and vice versa. Damage to other components of the motor system may produce not only paralysis but also tremor, incoordination of movements (ataxia), and loss of dexterity. Motor symptoms interfere with mobility as well as performance of self-care and other skilled tasks. In surveys of severe TBI patients assessed 1 to 6 years postinjury, roughly 30% to 45% reported difficulties with walking or running, and 20% to 30% endorsed trouble with basic activities of daily living such as toileting, grooming, and bathing (Dikmen, Machamer, Savoie, & Temkin, 1996).

Sensory impairments such as hemianesthesia or heminanopsia (blindness in one visual field) occur as a result of damage contralateral to the affected limb or visual field. Any sensory function (olfactory, tactile, auditory, etc.) may be diminished as a result of damage to a specific site in the brain or cranial nerves.

Language and Communication Impairments

Disorders of the oral-motor musculature create speech articulation difficulties called dysarthria. Impairment of expressive or receptive language, or aphasia, usually is a sign of damage to the left frontal and/or temporal lobes. Depending on the location of injury, aphasia may result in impaired word finding and grammatical expression of ideas or in impaired auditory comprehension, reading (dyslexia), and writing (dysgraphia) or in any combination of these disorders. Relatively few people with TBI have the pure aphasic syndromes often observed in stroke, but deficits in naming or word retrieval commonly occur. Many people with TBI who do not have focal language deficits are impaired in organization and coherence of verbal output and display diminished ability to comprehend complex material (Crosson, Cooper, Lincoln, Bauer, & Velozo, 1993; Prigatano et al., 1986).

Individuals with TBI may show nonverbal communication problems such as impaired capacity to convey and comprehend emotional meanings, as reflected in intonation of speech and facial expression. Thus, the person with TBI may not communicate feelings well or understand those communicated by others. Even subtle verbal and nonverbal communication problems affect social interaction and contribute to an erosion of relationships.

Visual-Perceptual Impairments

Visual perception includes the ability to recognize objects visually, to appreciate relationships among objects in space, and to organize elements in three dimensions. These abilities depend largely on the integrity of the right hemisphere, particularly the inferior temporal and parietal lobes. When deficits occur, as in cases of right hemisphere contusion or bullet wounds, they often result in disability. Functionally, visuospatial deficits may affect dressing, finding one's way around, meal preparation, interpretation of maps or drawings, and driving.

Attentional Impairments

There are several different attentional functions: maintaining optimal levels of arousal and alertness, maintaining task vigilance over time, registering new information as it is presented, filtering out distractions, and keeping track of multiple stimuli simultaneously. DAI and more focal lesions to the reticular activating system of the brain stem and frontal lobes contribute to attentional impairment (Mateer & Mapou, 1996; Whyte, 1992).

Severe deficits in basic arousal and alertness stemming from DAI may produce a temporary lack of conscious awareness or even a permanent vegetative state (Jennett, 1996). Milder injuries result in higher level attentional impairments, impacting on ability to perform complex tasks (Gronwall, 1989). Moderate to severe TBI typically produces slowing of reaction times and processing speed. Deficits in the capacity to handle two or more sources of information simultaneously—that is, divided attention—may interfere with performance in the presence of distraction or with the ability to do more than one thing at a time, such as listening and taking notes in school. Inadequate registration of material to be learned probably accounts in part for memory difficulty following TBI. One study found that over 60% of long-term survivors of severe TBI were observed to have attentional problems (Jacobs, 1988).

Memory Impairments

Memory impairments constitute a defining characteristic of TBI (Levin et al., 1982). After regaining consciousness, the person with TBI passes through a period of disorientation and confusion during which ongoing events are not encoded into memory. This severe impairment of new learning capacity is referred to as anterograde amnesia or posttraumatic amnesia (PTA). A period of retrograde amnesia (RA)—that is, inability to recall events that predate the injury—often accompanies anterograde amnesia. Figure 5.1 illustrates the temporal relationship of PTA and RA to the time of injury. Over time, RA usually shrinks so that preinjury memories are restored up until the minutes or hours immediately preced-

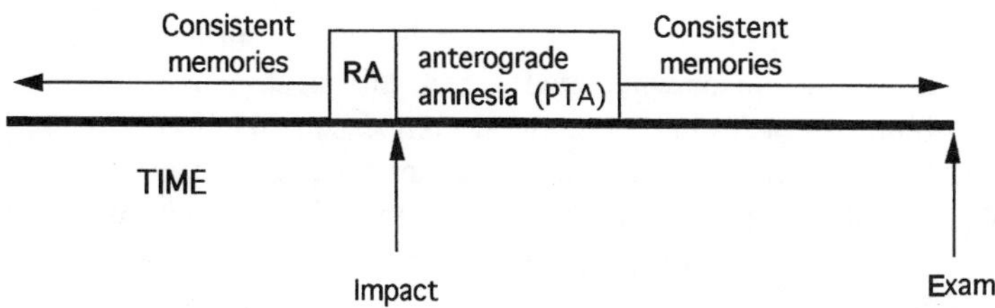

FIGURE 5.1 Temporal relationship between posttraumatic amnesia and retrograde amnesia (RA) following traumatic brain injury.

ing the time of impact. PTA, however, leaves a permanent gap in memory, lasting from minutes to weeks or longer and persisting after gross recall of daily events has returned. As we will discuss below, the duration of PTA reflects the severity of TBI. Focal brain injury from penetrating missile wounds may not produce PTA, but diffuse TBI almost always does to some extent.

TBI may entail chronic memory impairment following the acute resolution of PTA. In fact, trouble in remembering things is the single most common complaint noted by people with TBI and by their relatives (Jacobs, 1988; Oddy, Coughlan, Tyerman, & Jenkins, 1985). DAI, which affects registration of new material, and damage to the deep structures of the temporal lobes, which form the cerebral substrate for storing memories, contribute to the high frequency of memory disorders after TBI. Research has also demonstrated that TBI produces deficits in the ability to organize new information. These organizational problems may interfere with understanding the gist of new material or with knowing what information is important to recall. According to Levin (1997), approximately 40% of people with moderate to severe TBI recover normal functioning on general intellectual measures but still show disproportionately poor memory skills. From a practical standpoint, memory disorders undermine the continuity of day-to-day events and induce confusion as the injured person struggles to recall previous conversations, task instructions, schedules, the location of lost objects, and the like.

Executive Function Impairments

Executive functions refer to a group of skills that enable independent, purposeful, goal-directed activity in the service of long-term goals and projects. According to neuropsychological models of executive function, the frontal lobes act to form plans and intentions, then integrate and deploy subserving skills to carry out those plans and flexibly correct ongoing behavior to maintain effectiveness (Lezak 1995; Stuss & Benson, 1986). People with frontal and/or diffuse cerebral impairment due to TBI may display numerous intact skills in structured situations, such as the hospital unit or testing room, but decompensate in complex, unstructured situations because of their inability to sustain and regulate planful activity. Executive impairment sometimes leads to the perception that people with TBI lack judgment and common sense. Executive dysfunction may create long-term reliance on others for supervision and day-to-day guidance, as well as an unproductive lifestyle.

Personality and Emotional Consequences

Personality disturbances represent a common consequence of TBI and often comprise part of a larger pattern of impaired executive function. Thomsen (1984) reported that 80% of relatives who were interviewed 2.5 years after injury described their family member with a severe TBI as "another person." Other studies suggest that personality and behavioral changes appear in 30% to 50% of cases (Jacobs, 1988; Lezak, 1987). Table 5.2 lists commonly reported disturbances as documented by Prigatano (1992) in a comprehensive review of literature. Insufficient control of impulses, leading to behavioral excesses, or lack of drive, leading to behavioral deficits, appear as themes in clinical observation.

TABLE 5.2 Emotional and Motivational Disturbances Associated with TBI

Active types	Passive types
Irritability	Aspontaneity
Agitation	Sluggishness
Belligerence/anger	Loss of interest in environment
Impulsiveness	Loss of drive or initiative
Impatience	Tires easily
Restlessness	Depression
Inappropriate social responses	
Emotional lability	
Sensitivity to noise or distress	
Anxiety	
Suspiciousness or mistrust of others	
Delusional beliefs	
Paranoia	
Mania or manic-like states	

From Prigatano, 1992.

Prigatano (1992) distinguishes between direct and reactive emotional changes. More precisely, some difficulties such as impulsivity or loss of initiation may flow directly from the frontal/diffuse neuropathology of TBI, whereas problems such as irritability and depression may signify a normal psychological reaction to catastrophic loss. Understanding this distinction is clinically important because reactive emotional problems may be more amenable to psychotherapeutic treatment than neurologically based behavioral impairments.

Cognitive and emotional difficulties may interact with each other in a vicious cycle as depicted in Figure 5.2. For example, the slowing, decreased concentration and poor initiative that characterize depression may intensify cognitive losses resulting from brain damage. The intensified cognitive losses, in turn, serve as a focus for increased self-depreciation, depression, and anxiety.

Unawareness of Deficits

A significant proportion of persons with TBI who present with gross cognitive and behavioral difficulties report that they have nothing wrong with them. This impaired recognition of deficits is called anosognosia. Current theory holds that the capacity for self-awareness—the comparison of self against relevant standards—is the superordinate function of the frontal lobes (Stuss, 1991). People

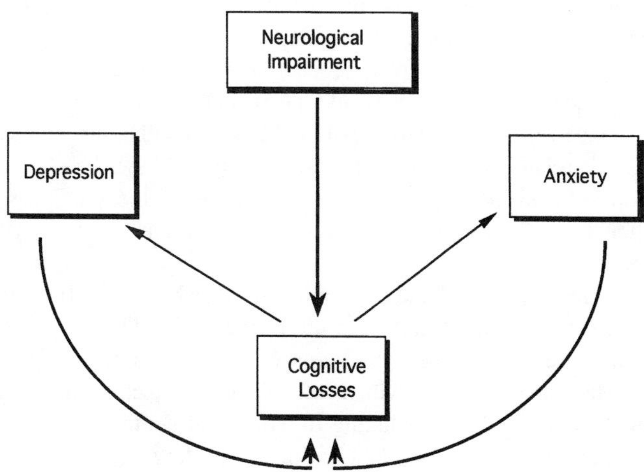

FIGURE 5.2 Relationship between neurocognitive losses and emotional functioning after brain injury.

with TBI, who often have frontal lobe involvement, are thus vulnerable to problems with awareness. Clinically, unawareness may result in choosing a level of work that is beyond their abilities or in not recognizing the negative impact that their behavior makes on others. Gently pointing out deficits creates temporary confusion or disbelief, but the feedback may be discounted later (Prigatano, 1991). Not all unawareness is neurologically based. Psychological denial for self-protective reasons also comes into play in the face of the painful flaws and shortcomings produced by TBI. Unawareness is the bane of rehabilitation, for people are less likely to cooperate with remediation of problems that, from their perspective, do not exist.

Continuum of Outcome and Measurement of Severity of TBI

TBI produces a wide continuum of outcomes, ranging from death to return of normal function, with varying degrees of disability in between. Criteria for assessing outcome include rating scales for specific functional abilities, neuropsychological tests, productivity/employment status, living arrangements after rehabilitation, social and emotional functioning, length of hospitalization, and cost of care (Hall & Johnston, 1994).

One widely used measure is the Glasgow Outcome Scale (GOS), which classifies outcome from TBI as follows: (1) death, (2) persistent vegetative state (i.e., no conscious awareness or purposeful activity), (3) severe disability (conscious but physically or cognitively dependent on others for daily care), (4) moderate disability (disabled but independent in self-care and basic access to community), and (5) good recovery (mild, persistent residual sequelae but capable of normal social life) (Jennett & Teasdale, 1981). The GOS has received justifiable criticism for its relative crudeness and insensitivity to higher level cognitive and emotional problems (Lezak, 1995). However, use of the GOS has provided valuable generalizations about the relationship between initial severity of TBI and long-term outcome.

Although many personal and environmental variables may affect brain injury recovery, research indicates that the initial severity of TBI, as determined by objective measures, is the best predictor of eventual outcome (Bond, 1990; Dikmen & Machamer, 1995; Levin, 1990). Several objective methods exist for grading the severity of TBI, including duration and depth of unconsciousness, length of posttraumatic amnesia, and radiologic findings.

Level of Coma

The Glasgow Coma Scale (GCS; Table 5.3) measures level of unconsciousness based on eye opening, capacity for purposeful movement, and verbalization

TABLE 5.3 Glasgow Coma Scale

Eye opening (E)	Spontaneous	4
	To speech	3
	To pain	2
	Nil	1
Best motor response (M)	Obeys	6
	Localizes	5
	Withdraws	4
	Abnormal flexion	3
	Extensor response	2
	Nil	1
Verbal response (V)	Oriented	5
	Confused conversation	4
	Inappropriate words	3
	Incomprehensible sounds	2
	Nil	1

Coma score (E + M + V) = 3 to 15.
From Jennet & Teasdale, 1981.

(Jennett & Teasdale, 1981). Scores vary from 3 (profound coma) to 15 (normal awareness and orientation). Initial GCS ratings in the range of 3–8 denote severe TBI; 9–12, moderate TBI; and 13–15, mild TBI. According to a review of nine large-scale studies, severe TBI (defined by GCS of 8 or lower at 6 hours or more postinjury) resulted in the following GOS classifications at 6 months: dead, 42%; vegetative, 3%; severe disability, 10%; moderate disability, 13%; and good recovery, 33% (Eisenberg, 1985).

Table 5.4 presents data on coma and outcome, showing that lower initial GCS scores are associated with greater mortality and disability. Initial GCS also predicts cognitive outcome. For example, one study found that 84% of subjects with less severe TBIs (GCS of 15-8) displayed minimal to no deficits on a cognitive test battery, whereas only 10% of those with more severe injuries (GCS of 3–4) presented with minimal to no deficits (Alexandre, Colombo, Nertempi, & Benedetti, 1983).

Duration of Coma

Another important outcome predictor, duration of coma, may be defined as the number of days that GCS remains below 9 or as the time to follow commands based on the motor subscale of the GCS (Dikmen, Machamer, Winn, & Temkin,

TABLE 5.4 Outcome Associated with Initial Glasgow Coma Scale (GCS) After TBI

GCS	*N*	Dead/vegetative (%)	Moderate disability/ good recovery (%)
> 11	57	7	87
8/9/10	190	27	68
5/6/7	525	53	34
3/4	176	87	7

From Jennett et al. (1979).

1995). Using the time to follow commands (TFC) criterion, Dikmen and her colleagues found that length of coma predicted both GOS and cognitive status at 1 year. People with TFC of less than 1 hour performed at the same level as controls on a neuropsychological test battery, but as TFC increased, so did cognitive impairment. Individuals with 1–13 days of coma showed selective impairments of cognitive functioning, whereas coma of 14 days or more predicted pervasive deficits. The chances of good recovery decrease with coma duration of 1 month or longer. A review of 434 TBI cases with coma duration of 1 month or longer found that only 7% eventually reached the good recovery classification on the GOS (Multi-Society Task Force on PVS, 1994).

Duration of PTA

Russell (1932) proposed the classic scheme for classifying severity of TBI according to duration of PTA:

PTA < 1 hour = mild brain injury

PTA 1–24 hours = moderate injury

PTA 1–7 days = severe injury

PTA > 7 days = very severe injury

Table 5.5 shows the relationship between PTA and outcome, illustrating that longer PTA corresponds with increased likelihood of severe disability. The clinician evaluating TBI months or years after injury may gain insight into the severity of injury by inquiring about the length of time before the person became truly oriented and able to recall daily events.

TABLE 5.5 Duration of Posttraumatic Amnesia (PTA) and Outcome at 6 Months

PTA	*n*	Severely disabled (%)	Moderately disabled (%)	Good recovery (%)
< 14 days	101	0	17	83
15–28 days	96	3	31	66
> 28 days	289	30	43	27

From Jennett & Teasdale, 1981.

Radiological Findings

Radiologic procedures such as computed tomography (CT) scanning and magnetic resonance imaging (MRI) offer information about severity, particularly in the acute stage of medical care. Severe brain injury, as measured by GCS, results in abnormal head CT scan findings in 95% of cases, whereas moderate TBI produces abnormal CT findings in only 25% of cases. Mild TBI seldom shows up on CT (Levin, Amparo, et al., 1987). MRI appears superior in detecting nonhemorrhagic white matter lesions occurring as a result of TBI and thus may have greater sensitivity to diffuse injuries that do not involve bleeding contusions or hematomas. The severity of DAI, estimated radiologically by determining the volume of fluid space within the brain, correlates fairly well with cognitive outcome. The presence of focal lesions contributes to residual problems as well, but the long-term effects of focal lesions do not appear as strong as those of diffuse damage (Levin, 1990). The increasing use of radiological measures of cerebral metabolism such as positron emission tomography may shed further light on the relationship between cerebral pathology and cognitive-behavioral impairments.

Limitations of Predictive Techniques

The generally positive statistical relationship between early measures of TBI severity and later outcome still is far from perfect. The terms mild, moderate, and severe applied at or near the time of the trauma are not intended to characterize subsequent disability in a simplistic, one-to-one manner. Indicators of severe brain injury—say, an initial GCS of 5 and PTA of 3 weeks—do not preclude the possibility of a favorable outcome in an individual case. By the same token, a mild brain injury may result in a poor outcome for a given person. Confusing initial severity with outcome may cause misconceptions in the study of milder injuries, where clinicians minimize or even dismiss the likelihood of complicated recovery (Dikmen & Levin, 1993).

Course and Mechanisms of Recovery After TBI

The natural history of TBI includes sudden onset, a variable length of unconsciousness and PTA, a period of recovery, and residual sequelae. The course of recovery generally follows a negatively accelerating curve, as depicted in Figure 5.3. People often make marked gains in the first several months after trauma, followed by a longer period of slowly tapering improvement (Levin, 1985). In general, the less severe the injury, the closer recovery may approximate preinjury functioning. For severe TBI, the phase of rapid improvement contains dramatic gains in basic attention, day-to-day memory, ambulation, and performance of basic activities of daily living. A longer stage follows that centers on reacquisition of complex cognitive and interpersonal skills.

Research reveals varying estimates for the time frame of recovery. For example, studies using the GOS have shown that 90% of people with TBI attain their ultimate outcome classification within 6 months. In contrast, more sensitive neuropsychological studies have documented functional improvement over 2 or 3 years (Levin, 1985). Thomsen (1984, 1990) followed a group of 40 persons with very severe brain injuries over a 10–15-year period, finding that a mixture of both positive and negative functional changes occurred during that time.

Neuroscience is beginning to unravel the mechanisms by which the brain heals itself following injury (Stein, Brailowsky, & Will, 1995). As evidenced by the many instances of remarkable recovery after TBI, the brain possesses resil-

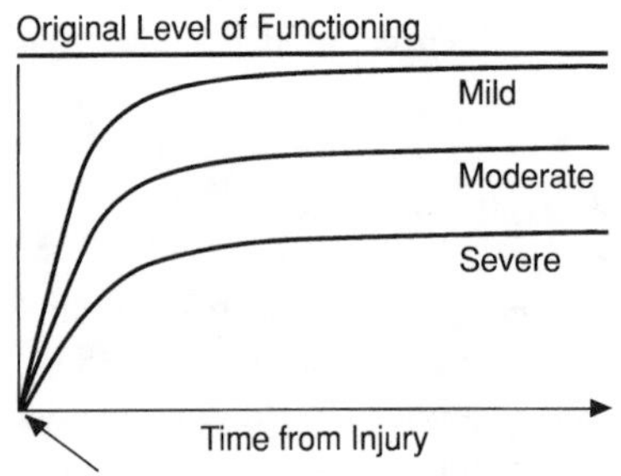

FIGURE 5.3 Negatively accelerating course of recovery following brain injury.

ience and plasticity. Research in animals has demonstrated that nerve cells may form new connections after injury by collateral sprouting of dendrites and thereby restore some lost function. Another recovery mechanism involves increased sensitivity of receptor sites so that neural circuits can work despite the absence of some neurons. Environmental context plays a role in these mechanisms because better recovery takes place in enriched environments than in deprived ones. The stimulation and challenge of rehabilitation activities after TBI likely facilitates neurological recovery, however incomplete. In the future, the true "cure" for TBI may center on the recruitment of restoration processes by means of pharmacological and environmental interventions.

Observations on Mild TBI

We wish to include a separate section on mild TBI because this disorder possesses unique features not covered by our previous discussion. Mild TBI is defined by (1) application of force to the head, (2) loss of consciousness for less than 30 minutes or simply dazed consciousness, (3) PTA not more than 24 hours, and (4) initial GCS of 13–15 within 30 minutes of injury (Evans, 1992). Neuroradiological findings are almost always normal. Commonly recognized early symptoms of mild TBI include headache, dizziness, fatigue, insomnia, memory difficulties, impaired concentration, ringing in the ears, sensitivity to lights and noises, depression, anxiety, and irritability (Lishman, 1987).

Mild TBI recently has attracted considerable interest (Alexander, 1995; Binder, 1997; Larrabee, 1997; Putnam, Millis, & Adams, 1996). Prospective clinical studies reveal that 85%–90% of individuals with mild TBI return to normal functioning with little or no intervention (Levin, Mattis, et al., 1987). However, a vigorous and sometimes partisan debate revolves around the topic of why certain people fail to recover. At issue is the relative contribution of neuropathology versus psychological factors such as posttraumatic stress, somatization, and impaired motivation in connection with pending personal injury litigation. The controversy is not merely an academic one, because if we assume that mild TBI results in disability even 10% of the time, then 40,000 people may suffer disabling mild TBIs each year (Kraus & Sorenson, 1994).

From our perspective, "minor" brain trauma is like minor surgery: it's only minor if it happens to somebody else. The etiology of mild TBI symptoms has both neurological and psychological components, and for each individual, multiple factors interact to produce dysfunction. Three lines of evidence implicate a neurological component for sequelae of mild TBI (Alexander, 1995). First, animal research models and human autopsy studies demonstrate that observable, permanent damage occurs to brain structure after "mild" trauma (Jane, Steward, & Gennarelli, 1985). Second, various forms of physical stress can unmask symptoms in otherwise asymptomatic cases (see Gronwall, 1989, for a review). For example, one study showed that college students who had sustained mild TBI and appeared to recover were abnormally prone to mental inefficiency when physiologically stressed by hypoxic conditions. Third, persons who suffer multiple mild TBIs, such as boxers or football players, eventually develop cognitive impairment. This observation suggests that mild TBI causes permanent damage that is unmasked by the cumulative effects of subsequent insults.

Effects of mild TBI that begin as neurological symptoms may be maintained by psychological variables long after the injury has resolved. Psychogenic factors contributing to mild TBI symptoms include preinjury personality and reactive emotional distress in connection with cognitive deficits. Individuals prone to somatization—that is, the expression of psychological stress in the form of physical symptoms—may be particularly vulnerable to chronic impairment. The symptoms of mild TBI are found among individuals who have been exposed to stressors but have never had a blow to the head. Accordingly, examination of mild TBI requires consideration of causes for complaint other than brain injury.

A relationship exists between involvement in litigation and symptom severity insofar as litigants are much more likely than nonlitigants to report persisting problems. Interestingly, the settlement of litigation generally does not improve symptoms, so simple desire for financial gain does not account for symptom formation in most cases (Rutherford, 1989). Nevertheless, because financial incentives are associated with successful litigation involving brain damage, a certain proportion of individuals who have been involved in an accident or assault may contrive or exaggerate deficits that they either never suffered or that have resolved to a greater extent than expressed at the time of clinical examination. Specialized techniques have been developed to detect malingering. Some research investigations indicate poorer performance by litigating mild TBI patients than by nonlitigating patients with severe brain injuries.

PSYCHOLOGICAL AND VOCATIONAL IMPLICATIONS OF TBI

Numerous investigations have clearly shown that people with TBI confront enormous difficulty in psychosocial functioning and that cognitive and behavioral disorders impair adaptation to a greater extent than physical problems do. This section provides an overview of psychosocial sequelae of TBI, including problems in psychological adjustment, impact on families, and vocational issues.

Psychological Adjustment

Prigatano (1994) uses the metaphor of life's journey to describe psychological adjustment after brain injury. A person who is progressing along a certain path through life and who suddenly has a TBI may wish to continue along the same road, even though this is no longer possible. Finding a new path (or failing to find one) defines the struggle of living with a brain injury. Prigatano also observes that people with TBI repeatedly confront three existential questions: (1) "Why did this happen to me?" (2) "Will I be normal again?" (3) "Is life worth living after brain injury?" (pp. 174–175). He believes that individuals with the internal resources to come to grips with their impairments and redefine themselves tend to become productive again.

Unfortunately, the empirical literature on psychosocial outcome following TBI suggests that many people fail to adapt successfully. The theme of loneliness and isolation emerges in studies of psychosocial sequelae (Morton & Wehman, 1995). People with TBI face a high risk of loss of relationships and social support, as evidenced by decreased number of friends, fewer social contacts, and less leisure activity in the community. Oddy et al. (1985) found that 50% of their sample of TBI survivors reported limited contact with friends, and 60% had no girlfriend or boyfriend. Individuals with more severe injuries tend to become more isolated because they may lack access to the community (e.g., not driving) and have more noticeable alteration in interpersonal skills. Jacobs (1988) noted that people who are single at the time of TBI tend to remain single, and divorce rates may increase. Negative changes in sexual behavior occur commonly, including decreased frequency of intercourse and decline in personal sex appeal (Kreutzer & Zasler, 1989; O'Carrol, Woodrow, & Maroun, 1991).

Not surprisingly, a parallel psychosocial theme is the development of emotional disorders such as anxiety and depression. Clinical studies suggest that approximately 15%–45% of people with TBI suffer anxiety symptoms, and 25%–50% suffer depressive disorders (Gualtieri & Cox, 1991; Taylor & Price, 1994).

Impact of TBI on Families

TBI poses enormous difficulty not only for the person who is injured but for the entire family (Dikmen et al., 1996; Kreutzer, Marwitz, & Kepler, 1992). Relatives typically experience stress and a sense of burden, beginning with the initial catastrophe of the injury and acute hospitalization and continuing long afterward. In cases of severe TBI, families often hear initial medical reports that their loved one may not live; great relief ensues when the person survives, followed by a long period of gradual understanding of residual problems. Research consistently has found that a significant proportion of family members report stress, anxiety, and depression. Some studies suggest that the perceived burden of caring for the person disabled by TBI increases over time. The level of emotional and behavioral disturbances shown by individuals with TBI may be a determinant of family response. Financial drain from the costs of TBI represents another source of stress. For example, Jacobs (1988) found that 34% of families reported mild to moderate financial drain and that some family members had to give up working in order to care for the individual with TBI or spend substantial sums on professional caregivers.

Return to Work After TBI

Although postinjury employment rates vary from sample to sample, research invariably shows that TBI results in an increase in unemployment (Sander, Kreutzer, Rosenthal, Delmonico, & Young, 1996). Two widely cited studies found that approximately 80% of persons with severe TBI were employed prior to injury but only 30% were able to resume working (Brooks, McKinlay, Symington, Beattie, & Campsie, 1987; Jacobs, 1988). According to the TBI Model Systems National Data Base, which contains information about individuals with moderate to severe TBI treated in urban centers, the rate of competitive employment decreased from 51% preinjury to 25% postinjury at the time of a 3-year follow-up (Sander et al., 1996). Many people with TBI who are able to return to work may have to change jobs in order to accommodate impaired abilities; job changes of this nature entail reductions in pay and status and engender resistance, anger, and feelings of loss.

The severity of TBI and associated neurobehavioral impairment have predictive value in determining the likelihood of vocational success. As problems with cognitive and interpersonal problems increase, the chances of successful employment generally decrease (Dikmen et al., 1996). However, other factors, such as level of job availability, employer attitudes toward disability, access to rehabilitation services, and transportation, play a role in employment. In many respects, vocational struggles exemplify the complex physical, cognitive, and interpersonal effects of brain injury on the purpose and efficacy of the individual.

ACKNOWLEDGMENT

The authors would like to thank Beth Gardini Dixon and Marjorie Batic for their editorial contributions to this chapter.

REFERENCES

Adams, J. H., Graham, D. I., & Gennarelli, T. A. (1985). Contemporary neuropathological considerations regarding brain damage in head injury. In D. P. Becker & J. T.

Povlishock (Eds.), *Central nervous system trauma status report* (pp. 65–77). Bethesda, MD: National Institutes of Health, NINCDS.

Alexander, M. P. (1995). Mild traumatic brain injury: Pathophysiology, natural history, and clinical management. *Neurology, 45,* 1253–1260.

Alexandre, A., Colombo, F., Nertempi, P., & Benedetti, A. (1983). Cognitive outcome and early indices of severity of head injury. *Journal of Neurosurgery, 59,* 751–761.

Binder, L. M. (1997). A review of mild head trauma. Part 2. Clinical implications. *Journal of Clinical and Experimental Neuropsychology, 19,* 433–458.

Bond, M. R. (1990). Standardized methods of assessing and predicting outcome. In M. Rosenthal, E. R. Griffith, M. R. Bond, & J. D. Miller (Eds.), *Rehabilitation of the adult and child with traumatic brain injury* (2nd ed., pp. 59–74). Philadelphia: F. A. Davis.

Brooks, N., McKinlay, W., Symington, C., Beattie, A., & Campsie, L. (1987). Return to work within the first seven years of severe head injury. *Brain Injury, 1,* 5–19.

Corrigan, J. D. (1995). Substance abuse as a mediating factor in outcome from traumatic brain injury. *Archives of Physical Medicine and Rehabilitation, 76,*302–309.

Crosson, B., Cooper, P. V., Lincoln, R. K., Bauer, R. M., & Velozo, C. A. (1993). Relationship between verbal memory and language after blunt head injury. *Clinical Neuropsychologist, 7,* 250–267.

Dikmen, S., & Levin, H. S. (1993). Methodological issues in the study of mild head injury. *Journal of Head Trauma Rehabilitation, 8,* 30–37.

Dikmen, S., & Machamer, J. E. (1995). Neurobehavioral outcomes and their determinants. *Journal of Head Trauma Rehabilitation, 10,* 74–86.

Dikmen, S., Machamer, J. E., Winn, H. R., & Temkin, N. R. (1995). Neuropsychological outcome at 1-year post head injury. *Neuropsychology, 9,* 80–90.

Dikmen, S., Machamer, J., Savoie, T., & Temkin, N. (1996). Life quality outcome in head injury. In I. Grant & K. M. Adams (Eds.), *Neuropsychological assessment of neuropsychiatric disorders* (2nd ed., pp. 532–576). New York: Oxford University Press.

Eisenberg, H. M. (1985). Outcome after head injury: Part 1. General considerations. In D. P. Becker & J. T. Povlishock (Eds.), *Central nervous system trauma status report* (pp. 271–280). Bethesda, MD: NIH/NINCDS.

Evans, R. W. (1992). Mild traumatic brain injury. *Physical Medicine and Rehabilitation Clinics of North America, 3,* 427–439.

Gronwall, D. (1989). Cumulative and persisting effects of concussion on attention and cognition. In H. S. Levin, H. M. Eisenberg, & A. L. Benton (Eds.), *Mild head injury* (pp. 153–163). New York: Oxford University Press.

Gualtieri, T., & Cox, D. R. (1991). The delayed neurobehavioral sequelae of traumatic brain injury. *Brain Injury, 5,* 219–232.

Hall, K. M., & Johnston, M. V. (1994). Outcomes evaluation in TBI rehabilitation. Part 2. Measurement tools for a nationwide data system. *Archives of Physical Medicine and Rehabilitation, 75,* SC10–SC18.

Harrison-Felix, C., Newton, C. N., Hall, K. M., & Kreutzer, J. S. (1996). Descriptive findings from Traumatic Brain Injury Model Systems National Data Base. *Journal of Head Trauma Rehabilitation, 11,* 1–14.

Jacobs, H. E. (1988). The Los Angeles Head Injury Survey: Procedures and initial findings. *Archives of Physical Medicine and Rehabilitation, 69,* 425–431.

Jane, J. A., Steward, O., & Gennarelli, T. (1985). Axonal degeneration induced by experimental noninvasive minor head injury. *Journal of Neurosurgery, 62,* 96–100.

Jennett, B. (1996). Clinical and pathological features of vegetative survival. In H. S. Levin, A. L. Benton, J. P. Muizelaar, & H. M. Eisenberg (Eds.), *Catastrophic brain injury* (pp. 3–13). New York: Oxford University Press.

Jennett, B., & Teasdale, G. (1981). *Management of head injuries*. Philadelphia: F. A. Davis.

Jennett, B., Teasdale, G., Braakman, R., Minderhoud, J., Heiden, J., & Kurze, T. (1979). Prognosis of patients with severe head injury. *Neurosurgery, 4,* 283–289.

Kraus, J. F., Black, M. A., Hessol, N., Ley, P., Rokaw, W., Sullivan, C., Bowers, S., Knowlton, S., & Marshall, L. (1984). The incidence of acute brain injury and serious impairment in a defined population. *American Journal of Epidemiology, 119,* 186–201.

Kraus, J. F., & Sorenson, S. B. (1994). Epidemiology. In J. M. Silver, S. C. Yudofsky, & R. E. Hales (Eds.), *Neuropsychiatry of traumatic brain injury* (pp. 3–41). Washington, DC: American Psychiatric Press.

Kreutzer, J. S., Marwitz, J. H., & Kepler, K. (1992). Traumatic brain injury: Family response and outcome. *Archives of Physical Medicine and Rehabilitation, 73,* 771–778.

Kreutzer, J. S., & Zasler, N. D. (1989). Psychosexual consequences of traumatic brain injury: Methodology and preliminary findings. *Brain Injury, 3,* 177–186.

Larrabee, G. J. (1997). Neuropsychological outcome, post concussion symptoms, and forensic considerations in mild closed head trauma. *Seminars in Clinical Neuropsychiatry, 2,* 196–206.

Levin, H. S. (1985). Outcome after head injury: Part 2. Neurobehavioral recovery. In D. P. Becker & J. T. Povlishock (Eds.), *Central nervous system trauma status report* (pp. 281–303). Bethesda, MD: National Institutes of Health, NINCDS.

Levin, H. S. (1990). Predicting the neurobehavioral sequelae of closed head injury. In R. L. Wood (Ed.), *Neurobehavioural sequelae of traumatic brain injury* (pp. 89–109). New York: Taylor & Francis.

Levin, H. S. (1997). Memory dysfunction after head injury. In T. E. Feinberg & M. J. Farah (Eds.), *Behavioral neurology and neuropsychology* (pp. 479–489). New York: McGraw-Hill.

Levin, H. S., Amparo, E. G., Eisenberg, H. M., Williams, D. H., High, W. M., McArdle, C. B., & Weiner, R. L. (1987). Magnetic resonance imaging and computerized tomography in relation to neurobehavioral sequelae of mild and moderate head injury. *Journal of Neurosurgery, 66,* 706–713.

Levin, H. S., Benton, A. L., & Grossman, R. G. (1982). *Neurobehavioral consequences of closed head injury*. New York: Oxford University Press.

Levin, H. S., Mattis, S. M., Ruff, R. M., Eisenberg, H. M., Marshall, L. F., Tabaddor, K., High, W. M., & Frankowski, R. F. (1987). Neurobehavioral outcome following minor head injury: A three center study. *Journal of Neurosurgery, 66,* 234–243.

Lezak, M. D. (1987). Relationships between personality disorders, social disturbances, and physical disability following traumatic brain injury. *Journal of Head Trauma Rehabilitation, 2,* 57–69.

Lezak, M. D. (1995). *Neuropsychological assessment* (3rd ed.). New York: Oxford University Press.

Lishman, W. A. (1987). *Organic psychiatry: The psychological consequences of cerebral disorder*. Oxford: Blackwell.

Mateer, C. A., & Mapou, R. L. (1996). Understanding, evaluating, and managing attention disorders following traumatic brain injury. *Journal of Head Trauma Rehabilitation, 11*, 1–16.

Max, W., MacKenzie, E. J., & Rice, D. P. (1991). Head injuries: Costs and consequences. *Journal of Head Trauma Rehabilitation, 6,* 76–87.

Miller, J. D., Pentland, B., & Berrol, S. (1990). Early evaluation and management. In M. Rosenthal, E. R. Griffith, M. R. Bond, & J. D. Miller (Eds.), *Rehabilitation of the adult and child with traumatic brain injury* (2nd ed., pp. 21–51). Philadelphia: F. A. Davis.

Morton, M. V., & Wehman, P. (1995). Psychosocial and emotional sequelae of individuals with traumatic brain injury: A literature review and recommendations. *Brain Injury, 9,* 81–92.

Multi-Society Task Force on PVS. (1994). Medical aspects of the persistent vegetative state. *New England Journal of Medicine, 330,* 1572–1579.

O'Carroll, R. E., Woodrow, J., & Maroun, F. (1991). Psychosexual and psychosocial sequelae of closed head injury. *Brain Injury, 5,* 303–313.

Oddy, M., Coughlan, T., Tyerman, A., & Jenkins, D. (1985). Social adjustments after closed head injury: A further follow-up seven years after injury. *Journal of Neurology, Neurosurgery, and Psychiatry, 48,* 564–568.

Prigatano, G. P. (1991). Disturbances of self-awareness of deficit after traumatic brain injury. In G. P. Prigatano & D. L. Schacter (Eds.), *Awareness of deficit after brain injury: Clinical and theoretical issues* (pp. 111–126). New York: Oxford University Press.

Prigatano, G. P. (1992). Personality disturbances associated with traumatic brain injury. *Journal of Consulting and Clinical Psychology, 60,* 360–368.

Prigatano, G. P. (1994). Individuality, lesion location, and psychotherapy after brain injury. In A. L. Christensen & B. P. Uzzell (Eds.), *Brain injury and neuropsychological rehabilitation: International perspectives* (pp. 173–186). Hillsdale, NJ: Lawrence Erlbaum Associates.

Prigatano, G. P., Fordyce, D. J., Zeiner, H. K., Roueche, J. R., Pepping, M., & Wood, B. C. (1986). *Neuropsychological rehabilitation after brain injury*. Baltimore: Johns Hopkins University Press.

Putnam, S. H., Millis, S. R., & Adams, K. M. (1996). Mild traumatic brain injury: Beyond cognitive assessment. In I. Grant & K. M. Adams (Eds.), *Neuropsychological assessment of neuropsychiatric disorders* (2nd ed., pp. 529–551). New York: Oxford University Press.

Russell, W. R. (1932). Cerebral involvement in head injury. *Brain, 55,* 549–603.

Rutherford, W. H. (1989). Concussion symptoms: Relationship to acute neurological indices, individual differences, and circumstances of injury. In H. S. Levin, H. M. Eisenberg, & A. L. Benton (Eds.), *Mild head injury* (pp. 217–228). New York: Oxford University Press.

Sander, A. M., Kreutzer, J. S., Rosenthal, M., Delmonico, R., & Young, M. E. (1996). A multicenter longitudinal investigation of return to work and community integration following traumatic brain injury. *Journal of Head Trauma Rehabilitation, 11,* 70–84.

Stein, D. G., Brailowsky, S., & Will, B. (1995). *Brain repair.* New York: Oxford University Press.

Stein, D. G., Glasier, M. M., & Hoffman, S. W. (1994). Pharmacological treatments for brain injury repair: Progress and prognosis. In A. L. Christensen & B. P. Uzzell (Eds.), *Brain injury and neuropsychological rehabilitation: International perspectives* (pp. 17–39). Hillsdale, NJ: Lawrence Erlbaum Associates.

Stuss, D. T. (1991). Disturbances of self-awareness after frontal system damage. In G. P. Prigatano & D. L. Schacter (Eds.), *Awareness of deficit after brain injury: Clinical and theoretical issues* (pp. 63–83). New York: Oxford University Press.

Stuss, D. T., & Benson, D. F. (1986). *The frontal lobes.* New York: Raven Press.

Symonds, C. P. (1937). Mental disorder following head injury. *Proceedings of the Royal Society of Medicine, 30,* 1081–1092.

Taylor, C. A., & Price, T. R. P. (1994). Neuropsychiatric assessment. In J. M. Silver, S. C. Yudofsky, & R. E. Hales (Eds.), *Neuropsychiatry of traumatic brain injury* (pp. 81–132). Washington, DC: American Psychiatric Press.

Thomsen, I. V. (1984). Late outcome of very severe blunt head trauma: A 10–15 year follow-up. *Journal of Neurology, Neurosurgery, and Psychiatry, 47,* 250–268.

Thomsen, I. V. (1990). Recognizing the development of behavior disorders. In R. Ll. Wood (Ed.), *Neurobehavioural sequelae of traumatic brain injury* (pp. 52–68). New York: Taylor & Francis.

Torner, J. C., & Schootman, M. (1995). Epidemiology of closed head injury. In M. Rizzo & D. Tranel (Eds.), *Head injury and postconcussive syndrome* (pp. 19–46). New York: Churchill Livingstone.

Walsh, K. (1994). *Neuropsychology: A clinical approach* (3rd ed.). Edinburgh: Churchill Livingstone.

Whyte, J. (1992). Attention and arousal: Basic science aspects. *Archives of Physical Medicine and Rehabilitation, 73,* 940–949.

Chapter 6

Burn Injuries

G. Fred Cromes, Jr., and Phala A. Helm

Annually, there are approximately 1.25 million persons in the United States who sustain burn injuries. Of these, about 5,500 do not survive, and 51,000 require hospitalization. House fires account for about 75% of deaths due to burn injury. There was a 50% decline in deaths from fire and burns from 1971–1991 (Brigham & McLoughlin, 1996). Persons whose burn injuries require hospitalization have about a 50% chance of sustaining temporary or permanent disability (Chocktaw, Eisner, & Wachtel, 1987; Rice & Mackenzie, 1989). The increased survival of persons with major burn injury has resulted in (a) more persons who require more intense and lengthy rehabilitative treatment and (b) an emphasis on treatment occurring in a well-coordinated, interdisciplinary environment. The most common part of the body involved in burn injury is an upper extremity, followed by the head and neck (Demling, 1989). Injury to these areas obviously affects function and appearance and can result in disability.

There is general agreement that 20%–25% of burn injuries occur in the workplace (Inancsi & Guidotti, 1989; Rossingnol, Locke, & Burke, 1989). About 50% of occupational burns require hospitalization and 20% result in permanent disability. These work-related burns more frequently involve men, particularly men employed in unskilled and semiskilled occupations. Skilled occupations that are vulnerable to burn injury include firefighters and electricians. There is a paucity of information on the vocational sequelae of burns that do not occur at work except that most burn injuries involve persons of working age.

Burn injury causes destruction of tissue, usually the skin, from exposure to thermal extremes (either heat or cold), electricity, chemicals, and/or radiation. Other tissue also can be injured. The mucosa of the upper gastrointestinal system (mouth, esophagus, stomach) can be burned with ingestion of chemicals. The respiratory system can be damaged if hot gases, smoke, or toxic chemical fumes are inhaled when a person is injured. In electrical injuries or prolonged thermal or chemical exposure, fat, muscle, bone, and peripheral nerves can be affected. If tissues other than skin are involved, the overall possible functional impairment from the injury is increased. Because the skin is the tissue most often affected by burn injury, it is important to understand its function and anatomy.

SKIN

The skin is the largest organ system in the human body. Its purpose is to maintain a balance (homeostasis) between the internal environment of the body and the impact of factors outside the body. More specifically, the skin serves to keep body fluids inside, regulate body temperature by controlling perspiration, prevent the invasion of bacteria, and reduce the effect of radiation from the sun.

The skin is composed of two layers, the outer *epidermis* and the *dermis*. The epidermis also has two layers, a basal layer called the *stratum germinativum* and a surface layer called the *stratum corneum*. The basal layer of the epidermis is where new skin cells form and then migrate to the surface layer. These cells contain the pigment (melanin) that produces skin color. As these new epidermal cells approach the surface, they undergo a process called keratinization by which they become more fibrous and form the outer protective layer of the skin. These cells eventually die and are sloughed off; they are replaced as new epidermal cell production proceeds. Epidermal cells also are found in the dermis, where they line the skin appendages (i.e., hair follicles, sweat glands, and sebaceous glands).

The dermis, which lies below the epidermis, is composed of connective tissue, capillaries, collagen, and elastic fibers. It provides structural and nutritional support to the epidermis and the skin appendages and contributes to the skin's elasticity.

Beneath the dermis is a layer of fat and connective tissue. Below this layer, which varies in thickness, are muscle, bone, and tendons. Peripheral sensory nerve endings are distributed throughout the skin and subcutaneous layer. Thus, burn injury may result in altered ability to sense pain, touch, and temperature.

BURN CLASSIFICATION

Burns are classified according to cause, depth, extent (total body surface area [TBSA]), and a combination of the above (American Burn Association [ABA]).

The importance of classifying burns is that treatment decisions, patient management, and prognosis are related to the type of burn injury.

Cause

The primary cause of burn injury is exposure to temperature extremes, heat or cold. Heat injuries are more frequent than cold injuries, and the most commonly occurring is exposure to hot liquids (water, steam, cooking oil, tar, etc.). Direct flame injuries are the second most common. Other sources of heat injury include contact with hot surfaces (irons, steam presses, household appliances, etc.). Cold injuries almost exclusively result from frostbite. Electrical and chemical injuries constitute 5%–10% of burn injuries and are largely the result of occupational accidents. Radiation burns are rare. In a 5-year survey of occupational injuries in a large metropolitan area, Inancsi and Guidotti (1987) found that flame burns resulted in the longest delay in returning to work and electrical burns in the longest initial hospitalization.

Depth

The depth of burn injury refers to what skin layers have been destroyed. The nomenclature for depth of burn injury includes an old and a new terminology. The old terminology is as follows:

1st degree—only the epidermis

2nd degree—epidermis and dermis, excluding all the dermal appendages

3rd degree—epidermis and all of the dermis

4th degree—epidermis, dermis, and subcutaneous tissues (fat, muscle, bone, and peripheral nerves)

The newer terminology parallels the old and is as follows:

Superficial—only the epidermis

Superficial partial thickness—epidermis and dermis, excluding the dermal appendages

Deep partial thickness—epidermis and most of the dermis

Full thickness—epidermis and all of the dermis

Because of the dynamic nature of burn injury pathophysiology, it is often difficult to determine the exact depth of burn injury for the first 3 to 5 days postinjury (Helm & Fisher, 1993).

Extent

Burn injuries also are classified in terms of the percentage of the skin surface injured (TBSA). Ideally, the percentage of partial- and full-thickness burn are indicated separately. A relatively simple but not totally accurate method for determining the extent of injury is the rule of 9s. In this system, the following body parts represent the TBSA indicated.

Head = 9%

Arms = 9% each

Legs = 18% each

Chest, stomach, and abdomen = 18%

Back = 18%

Perineum (genitals) = 1%

The ABA classification system describes burn injuries as mild, moderate, and major. In general, any burn classified as moderate or major requires hospitalization. Minor burns are defined as those of less than 15% TBSA partial thickness (10% for children) and less than 2% full thickness unless the eyes, ears, face, or perineum are involved. Moderate burns include 15%–25% TBSA (10%–20% for children) regardless of depth and 2%–10% full-thickness burns unless the eyes, ears, face, or perineum are involved. Major burns include greater than 25% partial-thickness burns (20% for children); greater than 10% full-thickness burns; all burns involving the face, eyes, ears, feet, and perineum; all burns that are electrical or involve inhalation injury; all burns with ancillary injury (fracture, tissue trauma, etc.); and all burns involving a person with factors that suggest poor risk secondary to age or illness.

PATHOPHYSIOLOGY OF BURN INJURY

Pathophysiology refers to the complex chain of mechanisms that occur in the skin (local effects) and in other organ systems (systemic effects) when a burn injury occurs, as well as what happens as the skin regenerates and heals. The initial response to a moderate or major burn injury can be life-threatening, and the mechanisms involved in skin regeneration and healing can cause functional and cosmetic problems. Information contained in the following synopsis of burn pathophysiology was taken from Dimick (1984), Helm and Fisher (1993), and Hunt (1984).

Local Effects

Superficial burns (like sunburns) affect only the epidermis and do not result in major clinical complications. Partial-thickness burns affect the dermis, but if skin appendages remain intact, new skin can regenerate. Full-thickness burns destroy all of the dermis and will not spontaneously regenerate skin. The initial response to partial- and/or full-thickness burn injury is constriction of blood vessels (capillaries). Within a few hours, these capillaries dilate, and plasma is released into the burn wound. By 24 hours, increased clotting begins, which can eliminate capillary blood flow. Without a blood supply, further cell death can occur. Because of this dynamic process, it can be difficult to judge the exact depth of burn for 3 to 5 days. During this process, massive fluid loss occurs through open wounds and from evaporation, resulting in heat loss, caloric drain, and increased metabolism.

With skin loss, there is no protection from bacteria. Bacteria enter the burn wound rapidly and cause local sepsis (infection). If this infection goes unchecked, the bacteria can destroy more tissue, and "conversion" from a partial-thickness to a full-thickness burn can occur, or the infection can become systemic and threaten life.

In partial-thickness burns, sensory nerve fibers are damaged but not destroyed. Thus, exquisite pain will accompany areas of partial-thickness injury. In contrast there is little pain associated with full-thickness burns because the nerve endings are destroyed.

Systemic Effects

The serious burn wound results in the loss of body fluids (hypovolemia) and causes a syndrome called burn shock. In addition to fluid loss from the wound, fluids also escape into surrounding tissues, causing edema (swelling). This edema results in stiffness, which reduces the ability to bend various joints (range of motion). It also causes pressure that can reduce blood flow to other tissues, with resultant cell death and damage to peripheral nerves and sensory and/or motor loss to areas of the body not burned.

The respiratory system also can be affected, with resultant hyperventilation and increased oxygen consumption. If there is inhalation of smoke or noxious gases, direct damage to the throat and trachea can occur, resulting in swelling and possible blockage of the upper airway. If the upper airway is injured, there is increased risk for pneumonia. Additional systemic effects involve the gastrointestinal and immune systems. Gastric dilation and gastrointestinal ileus (cessation of peristalsis) occur frequently. Suppression of the immune system increases risk for infection.

Skin Regeneration and Scarring

In partial-thickness burns, the epidermal cells lining the hair follicles and sweat glands in the deep dermis are intact. As a result, new cells are formed that eventually cover the burn wound in approximately 14 to 21 days, depending on the depth of the injury. The new skin formed resumes its role in temperature regulation and protection from bacteria. Despite the wounds being covered, healing continues until the skin is mature (6–24 months). During this time, nerves regenerate, and pigmentation gradually returns. As the skin heals, there is active deposition of collagen in the new skin, which is a major factor in scarring and tightness. This scarring and tightness can result in contractures (i.e., reduced joint mobility). Because there are active healing processes occurring for several months after wound coverage, rehabilitation continues until the skin is mature.

Healing can result in a special problem called hypertrophic scarring, which contributes to severe contracture and cosmetic deformity. If a burn wound loses its redness in 3 months, hypertrophic scarring usually does not result. Most deep partial- and full-thickness burns are grafted, but if not, the chances of hypertrophic scarring increase. The new cells in healing wounds deposit collagen, which takes on an abnormal configuration (i.e., instead of parallel, the fibers become nodular). As a result, large, lumpy scars (hypertrophic) form; they appear red and purple, firm, and warm to the touch and are hypersensitive.

Full-thickness burns require replacement of skin from unburned parts of the body (autografts). Skin grafting is discussed in the "Burn Treatment" section. The site from which these grafts are taken (donor site) is similar to a superficial partial-thickness burn and heals in similar fashion.

Electrical Burns

Injury caused by contact with electricity is relatively infrequent, accounting for less than 10% of burn admissions. Especially when an electrical injury involves contact with more than 1,000 volts, the consequences can be severe. The percentage of TBSA burned in electrical injury is relatively small, but there is deep tissue damage between entry and exit points (*contact points*) not overtly observable. The deep tissues affected may include nerve, blood vessels, muscle, tendon, cartilage, and bone. With very high voltages, the destruction of tissue at contact points can be massive. In addition to tissue destruction, the electrical current causes clotting, which deprives living tissue of a blood supply and results in tissue death. As a result, amputation may be necessary. Of all causes of burn injury, electrical injury results in the greatest frequency of amputation. The electric current can also affect cardiac functioning, resulting in immediate death or arrhythmias.

FUNCTIONAL IMPLICATIONS

Acute Limitations

Several functional problems occur during acute hospitalization. They are related to the intensive medical/surgical interventions that are necessary for survival and to the reactions of patients to the local and systemic effects of their burn injury. Because of burn shock, systemic infection, and/or medication, patients may experience delirium that precludes their participation in treatment. Edema, pain, bulky dressings, and immobilizing splints impair the patient's ability to perform usual activities like eating and other self-care. Sleep is frequently disrupted, which contributes to the already present anxiety and fear about survival, painful dressing changes, dependency, and long-term consequences. Although some of these functional problems may persist, they are less likely to result in permanent impairment and disability than are those that occur after hospital discharge (post-acute problems).

Postdischarge Limitations

The prevalence of long-term functional limitations of persons who have been burned is not well documented. The presence of limitations is, however, quite clear. The most frequent functional limitations of burn injury involve scarring and joint contracture. Scarring contributes to contracture and disfigurement. Contractures limit range of motion (i.e., ability to extend and/or flex joints normally). Disfigurement can affect self-concept, body image, comfort in interpersonal situations, and acceptance in the workplace. Sheffield et al. (1988) evaluated 212 moderate and major burns more than 12 months after injury. Of the patients studied, 18.4% had functional limitations due to range of motion (contracture), and 16.5% had limitations related to scarring. Deitch et al. (1983) studied 100 persons up to 2 years after being burned and found that 38 developed hypertrophic scarring and that incidence was greater in African American patients. In addition to scarring and contracture, there are a variety of other functional sequelae of burn injury, many of which result in permanent impairment (Helm & Fisher, 1993; Rivers, 1987), which can include the following:

1. Healed and/or grafted skin that is fragile, dry, inflexible, intolerant of heat and cold extremes, sensitive to chemicals and ultraviolet light, and hyper- or hypopigmented.
2. Pain and itching (pruritus).
3. Peripheral neuropathy with resultant sensory loss, reduced coordination, and/or muscle weakness.
4. Visual impairment due to corneal burns, complications of eyelid contractures, and/or cataracts (which occur after some electrical burns).
5. Hearing impairment, usually as a result of necessary antibiotics.
6. Reduced endurance and fatiguability resulting from peripheral neuropathy, deconditioning, respiratory problems, and/or cardiovascular status.
7. Disfigurement caused by scarring, contracture, amputation, and/or hair loss.
8. Emotional problems, including posttraumatic stress disorder; anxiety and/or depression in reaction to functional and/or cosmetic factors, family integrity, sexual functioning, ability to return to work, and resumption of recreational activities; and fear of the workplace or other situations that may be a reminder of the burn injury circumstances.
9. Central nervous system problems affecting cognitive capacity.
10. Disrupted sleep.

Cromes, Voege, Kowalske, and Helm (1997) studied persons with major burn injury with respect to changes over time in self-reported functional ability (standing up from a chair, climbing stairs, picking up something from the floor, driving a car, etc.) and community reentry (grocery shopping, social activity, household upkeep, family finances, etc.). The results indicated that functional ability was reported to have maximized at 2 months postdischarge and community reentry had maximized at 12 months postdischarge. It was also reported that functional ability was related to emotional distress at hospital discharge (lower ability—higher distress), but community reentry was not related to emotional distress at any time when tested. Thus, it appears that persons with major burn injuries resume basic functional abilities quickly but establish pre-burn community integration over a longer period.

When rehabilitation is completed, decisions arise regarding return to employment and/or permanent disability determination. Any of the above limitations could preclude return to employment, and reconstructive surgical procedures could be necessary that might delay return to employment. If return to one's pre-burn job is not feasible, consideration must be given to modifying that job; changing to a new job, which might require retraining; or accepting permanent disability. The criteria necessary to make such decisions and advise the burn patient depend on the patient's residual functional abilities relative to the demands of the job situation.

Major impediments to returning to work are often obvious, but the potential multisystem nature of burn injury can result in more subtle functional problems that must be considered. Among these are intolerance for heat and cold extremes, skin sensitivity to exposure to the sun or chemical agents, fatigability and reduced stamina, poor concentration, fear of the workplace, issues related to appearance, and overall psychological adaptation. Thus, though a person may appear to have the physical capacity to perform job tasks, there may be other factors that are significantly limiting.

BURN TREATMENT

Advances in knowledge of the pathophysiology of burn injuries have significantly reduced mortality and thus increased the number of persons who survive. Heimbach (1988) indicated that burn deaths in the United States decreased from 15,000 in 1970 to 6,000 in the mid-1980s. Survival of a 30% TBSA burn was 50% in 1970; now there is 50% survival of persons with 70% TBSA burns. In addition, approximately 90% of persons admitted to burn centers return to their pre-burn functional levels within 1 year. This resumption of functioning is related to advances in rehabilitation treatment that have paralleled medical breakthroughs.

Acute Medical–Surgical Burn Treatment

The first priority in the initial treatment of a moderate/major burn injury is to combat massive fluid loss (resuscitation) from capillary damage and evaporation. This is accomplished by intravenous replacement with electrolyte solutions in amounts that are related to the TBSA burn injury and the patient's weight. This procedure must be completed within 48 hours; if it is not successful, death can result from renal failure.

A secondary priority relates to the significant edema (swelling) that can compromise blood supply and injure peripheral nerves. This is a particularly important problem if the arms or legs are burned. It can also be an issue if edema across the chest interferes with breathing. The procedure used to acutely address these difficulties is called escharotomy. It involves an incision through the burned tissue that relieves tissue pressure by allowing trapped intercellular fluids to escape. As a result, extent of tissue damage is limited, and neurovascular complications are reduced.

If the burn injury involved smoke or toxic fume inhalation, immediate treatment is necessary to prevent death by asphyxiation. This treatment may require a tracheostomy. The next priorities in acute burn treatment involve prevention of infection and covering of open wounds. Following resuscitation, the burn wound is cleaned and dead tissue is removed. The removal of dead tissue is called debridement. Dead tissue is removed to a level where viable tissue exists. In some cases enzymes are used to debride wounds, but there are side effects and limitations. Surgical debridement is performed in a majority of cases. Surgical debridement occurs within 1–10 days post-burn and involves successively excising thin layers of tissue until viable tissue is evident. Once debridement is completed, spontaneous healing or skin grafting can proceed.

Once the partial-thickness burn wound is cleaned and dead tissue is removed, topical antibacterial creams are applied to combat infection. The wounds are redressed daily, and obvious remaining dead tissue can be mechanically debrided using scissors and/or forceps. In some cases debridement of partial-thickness wounds is accomplished by using wet-to-dry dressings. Coarse gauze, soaked with antibiotic solution or saline, is applied to the wound and allowed to dry. Then the dressing is moistened and removed, carrying with it dead tissue that has adhered. Other partial-thickness wounds are covered with temporary biological dressings. These include cadaver skin (homograft), human fetal membrane (allograft), and pigskin (heterograft or xenograft). These dressings contribute to debridement when removed and reduce pain as new skin generates underneath. They also are used to determine (in deep partial-thickness or full-thickness wounds) when definitive grafting can be performed; that is, if the biological dressing adheres to the wound, the wound is ready for grafting. Fluid loss and risk of infection are also reduced by using these biological dressings.

Full-thickness wounds require grafting. Deep partial-thickness wounds may require grafting, which can prevent the hypertrophic scarring that often occurs when the wound is allowed to heal spontaneously. Grafting involves use of skin from the patient's own body (autograft). Usually, split-thickness autograft is used (i.e., a graft including epidermis and part of the dermis). If extensive wound coverage is necessary and limited donor sites are available, this graft can be "meshed" and stretched to cover more area. This results in an X-shaped pattern in which there are areas not actually covered, and cosmetic results may not be ideal. Full-thickness allografts, or sheet grafts, are usually used for cosmetic purposes, particularly for grafts to the face and hands.

Since the mid 1980s, techniques have been developed to cover excised burn wounds with artificial skin. It is grown from the patient's own cells and results in a permanent skin replacement that includes a functioning dermis and epidermis. This procedure is often used in cases where a person has very large, full-thickness or deep partial-thickness burns and thus limited donor sites for grafting. It has its limitations, such as risk for contracture due to required immobility for 3 weeks and possible increased scarring (Tompkins & Burke, 1990).

Rehabilitation Treatment

Acute

Rehabilitation of the burn patient begins during acute hospitalization and may last for several months postdischarge. Rehabilitation personnel address such problem areas as wound care, positioning, splinting, exercise, and ambulation. These efforts continue after discharge, when the rehabilitation program increasingly focuses on independence in daily activities, increased physical conditioning, and psychological adaptation to burn sequelae. The general purpose of acute rehabilitation efforts is to prevent long-term problems of scarring and contracture.

During acute hospitalization, wound care is addressed by burn nurses, physicians, and rehabilitation personnel. Dressing changes, cleaning wounds, and debridement of dead tissue are performed daily, usually with hydrotherapy as an adjunct, to control infection and prepare wounds for the earliest possible spontaneous healing or autografting (Head, 1984).

Because wounds are actively healing and contracture dynamics are occurring, it is critical to try to prevent contracture formation by properly positioning patients' burned extremities while they are in bed or sitting. The position that is encouraged is extension. This contradicts the more comfortable flexed position of the extremities, which patients prefer and which contributes to contracture. Devices such as shoulder boards and splints may be necessary to maintain extension. In addition, pillows may be discouraged if there are burns to the neck and chest. If edema is present, extremities are elevated. These procedures can interfere with sleeping.

During hospitalization, extremities are passively stretched by the physical/occupational therapists in order to begin the process of preventing contracture. Active movement is stressed to involve the patient in the rehabilitation program. Patients also are encouraged to begin ambulation as soon as possible, using assistive devices (e.g., a walker) if necessary. Other devices may be provided to assist the patient in using the upper extremities for eating and grooming independently.

Postdischarge

When the burn patient is discharged, it is likely that some wounds are not completely healed. Therefore, wound care becomes one focus of outpatient rehabilitation. Hydrotherapy, debridement, and dressing changes are performed as needed, and when healing has progressed to where a few spotty areas remain, hydrotherapy is stopped. Attention is also directed to skin dryness, and appropriate lubricants are applied frequently. The new skin and scar tissue may require massage, which reduces sensitivity and improves flexibility.

If there is a risk of hypertrophic scarring or if it is already forming, continuous pressure applied to the area will prevent its progress. This pressure is applied progressively (Bruster & Pullium, 1983) until the skin is able to tolerate the increased pressure available in custom-made garments. These garments must be worn 20 hours per day for up to 1 year, that is, until skin is mature. The garments are uncomfortable, hot, and unattractive. Pressure for facial or neck hypertrophic scars is accomplished with custom-fitted clear plastic masks or with stretch garments.

Contracture control is another major concern. The physical or occupational therapist treats contracture by stretching the involved joints. Patients are encouraged to actively stretch their joints, but because of pain, they do not usually achieve the same extent of stretch. Often the joint or extremity is packed in paraffin prior to stretching. It has been found that greater range of motion can be achieved with this technique (Head & Helm, 1977). If a scar band involves more then one joint, the entire extremity must be stretched. This process continues until the skin is mature and loss of range of motion no longer occurs between therapy appointments or overnight.

Difficult contracture problems require specialized splints to maintain range of motion. Serial casting may be used for a contracture that resists improvement. In this procedure, the joint is casted in the maximum stretch position. After a few days the cast is removed, and the joint is stretched to maximum, where it is recasted (Bennett, Helm, Purdue, & Hunt, 1989).

Outpatient rehabilitation also involves reconditioning and strengthening. Thus, progressive resistive exercise and conditioning programs are indicated. Work simulators that test the patient's limits with respect to the demands of various vocational tasks also are employed.

Because of the pain, disrupted sleep, rigors of treatment, slowness of progress, interruption of lifestyle patterns, concern about physical and cosmetic outcomes, and not being able to work, as well as a host of other possibilities, the patient may display emotional difficulties. These problems may be overt or may be masked and appear as reduced compliance or acting out. They should be addressed by referral for assessment and possible counseling follow-up or involvement in a burn support group.

There are some cases in which functional or cosmetic deformity is not responsive to rehabilitation treatment. As a result, reconstructive surgery and follow-up outpatient rehabilitation therapy may be needed. Advances in rehabilitative therapy have reduced the percentage of patients readmitted for surgery.

Prasad, Bowden, and Thompson (1991), in a survey of 3,167 survivors of burn injury, indicated that 12.4% were readmitted for surgery from 1980 to 1985, compared with 30.5% from 1970 to 1975. In this study, the most common areas needing surgery were the hand and wrist, followed by the arm, forearm, face, and neck. The most common procedure was scar/contracture release and grafting.

PSYCHOLOGICAL AND VOCATIONAL IMPLICATIONS

Psychological Implications

Hospitalization for moderate to major burns is stressful. Initially, the burn patient may not be fully aware of what is occurring because of burn shock, delirium, and/or medication. As these factors resolve, the patient becomes aware of being dependent, not in control, in pain, and fearful of dying, feelings that may result in depression, agitation and acting out, and/or extreme anxiety. Posttraumatic stress disorder (PTSD) occurs with some frequency. In one survey, 30% of patients met the full criteria for PTSD sometime during hospitalization, but none did at discharge (Patterson, Carrigan, Questad, & Robinson, 1990). The investigators also found that PTSD was related to TBSA percentage burned, length of hospitalization, and lack of responsibility for the injury. Mancusi-Ungaro, Tarbox, and Wainwright (1986) suggest that PTSD and other significant emotional problems are more frequent in electrical injuries. Tucker (1987) indicates that the frequency of PTSD increases after discharge. This is consistent with delayed PTSD and is just one factor that points to the importance of consistent psychological follow-up.

As hospitalization proceeds and wounds are covered and/or healing, patient concerns turn to the potential impact of the burn on life after discharge. The stress of dressing changes, daily therapy, and pain continues. Giving patients control of appropriate options (type of medication, dressing change schedule, etc.) can facilitate the process of their becoming more responsible and independent in their care. Relaxation training may be employed to assist with pain tolerance and sleep disturbance. Individual and family counseling interventions may be more pertinent after discharge.

At discharge, there is usually ambivalence, that is, eagerness to get out of the hospital but anxiety about being on one's own. Emotional sequelae are focused on the time necessary for progress, social and family matters, appearance, and functional ability for resuming work or other valued activities.

Long-term emotional problems in burn patients are the exception. Browne et al. (1985) reported that 10% of 340 adults indicated emotional problems up to 12 years post-burn. These psychological adjustment problems were related to unemployment, reduced occupational status, avoidance behaviors, and reduced recreational activities. Other reports suggest that more severe burns are more likely to result in long-term quality-of-life problems with both physical and psychosocial aspects (Cobb, Maxwell, & Silverstein, 1990). Chang and Herzog (1976) indicate that emotional problems may be more frequent in persons with more than 30% TBSA burns or if the face and/or hands are involved. However, other research reports that TBSA percentage or location of burn injury are poor predictors of long-term emotional sequelae (Browne et al., 1985; Orr, Reznikoff, & Smith, 1989; Sheffield et al., 1988; Ward et al., 1987). Cromes et al. (1997) found that about 50% of persons with major burn injury had mild emotional distress up to 1 year postinjury.

Vocational Implications

A variety of functional limitations that may temporarily or permanently affect a burn patient's ability to return to work have been discussed previously. It has also been stated that vocational issues are often a major correlate of long-term psychological and emotional problems. It must be emphasized that many of these burn sequelae are not overtly apparent. If they are not recognized as valid, the rehabilitation counselor could very easily conclude that a person is malingering, whining, or unmotivated. When a question arises about return to work, a comprehensive medical evaluation by a burn rehabilitation specialist is necessary. Despite these considerations, most people who are employed when burned return to work. Inancsi and Guidotti (1989) indicated that of 115 hospitalized occupational burn injuries, 98 (85%) returned to work, and the remaining 17 (15%) were permanently disabled. Of the permanently disabled, 11 had electrical burns. For all of these hospitalized burn patients, the mean time from injury to return to work was 58 days. The authors point out that this is deceiving because of the length of time before return to work in some cases. Helm, Walker, and Peyton (1986) report that 54 of 70 persons with hand burns returned to work by 8 months postinjury, and the mean number of weeks off work was 19.

Other researchers have studied return-to-work latency and factors contributing to time off work. Engrav et al. (1987) found that 325 persons with an average 12% TBSA burn returned to work in an average of 13 weeks. Bowden, Thomson, and Prasad (1989) described a 63-day mean return-to-work interval in 155 patients. Helm and Walker (1992) found that 65 patients with 25% TBSA burns returned to work in an average 17 weeks. All of these studies suggest that size, depth, and location (hands) are factors that influence time to return to work. It is concluded that 70%–80% of working persons who have been burned return to work in an average of 10–20 weeks. It also must be considered that the seriousness of burn injury, etiology of burn injury, and site of burn injury can significantly affect return to work and how long it takes.

REFERENCES

Bennett, G. B., Helm, P. A., Purdue, F. G., & Hunt, J. L. (1989). Serial casting: A method for treating burn contractures. *Journal of Burn Care and Rehabilitation, 10,* 543–545.

Bowden, M. L., Thomson, P. D., & Prasad, J. K. (1989). Factors influencing return to employment after a burn injury. *Archives of Physical Medicine and Rehabilitation, 70*, 772–774.

Brigham, P.A., & McLoughlin, E. (1996). Burn incidence and medical care use in the United States: Estimates, trends, and data sources. *Journal of Burn Care and Rehabilitation, 17,* 95–107.

Browne, G., Byrne, C., Brown, B., Pennock, M., Streiner, D., Roberts, R., Eyles, R., Truscott, D., & Dabbs, R. (1985). Psychosocial adjustment of burn survivors. *Burns, Including Thermal Injury, 12*, 28–35.

Bruster, J. M., & Pullium, G. (1983). Gradient pressure. *American Journal of Occupational Therapy, 37,* 485–488.

Chang, F. C., & Herzog, B. (1976). Burn morbidity: A follow-up study of physical and psychological disability. *Annals of Surgery, 183,* 34–37.

Choctaw, W. F., Eisner, M. E., & Wachtel, T. L. (1987). Causes, prevention, prehospital care, evaluation, emergency treatment, and prognosis. In B. M. Achaver (Ed.), *Management of the burn patient* (pp. 4–5). Los Altos, CA: Appleton and Lange.

Cobb, N., Maxwell, G., & Silverstein, P. (1990). Patient perception of quality of life after burn injury: Results of an eleven-year survey. *Journal of Burn Care and Rehabilitation, 10*, 251–257.

Cromes, G. F., Voege, J., Kowalske, K. J., & Helm, P. A. (1997). Prospective changes in psychological, functional, and community integration measures at discharge and 2, 6, and 12 months post-discharge of persons with major burn injury [Abstract]. *Journal of Burn Care and Rehabilitation, 18*(pt. 3), p. 595.

Deitch, E. A., Wheelahan, T. M., Rose, M. P., Clothier, J., & Cotter, J. (1983). Hypertrophic burn scars: Analysis of variables. *Journal of Trauma, 23,* 895–898.

Demling, R. H. (1989). Preface. In C. LaLonde (Ed.), *Burn trauma* (p. x). New York: Thieme Medical Publishers.

Dimick, A. R. (1984). Pathophysiology. In S. V. Fisher & P. A. Helm (Eds.), *Comprehensive rehabilitation of burns* (pp. 16–27). Baltimore: Williams & Wilkens.

Engrav, L. H., Covey, M. H., Dutcher, K. D., Heimbach, D. M., Walkinshaw, M. D., & Marvin, J. A. (1987). Impairment, time out of school, and time off from work after burns. *Plastic and Reconstructive Surgery, 79*, 927–934.

Head, M. D. (1984). Wound and skin care. In S. V. Fisher & P. A. Helm (Eds.), *Comprehensive rehabilitation of burns* (pp. 148–176). Baltimore: Williams & Wilkens.

Head, M. D., & Helm, P. A. (1977). Paraffin and sustained stretching in the treatment of burn contractures. *Burns, 4,* 136–139.

Heimbach, D. M. (1988). American Burn Association 1988 presidential address: We can see so far because . . . *Journal of Burn Care and Rehabilitation, 9,* 340–346.

Helm, P. A., & Fisher, S. V. (1993). Rehabilitation of the patient with burns. In J. A. DeLisa (Ed.), *Rehabilitation medicine: Principles and practice* (2nd ed., pp. 1111–1130). Philadelphia: J. B. Lippincott.

Helm, P. A., & Walker, S. C. (1992). Return to work after burn injury. *Journal of Burn Care and Rehabilitation, 13,* 53–57.

Helm, P. A., Walker, S. C., & Peyton, S. A. (1986). Return to work following hand burns. *Archives of Physical Medicine and Rehabilitation, 67,* 297–298.

Hunt, J. L. (1984). Electrical injuries. In S. V. Fisher & P. A. Helm (Eds.), *Comprehensive rehabilitation of burns* (pp. 249–266). Baltimore: Williams & Wilkens.

Inancsi, W., & Guidotti, T. L. (1987). Occupation-related burns: Five-year experience of an urban burn center. *Journal of Occupational Medicine, 29,* 730–733.

Inancsi, W., & Guidotti, T. L. (1989). Return to work after occupation related burns: An exploratory study. *Canadian Journal of Rehabilitation, 2,* 169–174.

Mancusi-Ungaro, H. R., Tarbox, A. R., & Wainwright, D. J. (1986). Posttraumatic stress disorder in electric burn patients. *Journal of Burn Care and Rehabilitation, 7,* 521–525.

Orr, D. A., Reznikoff, M., & Smith, G. M. (1989). Body image, self esteem, and depression in burn-injured adolescents and young adults. *Journal of Burn Care and Rehabilitation, 10,* 454–461.

Patterson, D. R., Carrigan, L., Questad, K. A., & Robinson, R. (1990). Post-traumatic stress disorder in hospitalized patients with burn injuries. *Journal of Burn Care and Rehabilitation, 11,* 181–184.

Prasad, J. K., Bowden, M. L., & Thompson, P. D. (1991). A review of the reconstructive surgery needs of 3167 survivors of burn injury. *Burns, 17,* 302–305.

Rice, D. P., & MacKenzie, E. J. (1989). *Cost of injury in the United States: A report to Congress.* Atlanta: Centers for Disease Control.

Rivers, E. (1987). Vocational considerations with major burn patients. *Topics in Acute Care and Trauma Rehabilitation, 1,* 74–80.

Rossignol, A. M., Locke, J. A., & Burke, J. F. (1989). Employment status and the frequency and causes of burn injuries in New England. *Journal of Occupational Medicine, 31,* 751–757.

Sheffield, C. G., Irons, G. B., Mucha, P., Jr., Malec, J. F., Ilstrup, D. M., & Stonnington, H. H. (1988). Physical and psychological outcome after burns. *Journal of Burn Care and Rehabilitation, 9,* 172–177.

Tompkins, R. G., & Burke, J. F. (1990). Progress in burn treatment and the use of artificial skin. *World Journal of Surgery, 14,* 819–824.

Tucker, P. (1987). Psychosocial problems among adult burn victims. *Burns, Including Thermal Injury, 13,* 7–14.

Ward, H. W., Moss, R. L., Darko, D. F., Berry, C. C., Anderson, J., Kolman, P., Green, A., Nielsen, J., Klauber, M., & Wachtel, T. L. (1987). Prevalence of post burn depression following burn injury. *Journal of Burn Care and Rehabilitation, 8,* 294–298.

Chapter 7

Cancers

Ingrid Freidenbergs and Esin Kaplan

Psychologically, physically, and economically, the impact of cancer in the United States is staggering. New malignancies will develop in an estimated 1,228,600 individuals in 1998. This number does not include carcinoma in situ of any site except urinary bladder, and it does not include basal and squamous cell cancers, which will total over 1 million cases. The 1998 estimated cancer incidence by site and sex indicates that the most frequent site will be the breast (30%) in women and the prostate (29%) in men. Lung cancer will be by far the leading cause of cancer deaths in men (32%). In 1998 the leading cause of death for women will also be lung cancer (25%), surpassing even breast cancer (16%) (Landis, Murray, Bolden, & Wingo, 1998).

Cancer is not only a major problem in terms of the number of people afflicted, but it is a very complex management problem as well. Complicating matters is the fact that the etiology of cancer is generally unknown, the prognosis is often uncertain, and it is not even considered a single disease but rather a group of more than 100 different diseases.

The word *cancer* continues to evoke high levels of anxiety and fear. Why is this so? Susan Sontag (1979) has pointed out that, in this century, medicine's central promise is that all diseases can be cured. Cancer, however, still remains a disease that is not readily understood and is therefore mysterious, and it has even come to be used as a metaphor for what is socially or morally wrong. In addition, because cancer is so prevalent, all of us know someone with the disease, which may call forth many personal associations that can interfere with our role as "objective" helpers. Given the profound impact even the mere use of the word *cancer* holds for so many, it is imperative that the counselor have a clear understanding of both the physical nature and the emotional sequelae of the disease. Only in this manner can the myths surrounding the disease be dispelled and the patient helped to adjust.

DESCRIPTION OF MEDICAL CONDITION

There are more than 100 forms of neoplastic disease, with different biological and clinical manifestations. A neoplasm is defined as the growth of new cells proliferating without control and serving no useful function. Abnormal growth of a cell, with local tissue invasion and spread to other organ systems via the blood system or lymphatic channels, is typical for malignancies. The spread to other body parts is termed metastasis. Under the microscope, the actual cells may be classified as either well differentiated or undifferentiated. This distinction is important because well-differentiated cells offer a better prognosis than do undifferentiated ones. Cancers are further specified in terms of the type of tissue of origin: carcinoma (those tissues arising from epithelial cells), sarcoma (cancers arising from connective and supportive tissue), lymphoma (malignancies of lymphatic tissue), and leukemia (malignant transformation of white blood cells).

Because of the variety of cancers, it is most unlikely that a single causative factor will be identified. In fact, more than one factor most likely will be found that will convert a normal cell into a "cancerous" one. Epidemiological studies have shown environmental hazards, social practices, and heritable factors to play a part in the etiology of the various cancers. For example, smoking has been linked to lung cancer, alcohol and tobacco consumption to head and neck cancer, x-ray therapy to thyroid cancer, family history to breast cancer, diet to colon cancer, and the sun to melanoma and other skin cancers. Genetic as well as immunological factors may predispose one to acquiring cancer. Viruses, especially the DNA viruses, also play a role.

Cancer can develop at any age, in any tissue of any organ system. If it is detected at an early stage, it is potentially curable. About 40% of the cancer population is clinically cured with surgical treatment. Fifteen percent of the remaining 60% will survive at least another 15 years. The cancer warning signs include change in bowel or bladder habits, a sore that does not heal, unusual bleeding or discharge, a thickening or lump in breast tissue or elsewhere, indigestion or difficulty swallowing, an obvious change in a wart or mole, a nagging cough, and persistent fevers, sweats, pain, fatigue, or weight loss.

A detailed careful history and physical exam of all patients is essential. Screening tests for cancer detection include the routine use of the Pap smear, which has led to a significant decrease in mortality from cervical cancer. Breast self-examination and mammography may contribute to an early diagnosis and reduce mortality from breast cancer. Stool testing for occult blood may lead to an early diagnosis of colon cancer. Chest x-rays and a sputum exam are helpful in lung cancer diagnosis, especially for those with a history of heavy smoking and exposure to well-known carcinogenic agents.

Biopsy techniques include incisional biopsy, excisional biopsy, fine-needle biopsy, bronchial washes, and others. To determine the stage of the malignant process, diagnostic tests such as liver, spleen, bone, and brain scans are used. Magnetic resonance imaging is helpful for early metastatic detection in the various organ systems. The elevation of certain blood serum enzymes or chemistries is very specific for certain malignancies. Relatively recent tests include the CEA (carcinoembryonic antigen) for colon cancer, CA-125 for ovarian cancer, alpha-fetaprotein or beta human chorionic gonadotropin testing for testicular cancer, and serum immunoglobulins for multiple myeloma. Occasionally, the diagnosis of a metastatic cancer is made by biopsy without the presence of a primary site.

Age has a significant impact on both incidence and mortality. For example, certain cancers, such as prostate, stomach, or colon, reach a peak at ages 60–80, whereas others, such as acute lymphoma or acute lymphoblastic leukemia, peak at infancy to 10 years. Thus, if a mediastinal mass is found in a 20-year-old patient, the differential diagnosis would include Hodgkin's disease or non-Hodgkin's lymphoma, but the same mass in a 50-year-old would include lung cancer, non-Hodgkin's lymphoma, or thymoma (a malignancy of the thymus gland).

Treatment for cancer is directed at eradicating the primary tumor and any metastatic areas. The basic treatment modalities include surgery and radiation for regional control of disease and chemotherapy for systemic control. Other treatment modalities include immunotherapy, hormonal therapy, and hyperthermia.

Surgery is the oldest and still one of the most effective forms of cancer therapy. Cancers curable in the early stages with surgery alone include cancers of the oral cavity, larynx, lung, colon, prostate, kidney, testis, bladder, ovary, endometrium, cervix, and breast. Recently, laser beam techniques have been used in place of surgery to control regional disease.

Radiation therapy uses ionizing radiation, with radioactive cobalt usually being the source. Radiation generates a large amount of energy, which eradicates the localized population of neoplastic cells; the cell content is directly affected by changing the DNA structure. Radiation treatment is very effective with the non-Hodgkin's lymphomas and cancers of the testis, prostate, larynx, nasopharynx, cervix, and lung. Side effects may be systemic (e.g., nausea, vomiting, fatigue, bone marrow suppression) or local (e.g., skin or mucosal irritation). Long-term effects may include peripheral or central nervous system degeneration or the development of another malignancy.

Chemotherapy has become a powerful tool in reducing or controlling tumor activity. During recent years it has become more apparent that a combination of chemotherapy agents may potentiate a therapeutic effect. Chemotherapy agents include the alkylating agents, antimetabolites, plant alkaloids, antitumor antibodies, and enzymes. These agents affect cancer cell growth at various stages. Antineoplastic chemotherapy is considered curative of certain tumors, such as testicular tumors, acute leukemia, Burkitt's lymphoma, Hodgkin's and non-Hodgkin's lymphoma, and certain childhood tumors. Because all of the currently available antitumor drugs act on similar structures and metabolic pathways in both normal and neoplastic cells, the use of these agents is limited because of the toxic effect on normal tissue, such as bone marrow, liver, kidney, and the nervous system. In addition, many chemotherapeutic agents are carcinogenic as well. Side effects may include nausea, vomiting, bone marrow suppression, hair loss, mouth sores, and peripheral neuropathy or myopathy (Body, Lossignol, & Ronson, 1997; Colvin & Owens, 1988).

Cancer carries risks to the patient that extend over many years. Even though the primary disease may be cured, the patient may have functional or physical difficulties as a result of the medical treatments. When evaluating the functional status of patients, it is essential to determine the region of anatomical structure of the body that is affected, the type of tumor, the course the disease has taken, and the individual variables the patient presents. Because rehabilitation requires a holistic and comprehensive approach, the combined expertise of a multidisciplinary team is necessary. The following are examples of rehabilitation issues facing cancer patients (Kaplan & Gumport, 1988).

In treating tumors of the head and neck, functional and cosmetic deformities are frequently encountered. Because it has been noted that a history of alcohol and tobacco consumption is present in about 85% of patients, rehabilitation efforts are often made more difficult. Ninety percent of head and neck cancers are of the squamous cell type, the most common site being the larynx, followed by the tonsils and hypopharynx. The salivary glands, thyroid, and sinuses are less often involved. Depending on the source of the tumor and the extent of the disease, either surgical or radiation treatments, or both, are chosen. Many patients who have been treated for these tumors have had neck dissections. Physical limitation may include difficulties in opening the mouth, chewing or swallowing, speaking, or even breathing. Prostheses may be made to replace a lost body part. Head and neck prostheses include eyes, ears, nose, and even the palate.

The types of surgical treatments available for breast cancer include radical and modified-radical mastectomies and partial breast resection with axillary node dissections. During recent years immediate breast reconstructions have been more commonly performed, but these may be done at a later date as well. Depending on the extent of the disease, either radiation (which is mostly given to patients who undergo partial breast resection) or chemotherapy is the choice of treatment.

Currently, the use of the hormone tamoxifen is advocated as a treatment, especially in women with estrogen-receptor cells. After a mastectomy, instructions about postoperative arm positioning, exercises, and arm care are essential for the prevention of "frozen shoulder," pain syndromes, and lymphedema (swelling of the arm and hand). The prevention of lymphedema includes avoidance of obesity and minimizing any trauma, infection, or sunburn to the arm.

Soft-tissue tumors include those of connective tissue, blood and lymphatic vessels, smooth and striated muscles, fat fascia, and synovial structures. Treatment may range from a simple excision to amputation. Rehabilitation depends on the extent of the operative procedure as well as whether chemotherapy or radiation therapy is required. Adequate treatment of soft-tissue tumors may require removal of a large amount of muscle tissue. Splinting or supporting of major joints might be necessary to permit early resumption of daily living activities and ambulation. If amputation is to be done, preoperative consideration should be given to the level of amputation, type of prosthesis, and type of training that will make the postoperative transition easier.

Primary malignant tumors of the skeleton account for less than 1% of all tumors, with the greatest incidence found in children and young adults. Treatment may require amputation. Metastatic bone tumors stemming from the lung, breast, prostate, kidney, and thyroid gland are the most common malignancies affecting bones. The spine, pelvis, and long bones are the most common metastatic sites. General management includes steroids in high doses, radiation, surgical decompression, and stabilization. Appropriate external support is provided with braces and assistive devices to improve the patient's mobility, safety, and independence.

The most common primary malignant tumors of the central nervous system (CNS) are gliomas, which represent 45% of intracranial tumors. Malignant tumors of the CNS do not metastasize to other organ systems of the body, but they do spread within the CNS itself. Ten percent of CNS tumors are metastatic from other parts of the body. The most common site of the primary neoplasm is typically the lung. Almost any part of the brain may be involved in a metastatic process. The functional aftermath of CNS tumors includes paralysis, paresthesias, aphasia, memory impairment, confusion, and any other of the usual sequellae of brain damage.

PSYCHOLOGICAL IMPACT OF CANCER

It is safe to say that cancer may interfere with many daily activities and that the patient may react with anxiety, depression, loss of self-esteem, and a disruption of defense mechanisms. Many different types of fears can be activated: fears of loss of control, loss of independence, loss of privacy, loss of normal bodily functions, mutilation, isolation from family and friends, loss of income, pain, and death. However, it has been difficult to measure the actual psychosocial impact of the disease because study results vary according to such factors as site and histological type of cancer, staging of the disease, type of medical treatment administered, clinical course, functional impairment, cosmetic impairment, or the time interval separating cancer diagnosis and psychosocial assessment. Individual variables, such as the patient's age, gender, religion, socioeconomic status, living arrangements, and premorbid personality, also enter into consideration in determining one's response to cancer. Finally, the availability of rehabilitation services and psychological management by the medical team play important roles in influencing the impact of this disease.

When research on the actual emotional impact of cancer has been conducted, dysphoric reactions have been reported in roughly 4.5% to 50% of patients (Spiegel, 1996). For example, when the emotional status of 112 women with breast cancer was assessed, 50% admitted being either anxious or depressed. Derogatis et al. (1983) studied the prevalence of psychiatric disorders in 215 patients with cancer (varying sites) and found that 47% had some psychiatric disorder meeting DSM-III criteria. Of the total number of patients, only 11% had psychiatric problems prior to their illness. The remaining 36% exhibited disorders that were reactions to the disease or its treatment. Pasacreta and Massie (1990), in their study of 475 patients, found that 55% were perceived as having symptoms that required psychiatric consultation, situational depression and anxiety being the most common. Recent studies have shown fear of recurrence causes some patients to continue to suffer from affective disorders, particularly anxiety, despite the absence of disease (Thomas, Glynn-Jones, Chait, & Marks, 1997). These results indicate that, by and large, cancer patients do not suffer from psychiatric conditions other than those posed by the stresses of the disease and/ or its medical treatments.

Research studies have also centered on the impact of medical treatments on the cancer patient. For example, Peck and Boland (1972) used psychiatric interviews to study the affective reactions of patients undergoing radiation therapy. The most common affective responses were anxiety (98% of patients) and depression (75% of patients). Evans and Connis (1995) showed that both cognitive-behavioral and social support therapies resulted in fewer psychiatric symptoms and reduced maladaptive interpersonal relations in patients undergoing radiation therapy. When the effects of chemotherapy were examined, Carey and Burish (1988) noted that approximately 45% of adult cancer patients experience psychological side effects in the 24-hour period preceding treatment. These researchers state that such negative psychological symptoms are the product of both associative learning and the stress associated with chemotherapy and that those side effects can be ameliorated with psychological techniques.

Cancer patients have historically received a low priority for vocational rehabilitation services. Much has been written in the popular press about the prejudices that exist toward cancer patients when they apply for new job positions or when they return to work. In a study of 100 recovered cancer patients, the findings indicated that 13% of the patients were denied work because of their cancer history, 35% perceived some form of job-related discrimination, and 11% were excluded from group health benefits or had their previous benefits reduced (Feldman, 1978). Confirming that such discrimination still exists, a recent study of 422 cancer patients showed that although 76% of the respondents indicated that they were working at the time of diagnosis, only 56% were working at the time of the study. However, 82% stated that they wanted to work full- or part-time (Rothstein, Kennedy, Ritchie, & Pyle, 1995). Indeed, one of the most widespread consequences of having had cancer is the tendency to be locked into preexisting jobs; losing insurance coverage is too great a risk for patients to take.

Another area that is affected by cancer is sexuality. Cancer and its treatment can potentially damage sexual response by affecting emotions, central or peripheral components of the nervous system, the pelvic vascular system, and the hypothalamic-pituitary-gonadal axis (Lederberg, Holland, & Massie, 1989). Site of cancer has been found to be an important variable affecting sexual response, even in patients of comparable prognosis and treatment. For example, when patients with testicular cancer were compared to those with Hodgkin's disease, the former exhibited a greater degree of sexual dysfunction, as well as greater difficulty in the resolution of their sexual difficulties (Johnstone et al., 1989).

The psychosocial impact of cancer changes over time. Some researchers are of the opinion that there is a specific time-related pattern of patient response to the disease in which the emotional reactions of persons who have cancer evolve through the stages of denial, anxiety, regression, depression, and finally, realistic adaptation (Kübler-Ross, 1969). It is our experience that although these are generally typical behavioral responses of cancer patients, the sequence of such responses is not so neatly predictable. Even in the space of a single psychotherapy session, the patient's feelings may fluctuate among several different "stages." Furthermore, the disease is not static; there are certain crisis or transition points that exacerbate emotional upheaval. For example, the start of primary treatment, changing treatment modalities, and relapse are all points of stress at which one's response is often unpredictable. In a prospective study, Gordon et al. (1980) interviewed 308 patients over a 6-month period and noted that upon hospitalization the most frequent problems fell in the area of worry about disease. Immediately upon discharge, problems fell into the area of negative affect. Six months after discharge, problems were found to be more broadly distributed in the areas of physical discomfort, concern about medical treatment, dissatisfaction with health care services, mobility, financial concerns, family problems, social problems, worry about disease, experience of negative affect, and body image.

When gender differences in response to the disease were investigated in a group of advanced cancer patients, Leiber, Plumb, Gerstenzang, and Holland

(1976) noted that women patients were more depressed than their husbands, male patients, or the spouses of male patients. On the other hand, when Baider et al. (1989) studied 39 couples in which one partner had cancer of the colon, it was found that although male patients adjusted better than female patients did, male spouses adjusted far worse than female spouses and even worse than male patients. And in a study of the role of psychological variables in a group of 100 melanoma patients, Baider and her colleagues note that on all adjustment measures women did not do as well as men (Baider et al., 1997). Such findings suggest that more studies must be conducted on cultural, social, or intrapsychic factors that might influence differing gender responses to the disease and its ramifications.

One must consider age when evaluating the impact of the disease on the patient. Mages and Mendelsohn (1979) note that for young adults the experience of cancer tends to impede the development of self-sufficiency and results in delay and disruption in the establishment of adult roles. For midlife adults, the occurrence of cancer threatens to disrupt roles and important life tasks yet to be carried out. For older adults, cancer leads to an acceleration of the aging process and results in more rapid disengagement from work and social and leisure activities and a greater dependency on others. If the patient is a long-term survivor, difficulties in adjustment occur in that there is a fear of recurrence and often a permanent sense of physical vulnerability that may diminish self-assurance and confidence.

Once cancer has been diagnosed, are some patients more likely than others to develop psychosocial problems? Vulnerability factors, such as prior psychiatric problems, alcohol or drug abuse, depression, and chronic anxiety, are said to be strong predictors for poor adjustment (Lederberg et al., 1989). Morris, Greer, and White (1977) found that at-risk patients were those who were clinically depressed prior to surgery and who were emotionally labile as well. Craig and Abeloff (1974) divided a sample of 30 primary leukemia and lymphoma patients into high- and low-psychiatric-symptom subgroups. Patients in the high-symptom subgroup were younger, were more likely to be White females, were of higher socioeconomic level, had a higher degree of physical impairment, and had a poorer prognosis than did patients in the low-symptom group.

Whether cancer patients represent an increased risk for suicide compared to other patients also has been addressed. Recent studies have suggested that, although relatively few cancer patients actually commit suicide, they are nonetheless at greater risk (Breitbart, 1987). High suicide potential exists when the following factors are present: emotional stress, severe depression with feelings of hopelessness, anxiety, mood swings, low tolerance for pain and discomfort, chronic and poorly controlled pain, history of alcoholism or substance abuse, feeling of lack of support from family or medical team, and prior suicide threats or attempts.

Another area investigated is the patient's style of coping with cancer. Coping is seen as an extremely important variable in the patient's response to disease.

For example, it has been noted that it is not exposure to a stressor per se but the ability to cope with it effectively that is most likely to influence even the course of the disease itself. And when 53 cancer patients who dropped out of chemotherapy were compared to a group who completed their treatment, it was found that those who dropped out had more adjustment problems on every measure that was used (Gilbar & De-Nour, 1989). Weisman and Worden (1977) discuss coping strategies and state that coping and vulnerability have a reciprocal relationship. Vulnerability is an index of distress, whereas coping is what one does about the disease and its ramifications. They found that good copers face facts, find something favorable, and then confidently comply with their doctors' recommendations. In contrast, poor copers use suppression, passivity, and stoic submission.

Prior to the 1980s a common research topic involved the role of premorbid personality factors in the development of cancer. These early studies did not yield consistent results, and the quest for a cancer-prone personality diminished. There was then a shift in interest to consideration of the role that psychosocial factors play in the outcome of disease. For example, in a study conducted by Achterberg, Lawlis, Simonton, and Mathews-Simonton (1977), factors such as denial, a view of one's body as having little ability to fight disease, and a significant dependency on others proved to be predictors of poor prognosis. On the other hand, when testing the degree to which certain psychosocial factors predict survival and relapse, Cassileth, Lusk, Miller, Brown, and Miller (1985) reported contradictory findings. Three hundred fifty-one patients were investigated, using variables such as social ties and marital history, job satisfaction, use of psychotropic drugs, general life evaluation/satisfaction, degree of hopelessness/helplessness, subjective view of adult health, and subjective view of the amount of adjustment required to cope with the new diagnosis. The results indicated that none of these variables predicted longevity or survival. This well-designed study shows that in many cases the biology of the disease is the major factor determining the prognosis, "overriding the potentially mitigating influence of psychosocial factors." Richardson, Zarnegar, Bismo, and Levine (1990) examined 139 patients as to the effect on survival of depression, coping style, and locus of control. Again, none of these variables was found to be significantly related to survival. However, these same researchers have shown that factors such as compliance and the number of appointments kept are important predictors of survival. It is clear that many further studies are needed to answer adequately the question of the link between psychosocial status and outcome of disease.

Even more recently, there has been an expanding field of research on the connection between psychological events, endocrine secretion, and modulation of immunity (Kripke & Morison, 1984). A number of studies have shown that various stressors can adversely affect immune function and that there exists the possibility of a reciprocal relationship—the enhancement of immune function through psychological interventions (Kiecolt-Glaser & Glaser, 1992). When the effects of a structured group intervention program for patients with melanoma were studied, researchers found reduced psychological distress and significant immunological improvement in the control group (Fawzy et al., 1993). Similar effects were reported by Spiegel (1996), who studied the effects of group intervention in women with metastatic breast cancer. However, when Gellert, Maxwell, and Siegel (1993) followed up on the survival of breast cancer patients 10 years after they had received adjunctive psychosocial support, the results indicated that these patients did not live longer, on average, than did a comparable group of nonparticipants. Whether interventions that produce relatively small immunological changes can actually affect the incidence, severity, or duration of cancer is simply not yet known. Kiecolt-Glaser and Glaser (1992) suggest that the answer may depend on the type and intensity of the psychological intervention, degree of immune modulation, and the individual's own prior health status.

Although the effectiveness of psychological intervention on the outcome of disease is still in question, most researchers agree that, at minimum, adjunctive psychological interventions improve mood and enhance quality of life (Andersen, 1992; Cunningham & Edmonds, 1996). What is left to study are the classic questions of psychotherapy research, that is, what type of treatment should be administered and to whom, when should it occur, by whom should it be administered, and under what set of circumstances should it be conducted.

PSYCHOTHERAPY WITH CANCER PATIENTS

A variety of professionals (e.g., psychologists, social workers, psychiatrists, nurses) are involved in the psychosocial management of cancer patients. There are obviously separate areas of expertise that these professionals provide, but an overlapping of functions does exist. Therefore, team members must work closely and noncompetitively with each other. Self-help groups have become a modality for helping patients, with or without a professional facilitator. Such groups provide emotional support, a feeling of belonging, and even stress management and coping skills (Freidenbergs, 1997). More recently, patients have been receiving help by participating in computer-mediated support groups. This innovation allows patients to partake of psychological help without leaving home and with the option of remaining anonymous (Weinberg, Schmale, Uken, & Wessel, 1996).

In assessing the patient's reactions to cancer, the counselor should be well versed in both the physical and emotional consequences of the disease. Education is required to differentiate "normal" from "pathological" responses. When is a patient's negative response self-limited and when has it become pathological? For example, if depression is noted, is the depression reactive to the knowledge that one has cancer or is it a result of the toxin released by the disease itself? Is it a consequence of fatigue, or is it caused by a metabolic imbalance, nutritional deficiency, or infection? Is it a result of the medical treatment administered, or is it a result of the assault on body image? Or does it have nothing to do with the above but rather is caused by either a premorbid depressive pattern or some current interpersonal stress? Further, as Kübler-Ross (1969) has pointed out, there are two different depressive processes to consider: one, a reactive process involving mourning what has been lost, and the other, preparatory depression involving what is going to be lost. It is up to the counselor to determine what the cause of the patient's distress may be. In certain cases it is appropriate to allow patients to mourn their losses, whereas in other situations it might be advisable for the counselor to attempt amelioration of the distress through the counselor's own efforts or via referral to another resource.

Does the psychotherapy offered to cancer patients differ from the therapy offered to other types of patients? Although general principles of clinical psychotherapy remain the same, there are variations in approach that are necessary in treating the cancer patient. First, it is imperative to deal with physical issues relating to the disease and its various medical treatments. Table 7.1 contains a list of psychosocial intervention principles developed by the author and her colleagues (Freidenbergs, Gordon, Hibbard, & Diller, 1980). As can be seen from this list, great emphasis is placed on educating patients, both about their medical condition and about the emotional reactions one may have in response to the disease. Another variation in psychotherapeutic principles involves the timing of interventions. In some cases psychological interpretation must be hastened; in other cases, delayed. Although countertransference is present in all clinical work, the cancer patient may pose even more challenges to the counselor. One should be especially sensitive to emotional fatigue and burnout and seek help quickly if one notices such feelings in oneself.

When working with cancer patients, counselors must allow them to express their feelings about their illness. One has to explore with patients what they think their cancer may signify, what they have been told of the nature of their disease by other medical personnel, and what impact they believe the disease may have on their lives. Patients' efforts at coping should be viewed in the context of their personal backgrounds, experiences, strivings, guilt, fears, and antecedent personalities. Because patients tend to engage in medical "role modeling" (i.e., comparing themselves with other people who have had similar diseases), it is advisable to ask if any family members or friends have had cancer, what kind it was, what course it took, how it was managed medically, and how the condition was coped with.

In reporting on research suggesting that psychological attitudes affect the development, course, and outcome of cancer, the popular media has contributed to many patients' feeling that they have brought on their own disease because of their "negative personality" or that they can improve their prognosis by improving their "mental outlook." It is the counselor's role to make clear that self-

TABLE 7.1 Psychosocial Intervention Principles

Educational	
(Ed 1)	Clarifying/giving information about the medical system—e.g., explaining hospital procedures, teaching patients' rights, informing patients of existing outpatient services
(Ed 2)	Clarifying the patients' own medical condition—e.g., what type of cancer the patient has, the meaning of test results
(Ed 3)	Teaching about cancer and its side effects—e.g., the side effects to be expected from treatment, what the norms are regarding resumption of activities
(Ed 4)	Teaching what to do to relieve physical discomfort, emotional discomfort, etc., e.g., relaxation training, self-hypnosis
(Ed 5)	Reinforcing what *other* medical personnel have said—i.e., helping patients comply with prescribed medical regimen—e.g., reinforcing the necessity of medical treatment, reinforcing MD statements about the medical condition or treatment
(Ed 6)	Teaching about the emotional reactions to cancer—e.g., what emotional responses can be expected by the patient himself/herself, what reactions can he/she expect from others
Counseling	
(C1)	Allowing or encouraging the patient to vent feelings
(C2)	Offering the patient reassurance or verbal support
(C3)	Helping the patient clarify own feelings and interpreting thoughts, feelings, and behavior in more psychodynamic terms to patient
(C4)	Encouraging the patient to act on his/her environment—e.g., urging patient to speak to medical personnel and to family, urging patient to ask questions
(C5)	Exploring the patient's past and/or current situation.
(C6)	Offering indirect support, e.g., by listening to patient, chatting with patient about events unrelated to medical condition
Environmental	
(Ev 1)	Speaking with health care personnel about the patient
(Ev 2)	Making a formal health service referral

blame is counterproductive and at times even clinically harmful. The counselor needs to stress that at this point we still do not know what the relationship between psychological factors and the course of the disease may be, and we do not know whether stress is necessarily always harmful (Freidenbergs, 1991).

When viewing the coping strategies patients use, the counselor needs to focus not on whether the strategy is "good" or "bad" but rather whether or not it is appropriate to the situation. For example, active attempts to deal with cancer, such as seeking information about the illness, can reinforce a patient's sense of control while reducing feelings of helplessness. However, delaying needed treatment because one is continuously seeking information is obviously inappropriate. Denial may be an adaptive defense in temporarily rescuing patients from overwhelming anxiety, or it can be pathological in that it prevents the patient from being alert to possible symptoms of recurrence. Being aware of both the positive and negative effects of psychological defenses can thus be critical in treating the cancer patient.

SOME SPECIFIC THERAPEUTIC ISSUES

Cancer may assault body image in a multitude of ways. Amputation of limbs may result from osteosarcoma; mastectomies, from breast carcinoma; wide and deep scars, from malignant melanoma; and loss of parts of the face, from skin tumors. Chemotherapy may cause hair loss, mouth sores, and weight loss or gain. Radiation may cause skin changes such as puckering and hardening in addition to a blistering redness. The disease may also cause a generalized weakening of muscles, a premature aged look, bloating of the stomach, and a host of other bodily assaults. It is the task of the counselor to assess the psychological effect that such assaults may cause and to provide support throughout the many physical changes the patient may undergo. It must be kept in mind that there is a process of readjustment to any change in one's appearance. Each change, however minor, may provoke disturbance in the body image equilibrium. Equipped with the knowledge that any change in appearance (for better or for worse) will require a period of adjustment, the counselor may then be more able to sensitively assist the patient (Freidenbergs, 1991).

Surgical procedures such as mastectomies, oophorectomies, laryngectomies, thyroidectomies, or colostomies are common in the treatment of cancer. When patients face such surgeries, many fears are encountered (e.g., fear of loss of control, of the unknown, or even of death). The counselor may help by encouraging the verbalization of these fears, by exploring any personal experiences the patient may have had with surgery, and by providing objective information and emotional support. Mental rehearsal of upcoming medical procedures may be particularly helpful in alleviating anxiety. Some common postsurgical reactions, such as shock followed by emotional numbness and a feeling of derealization, should be discussed. It should also be noted that patients may experience mood swings and difficulty in concentrating, sleeping, or eating. It should be explained that these symptoms are temporary and usually subside quickly. If there is any residual discomfort following surgical intervention, it should be explored in depth. Furthermore, the approach the patient is taking to alleviate this discomfort, as well as whether or not it is effective, also should be discussed.

Counselors must clarify the misunderstanding, confusion, and fear of the unknown that patients often feel when facing radiation therapy. This is especially true given the context of the public's long-held fear of radiation's harmful effects. The effect of radiation is often progressive, and side effects may increase as the cumulative dose of radiation is increased. Patients, therefore, should be advised about the changing nature of the treatment. Patients also may be helped by knowing that even after the radiation treatments have stopped there may be a worsening of side effects prior to resolution.

When patients are undergoing chemotherapy, they often have to balance toxicity against benefits. Open communication with oncologists should be encouraged so that patients can make psychologically sound decisions. It is extremely important that patients be made aware that all chemotherapies are not the same and that it is not helpful to compare oneself to others. Even if the chemotherapy protocols are the same, the "host"—namely, the patient—differs biologically from all other patients and therefore may respond in a different manner. In addition to reassuring the patient regarding anticipated nausea and vomiting, preparing the patient for hair loss is critical. This bodily change may provoke a severe psychological reaction in both male and female patients. This reaction is not abnormal as it occurs too regularly in too many patients to be considered as such. Therefore, much reassurance before, during, and after chemotherapy is required. As hair does not often grow back for many weeks following the last chemotherapy treatment, the counselor should be giving support throughout what may appear to be an endless period for the patient. Finally, completion of chemotherapy may be experienced by some patients as a mixed blessing in that stopping treatment might imply the regrowth and relapse of disease.

Much attention has been focused on the terminally ill patient, and in-depth discussions can be found by Chochinov and Holland (1989) and Osterweis, Solomon, and Green (1984). Open discussion of reactions to approaching death may allow for less emotional distress. Grief also may be tolerated better when the loss is expected and there has been some psychological preparation. However, as with all issues, individual differences predominate, and the counselor must be sensitive to just how much reality can be absorbed by patients and family members at any time. Duration of grieving when a family member dies also varies tremendously. A close, trusting, and supportive relationship with caregivers is important at whatever stage grief is encountered.

REFERENCES

Achterberg, J., Lawlis, G. F., Simonton, O. C., & Mathews-Simonton, S. (1977). Psychological factors and blood chemistries as disease outcome predictors for cancer patients. *Multivariate Experimental Clinical Research, 3,* 107–122.

Andersen, B. L. (1992). Psychological interventions for cancer patients to enhance the quality of life. *Journal of Consulting and Clinical Psychology, 60,* 552–568.

Baider, L., Perez, T., & De-Nour, A. T. (1989). Gender and adjustment to chronic disease: A study of couples with colon cancer. *General Hospital Psychiatry, 11,* 1–8.

Baider, L., Perry, S., Sison, A., Holland, J., Uziely, B., & DeNour, A. K. (1997). The role of psychological variables in a group of melanoma patients. *Psychosomatics, 38,* 45–53.

Body, J,, Lossignol, D., & Ronson, A. (1997). The concept of rehabilitation of cancer patients. *Current Opinion in Oncology, 9,* 332–340.

Breitbart, W. (1987). Suicide in cancer patients. *Oncology, 1,* 49–54.

Carey, M. P., & Burish, T. G. (1988). Etiology and treatment of the psychological side effects associated with cancer chemotherapy: A critical review and discussion. *Psychological Bulletin, 104,* 307–325.

Cassileth, B. R., Lusk, E. J., Miller, D. S., Brown, L. L., & Miller, C. (1985). Psychosocial correlates of survival in advanced malignant disease. *New England Journal of Medicine, 312,* 1551–1555.

Chochinovar, H., & Holland, J. C. (1989). Bereavement: A special issue in oncology. In J. C. Holland & J. H. Rowland (Eds.), *Handbook of psychooncology* (pp. 612–627). New York: Oxford University Press.

Colvin, M., & Owens, A. H. (1988). Neoplastic diseases. In. A. M. Harvey, R. J. Johns, V. A. McKusick, A. H. Owens, & R. S. Ross (Eds.), *The principles and practices of medicine* (pp. 384–449). East Norwalk, CT: Appleton & Lange.

Craig, T. J., & Abeloff, M. D. (1974). Psychiatric symptomatology among hospitalized hospital patients. *American Journal of Psychiatry, 131,* 1323–1327.

Cunningham, A. J., & Edmonds, C. V. (1996). Group psychological therapy for cancer patients: A point of view, and discussion of the hierarchy of options. *International Journal of Psychiatry in Medicine, 26,* 51–82.

Derogatis, L. R., Morrow, G. R., Fetting, J., Penman, D., Piasetsky, S., Schmale, M., Hendricks, M., & Carnicke, C. (1983). The prevalence of psychiatric disorders among cancer patients. *Journal of the American Medical Association, 249,* 751–757.

Evans, R. L., & Connis, R. T. (1995). Comparison of brief group therapies for depressed cancer patients receiving radiation treatment. *Public Health Reports, 110,* 306–311.

Fawzy, F. I., Fawzy, N. W., Hyun, C., Elashoff, R., Guthrie, D., Fahey, J. L., & Morton, D. L. (1993). Malignant melanoma: Effects of an early structured psychiatric intervention, coping, and affective state on recurrence and survival 6 years later. *Archives of General Psychiatry, 50,* 681–689.

Feldman, F. L. (1978). *Work and cancer related histories.* New York: American Cancer Society.

Freidenbergs, I. (1991). Psychological understanding and management of the skin cancer patient. In R. J. Friedman, D. S. Rigel, A. W. Kopf, M. N. Harris, & D. Baker (Eds.), *Cancer of the skin* (pp. 580–588). Philadelphia: W. B. Saunders.

Freidenbergs, I. (1997). How support groups benefit melanoma patients. *Skin Cancer Foundation Journal, 15,* 43–44.

Freidenbergs, I., Gordon, W., Hibbard, M. R., & Diller, L. (1980). Assessment and treatment of psychosocial problems of the cancer patient: A case study. *Cancer Nursing, 3,* 111–119.

Gellert, G. A., Maxwell, R. M., & Siegel, B. S. (1993). Survival of breast cancer patients receiving adjunctive psychosocial support therapy: A 10-year follow-up study. *Journal of Clinical Oncology, 11,* 66–69.

Gilbar, O., & De-Nour, A. K. (1989). Adjustment to illness and dropout of chemotherapy. *Journal of Psychosomatic Research, 33,* 1–5.

Gordon, W. A., Freidenbergs, I., Diller, L., Hibbard, M., Wolf, C., Levine, L., Lipkins, R., Ezraschi, O., & Lucido, D. (1980). Efficacy of psychosocial intervention with cancer patients. *Journal of Consulting and Clinical Psychology, 48,* 743–759.

Johnstone, B. G., Silberfeld, M., Chapman, J., Phoenix, C., Sturgeon, J., Till, J. E., & Sutcliffe, S. B. (1989). Heterogeneity in responses to cancer: Part 2. Sexual responses. *Canadian Journal of Psychiatry, 36,* 182–185.

Kaplan, E., & Gumport, S. L. (1988). Cancer rehabilitation. In J. Goodgold (Ed.), *Rehabilitation medicine* (pp. 285–297). St. Louis: C. V. Mosby.

Kiecolt-Glaser, J. K., & Glaser, R. (1992). Psychoneuroimmunology: Can psychological interventions modulate immunity? *Journal of Consulting and Clinical Psychology, 60,* 569–575.

Kripke, M. L., & Morison, W. L. (1984). Immunology of skin cancer. In R. Fleishmajor (Ed.), *Progress in diseases of the skin* (pp. 31–51). New York: Grune and Stratton.

Kübler-Ross, E. (1969). *On death and dying.* New York: Macmillan.

Landis, S. H., Murray, T., Bolden, S., & Wingo, P. A. (1998). Cancer statistics, 1998. *CA: A Cancer Journal for Clinicians, 48*(1), 6–30.

Lederberg, M. S., Holland, J. C., & Massie, M. (1989). Psychologic aspects of patients with cancer. In V. T. De Vita (Ed.), *Cancer: Principles and practice of oncology* (pp. 2191–2204). Philadelphia: J. B. Lippincott.

Leiber, L., Plumb, M. M., Gerstenzang, M. L., & Holland, J. (1976). The communication of affection between cancer patients and their spouses. *Journal of Psychosomatic Medicine, 38,* 379–389.

Morris, T., Greer, H. S., & White, P. W. (1977). Psychological and social adjustment to mastectomy. *Cancer, 40,* 2381–2387.

Osterweis, M., Solomon, F., & Green, M. (Eds.). (1984). *Bereavement reactions, consequences and care.* Washington, DC: National Academy Press.

Pasacreta, J. V., & Massie, M. (1990). Nurses' reports of psychiatric complications in patients with cancer. *Oncology Nursing Forum, 17,* 347–354.

Peck, A., & Boland, L. (1972). Emotional reaction to having cancer. *American Journal of Roentgenology, Radiation Therapy and Nuclear Medicine, 114,* 591–599.

Richardson, J. L., Zarnegar, Z., Bismo, B., & Levine, A. (1990). Psychosocial status at initiation of cancer treatment and survival. *Journal of Psychosomatic Research, 34*(2), 189–301.

Rothstein, M. A., Kennedy, K., Ritchie, K. J., & Pyle, K. (1995). Are cancer patients subject to employment discrimination? *Oncology, 9,* 1303–1306.

Sontag, S. (1979). *Illness as metaphor.* New York: Vintage Books.

Spiegel, D. (1996). Cancer and depression. *British Journal of Psychiatry, 168*(30), 109–116.

Thomas, S. F., Glynn-Jones, R., Chait, I., & Marks, D. F. (1997). Anxiety in long-term cancer survivors influences the acceptability of planned discharge from follow-up. *Psycho-Oncology, 6,* 190–196.

Weinberg, N., Schmale, J., Uken, J., & Wessel, K. (1996). Online help: Cancer patients participate in a computer-mediated support group. *Health and Social Work, 21*(1), 24–29.

Weisman, A. D., & Worden, J. W. (1977). *Coping and vulnerability in cancer patients* (Research report). Washington, DC: National Cancer Institute.

Chapter 8

Cardiovascular Disorders

Mariano J. Rey

Cardiovascular diseases represent the major health epidemic of the 20th century. In the United States and in most other industrialized countries nearly two thirds of all deaths are caused by cardiovascular disorders. One person dies every minute from cardiovascular disease in the United States. In countries of the developing world, cardiovascular disease accounts for a quarter of all deaths, and this number increases with increasing economic development. It is estimated that cardiovascular disease will be the major killer in the world by the year 2025 as infectious diseases are brought under better control and as the unhealthy lifestyles of Western society spread across the globe.

Cardiovascular diseases also represent the most common cause of disability in the United States. It is estimated that in 1990 alone about 1 million Americans survived an acute, discrete, major cardiac event or intervention (500,000 Americans suffered heart attacks, about 250,000 underwent coronary artery bypass surgery, and another 250,000 underwent coronary artery angioplasty). In addition, at any given time there are about 6 million Americans with symptoms of cardiovascular disease. The prevalence of chronic atrial fibrillation is on the rise as the average age of the American population increases and a greater number of individuals live beyond the age of 80 years. During this decade congestive heart failure became the most common diagnosis on discharge from United States hospitals. Such is the magnitude of the cardiac disease epidemic that it is a rare to find an American family that is not affected by its mortality and morbidity.

Cardiovascular diseases constitute the major health challenge to all providers of medical, psychological, rehabilitative, and vocational services. A comprehensive review of the cardiovascular system and its diseases is therefore imperative for all health professionals.

DISEASES OF THE HEART

Cardiovascular diseases are those that affect the heart and the vascular system. By structural and functional criteria (or by anatomy and physiology) the heart has five components: the coronary arteries, the pericardium, the myocardium, the endocardium, and the electrical conduction system.

THE CORONARY ARTERIES

The coronary arteries can be deemed to be the most important blood vessels in the body—for they supply the heart itself. Without normal coronary blood flow the heart cannot carry out its function of supplying blood to the rest of the body. There are two coronary arteries: the left coronary artery and the right coronary artery. The left coronary vessel, after a short main segment, bifurcates into two branches. One branch is the left anterior descending coronary artery, which brings blood to the septum (the muscle between the two ventricles) and to the anterior wall of the left ventricle; the other branch is the circumflex coronary artery, which brings blood to the lateral wall of the left ventricle. The right coronary vessel supplies blood to the right ventricle and to the inferior wall of the left ventricle. In any individual, the blood supply to the posterior wall of the left ventricle can originate from either the circumflex or the right coronary artery, or from both.

Disease Description

The story of cardiovascular disease in the latter half of the 20th century is basically the story of coronary artery disease. In turn, the story of coronary artery disease is that of the pathological process of atherosclerosis. Over 90% of all of the mortality and morbidity of cardiovascular disease at present is from coronary atherosclerosis. Any heart disease that results from disorders of the coronary arteries is known as coronary heart disease. The most common clinical syndromes of coronary heart disease are stable angina pectoris, unstable angina pectoris, acute myocardial infarction, sudden death, and congestive heart failure.

The cause of coronary heart disease can be best described as biopsychosocial failure (Medallie, 1990). It is a complex constellation of biological, psychological, and social factors that have resulted in the epidemic of coronary heart disease. The risk factors for coronary atherosclerosis are elevated blood cholesterol, high blood pressure, cigarette smoking, diabetes, and a sedentary but stressful lifestyle. These risk factors, alone or in several combinations, create the initial lesion of coronary heart disease, the atherosclerotic plaque, or atheroma.

The pathophysiological process is one in which the endothelium, the single-cell thick lining of the inner surface of the coronary arteries, becomes structurally or functionally damaged. The injury to the endothelial cell is directly or indirectly caused by one of the risk factors for atherosclerosis. Once this endothelial barrier is broken, there is deposition of cells, fats, calcium, and amorphous debris inside the arterial wall. Eventually, the atherosclerotic plaques create rigid arterial walls and lead to progressive narrowing of the arteries—which is termed coronary stenosis. Once the coronary vessel has a 70% stenosis, the reduced blood flow may still meet the metabolic needs of the heart when the individual is at a state of rest. Such a narrowing can no longer allow an increase in blood flow to meet the tissue's increased metabolic and oxygen needs during a state of exercise, however. Such an imbalance between oxygen demand and supply, which results in metabolic derangement of heart cells, is called myocardial ischemia. Coronary artery disease is therefore also known as ischemic heart disease.

Furthermore, the atherosclerotic plaque is an unstable structure that can easily become damaged. At the site of such an ulcerated or fissured plaque there is a tendency to form a clot, or thrombus, and to have arterial spasm. Alone or in combination, thrombus and spasm lead to more severe stenosis and at times to a total, or 100%, occlusion of the artery, with complete cessation of all blood flow to the segment of heart muscle supplied by that artery. The understanding of the clinical presentations of coronary heart disease must be based on this understanding of atheroma pathophysiology.

Ischemic chest pain, or angina pectoris, is the only cardiac symptom in the relatively fortunate group of cardiac patients who have stable atheromas that result in coronary narrowing greater than 70% but in less than a total occlusion. Angina pectoris is described as a visceral pain because it is usually felt deeply, rather than superficially, in the chest. The angina sufferer describes the discomfort as squeezing, pressing, or crushing, or as heaviness or a dull ache. Angina is usually felt in the midchest or sternal area. It often radiates to the left arm or the jaw. It is brought on by physical exertion or by mental stress. It is relieved by the cessation of the activity that caused it. Angina usually lasts less than 5 minutes. Patients with this typical pattern are said to have the clinical syndrome of stable angina. It is estimated that at any given time there are about 5 million Americans with stable angina pectoris.

Angina that occurs at rest, without obvious provocation, or with less effort than usual, is unstable angina. This syndrome is usually a manifestation of an unstable atheroma, which has a superimposed thrombus and spasm that has caused further acute stenosis of the coronary artery. When such unstable angina is severe in intensity or sustained in duration, it is termed preinfarction angina. It may be an indication that a 100% coronary artery occlusion is taking place.

If there is total blood flow cessation for 30 minutes or more, the usual consequence is death to the segment of heart muscle supplied by the occluded artery. This muscle death is a myocardial infarction, popularly known as a heart attack. The main presenting symptom of an acute myocardial infarction is angina that is much more severe in intensity and that lasts for a much longer time than the typical episode of stable angina syndrome. The pain often occurs in the context of generalized symptoms such as weakness, sweating, and anxiety. Many victims have a sense of impending doom—they feel they are going to die. Contrary to popular misinformation, myocardial infarctions are seldom a result of physical activity. They nearly always strike at rest and most often during the early morning hours, shortly after awakening. The timing of the event reflects its pathophysiology. Myocardial infarctions are not a consequence of the increased myocardial demand of exercise outstripping a compromised blood supply; they are caused by the sudden thrombus formation on an unstable atheroma, which then totally occludes the atherosclerotic coronary artery.

Over the last decade, aggressive treatment of hospitalized myocardial infarction patients, with acute thrombolytic (clot-dissolving) therapy and with beta-receptor blockers, has drastically reduced both the in-hospital death rate and the 1-year death rate to less than 10% for treated patients. Unfortunately, about 60% of all deaths from an acute infarction occur within 1 hour after the onset of symptoms. Half of all individuals die before they reach the hospital and before they can receive the benefits of these new therapies. Yearly, about 500,000 Americans have myocardial infarctions, and in spite of all recent advances, these acute myocardial infarctions still cause 25% of all deaths in the United States every year.

Sudden cardiac death is best defined as an unexpected demise with a lack of warning symptoms or prodrome. About 80% of victims of sudden death have coronary heart disease. Sudden death is usually the result of a lethal ventricular rhythm disturbance that has its origin in the unstable electrical milieu of heart muscle cells that are affected by ischemia or that are adjacent to an area of scar caused by a prior myocardial infarction. Some persons are fortunate to have the benefit of prompt cardiopulmonary resuscitation within a few minutes of being stricken. They are said to be sudden-death survivors. Their long-term prognosis is poor, with a chance of about 50% of a subsequent fatal event within a year or 2. It is estimated that there are about 300,000 sudden cardiac deaths in the United States yearly. They account for about 50% of all the deaths from cardiovascular diseases.

Two recent developments may help decrease the frequency of sudden electrical cardiac death. One is the creation of small defribillators (about the size of the better known pacemakers) that can be permanently implanted within the chest wall of survivors of sudden death (or of those deemed susceptible to such a tragic event). These devices can deliver a resuscitative electric shock to the heart whenever a potentially lethal arrhythmia occurs. The other development is the more extensive availability of external defibrillators in public places such as airports and train and bus stations—so that victims of severe arrhythmias can be quickly brought back to stable rhythms and to life itself.

The concept of silent myocardial ischemia is relatively new. It is based on the observation that the cardiac muscle can be ischemic (or even infarcted) without any symptoms. Such silent ischemia has been detected by electrocardiogram (ECG) changes in 24-hour ambulatory recordings by Holter monitors and described in the findings of the Framingham Study and other investigations that show that as many as 25% of all myocardial infarctions can be silent. Such individuals with silent ischemia and infarction can have as their first presentation sudden cardiac death. They can also present with an ischemic cardiomyopathy, a heart that has suffered small multiple silent infarctions and has become boggy and dilated. Their symptoms will be those of congestive heart failure.

Every year in the United States about 1 million men in the total male population older than 30 years of age manifest symptomatic coronary heart disease for the first time. About 40% present with angina pectoris; another 40% with an acute myocardial infarction; and another 10% have sudden death as their first, last, and only symptom. In the remaining 10%, the first symptoms are those of heart failure, or of palpitations, or of syncope, the sudden loss of consciousness.

One should not adopt the common misconception that coronary heart disease afflicts only men. Coronary atherosclerosis and its clinical syndromes affect just as many women as men. On average, however, women experience their clinical coronary heart disease 10 years later than men do. For example, women in their 60's have an incidence of coronary syndromes similar to that of men in their 50's. This is because of the loss of the protective effect of the female hormones, mainly estrogens, whose production is greatly decreased at the onset of menopause.

Function and Disability

The major determinant of impaired function and disability in coronary heart disease is angina. Coronary artery atherosclerosis is not a stable condition. For a myriad of reasons, the tonicity of the muscles in the vessel wall varies during any given time interval and so does the percentage of coronary artery diameter stenosis. Thus, an individual patient's angina pattern may have minor weekly, and even daily, variations in severity, frequency, and the level of exertion needed to provoke it. Nonetheless, the typical patient with a typical stable angina syndrome usually has a predictable functional impairment. That is, a similar number of blocks walked on a level surface or on an incline, a similar number of flights of stairs climbed, a similar weight that he lifted or carried, will reproducibly, time after time, result in the same intensity and duration of angina pectoris. The functional impairment and disability can be best determined based on a careful history, which is unique for each individual. Based on this unique individual history medical therapy can be instituted, referral to surgical intervention can be made, and rehabilitation protocols can be carried out.

The estimated functional capacity and subsequent disability of an individual with angina can be confirmed by exercise stress testing. Exercise tests, whether performed on a treadmill or on a bicycle, approximate the exertion of normal activities of daily living. The goal of all stress testing is to increase the work of the heart and its muscle oxygen demand by increasing the exerciser's heart rate and systolic blood pressure. The age-adjusted target heart rate is roughly the number 220 minus the patient's age. For example, the exercise target heart rate of a 40-year-old is 180 beats per minute; that of a 60-year-old, 160 beats per minute. The systolic blood pressure should rise about 60 mmHg from the rest level to the peak exercise level, and the diastolic blood pressure should drop slightly or remain unchanged. The increasing heart rates and blood pressures are achieved by increasing the workload. On a treadmill, workload is increased by a progressively faster speed and higher incline and on a bicycle, by gradual greater pedal resistance.

The most widely used treadmill protocol for establishing functional capacity, as well as diagnosis and prognosis is the Bruce protocol. For patients who are undergoing evaluation before or after a program of cardiac rehabilitation and for individuals in whom gas-exchange metabolic evaluation is also being performed, we prefer to use the Bensen protocol at our institution. This is a gentler protocol of 2-minute stages, with energy expenditure increases in each stage of only 25% over the prior stage. By comparison, the Bruce protocol elicits more demanding increases of 50% in work with each successive stage.

Heart-imaging techniques with exercise, such as thallium myocardial perfusion scanning, nuclear ventriculograms, and most recently, echocardiography, have independent value in establishing diagnosis and prognosis and give insightful understanding of the anatomical and physiological basis for an individual's exercise tolerance and functional capacity.

Whenever possible, as determined by the information gained by a medical history, a physical exam, and an exercise stress test, the functional capacity of the individual with heart disease should be described according to the classification system of the New York Heart Association (NYHA). This system establishes four functional classes: Class IV—symptomatic at rest (no effort); Class III—symptomatic with minimal effort; Class II—symptomatic with moderate effort; Class I—asymptomatic at any effort level. This traditional functional classification is useful because it provides a common language and point or reference for all health professionals.

Treatment and Prognosis

The definite and ultimate treatment of coronary artery disease is the radical correction of the biopsychosocial failure that is at its root. Primary prevention (i.e., before any clinical event has taken place) of coronary heart disease should be a main mission of all health professionals and can be accomplished by the reduction or the elimination of all of the risk factors for atherosclerosis.

An elevated serum cholesterol level is considered by some investigators to be the primary culprit in atherosclerosis. Some families have an autosomal dominant genetic condition called familial hypercholesterolemia. Patients who are homozygous for the gene have serum cholesterol levels as high as 1,000 mg/dl and have severe coronary and peripheral atherosclerosis in childhood and adolescence. Heterozygous individuals have a serum cholesterol level that ranges from 300 to 500 mg/dl. They also have premature and severe atherosclerosis. Homozygous individuals are only about one per million and heterozygous only about 2% of the U.S. population, however.

Thus, the atherosclerosis epidemic is not the result of an unalterable genetic disorder but is the consequence of an atherogenic lifestyle that can be altered. It has been recently shown that chronic mental and emotional stress can elevate cholesterol. Numerous epidemiological and population studies, human trials of dietary intervention, and experimental animal investigations have shown the high causative correlation between an elevated serum cholesterol and atherosclerosis. Cholesterol can be lowered below the recommended 200 mg/dl by weight loss and by reducing the consumption of animal fats that contain cholesterol and of saturated fats in general. It is now well documented that one of the lipoproteins that carry cholesterol in the blood, high-density lipoprotein (HDL), has an opposite and protective effect by scooping up circulating cholesterol and bringing it to the liver for degradation. HDL cholesterol can be raised by frequent exercise and by the judicious moderate daily drinking of alcoholic beverages.

Hypertension can be lowered by weight loss, exercise, and a diet low in salt. When these natural measures are not successful, or while they are being undertaken, aggressive control of the elevated blood pressure with medication is indicated. Few are the individuals who cannot attain blood pressure control by a combination of interventions.

Most adult-onset diabetic patients have their metabolic disease because of obesity. Weight reduction significantly lowers serum glucose levels in these patients, even to normal levels. It is still controversial whether obesity by itself is an independent risk factor. There can be no argument, however, that obesity has a causative relation with all of the atherosclerotic risk factors—except for smoking. The smoking of cigarettes doubles the risk of coronary heart disease. Beyond being a causative factor for atherosclerosis, it may constitute an additional separate risk for myocardial infarction. The reduction of risk for infarction may be an astounding 50% within only 1 year after complete smoking cessation.

Multiple studies have shown that exercise, through many mechanisms, results in reduced atherosclerosis and in a lower risk of clinical events if atherosclerosis is already present. Coronary heart disease, however, is usually first treated with medications. The medical therapy of stable angina pectoris is based on an understanding of its pathophysiological basis: ischemia from an increased metabolic demand that cannot be met by a fixed supply. Pharmaceutical intervention has as its goal the reduction or prevention of that ischemia through two main pharmacological means: an increased supply of blood to the heart muscle and a decreased demand of the heart muscle for that blood. These desired effects are accomplished by the three principal classes of cardiac pharmaceutical agents: nitrates, beta-receptor blockers, and calcium channel blockers.

Nitrates are vasodilators. They exert their beneficial effects by dilating coronary arteries directly, thus increasing blood flow to the heart muscle. They also dilate peripheral veins, resulting in the peripheral pooling of blood, with a subsequent reduction in blood return to the heart, with less stress on the heart wall, and finally a decreased need for oxygen. Beta-receptor blockers reduce oxygen demand by lowering the heart rate, or chronotropy, and are termed negative chronotropic agents. Calcium channel blockers combine the effects of the nitrates and the beta-blockers. Most of the calcium channel blocker agents now commercially available have both vasodilatory and negative chronotropic properties.

Most patients with a stable angina pectoris syndrome can have their angina controlled and their functional impairment and disability eradicated or significantly reduced with the use of one of these agents alone or with some combination of all three. Unless a contraindication exists, patients with coronary heart disease, and also perhaps asymptomatic individuals with atherosclerosis risk factors, should take low-dose prophylactic daily aspirin.

Patients with unstable angina pectoris require immediate hospitalization because they are at a high risk for an acute myocardial infarction. The treatment of unstable angina is based on an understanding of its pathophysiological basis: An unstable atherosclerotic plaque that creates a substrate for new thrombus formation and artery spasm, which in turn may result in total vessel occlusion and heart muscle death. Treatment with intravenous heparin is directed at the inhibition of further thrombus formation. Treatment with intravenous nitrates aims to reduce and prevent arterial spasm.

Patients with an acute myocardial infarction should receive immediate intravenous thrombolytic therapy with either streptokinase or tissue plasminogen activator (TPA). The prompt breaking up of the occluding thrombus results in restoration of blood flow. If this is done within the first hour or two after the onset of symptoms there is considerable myocardial salvage. The earlier these agents are administered, the greater is the rescue of heart muscle and the patient's chance of survival.

Nonmedical therapy of coronary heart disease is percutaneous transluminal coronary angioplasty (PTCA) and coronary artery bypass grafting (CABG). About an equal number of these procedures (about 250,000) are now performed in the United States yearly. Several randomized studies comparing the efficacy of each treatment are currently under way and preliminary reports indicate no clear superiority of one treatment modality over the other. In PTCA, a balloon-tipped catheter is introduced through a peripheral artery and then manipulated around the aortic arch and inserted into the coronary artery that has the occluding atheroma. The balloon inflation causes an increase of the overall vessel diameter and increased blood flow by the process of atheroma fracture and compression and by stretching of the vessel wall. The initial success rate is now greater than 90%, but restenosis occurs at a rate of about 25% within 1 year of the procedure. The recent development of stents—cylindrical rigid metal devices that are placed within a coronary artery at the site of an angioplasty—has decreased the frequency of post-PTCA restenosis.

In CABG, saphenous veins from the legs (or an internal mammary artery from inside the chest wall) are used as conduits to restore blood flow by bypassing the site of the atherosclerotic plaque. CABG is performed at present with an operative mortality rate approaching only 1%. More than 90% of operated patients achieve total or significant symptom relief. Progressive atherosclerotic occlusion of the vein grafts, through the same process that affected the native coronary arteries, is likely to occur within 10 years of surgery if the treated individuals do not change their lifestyles to reduce the risk factors for atherosclerosis.

Both procedures are indicated in the patients with stable angina pectoris who cannot obtain symptom relief with medical therapy. Emergency PTCA should also be performed when medical treatment alone does not appear to arrest ongoing cardiac muscle damage in unstable angina or in acute myocardial infarction. Bypass surgery is indicated, regardless of symptoms, in patients who are found, by coronary angiography, to have significant disease of the main left coronary artery segment or to have severe triple-vessel disease, especially if they have impaired left ventricular function. Several studies have shown improved survival with surgical (compared to medical) therapy in these patient subgroups with more extensive coronary heart disease.

Newer alternative revascularization techniques include removal of the coronary atheroma by mechanical excision (coronary atherectomy) or by ablation using laser energy (laser angioplasty). Both procedures are considered experimental, but they hold great promise because both may supplant the major surgical procedure of coronary artery bypass surgery and solve the problem of restenosis in coronary angioplasty. Perhaps the most recent significant development in the management of coronary heart disease is the evidence that coronary atherosclerosis is reversible (Blankenhorn, Aulaupovic, Wickhan, Chin, & Azen, 1990). It has now been convincingly shown by coronary angiography studies that coronary atherosclerosis can be reversed by lowering cholesterol with lipid-lowering agents or with changes in lifestyle (Ornish et al., 1990).

The major determinants of prognosis in coronary heart disease are the extent and severity of the coronary atherosclerosis and of the ventricular dysfunction. Coronary artery disease can be best diagnosed and evaluated by exercise stress tests and by cardiac catheterization with coronary angiography. Echocardiography and nuclear ventriculography can assess the ventricular function. The lower the left ventricular ejection fraction (the percentage of blood in the left ventricle ejected with each heart beat, normal being 50% or higher), the worse the prognosis.

Even though the atherosclerotic epidemic still rages, there has been a significant decline in the age-adjusted mortality from all cardiovascular diseases over the past 20 years. The death rate from myocardial infarction alone declined by about 30% during the 1980s. This reduction in mortality is partly accounted for by the creation of hospital coronary care units, the development of sophisticated diagnostic tools, and the advances in medical and surgical therapies. Most of the reduction is the result of changes in lifestyle, however (Goldberg, 1989).

Psychological and Vocational Implications

There is an undisputed relationship between coronary heart disease and psychological disorders. Psychological disorders are definite contributors to atherosclerosis and the clinical syndromes of coronary artery disease. In turn, the diagnosis and treatment of coronary heart disease may create or worsen psychological disorders (Ben-Sire & Eliezer, 1990).

The mechanisms whereby psychological disorders cause or accelerate coronary atherosclerosis have not been well defined. Psychosocial stresses result in increased sympathetic nervous system activity, however, with a greater release of circulating catecholamines (epinephrine and norepinephrine). These, in turn, lead to elevated heart rates, elevated systemic blood pressures, and elevated cholesterol levels and also perhaps to enhanced platelet aggregation and thrombus formation. High catecholamine levels also lower the triggering threshold for ventricular arrhythmias.

Recent primate experiments appear to indicate that atherosclerotic vessels may respond with vasoconstriction when the experimental subjects are exposed to several psychosocial stresses (Williams, Vita, Manuck, Selwyn, & Kaplan, 1991). Moreover, far too many individuals in our society respond to mental or emotional stress by resorting to the immediate oral gratification of smoking or overeating. The poor dietary habits, with the wrong quality and quantity of foods, lead indirectly through obesity—and directly through elevated cholesterol, sugar, and salt intake—to a worse atherosclerosis risk profile.

More specifically, several studies have shown that emotional or mental stress precedes the clinical manifestations of coronary heart disease (Appels, 1990). There seems to be a positive correlation between an exacerbation of anxiety or of depression just before the onset of the symptoms of stable angina and of unstable angina, and prior to the occurrence of both fatal and nonfatal myocardial infarction and of sudden electrical death (Rosengren, Tibblin, & Wilhelmsen, 1991). Psychiatric patients with previously diagnosed depression have been shown to have a much greater mortality from coronary heart disease than the general population. Social isolation, both of individuals and of large populations, seems to result in higher rates of sudden death.

Over the past 30 years perhaps the most studied relationship between the mind and the heart has been Type A behavior. Excessive drive, competitiveness, an exaggerated sense of time urgency, and free-floating hostility characterize this behavior. The earlier data seemed to support the thesis that such behavior was a significant independent risk factor for coronary heart disease. Then over the past decade, several major studies found no correlation. One investigation even suggested that Type A behavior may confer a survival advantage by reducing the death rate in survivors of myocardial infarction. Recently, a consensus seems to be developing that the subset of patients with Type A behavior who show cynical hostility and suppressed anger may be the only ones at risk for coronary disease (Hartel & Chambless, 1989). The conflicting findings may be a consequence of the differing methods (self-administered questionnaires, structured interviews, videotaped observation of subjects) used in defining the behavior and evaluating the individuals who display it. The issue remains controversial (Evans, 1990).

Coronary heart disease leads to psychological distress and the development of psychiatric symptoms (Cone, Taylor, & Wiman, 1991). Denial, a useful defense mechanism in some circumstances, may be injurious when it leads to self-destructive behavior—such as a delay in getting to the hospital after the first symptoms of a myocardial infarction. Denial is an acute adaptive and beneficial reaction during hospitalization, but when chronic it can be maladaptive and detrimental because it may lead to noncompliance with prescribed medical therapy or risk factor modification (Ladwig, Kieser, Kronig, Breithardt, & Borggrefe, 1991). Anxiety, as both an appropriate response and as an inappropriate one when excessive, is seen during most diagnostic cardiac procedures from the most innocuous, such as echocardiography, to the most tedious and dangerous, such as electrophysiology testing.

An additional interface of psychological disorders and coronary heart disease occurs with the presentation of primary psychiatric disorders as cardiac disease when no cardiac disease exists. Such cardiac presentations are most commonly seen in patients who carry psychiatric diagnoses of hypochondriasis, chronic depression, and chronic anxiety. It is of interest that whereas in the United States anxiety disorders have a prevalence of about 10% in the population, a higher percentage of patients with anxiety disorders consult cardiologists. Specifically, patients with panic attacks are frequent visitors to emergency rooms and the offices of cardiologists. These patients can have many of the symptoms of an acute myocardial infarction: chest pain, palpitations, shortness of breath, dizziness, nausea, sweating, and a sense of impending doom. Many of them are treated erroneously, as if they had coronary heart disease. Indeed, as many as a third of all patients with chest pain syndromes referred for diagnostic coronary angiography who are found to have normal coronary arteries have a panic attack syndrome.

Coronary heart disease has significant vocational implications. Coronary heart disease causes more economic loss in the United States than any other disease or disorder. Millions of Americans are unemployed or underemployed because of the effects of coronary heart disease. The vocational counselor should consider, however, the magnitude of the problem in the context of the fact that the energy requirements of work have decreased in industrialized countries in this century. This is a result of the mechanization, automation, and computerization of labor. In 1950, 65% of all work was considered heavy labor, in 1990 only 5% was.

Therefore, through creative vocational counseling, if the economy and the job market allow, many now unemployed cardiac patients could rejoin the work force. The vocational counselor should take into account the individual's cardiac diagnosis; his or her functional capacity as determined by a careful history, personal observation, and the results of the exercise stress test; and an occupational history that incorporates physical, mental, emotional, and environmental job requirements. Whenever possible, the functional status should be expressed as an NYHA class.

Both the exercise tolerance on the stress test and the energy costs of work or other physical activities should be expressed in metabolic equivalents (METs). One MET is defined as the amount of oxygen consumed by an awake individual at rest. It is equivalent to 3.5 cc of oxygen per kilogram of body weight per minute. Stages of exercise and many vocational and recreational activities have been traditionally classified in terms of how many METs or multiples of the resting oxygen consumption are required by the activity. By the use of this method, results of the exercise stress test can be translated, though not precisely, to the level of exertion at work that the individual may safely perform.

Rates of return to work after a cardiac event or procedure have a wide range of 35% to 95% (Shanfield, 1990). Factors associated with a lower likelihood of reemployment are severity of the cardiac condition; older age of the patient; a lower salary, social class, or educational level; coexisting psychological conditions; and a family environment that is either not supportive or too protective. After a myocardial infarction men return to work at a rate of about 75% (Abbott & Berry, 1991). Women have a lower rate of reemployment (Hamilton, 1990). Surprisingly, the rate for patients after coronary bypass surgery is lower at about 60% (Rogers et al., 1990). This is paradoxical because 100% of patients have a reduced myocardial function after an infarction, and 90% of patients have improved myocardial blood flow after bypass surgery. The explanation appears to be that a greater number of patients will perceive themselves as disabled, even though they are not, after heart surgery than after a heart attack. PTCA, perhaps because it is a less traumatic and dramatic intervention than CABG, appears to result in a higher rate of return to work, as high as 90% in patients who are asymptomatic after the procedure (Allen, Fitzgerald, Swank, & Becker, 1990).

Formal rehabilitation programs with a multidisciplinary approach that incorporate supervised exercise, education, and nutritional and psychological counseling are increasingly proving to be beneficial in many aspects (Squires, Gerald, Miller, Allison, & Lavie, 1990). They provide an excellent environment for the effective modification of atherosclerotic risk factors, they improve psychological status, they increase rates of return to work. Moreover, several recent meta-analytic studies (in which data from similar randomized controlled studies are pooled and analyzed) indicate a secondary-prevention (the avoidance of a subsequent cardiac event) benefit of increased survival and decreased cardiovascular complications (O'Connor et al., 1989).

THE PERICARDIUM

The pericardium is the sac that contains the heart. It helps to fix the heart inside the thorax, protecting it from excessive movement. It prevents direct contact with other organs in the chest, reducing friction during constant cardiac motion. It perhaps slows the spread of infection to the heart from other organs such as the lungs. Lack of a pericardium is quite compatible with life, however, and if removed, there are usually no clinical consequences.

Disease Description

The most common pericardial disease is pericarditis, or inflammation of the pericardium. This can be caused by infections with tuberculosis, bacteria, or viruses. Other causes are trauma, metabolic or autoimmune diseases, and adverse reactions to medications. Pericarditis can result in the accumulation of fluid, within the two layers that make up the pericardium, termed pericardial effusion. When severe, it may result in cardiac tamponade—a choking of the heart that prevents its proper filling and emptying and may result in death. Tumors in the pericardium, there either by adjacent spread or by metastasis from a distant site, can also cause pericardial effusion. Months after the acute episode of pericarditis, some patients, especially those with tuberculous pericarditis, may develop chronic constrictive pericarditis. As the inflamed pericardium heals, it scars, contracts, and constricts the heart, resulting in a condition similar to cardiac tamponade. The pericardium can be best visualized, and pericardial diseases diagnosed and evaluated, with echocardiography.

Function and Disability

Functional impairment and disability are usually not considerations in individuals with acute pericarditis because it is a short, limited process without sequelae. The most common symptom in the individual with acute pericarditis is chest pain, quite similar to that of angina pectoris. But it is usually the so-called pleuritic kind because, just as with inflammations of the pleura (the lining of the lungs), the pain comes about at rest, is of a sharp quality, and is worsened by motion, breathing, or coughing. Cardiac tamponade's main symptoms are similar to those of congestive heart failure. Chronic constrictive pericarditis presents with symptoms similar to tamponade, but its time course is more insidious. The patient may be ill for months, even years, and may appear emaciated, as if suffering from terminal cancer.

Functional impairment and disability in chronic constrictive pericarditis are similar to those of myocardial failure, with the notable exception that in chronic pericarditis the complete elimination of the functional impairment or disability may be possible by surgical excision of the constricting pericardium.

Treatment and Prognosis

The treatment of acute pericarditis is the direct treatment of the underlying disease causing the inflammation or infection. The threatening fluid of pericardial effusion or cardiac tamponade can be removed by inserting a small needle in the pericardial space. This procedure is called pericardiocentesis. A persistent or recurrent pericardial effusion of physiological import can be eradicated by the definitive curative procedure of surgical resection of the pericardium. This is also the treatment for chronic constrictive pericarditis. Great care must be taken that a patient with constrictive pericarditis not be medically managed as if ventricular failure was present. Such treatment may cause fluid depletion and dehydration and further decrease cardiac output, which will worsen symptoms and even lead to death.

Prognosis for patients with pericarditis is excellent; it depends on the nature of the condition causing the pericardial inflammation. Proper management of the acute condition, prompt recognition and drainage of pericardial fluid, and correct diagnosis and management of chronic constrictive pericarditis should result in a normal life span.

Psychological and Vocational Implications

The psychological and vocational implications of pericardial disease are not well studied or described. This is mainly because pericardial disorders are neither common nor chronic. The most usual psychological manifestation is the anxiety provoked by the pain of pericarditis because it is confused by the patients, their families, and even by health professionals, with the ischemic pain of angina or of an acute myocardial infarction. This situation is particularly devastating because the majority of patients with viral or traumatic pericarditis are young people. Patients with chronic constrictive pericarditis often suffer from clinical chronic depression. Their vocational evaluation should include both physiological and psychological factors.

THE MYOCARDIUM

The myocardium is the heart muscle itself. It is divided into the left ventricle and the right ventricle. The left ventricle receives oxygenated blood from the lungs, via the left atrium, and then pumps that blood to the body, via the aorta and its branches. The right ventricle receives deoxygenated blood from the body, via the right atrium, and then delivers that blood to the lungs for reoxygenation, via the pulmonary artery.

Disease Description

Diseases of the myocardium are termed cardiomyopathies. There are three anatomical and physiological categories of cardiomyopathies: dilated (an enlarged heart with a thin or normal-thickness muscle wall), hypertrophic (a normal-size or only slightly enlarged heart with a thick muscle wall), and restrictive (a normal-size heart with a thick or normal muscle wall of increased rigidity). The cardiomyopathies are best diagnosed and evaluated with echocardiography.

In the United States dilated cardiomyopathies are usually caused by alcoholism, diabetes, and, principally, by coronary heart disease (ischemic cardiomyopathy). Another cause of dilated cardiomyopathy is inflammation of the myocardium, or myocarditis. This is most frequently caused by a viral infection and unfortunately occurs in young individuals. Some cardiomyopathies that were previously deemed idiopathic, or of unknown cause, are probably viral in origin.

Hypertrophic cardiomyopathies are most often the result of chronic untreated or improperly treated elevated blood pressure, or hypertension. These myopathies secondary to pressure overloads usually result in a symmetrical or concentric type of hypertrophy. A different type, asymmetric hypertrophy, which includes idiopathic hypertrophic subaortic stenosis (IHSS), has an unknown etiology, is often familial, and is associated with sudden death in young people.

Restrictive cardiomyopathies are the least common in the United States. The infiltration or deposition of extraneous material in the heart muscle causes them. In the case of patients with metabolic diseases or multiple blood transfusions, iron is an example of such extraneous material, as is amyloid in the case of those with chronic infections.

Function and Disability

The major determinant of impaired function and disability in myocardial disease is the degree of myocardial dysfunction. All of the cardiomyopathies, by definition, entail myocardial dysfunction. In dilated cardiomyopathies there is impaired ventricular contraction, or systole. In the hypertrophic and restrictive cardiomyopathies the initial dysfunction is in ventricular relaxation, or diastole. In their advanced stages, the latter two myopathies may also exhibit systolic dysfunction and cardiac dilation and may progressively begin to resemble, anatomically and physiologically, a dilated cardiomyopathy. All of the cardiomyopathies may create a decreased cardiac blood output state that is insufficient to meet the metabolic needs of the peripheral tissues. This altered physiological state is called congestive heart failure. Congestive heart failure is usually the pathophysiological endpoint of most cardiovascular diseases because eventually the myocardium is affected. Therefore, whether the initial disorder originated in the coronary arteries or in the cardiac valves or whether it was the result of a systemic condition such as diabetes or hypertension, it is myocardial failure that produces the symptoms that determine functional capacity and disability.

The decreased blood flow in congestive heart failure signals the kidneys to retain fluid. When the excess fluid accumulates in the lungs, it causes the most common symptom of heart failure: difficult breathing, or dyspnea. In the beginning stages of heart failure, when there is only mild impairment, dyspnea occurs only with significant exertion. As the condition becomes more severe and the ventricular function deteriorates, the dyspnea may occur with minimal effort and even at rest. When dyspnea occurs while the patient is lying down, it is termed orthopnea; when it suddenly wakens a patient, it is called paroxysmal nocturnal dyspnea. The excess fluid may also cause abdominal distension, or ascites. It may cause the liver to be enlarged, a condition called hepatomegaly. The fluid deposition in the legs, which usually begins about the ankle area, is termed edema. The symptoms of weakness, fatigue, and lethargy indicate even more severe heart failure and reflect a greatly decreased cardiac blood output.

Functional impairment and disability are best defined by placing a patient in an NYHA class. This can be done by a careful interview, with special attention given to the patient's daily activities. Treadmill exercise stress testing can be useful in determining functional capacity in patients with cardiomyopathies and are of greatest help in those with dilated cardiomyopathies. They are not particularly useful in patients with restrictive cardiomyopathies because often their primary disease is the major contributor to their functional impairment and disability. Moreover, it must be specifically emphasized that patients with ideopathic hypertrophic subaortic stenosis (IHSS) should not (as a rule with occasional exceptions) undergo exercise stress testing. In the natural history of their disease, these individuals can have syncope and sudden death with exercise. To exercise them on purpose is a risk. This is particularly true if their intraventricular obstruction to blood flow is physiologically significant.

For the assessment of functional capacity in the patient with a dilated cardiomyopathy, a gentler exercise test using the Modified Bruce or the Bensen protocols is recommended. Before the test, it should be absolutely determined by interview and careful physical exam that the individual does not have active or decompensated congestive heart failure. Particularly useful and informative in these patients are exercise tests that use imaging of ventricular function such as nuclear ventriculograms or echocardiograms. The patient's ventricular function, including global ejection fraction and segmental wall motion, at rest and with exercise, can be easily, objectively, and safely determined with both techniques. Individuals whose ventricular function worsens with exercise are evidently more functionally limited and more likely to be disabled.

It is of great interest that a low left ventricular ejection fraction at rest, without question the best predictor of prognosis in any cardiovascular disorder, may not be predictive of functional capacity. Some patients with ejection fractions below 30% can have a normal exercise tolerance, whereas some patients with normal ejection fractions of greater than 50% can have a markedly reduced exercise tolerance. This seeming paradox is accounted for by the differing peripheral adaptations in different individuals. Those with higher exercise tolerance and greater functional capacity are more physically fit individuals because of their more efficient skeletal musculature and greater oxygen extraction capability.

Treatment and Prognosis

In the medical management of the patient with myocardial failure it is important to consider first the elimination of any conditions that might have helped to precipitate the failure. Such conditions may be internal stresses (e.g., anemia, fevers, infection, rhythm disturbances, and thyroid disorders) or they may be environmental stresses (e.g., high altitudes or excessive heat or cold). After such contributing factors are eradicated, therapy is aimed at creating the optimal hemodynamic milieu for myocardial function. This milieu can be best created by positively intervening in three components of myocardial mechanics and of congestive heart failure pathophysiology. This is accomplished by increasing inotropy, or myocardial contractility; by decreasing preload, or diastolic ventricular volume; and by decreasing afterload, or the stress or tension of the heart muscle wall during the ejection of blood. By improving one of the three, the two others are also improved.

Specific treatment includes nitrates to directly decrease preload, diuretics to eliminate excess fluid and indirectly reduce preload, digitalis to directly increase inotropy, and after-load reducing agents such as direct vasodilators or angiotensin converting enzyme (ACE) inhibitors. Most patients are also advised to restrict their salt intake because excessive dietary salt will cause fluid retention. There is no definite cure for myocardial failure other than complete cardiac transplantation. Patients referred for cardiac transplantation are those who prove refractory to the best possible combination of medical therapy and are in an NYHA Class IV functional status. Without transplantation, some of these individuals may have as high as a 90% 1-year mortality. This mortality is to be compared to the survival rates of transplantation, which are currently about 85% in 1 year and about 70% in 3 years.

The prognosis of patients with cardiomyopathies depends on the kind of cardiomyopathy and the degree of myocardial dysfunction and congestive heart failure present. Patients with a dilated cardiomyopathy have the worst average prognosis of all cardiomyopathies. Within that group, the individuals with the ischemic cardiomyopathies fare the worst. As a general rule, the worse the ventricular function, as assessed by resting left ventricular ejection fraction, the worse the prognosis and the greater the likelihood of death from end-stage congestive heart failure, cardiovascular collapse, and shock. Rheumatic fever, a result of the body's immune response against a streptococcal infection, can result in both valvular insufficiency and valvular stenosis or "tight" valves. With the introduction of penicillin and other antibiotics, the incidence of rheumatic heart disease, and of valvular disease in general, has progressively and significantly decreased over the past half-century. This decrease, at the same time that coronary atherosclerosis was on the increase, has limited endocardial and valvular disease to less than 10% of all cardiovascular disease. Valvular heart disease is best diagnosed and evaluated with echocardiography and intracardiac Doppler studies.

Mitral stenosis, with very few exceptions, is always secondary to rheumatic heart disease. About 70% of patients with mitral stenosis are women. Even though the left ventricle is usually normal in mitral stenosis, symptoms similar to those of congestive heart failure, such as dyspnea and orthopnea, begin in these patients when they are in their 40's or 50's. The elevated pressures in the left atrium and the pulmonary vasculature that must be generated to force the blood through the stenotic mitral valve cause these symptoms. Complications of mitral stenosis such as arrhythmias can lead to symptoms of palpitations.

Mitral regurgitation is caused in 50% of cases by rheumatic fever. Pure rheumatic mitral regurgitation is more common in men than in women. Infective endocarditis, which preferentially attacks valves previously damaged by rheumatic disease, also leads to mitral regurgitation. Causative are also a variety of conditions that affect the supporting structures of the valve. There can be dilation or calcification of the mitral annulus, the ring-like orifice between the left atrium and ventricle that the valve occupies. Also there can be fibrosis of the papillary muscles, which through the netlike chordae tendinea, attach the valve leaflets to the left ventricle. A unique disease entity of the mitral valve is the mitral valve prolapse syndrome. In this condition, the leaflets of the mitral valve prolapse into the left atrium during valve closure. Echocardiographic studies have suggested that the incidence of this condition may be about 5% in the female population.

Aortic stenosis may be caused by rheumatic fever, by degenerative calcification of the cusps, or by a congenital condition called bicuspid aortic valve. A bicuspid aortic valve is abnormal because it has two instead of three cusps. This abnormality, the most common congenital cardiac abnormality, occurs in about 2% of the population. In only a small portion of that group does this congenital condition result in clinical disease, however. As opposed to stenosis of the mitral valve, where mainly women are affected, about 80% of adult patients with aortic stenosis are men.

Aortic regurgitation is mainly rheumatic in origin, especially when found in combination with mitral valve disease. Nearly 80% of patients with pure aortic regurgitation are men. Women are the majority of those who have concomitant mitral disease. A bicuspid aortic valve can also become insufficient. An increasing incidence of aortic regurgitation is caused by infective endocarditis. Diseases that result in the dilation of the aorta itself may also dilate the aortic valve annulus and lead to secondary aortic insufficiency.

Disorders of the valves of the right side of the heart are far less common than those of the valves of the left side of the heart. Tricuspid stenosis is very uncommon and is usually secondary to rheumatic heart disease and found in association with disease of the other valves. Tricuspid insufficiency is more common than stenosis and results from either infective endocarditis in users of intravenous drugs or from right ventricular enlargement and accompanying tricuspid ring dilation. Of all valvular disorders, those of the pulmonic valve are the rarest. The most common pulmonic valve disorder is insufficiency secondary to pulmonary hypertension.

Function and Disability

The major determinant of impaired function and disability in endocardial disease is the severity of the valvular stenosis or insufficiency and the degree of secondary myocardial dysfunction. Valvular insufficiency and valvular stenosis both interfere with normal intracardiac blood flow. Valvular insufficiency leads to a volume overload and eventual dilation of the cardiac chambers. Aortic and pulmonic stenosis lead to a pressure overload and ventricular hypertrophy and atrial dilation. These overloads, if severe and if left untreated, will invariably lead to congestive heart failure. The time to onset of symptoms is related to the severity of the valvular lesion and also to the age and physical fitness of the individual. Most patients with mitral valve prolapse are asymptomatic. They can have the following symptoms, however: chest pain that has some of the features of angina pectoris, palpitations from both atrial and ventricular arrhythmias, and dyspnea when mitral regurgitation is present. In addition to the symptoms of congestive failure, patients with aortic stenosis can also have chest pain indistinguishable from angina pectoris and can also have sudden death as their only presentation.

Functional classification is similar to that of the patient with coronary heart disease or with a cardiomyopathy. If an appropriate functional history cannot be obtained, exercise stress testing is a good objective indicator of function in these patients. It should be noted, however, that exercise testing is relatively contraindicated in patients with mild to moderate mitral stenosis and aortic stenosis and absolutely contraindicated when the stenoses are severe. With exercise testing, those with mitral stenosis may develop acute pulmonary edema and those with aortic stenosis may have syncope.

Treatment and Prognosis

Treatment is the surgical replacement of the diseased valve with either a porcine (pig) valve or a metal valve prosthesis. The use of porcine valves is rapidly falling into disfavor because it is becoming evident that they may become dysfunctional about 10 years after implantation. Valves resulting in regurgitant lesions can at times be surgically repaired, rather than replaced, in what is essentially plastic surgery of the heart. Patients with valvular stenosis can have significant relief of their symptoms with valvuloplasty. This recently developed procedure, the dilation of the stenosed orifice with a balloon inserted through the peripheral vasculature, obviates the need for surgery.

The treatment of patients with mitral valve prolapse is mainly reassurance that they have a good prognosis. Medical treatment with beta-blockers may be necessary to treat symptoms of palpitations from their benign yet symptomatic arrhythmias. A mitral valve prolapse patient with significant mitral regurgitation, like all other patients with valvular disease or with prosthetic valves, should have antibiotic prophylaxis before dental work or before surgery to prevent acquiring endocarditis from the bacteremia (the introduction of bacteria into the blood) that may happen with such procedures.

The prognosis of patients with valvular heart disease is excellent as long as replacement, repair, or valvuloplasty is performed before there is damage to the ventricles, the atriae, or the pulmonary vasculature. Once the chronic volume or pressure overloads have irreversibly damaged these structures, the surgical mortality is markedly increased, from about 1% in uncomplicated cases to greater than 15% in those with failing ventricles. These unfortunate individuals have a decreased life span even if the surgery is successful and the prosthetic valve has perfect function. Severely dysfunctional cardiac valves, if not repaired or replaced, will lead to death within 5 years.

Psychological and Vocational Implications

In many respects, the psychological and vocational implications of endocardial and valvular heart disease are the same as those of the dilated cardiomyopathies, especially when secondary ventricular dysfunction exists. Unique psychological situations in the valvular diseases arise because many of the patients with rheumatic valvular disease are young women of child-bearing age. Often, some patients who are childless must make a decision as to whether to become pregnant even though pregnancy could worsen their cardiac condition and lead to a risk of death. At times, the stress-laden decision is not whether to become pregnant but whether to terminate an advanced wanted pregnancy. Psychological intervention and support is needed before, during, and particularly after the time of decision making. Patients with mitral valve prolapse present a difficult challenge to the psychologist. These individuals, with cardiac symptoms but with a good prognosis, are often disabled for psychological, not physiological reasons. A team approach, with the cardiologist, the psychologist, and other caregivers working together, is often more effective than an uncoordinated approach that often confuses the patient and results in further disabling distress.

Unique vocational implications exist with patients with valvular heart disease because this is the only group of cardiovascular diseases in which women constitute a majority. Patients with mitral valve prolapse and rheumatic mitral valve disease are often young women who have to care for a family and work outside the home in the context of their mitral disease. Surgical valve replacement often occurs in older women in their late 50's or early 60's who are near retirement age. Many do not return to work after the surgery. Many live alone because they have survived their husbands, who have already died from their own coronary heart disease. The rehabilitative and vocational challenges are great in this group of patients.

THE ELECTRICAL CONDUCTION SYSTEM

The cardiac conduction system, made of specialized fibers, has two functions. The main cardiac pacemaker, the sinus, or sinoatrial (SA) node, generates the rhythmic electrical impulse that is the basis of life. The other parts of the system include the atrioventricular (AV) node (the backup or auxiliary pacemaker), the bundle of His, the bundle branches, and the Purkinje fibers. They all ensure the sequential and uniform propagation of the electrical current so that the cardiac cycle of ventricular systole and diastole is an organized and effective activity.

Disease Description

Disorders of the electrical system can result in bradycardia (slow rates of less than 60 beats per minute), tachycardia (fast rates at greater than 100 beats per minute) or arrhythmias or dysrhythmias (irregular rhythms). Arrhythmias of a slow rate are brady-arrhythmias and those of a fast rate are tachy-arrhythmias. Dysrhythmias can be further classified as those with an abnormal current originating from the atriae, or supraventricular arrhythmias, or those with an abnormal origin in the ventricles, or ventricular arrhythmias. They are usually tachy-arrhythmias. Arrhythmias are best diagnosed and evaluated with resting ECGs, 24-hour ambulatory ECGs (Holler monitoring), exercise ECGs, and invasive electrophysiological studies.

Supraventricular arrhythmias are paroxysmal atrial tachycardia (PAT), atrial flutter, atrial fibrillation, and multifocal atrial tachycardia (MAT). Although the atrial rates vary, the ventricular rate in these arrhythmias, even if untreated, is generally relatively slow, about 150 beats per minute, because the impulses are slowed or blocked at the level of the AV node and the His bundle. MAT occurs mostly in patients with pulmonary disease. PAT can occur in normal persons without heart disease and is most commonly precipitated by anxiety or by the ingestion of irritants such as alcohol and caffeine. Atrial flutter and fibrillation happen in patients with atriae that are enlarged either because of ventricular dysfunction or mitral or tricuspid valvular disease. An overly active thyroid gland, or hyperthyroidism, may cause atrial fibrillation.

Ventricular arrhythmias are evident in ventricular tachycardia, and ventricular fibrillation. Ventricular tachycardia and fibrillation usually occur in patients with a dilated cardiomyopathy or a prior myocardial infarction. They are rare, but do occur, in people with normal ventricles.

A rare congenital anomaly of the conduction system occurs in the presence of an accessory pathway, an extra bundle with conduction properties akin to those of the conduction system. Such a bundle allows the electrical activity from the atriae to the ventricles to bypass the AV node and the bundle of His. Patients with these abnormalities, called preexcitation syndromes, are usually young, are prone to episodes of PAT, and can have very fast ventricular rates with atrial fibrillation. There are two types of preexcitation syndromes: Wolff-Parkinson-White (WPW) syndrome and Lown-Ganong-Levine (LGL) syndrome.

Cardiac electrical block is said to occur when either of the two cardiac pacemakers cannot generate a normal electrical impulse or when a normal impulse is not conducted correctly through the conduction system. Fibrosis of the conduction system, which is part of the aging process, is a cause of electrical blocks in the elderly. Most blocks, however, like most arrhythmias, are the result of coronary heart disease.

Function and Disability

The functional impairments and disabilities that result from the cardiac arrhythmias fall into two major categories. One is the physiologic disability from the ineffective ventricular contractions and decreased cardiac output that are secondary to a chronic arrhythmia that is too slow, too fast, or too disorganized. (Atrial fibrillation is the prototype and its symptoms place the functional considerations of this arrhythmia with those of congestive heart failure.) The other is the psychological disability secondary to an arrhythmia that is not chronic but acute. Such an arrhythmia is unpredictable. It arrives suddenly and without any warning. Ventricular tachycardia is the prototype. The individual may have no physiological functional limitation or disability with the activities of daily life yet may refrain from work because of the fear of precipitating the arrhythmia with activity.

Patients with supraventricular arrhythmias have palpitation as their most common symptom. PAT and atrial flutter are acute and not chronic arrhythmias and therefore have no functional or disability implications when they are not present. Those with atrial flutter or fibrillation may develop syncope or symptoms of congestive heart failure especially if they have the arrhythmias in the context of impaired ventricular function. Those with coexisting coronary artery disease may develop angina pectoris because the fast heart rates of the arrhythmias create metabolic demands that cannot be met by the compromised blood supply through the obstructed coronary arteries. Patients whose heart rate in atrial fibrillation is controlled at rest can still have exertional dyspnea, as in this condition the heart rate may rapidly increase with little exertion.

The chaotic atrial electrical activity of atrial fibrillation creates a combination of turbulence and stasis of blood in the atriae. This can lead to the complication of thrombus formation in the atriae. These thrombi can dislodge and be carried by the circulation to other parts of the body. Such a traveling thrombus, or embolus, may cause obstruction of blood flow to the eyes, leading to blindness, or to the kidneys, causing renal failure. When carried to the brain, it may result in cerebral infarction, or stroke.

If ventricular tachycardia is of a short duration (a few seconds), the patient may experience palpitation. If of a longer duration (a few minutes), syncope may occur. If sustained beyond a few minutes, degeneration to ventricular fibrillation is likely, and sudden death may ensue.

Individuals with the accessory pathway syndromes will experience palpitation when PAT is their acute arrhythmia. In them, atrial fibrillation, if of prolonged duration and of a very fast ventricular rate, may degenerate into ventricular fibrillation and lead to sudden cardiac death. The health professional should not be deceived into complacency because the patient looks young, healthy, and vigorous. Atrial fibrillation in a patient with a preexcitation syndrome is a dire medical emergency.

Severe bradycardias or high degrees of block, resulting in heart rates of less than 30 beats per minute, can cause fatigue and dizziness because of the decreased cardiac output, and the resultant diminished cerebral perfusion. When the effective rate is even slower or when the bradycardia is sudden in onset, syncope may occur.

Treatment and Prognosis

The treatment of supraventricular arrhythmias involves their prevention, their quick termination, or the prompt and effective control of their fast rate. Avoiding stressful situations and the ingestion of alcohol or stimulants such as caffeine and antihistamines can prevent supraventricular arrhythmias. If the initiation of the arrhythmia is not preventable, then it may be terminated, or its fast rate controlled, by medications that slow electrical conduction through the AV node such as digitalis, beta-blockers, and calcium channel blockers. Individuals whose atrial fibrillation is chronic or recurrent (paroxysmal atrial fibrillation) need to take such medications for life to control their heart rates. Most of them will also require lifelong anticoagulation with warfarin (Comedian) to prevent thrombus formation and embolization. If medication fails to abolish the arrhythmia or if the patient is severely ill because of angina pectoris, severe congestive heart failure, or shock, then prompt electrical cardioversion to a normal sinus rhythm is indicated.

The treatment of sustained ventricular tachycardia and of ventricular fibrillation should be prompt electrical cardioversion to a normal rhythm. Only younger individuals with normal ventricular function can tolerate sustained ventricular tachycardia. Ventricular fibrillation is not compatible with life. Antiarrhythmic agents to prevent these ventricular arrhythmias should be prescribed only by expert cardiologists who have evaluated the arrhythmia with invasive electrophysiological studies. It is no longer acceptable to treat such patients empirically, as these agents have been found to have a high proarrhythmic potential. In as high as 25% of the cases, they can precipitate the very arrhythmia they are supposed to prevent or even make it worse.

Patients with ventricular arrhythmias who do not respond to medical therapy may require surgical ablation of the myocardial focus from which the arrhythmia originates. Some, with recurrent episodes of ventricular fibrillation, may require the chronic implantation of an antiarrhythmia device, similar to a pacemaker, called an implantable automatic defibrillator, to deliver an electric shock whenever ventricular fibrillation occurs. The ultimate treatment of ventricular arrhythmias, however, lies in the prevention of coronary heart disease, which is present in about 80% of patients with malignant ventricular arrhythmias and sudden electrical death.

The treatment of patients with the preexcitation syndromes is similar to that of those with supraventricular arrhythmias. Great caution is needed when giving antiarrhythmic agents to these patients because a paradoxical effect may result, however, that is, the arrhythmia may be made worse and faster rates may obtain if agents that would normally control the arrhythmia or slow down its rate are administered. In patients whose arrhythmia is refractory to medical therapy or those who have the lethal trial fibrillation with a very rapid ventricular rate, ablation of the accessory pathway, possible nowadays by different techniques, is recommended.

Cardiac electrical blocks and symptomatic bradycardias are treated with the implantation of permanent pacemakers that substitute for the heart's own pacemakers and conduction system. In recent years, technology has led to the development of ever-more sophisticated and smaller pacing devices that nearly duplicate the heart's electrophysiological mechanisms and allow for nearly normal ventricular hemodynamics.

The prognosis for patients with supraventricular arrhythmias under appropriate medical care is excellent. Their mortality depends on the physiological cause of the arrhythmia rather than on the arrhythmia itself. For example, those with normal hearts or with hyperthyroidism have a much better prognosis than do those whose arrhythmias are complications of structural heart disease, such as mitral stenosis or myocardial dysfunction.

The prognosis for the patient who is a survivor of sudden death and who has recurrent episodes of ventricular fibrillation or ventricular tachycardia is dismal. This is particularly the case for those with a dilated cardiomyopathy and a left ventricular ejection fraction of less than 20%. This poor prognosis has been ameliorated by the practice of medical therapy guided by electrophysiolo-gieal testing, by the newer surgical techniques, and by the use of the implantable defibrillators.

The prognosis in patients with preexcitation syndrome is excellent because they usually have otherwise normal hearts. If the correct diagnosis is made and expert prompt treatment is rendered the few times it is needed, these individuals will have normal life spans. The prognosis of patients requiring pacemakers is excellent if the ventricular function is normal. If pacing was necessary because of severe coronary heart disease, however, then the prognosis is poor. These patients will die from myocardial disease or from a ventricular tachyarrhythmia with a normally functioning pacemaker in place.

Psychological and Vocational Implications

The psychological implications of cardiac arrhythmias are significant. Not only is the psychologist confronted with the psychological consequences of the arrhythmias, but perhaps more important, psychological disorders may trigger lethal arrhythmias.

As mentioned, a chronic depression or anxiety syndrome that may develop over time after repeated episodes of their sudden and unexpected tachyarrhythmias may disable patients with paroxysmal atrial fibrillation, PAT, and recurrent ventricular tachycardia and fibrillation. They may progressively and drastically curtail their range of activities as they associate the onset of their arrhythmias with particular events, places, or times. Phobias and a repertoire of superstitious behaviors may develop in many of these individuals. Intensive yet nonthreatening psychological interventions are often necessary.

Particularly difficult is the control and prevention of the psychological precipitants of the arrhythmias. It is well documented that about 1% of all patients with malignant ventricular arrhythmias have no demonstrable structural heart disease, and the only causative factor for their arrhythmia is psychological. An even greater percentage of patients with known heart disease have their potentially lethal arrhythmias triggered by psychological factors. A few medical centers specialize in the careful search and discovery of the precise feelings and the specific thoughts, ideas, or mental images that trigger the arrhythmias in a particular individual.

The judicious use of antiarrhythmic agents, in combination with beta-blockers and directed and focused psychological intervention, has proved quite successful in preventing or reducing the frequency of arrhythmias in such patients. The vocational implications of cardiac arrhythmias are also significant. The vocational counselor must undertake a careful evaluation of the work situation, with special attention given to any environmental, emotional, or mental stress that may precipitate or aggravate the arrhythmia.

DISEASES OF THE VASCULAR SYSTEM

The vascular system, also known as the peripheral vascular system, is responsible for the circulation of blood from the heart to the rest of the body and back again to the heart. Its components are the aorta, the arteries, the arterioles, the capillaries, and the veins. In this chapter, only diseases of the aorta will be considered. Disease of specific vessels and of the smaller vasculature will be covered in other chapters.

THE AORTA

The aorta, the largest artery in the body, receives the blood from the heart and then, through its branches, delivers that blood to the rest of the body. Because of its large size and its unique function as the receiving conduit for blood directly from the left ventricle, the walls of the aorta experience greater tension and stress than do other blood vessels. Therein lies the anatomical and physiological substrate for its diseases.

Disease Description

Arteriosclerosis develops in the aorta just as it does in the coronary arteries. Such is the extent of the process that nearly all adults in the United States are believed to have some measure of aortic arteriosclerosis. Even children and adolescents have been shown to have aortic fatty streaks, the earliest lesion of aortic arteriosclerosis. The vast majority of patients with clinical aortic disease are hypertensive men who smoke cigarettes. There are three main diseases of the aorta: aneurysms, dissections, and obstructive disease. Disease of the aorta and its branches are best evaluated by angiography. The new technique of transesophageal echocardiography (TEE) is particularly useful for the evaluation of diseases of the thoracic aorta.

An aortic aneurysm is an abnormal dilation of the aorta that is susceptible to acute rupture. Aneurysms can be found in the thoracic aorta (in both its ascending and descending segments) and also in the abdominal aorta. Ascending aortic aneurysms are the ones that are least likely to be caused by arteriosclerosis.

Before our age of antibiotics and organized prevention of sexually transmitted diseases, ascending aortic aneurysms were mainly caused by syphilis. At present the most common cause of ascending aneurysms is damage of the middle layer of the aortic wall, the media. This condition is termed cystic medial necrosis and is of unknown etiology. Aneurysms of the descending thoracic aorta and of the abdominal aorta are nearly all caused by arteriosclerosis. Many patients who have thoracic aneurysms also have abdominal aneurysms, and about 10% of those with abdominal aneurysms have more than one.

Aortic dissections can occur anywhere in the aorta. A dissection takes place when the innermost of the three layers of the wall of the aorta, the intima, breaks and allows blood to flow into the wall of the aorta itself. The pressure of the blood separates the layers of the aorta. Hypertension plays a significant role in aortic dissections regardless of their location. Surgeons categorize dissections into three types: Type I dissection involves the entire aorta, from its ascending portion, around the arch, and into the abdominal aorta; Type II dissection is limited to the ascending aorta; and Type III dissection is limited to the descending aorta. Aortic obstructive disease, like coronary artery obstructive disease, impedes the adequate flow of blood. Obstruction in the aorta is most frequently noted in its terminal portion, usually at its bifurcation into the iliac and femoral arteries, the vessels that supply the lower extremities.

Function and Disability

Most patients with aortic aneurysms and dissections are free of functional impairments and disability because they are asymptomatic until the moment of the acute event. Aortic aneurysms are most often found on routine abdominal physical exam or by x-rays. Symptoms, when they do exist, may be only those of a lower back pain syndrome. Some patients may actually have been misdiagnosed as having lumbar vertebral disease.

Obstructive aortic disease does cause disability and chronic functional impairment. The most common symptom is claudication. This is pain of one or both leg calves with walking. Patients may be able to walk only a few feet before disabling pain impedes further walking. They may also have pain of the thighs and buttocks with walking and at rest. They often have impotence. The functional capacity of patients with claudication and the degree of their vascular stenosis can be evaluated by Doppler ultrasound of the legs. This is performed before and after treadmill walking, using special test protocols different from those used for the evaluation of the impairment in coronary heart disease.

Treatment and Prognosis

The treatment of aortic aneurysms, of dissections, and of severe obstructive disease is always surgical. The acute rupture of an aortic aneurysm is nearly always a fatal event. When an abdominal aneurysm has a diameter of less than 6 cm, the probability of rupture is about 15% over a 10-year period, but if the diameter is 6 cm or greater, there is a 50% probability of rupture. The operative mortality of elective abdominal aneurysm resection is less than 10%. Resection of aneurysms of the ascending aorta or of the aortic arch carries a greater operative mortality. There is about a 20% mortality in the surgical treatment of aortic dissections. The surgical treatment of obstructive disease is aortic–femoral bypass grafting, using synthetic conduits to restore circulation to the legs. Excellent results are achieved with little mortality and morbidity, and claudication is abolished or decreased in about 90% of patients. As in coronary disease, an alternative treatment is percutaneous balloon angioplasty. This procedure is particularly feasible in discrete lesions of the iliac arteries.

The prognosis of patients with any type of arteriosclerotic aortic disease can be determined only in the context of their coexisting coronary artery arteriosclerosis. It is the extent and severity of that coronary disease that is the major determinant of both the operative mortality and of the long-term survival of patients who survived successful aortic surgery.

Psychological and Vocational Implications

There are usually no psychological implications in aortic disorders before the acute events of aortic aneurysm rupture and of aortic dissection because the patients are usually asymptomatic up to that time. Most of these patients had denied the potential consequences of their smoking or of their uncontrolled hypertension. The acute event has perhaps no match in all of medicine as a truly terrifying experience. Most survivors of the event, and the subsequent surgery, experience a reversal of their preevent psychological mind-set and become acutely aware of their mortality and may develop chronic depression and even excess anxiety and an overvigilant state. Such individuals can benefit from psychological intervention. A group of patients with a similar problem are those who are informed of the presence of an abdominal aortic aneurysm that is still too small to undergo surgical resection. They may spend months or even years in watchful waiting before surgery is finally indicated. Psychological implications in patients with obstructive aortic disease usually focus on their loss of self-esteem because of their inability to walk and work and principally because of impotence.

There are important vocational implications in aortic diseases. The patients who have had surgical repair of an aortic aneurysm or dissection have an even lower rate of return to work than do those who had coronary bypass surgery. This may be due to the advanced age of these patients, most of whom are in their 60's and 70's. It may also be because the surgical procedure that was performed on them is perceived as, and is in fact, more complex than coronary bypass surgery. Patients with occlusive disease have specific vocational considerations because they are unable to perform most work activity that entails walking. They may be employed in jobs that require the performance of arm work while sitting and only infrequent walking for short distances.

SUMMARY

The challenge of cardiovascular disorders will continue to grow as long as their prevention is not given emphasis and priority. If present trends continue, the diagnostic and therapeutic advances of the past decades may reduce cardiovascular mortality without a reduction of the prevalence of cardiovascular disease and its attendant functional limitation and disability. The need of individuals with cardiovascular disease for medical, psychological, rehabilitative, and vocational services may be greater than ever.

REFERENCES

Abbott, J., & Berry, N. (1991). Return to work during the year following first myocardial infarction. *British Journal of Clinical Psychology, 30,* 268–270.

Allen, J. K., Fitzgerald, S. T., Swank, R. T., & Becker, D. M. (1990). Functional status after coronary artery bypass grafting and percutaneous transluminal coronary angioplasty. *American Journal of Cardiology, 66,* 921–925.

Appels, A. (1990). Mental precursors of myocardial infarction. *British Journal of Psychiatry, 156,* 465–471.

Ben-Sira, Z., & Eliezer, R. (1990). The structure of readjustment after heart attack. *Social Science and Medicine, 30,* 523–536.

Blankenhorn, D. H., Aulaupovic, P., Wickhan, E., Chin, H. P., & Azen, S. P. (1990). Prediction of angiographic changes in native human coronary arteries and bypass grafts. *Circulation, 81,* 470–476.

Conn, V., Taylor, S. G., & Wiman, P. (1991). Anxiety, depression, quality of life, and self-care among survivors of acute myocardial infarction. *Issues of Mental Health in Nursing, 12,* 321–331.

Evans, P. D. (1990). Type A behavior and coronary heart disease: When will the jury return? *British Journal of Psychology, 81,* 147–157.

Goldberg, A. P. (1989). Aerobic and resistive exercise modify risk factors for coronary heart disease. *Medical Sciences and Sports, 21,* 669–674.

Hamilton, G. A. (1990). Recovery from acute myocardial infarction in women. *Cardiology, 77*(Suppl. 2), 58–70.

Hartel, U., & Chambless, L. (1989). Occupational position and type A behavior. *Social Sciences and Medicine, 29,* 1367–1372.

Ladwig, K. H., Kieser, M., Kronig, J., Breithardt, G., & Borggrefe, M. (1991). Affective disorders and survival after acute myocardial infarction: Results from the post-infarction late potential study. *European Heart Journal, 12,* 959–964.

O'Connor, G. T., Buring, J. E., Yusuf, S., Goldheber, S. Z., Olmstead, E. M., Paffenbarger, R. S., Jr., & Hennekens, C. H. (1989). An overview of randomized trials of rehabilitation with exercise after myocardial infarction. *Circulation, 80,* 234–244.

Ornish, D., Brown, S. E., Scherwitz, L. W., Billings, J. H., Armstrong, W. T., Ports, T. A., McLanahan, S. M., Kirkeeide, R. L., & Brand, R. J. (1990). Can lifestyle changes reverse coronary heart disease? The Lifestyle Heart Trial. *Lancet, 336,* 129–133.

Rogers, W. J., Coggin, C. J., Gersh, B. J., Fisher, L. D., Myers, W. O., Oberman, A., & Sheffield, L. T. (1990). Ten year follow-up of quality of life in patients randomized to receive medical therapy or coronary artery bypass graft surgery: The Coronary Artery Surgery Study (CASS). *Circulation, 82,* 1647–1658.

Rosengren, A., Tibblin, G., & Wilhelmsen, L. (1991). Self-perceived psychological stress and incidence of coronary disease in middle age men. *American Journal of Cardiology, 68,* 1171–1175.

Shanfield, S. B. (1990). Return to work after an acute myocardial infarction: A review. *Heart and Lung, 19,* 109–117.

Squires, R. W., Gerald, G. T., Miller, T. D., Allison, T. G., & Lavie, C. J. (1990). Cardiovascular rehabilitation: Status 1990. *Mayo Clinic Proceedings, 65,* 731–755.

Williams, J. K., Vita, J. A., Manuck, S. B., Selwyn, A. P., & Kaplan, J. R. (1991). Psychosocial factors impair vascular responses of coronary arteries. *Circulation, 84,* 2146–2153.

Chapter 9

Chronic Pain Syndromes

Andrew R. Block, Edwin F. Kremer, and
Craig C. Callewart

One of America's most significant health problems is chronic pain, that is, pain lasting 6 months or more. Approximately 30% of the U.S. population experiences such protracted painful conditions (Bonica, 1990). Frymoyer and Durett (1997) estimate that over $125 billion is expended annually on hospital and medical treatment of chronic pain. Approximately 50 million Americans are partially or totally disabled by chronic pain, with the disability lasting from weeks to permanently.

Chronic pain is associated with a tremendously wide variety of medical conditions and can affect every organ system in the body. The International Association for the Study of Pain has developed the *Classification of Chronic Pain* (Merskey & Bogduk, 1994), which lists literally hundreds of different chronic pain syndromes, divided by the body region affected: head, neck, shoulder and upper limbs, chest, abdomen, lower back, lower legs, pelvis, anal and genital region, and generalized syndromes (affecting more than three sites). With such a plethora of conditions it is obvious that no one chapter can hope to provide complete coverage. However, by examining some more common syndromes, much can be learned about the assessment and treatment of chronic pain in general.

INCIDENCE OF CHRONIC PAIN

Large-scale epidemiological research on chronic pain demonstrates several prevalent syndromes. The two most common syndromes are chronic back pain and headaches. Research by Von Korff, Dworkin, LeResche, & Kruger (1988) of HMO enrollees found that between 33% and 51% of participants reported an episode of significant back pain within a 6-month period. Generally, the incidence of back pain increased with age and was higher among women than among men. Others studies have shown similar (Walsh, Cruddas, & Connon, 1992) or slightly lower rates (Croft & Rigby, 1994). Headaches are even more prevalent than back pain. Migraine headache 1-year prevalence rates range from 12.9% to 17.6% in women and from 3.4% to 6.1% in men (see Stewart, Shechter, & Rasmussen, 1994, for a review). Tension-type headaches are even more frequent, occurring each year in up to 92% of women (aged 25–34) and 49% of older men (aged 55–64).

Several other pain syndromes occur with lesser but still significant frequency. Pain in the area of the temporomandibular joint, including the "jaw joint" and muscles of mastication, occurs in 3% to 10% of men and 6% to 15% of women, and prevalence rises with age (LeResche, Saunders, Von Korff, Barlow, & Dworkin, 1997). Abdominal pain has a 6-month prevalence rate of approximately 14% in 18–24-year-old men and 31% in women of that age group, decreasing to 7% among men and 12% among women aged 65 and older (Von Korff et al., 1988). Finally, a condition known as chronic widespread pain is also quite common. This condition is defined as pain of longer than 3 months duration, occurring in two contralateral quadrants of the body. When widespread pain is accompanied by tenderness to palpation in at least 11 of 18 specific physical sites, the syndrome is known as fibromyalgia. Wolfe, Ross, Anderson, Russell, and Herbert (1995) conducted a random survey of 3,006 individuals in Witchita, Kansas, and found that widespread pain was lowest in 18–29-year-old men (3%) and women (6%) and peaked among 60–69-year-old men (13%) and women (22.5%), dropping thereafter. Fibromyalgia rates were lower but still significant (7.4%) in women aged 70–79.

BIOPSYCHOSOCIAL MODEL OF CHRONIC PAIN

Each pain syndrome is unique, involving different body regions and underlying disturbed physical conditions (pathophysiology). These pathophysiological conditions provide the basis for the development of a multitude of psychological difficulties. It is now widely accepted that chronic pain is a biopsychosocial disorder (see Figure 9.1). The biopsychosocial model (Loesser, 1982) views nociception (the stimulation of pain receptors due to pathophysiology) as the ground on which other aspects of the pain experience are laid. Pain perception, suffering, and pain behavior can grow well beyond the initial pathophysiology, to encompass a great portion of the patient's life. Thus, patients may come to

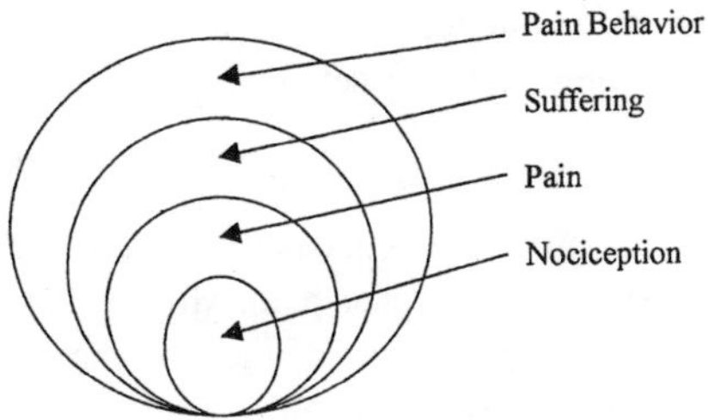

FIGURE 9.1 The biopsychosocial model of chronic pain (adapted from Loeser, 1982).

experience high levels of pain and display large amounts of pain behavior, even with minimal tissue damage.

The biopsychosocial model has significant implications for the evaluation and treatment of chronic pain. First, the model points to the importance of examining psychological factors associated with excessive pain behavior, emotional distress, and poor treatment. Further, the model implies that successful treatment of chronic pain focuses not only on ameliorating the pathophysiological condition underlying pain, but also must address the psychosocial sequelae of the protracted suffering.

LOW BACK PAIN

Chronic pain syndromes are extremely diverse, so no one chapter can provide adequate coverage of pathophysiological conditions (for comprehensive treatments of chronic pain, see Block, Kremer, & Fernandez, 1998; Bonica, 1990). To illustrate both the physical basis of chronic pain and the utility of the biopsychosocial model, the current chapter will examine two archetypal syndromes: low back pain and functional gastrointestinal pain.

One model for understanding the pathological anatomy of low back pain is termed the cascade of degeneration. The spinal column is composed of segments, each containing two adjoining bones, the vertebrae. The vertebrae are joined in front by a cartilaginous joint, the disc, and in back by two bony joints, the facets. Together these joints form a three-pronged connection, much like a stool with three legs. On the back or posterior side of the vertebra, bony protrusions known as spinous processes provide the location for muscular attachments. The muscles can move the vertebral bodies in order to twist, turn, and bend. Pain usually arises in the spine beginning with the front of the disc, and later involving the facets. It is this progression of derangement in the spinal column, beginning in the discs and proceeding to the facet, that has come to be known as the degenerative cascade.

Some spinal pain does not fit this model. There are numerous other causes, including cancer, visceral problems (e.g., pancreatitis), vertebral fractures, and some congenital conditions that can cause pain. Most spinal conditions, however, can be classified as derangements of one of the structures. Derangements in the front, or anterior, of the spine often begin as a prolapse or displacement of the internal gel-like substance. Known as disc herniation, this gel may directly compress peripheral nerves in the spinal column and cause back and lower extremity pain. Additionally, disc herniation often elicits an inflammatory response, producing more pain. Removal of the displaced gel, through a procedure known as discectomy, eliminates the compression of nerves and reduces the inflammatory response. In a discectomy procedure only the 5%–10% displaced portion will be removed, with the remaining stable portion left undisturbed. Laminectomy/discectomy represents the most common of surgical spinal treatments. Taylor, Deyo, Cherkin, and Kreuter (1994) report that of the approximately 280,000 spine surgeries performed in the United States during 1990, approximately 200,000 involved discectomy. Unfortunately, discectomy is not always successful, and the inflammation may persist for reasons poorly understood, becoming a contributor to back pain syndromes.

Sometimes the degenerative cascade continues, and the disc space diminishes in height, collapsing to rest on the two posterior facets. In turn, these facets can become painful because they are forced to carry a disproportionate load. If this occurs, the facets may enlarge in response to the increased mechanical stress and block the opening for nerves to exit the spinal column, leading to nerve root compression and pain. This process is known as stenosis. Its surgical treatment is more radical than a simple discectomy and involves removing part of the facet and part of the disc, in a procedure known as decompression. The goal is to free all compressed neural structures.

Finally, the degeneration may progress sufficiently that the normal alignment of the spine is disturbed. When the spine becomes misaligned in the forward or lateral planes, the condition is termed spondylolisthesis. If the spine is also twisted, the condition is known as scoliosis. As the vertebrae become misaligned, nerves in the spinal column are compressed or stretched. Surgery is performed to prevent further slippage or misalignment of the vertebrae. This is accomplished by surgically constructing a bridge between the vertebrae, in a procedure known as spinal fusion. To accomplish the fusion, bone is typically scraped from the pelvis and placed between the vertebral bodies. To correct alignment, hooks, screws, and/or rods are permanently implanted in to the spine. As the fusion develops, a mass of bone eventually grows over these implants.

The term "failed spine syndrome" is applied to the patient who continues to experience disabling pain symptoms despite surgical treatment. Various factors lead to failed spine syndrome, such as infection, vascular event, or damage to the neural structures during decompression. Additionally, sometimes the spinal fusion may fail to consolidate (much like concrete must set), causing pain. Inability to fully decompress the nerve is also a common cause of failure. Many patients develop failed spine syndrome as a result of inadequate postoperative rehabilitation. For many nonresponsive patients, it is the impact of psychosocial factors on pain that militates against recovery.

Only about 1% of back pain sufferers actually require surgery (Spitzer, 1987). Most recover with just 2–3 days of bed rest and antiinflammatory medication (Deyo, Diehl, & Rosenthan, 1986). However, a small proportion of patients are responsible for a great deal of difficulty in managing low back pain. Leavitt, Johnson, and Beyer (1971) found that 25% of patients with job-related injuries were responsible for 87% of total treatment costs. Similarly, Spitzer (1987) found that 7.4% of all industrial back claims were responsible for 86% of total costs. Many of these patients have no identifiable basis for pain (termed nonspecific low back pain) or have pathophysiology that could not be expected to respond to surgery. In such cases, patients frequently go on to be treated at multidisciplinary pain programs (see below). However, as is the case with the failed back surgery patient, the nonoperative back pain patient who fails to recover may also have significant psychosocial issues that influence both the perception of pain and its influence on behavior.

FUNCTIONAL GASTROINTESTINAL PAIN SYNDROMES

A very different type of chronic pain disorder is seen in patients with functional gastrointestinal pain syndromes, including irritable bowel syndromes (IBS), noncardiac chest pain (NCCP), and nonulcer dyspepsia (NUD). For most patients with these syndromes, pathophysiology is not evident (Crowell & Barofsky, 1998). These patients most frequently present to the physician with complaints of nausea, vomiting, bloating, altered bowel patterns, and most commonly, chronic intermittent pain. Research has shown that such patients may be hypersensitive to pain signals arising from the gut. For example, Barish, Castell, and Richter (1986) utilized balloon distention of the esophagus in patients with NCCP and found that distention caused pain in 56% of patients, compared with 20% of normal controls (see also Deschner, Maher, Cattau, & Benjamin, 1990). Similarly, Coffin, Azpiroz, Guarner, and Malagelada (1994) found that patients with NUD demonstrated greater sensitivity to balloon distention of the stomach than do normals, and patients with IBS are more sensitive than normals to distention of the colon (Whitehead et al., 1990) and of the small bowel (Moriarty & Dawson, 1982).

Research on functional gastrointestinal pain syndromes has demonstrated that such difficulties can be best explained by a reliance on the biopsychosocial model. That is, to fully appreciate these syndromes one must understand both the pathophysiological basis of the pain and the influence of psychosocial factors in magnifying and maintaining pain symptoms. The key to understanding the nociceptive process in gastrointestinal syndromes is an appreciation of the nature of pain receptors in the gut. Essentially, there are three types of receptors (see Crowell & Barofsky, 1998, for a more complete understanding). First, there are low-threshold intensity-coding neurons, which identify and send information about regulatory functioning and nonpainful stimulation of the gut to the brain. These fibers seem to provide important information from both the stomach and colon and show gradations in sensation and perception, from mild distention, to fullness, to intense pain. Second, there are high-threshold intensity-coding neurons, also known as dedicated nociceptors, that are activated only when the intensity of stimulation in the low-threshold receptors exceeds a predefined level, indicating actual damage to an organ. Finally, a third type of neuron, the silent nociceptor, is generally quiet, providing neither regulatory nor nociceptive information. However, the silent nociceptor can become activated through injury or inflammation and, once sensitized, can respond to even mild stimulation. Thus, the sensitized silent nociceptor can transmit pain signals in response to even normal regulatory activity in the gut and may provide the mechanism for persistent pain, even in the absence of identifiable pathophysiology.

Altered nociceptive input is only the beginning of a series of factors militating the maintenance of chronic gastrointestinal pain. As is the case with failed back pain patients, psychosocial factors may lead to misinterpretation of bowel pain signals. For example, Whitehead, Crowell, and Heller (1994) have shown that reinforcement of gastrointestinal symptoms in childhood is associated with IBS as an adult. Drossman et al. (1990) have shown that sexual and physical abuse in childhood is associated with the development and severity of gastrointestinal symptoms and negatively influences treatment outcome.

Generally, treatment of patients with functional gastrointestinal pain syndromes also follows from a biopsychosocial model, which recognizes that "psychosocial factors such as depression and anxiety may influence visceral perception through brain-gut neurotransmitters and modulate descending pathways to increase or decrease pain perception" (Crowell & Barofsky, 1998). The specific types of interventions used depend on the severity of the patient's symptoms. In mild cases, patients may benefit from educational efforts, reassurance, and dietary or medication changes. For patients with moderate symptoms, pharmacotherapy, relaxation exercises, biofeedback, and psychotherapy are often utilized. Patients with intractable symptoms are treated through a combination of social support;

realistic goal setting; changing expectations, to teach the patient to cope with pain as a long-term problem; and the elimination of unnecessary tests.

PSYCHOLOGICAL ASPECTS OF CHRONIC PAIN

The two archetypal syndromes of low back pain and functional gastrointestinal pain exemplify the diversity of the pathophysiological processes underlying pain. As research on both these and other pain syndromes make clear, it is the psychosocial aspects of each individual's case that influence, in large part, both pain perception and functional ability. This section details some of the psychosocial factors that occur in a broad range of chronic pain problems.

Emotional Aspects

Depression. All chronic pain syndromes can be associated with significant emotional disturbance. The most frequent emotional difficulty is depression. A widely cited study by Lindsey and Wyckoff (1981) found that up to 85% of chronic pain patients fit the diagnostic criteria for clinical depression. Depression, however, may have multiple roots in chronic pain patients. A study by Polatin, Kinney, Gatchel, Lillo, and Mayer (1993) found that up to 39% of chronic pain patients have a history of depression that predates the onset of pain. Therefore, the depression experienced by many chronic pain patients may be an exacerbation of a preexisting emotional difficulty. Further complicating consideration of the etiology of depression is the fact that there is a great overlap in many of the symptoms of depression and chronic pain, including sleep disturbance, impaired appetite, difficulty with concentration, and social withdrawal (Cavanaugh, Clark, & Gibbons, 1983). It therefore appears that depression and pain interact, leading a vulnerable patient into a downward spiral of emotional difficulty, decreased physical functioning, and consequent lowered self-esteem.

Anger. Another common emotional difficulty experienced by chronic pain patients is intense anger. Fernandez, Clark, and Ruddick-Davis (1998) report that 86% of outpatient chronic pain patients experience anger and that this anger is of greater intensity than that reported by age-matched pain-free individuals. This and subsequent research has found that the anger was directed primarily at the health care system and insurance companies. The target of the pain patient's anger is significant, for it may influence treatment outcome. DeGood and Kiernan (1996) found that chronic pain patients who placed blame for the injury on the employer had poorer pain treatment outcomes, as well as higher levels of mood disturbance, than those who did not make such attributions. Turk and Fernandez (1995) have suggested that patients who are angry, blame others for their difficulties, and are rebellious toward authority figures may respond more poorly to treatment because they fail to form a therapeutic alliance with the health care team.

Pain Sensitivity. The most problematic emotional factor associated with chronic pain is pain sensitivity (also known as somatization). It has long been felt that chronic, unremitting physical complaints, especially when associated with minimal identifiable physiological problems, are the result of psychological difficulties. Freud (Breuer & Freud, 1895) and neo-Freudians (Engle, 1959) consider that such protracted physical complaints arise from the conversion of unconscious psychological conflicts into physical symptomatology. Although there is little direct evidence to support such a contention (Gamsa, 1994), there is a converging body of evidence demonstrating that at least a large portion of chronic pain patients may be excessively sensitive to pain. First, research using the Minnesota Multiphasic Personality Inventory (MMPI) indicates that the most common personality profile for chronic pain patients involves elevations on the Hypochondriasis and Hysteria scales (Keller & Butcher, 1991), scales that assess disease conviction, sensitivity to physical symptoms, and denial of psychological problems (Graham, 1990). Patients with such MMPI profiles respond poorly to both conservative treatment for chronic pain (Klinke & Spangler, 1988), and surgical intervention (Block, 1996; Riley, Robinson, Geisser, Wittmer, & Smith, 1995). Second, controlled research has documented excessive pain sensitivity in chronic pain patients. Schmidt (1987; Schmidt & Brands, 1986), for example, subjected chronic low back pain patients to cold pressor tests (immersion of the forearm into an ice water bath). Results showed that the patients both reported higher pain levels and tolerated the ice water for a shorter period of time than did a control, nonpatient group. In our own laboratory we have found that MMPI Hysteria and Hypochondriasis elevations are associated with false-positive reports of pain in patients undergoing discography, a presurgical diagnostic test for disc herniation (Block, Vanharanta, Ohnmeiss, & Guyer, 1996). If chronic pain patients display such pain sensitivity, it is not surprising that their pain conditions should be so protracted.

Behavioral Factors

Beginning with Fordyce's (1976) pioneering text, *Behavioral Methods in Chronic Pain and Illness*, chronic pain has been conceptualized from a behavioral perspective. According to this approach, while chronic pain *sensation* arises from the nociception associated with a pathophysiological process, chronic pain *behaviors* may be maintained by reinforcement. That is, behaviors such as limping or groaning, disability from work, and decreased sexual activity lead to certain desirable consequences. For example, the spouse may bring the patient medication whenever pain is apparent. Similarly, a victim of a motor vehicle accident may receive financial compensation for prolonged pain. According to the behavioral perspective explored by Fordyce, such reinforcement is sufficient to maintain the pain "long after the original nociceptive stimulus has been resolved" (p. 59). Indeed, there appears to be some support for such speculations.

Spousal Reinforcement. The power to influence chronic pain behaviors rests perhaps most strongly with the patient's spouse or significant other. It is the spouse with whom the patient interacts most and the spouse who can provide the reinforcement for pain in addition to discouraging alternative well behaviors. Research in our laboratory has demonstrated that spousal reinforcement may strongly affect pain behaviors. In this study (Block, Kremer, & Gaylor, 1980), chronic pain patients were given a questionnaire assessing spousal reinforcement of pain behavior and were divided into high and low reinforcement groups. Patients with highly solicitous spouses reported higher pain levels in the presence of their spouse than in the presence of the ward clerk, whereas the opposite result obtained for patients with minimally solicitous spouses. This result demonstrated that the solicitous spouse could act as a discriminative stimulus for the patient to display an increase in pain behavior. More recent research has demonstrated that spouses who view themselves as solicitous may influence actual pain behavior (Lousberg, Schmidt, & Groenman, 1992). In the presence of such solicitous spouses patients show decreased walking time on a treadmill and have greater pain reports than do patients with nonsolicitous spouses (see also Romano et al., 1995).

Vocational Factors. Aspects of the patient's employment situation may act in a number of ways, both to maintain pain behavior and as a disincentive to recovery. First, vocational attitude may influence the onset of pain. A classic prospective study of 3,000 aircraft workers by Bigos et al. (1991) found that workers who reported a high level of job dissatisfaction were 2.5 times more likely to incur a job-related back injury than were workers who enjoyed their work. Once back pain occurs, patients who blame the employer for the original injury have been shown to have a higher level of mood disturbance and poorer outcome of treatment for chronic pain than do patients who place blame on other individuals, on themselves, or on no one in particular (DeGood & Kiernan, 1996). Finally, the occurrence of a job-related injury often is directly associated with at least some disincentives for improvement. Patients injured on the job frequently receive worker's compensation benefits, medical coverage for their injury, and at least partial replacement of lost wages if they are unable to work due to the injury. Patients receiving such worker's compensation payments have been found to have poorer outcome of treatment for pain (Davis, 1994; Hudgins, 1976), leading Frymoyer and Cats-Baril (1987) to conclude that "compensability" is one of the strongest predictors of excessive disability among chronic pain patients. It should be noted, however, that the factors in a worker's compensation case militating against recovery may not be as simple as mere financial disincentives.

R. Dworkin et al. (Dworkin, Handlin, Richlin, Brand, & Vannucci, 1985) examined the relationships among compensation, litigation, and employment status in chronic pain patients. Using a multiple regression analysis, these researchers found that poor treatment outcome was predicted only by length of time off work, not simply by worker's compensation status. Thus, the influence of financial disincentives for improvement in job-related injuries is complicated by the "deconditioning" (Mayer et al., 1987) that can occur when many patients are unable to work for protracted periods because of their pain.

Cognitive Factors

The behavioral model of chronic pain emphasizes the relationship between overt manifestations of pain (pain behaviors) and the response of others in the patient's environment to such behaviors. This model does not incorporate any aspects of the patient's thought process. An alternative approach, the cognitive-behavioral model, focuses on the influence of the patient's *beliefs* about pain and *coping strategies* for dealing with pain. According to this model, such cognitive factors can serve to either minimize or magnify the impact of pain on behavior, mood, and recovery.

According to the cognitive-behavioral model, some patients hold *irrational* beliefs about pain. In considering pain, such patients may "catastrophize" (believe that a minor setback indicates the occurrence of a major injury), "personalize" (inappropriately believe that they are the cause of injury or continued pain) or have "emotional reasoning" (believe that their feelings about the pain must be true). Such irrational beliefs have been found to be predictive of high pain levels and poor treatment outcome. For example, Keefe, Brown, Wallston, and Caldwell (1989) found that, among arthritis patients, catastrophizing was associated with high pain intensity, high levels of depression, and low physical functioning. Similarly, Gil, Abrams, Phillips, and Keefe (1990), examining sickle cell, rheumatoid arthritis, and mixed chronic pain patients found that higher reports of negative self-statements (such as "I am a burden on my family" or "I am useless") were associated with greater pain and greater psychological distress.

Coping strategies are the second set of cognitive factors that have been the focus of a great deal of attention among researchers in chronic pain. Coping strategies refer to specific thoughts or behaviors that people use to manage their pain or emotional reactions to pain (Brown & Nicassio, 1987). The Coping Strategies Questionnaire (CSQ; Rosensteil & Keefe, 1983) is the most widely used questionnaire for assessing these strategies. The CSQ contains three basic dimensions (Lawson, Reesor, Keefe, & Turner, 1990): conscious cognitive coping (including ignoring the pain and coping self-statements), self-efficacy (including the ability to control and the ability to decrease pain), and pain avoidance (including diverting attention and hoping and praying). Research on the CSQ has found that higher self-efficacy is frequently associated with lower pain intensity and greater physical functioning (Jensen, Turner, Romano, & Karoly, 1991). Research on the CSQ, as well as the Fear-Avoidance Beliefs Questionnaire (Waddell, Newton, Henderson, Sommerville, & Main, 1993) has shown that pain avoidance, especially through hoping and praying, is maladaptive and leads to poorer pain treatment outcome (Rosensteil & Keefe, 1983). These results, together with other research on cognitive factors in chronic pain, indicate that patients' thoughts and beliefs, as well as incentives in the patients' environment, can serve to magnify pain sensation and decrease the ability of the chronic pain patient to function and recover.

MULTIDISCIPLINARY PAIN TREATMENT

The earliest modern attempts to treat chronic pain patients were made by John Bonica (1985), who described his great frustration in attempting to treat chronic pain in the military during World War II. There was no coherent literature addressing the treatment of pain, treatment efforts were piecemeal, and communication among the various treatment providers was sporadic. It was during this time that Bonica developed the concept of multidisciplinary treatment for chronic nonmalignant pain. All clinical specialties would be physically located in a single clinical setting, thereby optimizing communication among specialists and coordination of care.

It was not until 1961, however, that Bonica and Lowell White, a neurosurgeon, established the first multidisciplinary pain treatment program at the University of Washington in Seattle (Bonica, 1975). In following years, Wilbert Fordyce, PhD, joined the program. As already noted, Fordyce's (1976) text, describing the application of behavioral principles to the treatment of chronic pain, served as the philosophical underpinnings of the program. Fordyce argued that the disease model in medicine, though perhaps appropriate for infectious disease, was not particularly helpful in providing guidance in the care of chronic pain. In the disease model, observed symptoms reflect some underlying pathology. Treatment, in turn, is directed at the underlying pathology. In contrast, it had already been well established that pain behavior is "subject to influence by a host of factors besides so-called underlying pathology" (Fordyce, 1976, p. 33). Further, there are instances, such as nonspecific low back pain, where a pain generator cannot be identified. Alternatively, a pain generator may be identified, but the pain complaint is far out of proportion (i.e., somatoform pain disorder). Finally, even in the presence of obvious, objectively confirmed pathophysiology, psychosocial factors may exert a significant influence on pain perception and response to treatment. For Fordyce, the salient relationship in chronic pain is between pain behavior and its consequences, rather than between pain behavior and some putative pain generator.

Multidisciplinary Behavioral Treatment

Fordyce (1976) applied a richly developed literature in learning theory to patients with chronic pain syndrome. This syndrome can be defined as excessive pain behavior, overuse of pain medications, overutilization of the health delivery system, and a low level of activity. Treatment in an inpatient setting was designed to maximize control over stimuli and reinforcers; pain behaviors were no longer rewarded; and well behaviors such as walking to a quota distance, were rewarded. Spouses and families were educated to discontinue often unwitting reinforcement of pain behavior and disability. Medications were scheduled on a time basis rather than *prn*, as the latter protocol creates a reinforcement contingency between pain complaint and medication. Problem medications, such as narcotic analgesics and minor tranquilizers, were placed in a "cocktail" to maintain stimulus constancy and gradually tapered over time. Careful and detailed record-keeping was required so that patients could track their progress and benefit from the motivational effects of that progress.

Fordyce had already published outcome data demonstrating the efficacy of behavioral treatment of chronic pain, and his book presented numerous case studies also reflecting the success of this approach. The 1970s and 1980s witnessed the development of numerous pain programs based on Fordyce's model. Flor, Fydrich, and Turk (1992) conducted a meta-analytic analysis of a number of studies reporting outcome of treatment in multidisciplinary pain treatment programs based at some level on the Fordyce's model. The results of the analysis provide clear evidence as to the efficacy of this approach.

Cognitive-Behavioral Treatment

Paralleling the application of behavioral principles to the evaluation and treatment of chronic pain, cognitive learning theory was demonstrating greater heuristic value than traditional learning theory. Not surprisingly, the application of cognitive psychology to the clinical enterprise occurred in short order in the development of cognitive-behavioral therapy. Turk, Meichenbaum, and Genest (1983) cogently synthesized these various influences in their work, *Pain and Behavioral Medicine: A Cognitive-Behavioral Perspective*. Behavior and behavioral change are seen as end products of cognitive events, affect, behavior, and consequences. Cognitions can be changed by reframing or reconceptualizing a problem for the patient, by teaching problem-solving skills, and by education. Behavior can be changed by altering consequences, working to quotas, modeling, and rehearsal. As patients successfully perform target behaviors, they become increasingly confident and develop feelings of self-efficacy and self-control (Bandura, 1977). Faced with a situation that once was overwhelming and impossible to manage, patients can acquire the skills and problem-solving ability to control the situation.

The case of John exemplifies the cognitive-behavioral approach to chronic pain. John is a 30-year-old engineer who is beginning a new job. Understandably, he is concerned about his performance and about making a good impression. John has a history of migrainous headaches, and these headaches are more frequent and more intense when he is under stress. John worries that he will have a headache, miss work, and make a bad first impression. He has had this problem in the past. He also knows that medication cannot entirely rescue him from his dilemma as it dramatically reduces his performance.

In a cognitive-behavioral intervention, John first has to be educated to the fact that many migraine headache sufferers can learn to control their headaches. At present, if he begins to feel the early signs of a headache, he worries that it will escalate and cause him to miss work. He knows there is nothing he can do to control the course of the headache. Worry and defeat are cognitions that can increase activity in the sympathetic nervous system and thereby promote headache. John can be taught relaxation exercises and imagery or be trained with biofeedback to acquire skills that can decrease activity in the sympathetic nervous system and abort headaches. Further, he can learn to be problem- or solution-focused in his thinking rather than emotion focused. As John acquires headache control skills and is successful in aborting headaches, he worries less about missing work. This reduces the stress and worry of a bad first impression, further decreasing the likelihood of headache.

Turk et al. (1983) noted the effectiveness of application of cognitive-behavioral therapy not only to pain treatment but also to risk factors such as essential hypertension, type-A coronary-prone behavior patterns, obesity, smoking, and alcoholism, as well as disease areas such as cancer and diabetes mellitus. More recent work, such as that by Bradley (1996) and Turk (1996), underline the continued applicability of cognitive-behavioral therapy as well as its clinical effectiveness.

Functional Restoration Model

The most recent development in the evolution of multidisciplinary treatment of chronic nonmalignant pain is the functional restoration model (Mayer & Gatchel, 1988). While incorporating many aspects of Fordyce's model and of cognitive-behavioral therapy, the functional restoration model specifically focuses on the use of sports medicine technology to assess physical capability and to design treatment protocols to enhance functional capability, the most common goal being return to work.

Mayer et al. (1987) described the functional restoration program at the Productive Rehabilitation Institute of Dallas for Ergonomics (PRIDE). Staffing comprises a directing physician, a physical therapist, an occupational therapist, a psychologist, and a nurse. As with the Fordycian model, evaluation and treatment in a single clinical setting is critical. Beyond this, functional restoration focuses on objective, quantifiable measures of both physical and psychosocial function that are relevant to the functional goal. Development of measures with such parameters allows a more or less precise definition of the patient's capability and a comparison of this capability to the rational standard of a normative database. The remaining consideration in measurement of performance is an "effort factor" so that suboptimal effort is not confused with the patient's true level of ability or disability.

Obviously, the focus of each discipline is somewhat different, although the overall functional goal is the same. The physical therapist is responsible for supervision of the patient's individualized physical therapy program, which is designed to treat the specific injuries and hence enhance functional capability. Occupational therapy focuses on functional tasks through work hardening and work simulation. In this program the occupational therapist also addresses any financial, legal, or work-related barriers to successful return to work. The psychologist addresses psychosocial and behavioral issues through a MultiModal Disability Management Program (MDMP). This program is individualized but can consist of group and family counseling, behavioral stress management training (including relaxation training and biofeedback), and cognitive-behavioral skills training. The nurse serves as an extension of the physician, checking and ordering medications and injections and making a preliminary evaluation of medical problems affecting a patient's ability to participate in the physical reconditioning program. Team members confer on a biweekly basis to ensure a high level of communication.

There are four phases in the treatment. The preprogram phase can be of a varying number of sessions; it addresses issues of compliance, motivation, and other barriers to functional recovery. The core program consists of 3 weeks of daily 10-hour sessions. The follow-up phase is 0–20 sessions over 0–6 weeks and consists of a variety of interventions to reinforce and maintain the pain management habits and functional skills acquired during the first two phases of the program. Finally, the outcome tracking phase can consist of periodic, repeated quantitative functional evaluations (QFEs), structured phone contact, and an annual interview.

Hazard (1993) reviewed outcome data for patients treated at the PRIDE program by Dr. Mayer and his team. He also reported outcome data of his own functional restoration program at the New England Back Center (NEBC). Using return to work as an index of success, at 1 year posttreatment the PRIDE program had 86% of their treated patients at work or in training, and the NEBC had 81% of their patients working. These outcomes were compared to various control groups where return-to-work rates varied between 20% and 45%. At 2-year follow-up, the PRIDE program found its success rate maintained, with 85% of program graduates at work. For both programs, significantly fewer treated patients had additional surgery, compared to controls. Also, the PRIDE-treated patients had significantly fewer visits to health professionals than comparison patients at both 1- and 2-year follow-up.

Though the functional restoration model described by Mayer and Gatchel (1988) is focused specifically on patients with disorders of the spine, the model obviously can and should be applied to other chronic pain diagnoses. The overall conceptual model is biopsychosocial and has been well elaborated (see, for example, Turk, 1996). Some of the unique aspects of the model are its focus on objective, valid, and reliable measures; functional improvement; and return to work. Headache treatment programs described by Scharff and Marcus (1994) and Kremer, Hudson, and Schreiffer (1998) are reasonable examples of the application of functional restoration principles within the parameters of at least some headache diagnoses. For other chronic pain syndromes, such as functional gastrointestinal pain syndrome, such programs, with their focus on return to work, may have to be modified to incorporate a focus on more subtle aspects of pain and its effects.

ISSUES FOR THE FUTURE

As Kulich and Lande (1997) have noted, the advent of managed care has not proved to be a congenial environment for multidisciplinary pain treatment. Some managed care organizations (MCOs) simply do not provide programmatic care as a covered service; some consider chronic pain a mental health benefit, greatly reducing coverage; still others provide piecemeal service, such as sending social workers or psychologists to primary care physician's offices to counsel chronic pain patients.

As the studies reviewed in the current chapter indicate, programmatic care has been shown to be efficacious (Flor et al., 1992), and approaches that focus on functional restoration result in greater than 80% of treated patients returning to work (Hazard, 1993). Multidisciplinary treatment, especially if it is "customized" to each patient's problems and personality (Turk, 1990), offers to the patient and insurer alike the possibility of substantial reduction in cost, total treatment time, and redundant medical care. For example, there is substantial documentation that multidisciplinary programs are more cost-effective than other treatment strategies, such as surgery or piecemeal, unorganized treatment (Okifuji,

Turk, & Kalauokalani, 1998). Further it has been shown that calculable cost savings follow such treatment (Caudill, Schnoble, Zuttermeister, Benson, & Friedman, 1991). Refinement of treatment programs and continued demonstrations of the cost-effectiveness of pain intervention based on the biopsychosocial model should overcome the reluctance of managed care to embrace the field of pain management.

REFERENCES

Bandura, A. (1977). Self-efficacy: Toward a unifying theory of behavior change. *Psychological Review, 84,* 191–215.

Barish, C. F., Castell, D. O., & Richter, J. E. (1986). Graded esophageal balloon distention: A new provocative test for noncardiac chest pain. *Digestive Diseases and Sciences, 31*, 1292–1298.

Bigos, S. J., Battie, M. C., Spengler, D. M., Fisher, L. D., Fordyce, W. E., Hansson, T., Nachemson, A. L., & Worthly, M. D. (1991). A prospective study of work perceptions and psychosocial factors affecting the report of back injury. *Spine, 16,* 1–6.

Block, A. R. (1996). *Presurgical psychological screening in chronic pain syndromes: A guide for the behavioral health practitioner.* Mahwah, NJ: Lawrence Erlbaum Associates.

Block, A. R., Kremer, E. F., & Fernandez, E. (1998). *Handbook of pain syndromes: Biopsychosocial perspectives*. Mahwah, NJ: Lawrence Erlbaum Associates.

Block, A. R., Kremer, E. F., & Gaylor, M. (1980). Behavioral treatment of chronic pain: The spouse as a discriminative cue for pain behavior. *Pain, 9,* 243–252.

Block, A. R., Vanharanta, H., Ohnmeiss, D., & Guyer, R. D. (1996). Discographic pain report: Influence of psychological factors. *Spine, 21* , 334–338.

Bonica, J. J. (1975). Organization and function of a multi-disciplinary pain clinic. In M. Weisenberg & B. Tersky (Eds.), *Pain: New perspectives in therapy and research.* New York: Plenum Press.

Bonica, J. (1985). History of pain concepts and pain therapy. *Seminars in Anesthesia, 3,* 189–208.

Bonica, J. J. (Ed.) (1990). *The management of pain* (2nd ed.). Philadelphia: Lea & Febiger.

Bradley, L. A. (1996). Cognitive-behavioral therapy for chronic pain. In R. J. Gatchel & D. C. Turk (Eds.), *Psychological approaches to pain management: A practitioner's handbook.* New York: Guilford Press.

Breuer, J., & Freud, S. (1895). *Studies in hysteria.* New York: Basic Books.

Brown, G. K., & Nicassio, P. M. (1987). Development of a questionnaire for the assessment of active and passive coping strategies in chronic pain patients. *Pain, 31,* 53–64.

Caudill, M., Schnoble, R., Zuttermeister, P., Benson, H., & Friedman, R. (1991). Decreased clinic use by chronic pain patients: Response to behavioral medicine intervention. *Clinical Journal of Pain, 1,* 305–310.

Cavanaugh, S., Clark, D. C., & Gibbons, R. D. (1983). Diagnosing depression in the hospitalized medically ill. *Psychosomatics, 24*, 809–815.

Coffin, B., Azpiroz, F., Guarner, F., & Malagelada, J. R. (1994). Selective gastric hypersensitivity and reflux hyporeactivity in functional dyspepsia. *Gastroenterology, 107,* 1345–1351.

Croft, P. R., & Rigby, A. S. (1994). Socioeconomic influences on back problems in the community in Britain. *Journal of Epidemiology and Community Health, 48,* 166–170.

Crowell, M. D., & Barofsky, I. (1998). Functional gastrointestinal pains syndromes. In A. R. Block, E. F. Kremer, & E. Fernandez (Eds.), *Handbook of pain syndromes: Biophysical perspectives.* Mahwah, NJ: Erlbaum.

Davis, R. A. (1994). A long-term outcome analysis of 984 surgically treated herniated lumbar discs. *Journal of Neurosurgery, 80,* 514–421.

DeGood, D. E., & Kiernan, B. (1996). Perception of fault in patient with chronic pain. *Pain, 64,* 153–159.

Deschner, W. K., Maher, K., Cattau, E. L., & Benjamin, S. (1990). Intraesophageal balloon distention versus drug provocation in the evaluation of noncardiac chest pain. *American Journal of Gastroentology, 85,* 938–943.

Deyo, R. A., Diehl, A., & Rosenthan, M. (1986). How many days of bedrest for acute low back pain? *New England Journal of Medicine, 315,* 1064–1070.

Drossman, D. A., Leserman, J., Nachman, G., Zhiming, L., Gluck, H., Toomey, T. C., & Mitchell, C. M. (1990). Sexual and physical abuse in women with functional or organic gastrointestinal disorders. *Annals of Internal Medicine, 113,* 828–833.

Dworkin, R. H., Handlin, D. S., Richlin, D. M., Brand, L. & Vannucci, C. (1985). Unraveling the effects of compensation, litigation and employment on treatment response in chronic pain. *Pain, 23,* 49–59.

Engle, G. L. (1959). "Psychogenic" pain and the pain-prone patient. *American Journal of Medicine, 26,* 899–918.

Fernandez, E., Clark, T. S., & Ruddick-Davis, D. (1998). A framework for conceptualization and assessment of affective disturbance in pain. In A. R. Block, E. F. Kremer, & E. Fernandez (Eds.), *Handbook of pain syndromes: Biopsychosocial perspectives.* Mahwah, NJ: Lawrence Erlbaum Associates.

Flor, H., Fydrich, T., & Turk, D. C. (1992). Efficacy of multidisciplinary pain treatment centers: A meta-analytic review. *Pain, 49,* 221–230.

Fordyce, W. E. (1976). *Behavioral methods in chronic pain and illness.* St. Louis: C. V. Mosby.

Frymoyer, J. W., & Cats-Baril, W. L. (1987). An overview of the incidences and cost of low back pain. *Orthopedic Clinics of America, 22,* 263–271.

Frymoyer, J. W., & Durett, C. L. (1997). The economics of spinal disorders. In J. W. Frymoyer et al. (Eds.), *The adult spine* (2nd ed., pp. 143–150). Philadelphia: Lippincott-Raven.

Gamsa, A. (1994). The role of psychological factors in chronic pain: 2. A critical appraisal. *Pain, 57,* 17–29.

Gil, K. M., Abrams, M. R., Phillips, G., & Keefe, F. J. (1990). Sickle cell disease pain: Relation of coping strategies to adjustment. *Journal of Consulting and Clinical Psychology, 57,* 725–731.

Graham, J. R. (1990). *The MMPI-2: Assessing personality and psychopathology.* New York: Oxford University Press.

Hazard, R. G. (1993). Functional restoration treatment outcomes. In T. J. Mayer, V. Mooney, & R. J. Gatchel (Eds.), *Contemporary conservative care for painful spinal disorders*. Philadelphia: Lea & Febiger.

Hudgins, W. R. (1976). Laminectomy for treatment of lumbar disc disease. *Texas Medicine, 72*, 65–69.

Jensen, M. P., Turner, J. A., Romano, J. M., & Karoly, P. (1991). Coping with chronic pain: A critical review of the literature. *Pain, 47,* 249–283.

Keefe, F. J., Brown, G. K., Wallston, K. A., & Caldwell, D. S. (1989). Coping with rheumatoid arthritis pain: Catastrophizing as a maladaptive strategy. *Pain, 37,* 51–56.

Keller, L. S., & Butcher, J. N. (1991). *Assessment of chronic pain patients with the MMPI-2* (MMPI-2 Monographs, Vol. 2). Minneapolis: University of Minnesota Press.

Kleinke, C. L., & Spangle, A. S. (1988). Predicting treatment outcome of chronic back pain patients in a multidisciplinary pain clinic. Methodological issues and treatment implications. *Pain, 33,* 41–48.

Kremer, E. F., Hudson, J., & Schreiffer, T. (1998). Headache. In A. Block, E. Kremer, & E. Fernandez (Eds.), *Handbook of pain syndromes: Biopsychosocial perspectives.* Mahwah, NJ: Lawrence Erlbaum Associates.

Kulich, R., & Lande, S. D. (1997). Managed care: The past and future of pain treatment. *American Pain Society Bulletin, 7,* 1–5.

Lawson, K., Reesor, K. A., Keefe, F. J., & Turner, J. A. (1990). Dimensions of pain-related cognitive coping: Cross validation of the factor structure of the Coping Strategy Questionnaire. *Pain, 43,* 195–204.

Leavitt, S. S., Johnson, T. L., & Beyer, R. D. (1971). The process of recovery patterns in industrial back injury: Costs and other quantitative measures of effort. *Industrial Medicine and Surgery, 40,* 7.

LeResche, L., Saunders, S., Von Korff, M., Barlow, W., & Dworkin, S. (1997). Use of exogenous hormones and risk of temporomandibular disorder pain. *Pain, 69,* 153–160.

Lindsay, P., & Wyckoff, M. (1981). The depression-pain and its response to antidepressants. *Psychosomatics, 22,* 571–577.

Loeser, J. D. (1982). Concepts of pain. In M. Stanton-Hicks & R. Boas (Eds.), *Chronic low back pain.* New York: Raven Press.

Lousberg, R., Schmidt, A. J., & Groenman, N. H. (1992). The relationship between spouse solicitousness and pain behavior: Searching for more evidence. *Pain, 51,* 75–79.

Mayer, T., & Gatchel, R. (1988). *Functional restoration for spinal disorders: The sports medicine approach.* Philadelphia: Lea and Febiger.

Mayer, T. G., Gatchel, R. J., Mayer, H., Kishino, N. D., Keeley, J., & Mooney, V. (1987). A prospective two-year study of functional restoration in industrial low back injury. *Journal of the American Medical Association, 258,* 1763–1768.

Merskey, H., & Bogduk, N. (Eds.). (1994). *Classification of chronic pain* (2nd ed.). Seattle: IASP Press.

Moriarty, K. J., & Dawson, A. M. (1982). Functional abdominal pain: Further evidence that the whole gut is affected. *British Medical Journal, 284*, 1670–1672.

Okifuji, A., Turk, D., & Kalauokalani, D. (1998). Clinical outcome and economic evaluation of multidisciplinary pain centers. In A. Block, E. Kremer, & E. Fernandez (Eds.), *Handbook of pain syndromes: Biopsychosocial perspectives.* Mahwah, NJ: Lawrence Erlbaum Associates.

Polatin, P. B., Kinney, R. K., Gatchel, R. J., Lillo, E., & Mayer, T. G. (1993). Psychiatric illness and chronic low-back pain. The mind and the spine—which goes first? *Spine, 18,* 66–71.

Riley, J. L., Robinson, M. E., Geisser, M. E., Wittmer, V. T., & Smith, A. G. (1995). Relationship between MMPI-2 cluster profiles and surgical outcome in low-back pain patients. *Journal of Spinal Disorders, 8,* 213–219.

Romano, J. M., Turner, J. A., Jensen, M. P., Friedman, L. S., Bulcroft, R. A., Hops, H., & Wright, S. F. (1995). Chronic pain patient-spouse interactions predict patient disability. *Pain, 63*, 353–360.

Rosensteil, A. K., & Keefe, F. J. (1983). The use of coping strategies in chronic low back pain patients: Relationship to patient characteristics and current adjustment. *Pain, 17,* 33–44.

Scharff, L., & Marcus, D. A. (1994). Interdisciplinary outpatient group treatment of intractable headache. *Headache*, *34*, 73–78.

Schmidt, A. J. M. (1987). The behavioral management of pain: A criticism of a response. *Pain, 30,* 285–291.

Schmidt, A. J. M., & Brands, A. E. F. (1986). Persistence behavior of chronic low back pain patients in an acute pain situation. *Journal of Psychosomatic Research, 30,* 339–346.

Spitzer, W. O. (1987). Scientific approach to the assessment and management of activity-related spinal disorders. *Spine, 12*(Suppl.), 1.

Stewart, W. F., Shechter, A., & Rasmussen, B. K. (1994). Migraine prevalence: A review of population-based studies. *Neurology, 44*(Suppl. 4), S17–S23.

Taylor, V. M., Deyo, R. A., Cherkin, D. C., & Kreuter, W. (1994). Low back pain hospitalization: Recent United States trends and regional variations. *Spine, 19,* 1207–1212.

Turk, D. C. (1990). Customizing treatment for chronic pain patients: Who, what and why. *Clinical Journal of Pain*, *6*, 255–270.

Turk, D. C. (1996). Biopsychosocial perspective on chronic pain. In R. J. Gatchel & D. C. Turk (Eds.), *Psychological approaches to pain management: A practitioner's handbook* (pp. 3–32). New York: Guilford Press.

Turk, D. C., & Fernandez, E. (1995). Personality assessment and the Minnesota Multiphasic Personality Inventory in chronic pain: Underdeveloped and overexposed. *Pain Forum, 4*(2), 104–107.

Turk, D. C., Meichenbaum, D., & Genest, M. (1983). *Pain and behavioral medicine: A cognitive-behavioral perspective*. New York: Guilford Press.

Von Korff, M., Dworkin, S. F., LeResche, L., & Kruger, A. (1988). An epidemiologic comparison of pain complaints. *Pain, 32*, 173–183.

Waddell, G., Newton, M., Henderson, I., Sommerville, D., & Main, C. J. (1993). A Fear-Avoidance Beliefs Questionnaire (FABQ) and the role of fear-avoidance beliefs in chronic low back pain and disability. *Pain, 52,* 157–168.

Walsh, K., Cruddas, H., & Connon, D. (1992). Low back pain in eight areas of Britain. *Journal of Epidemiology and Community Health, 46*, 227–230.

Whitehead, W. E., Crowell, M. D., & Heller, B. R. (1994). Modeling and reinforcement of the sick role during childhood predicts adult illness behavior. *Psychosomatic Medicine, 6*, 541–550.

Whitehead, W. E., Holtkotter, B., Enck, P., Hoelzl, R., Holmes, K. D., Anthony, J., Shabsin, H. S., & Schuster, M. M. (1990). Tolerance of rectosigmoid distention in irritable bowel syndrome. *Gastroenterology, 98*, 1187–1192.

Wolfe, F., Ross, K., Anderson, J., Russell, I. J., & Herbert, L. (1995). The prevalence and characteristics of fibromyalgia in the general population. *Arthritis and Rheumatism, 38*, 19–28.

Chapter 10

Diabetes Mellitus

John C. Guare, Greg A. Myers, and
David G. Marrero

Diabetes is a major health problem. Current estimates indicate that 16 million people in the United States have the disease (American Diabetes Association [ADA], 1996). Diabetes is considered the seventh leading cause of death, and the sixth leading cause of death by disease (National Institutes of Health [NIH], 1995). Individuals with diabetes are significantly more likely than their nondiabetic peers to develop macrovascular (large blood vessel) disease as well as the microvascular problems of retinopathy, neuropathy, and nephropathy. Such multiple morbidity problems can lead to various forms of functional limitation and disability. The combined direct and indirect costs attributable to diabetes care in 1997 were estimated at $98 billion (ADA, 1998a).

Diabetes is most accurately viewed as a family of diseases characterized by the body's inability to effectively metabolize glucose. This inability is the result of defects in insulin secretion and/or insulin action. The result is chronic hyperglycemia (elevated blood glucose). The chronicity and degree of elevated glucose is associated with many of the long-term diabetes-related health problems (Eastman, 1995; Klein & Klein, 1995).

CLASSIFICATION OF DIABETIC CONDITIONS

The National Diabetes Data Group (NDDG, 1979) and the World Health Organization (WHO, 1980) made similar recommendations for a system of classification and nomenclature of diabetes. The result of their work was a general agreement on five types of diabetes: insulin-dependent diabetes mellitus (IDDM or type I diabetes), noninsulin-dependent diabetes mellitus (NIDDM or type II diabetes), gestational diabetes mellitus (GDM), malnutrition-related diabetes mellitus, and other types. Each is characterized by fasting hyperglycemia or elevated glucose concentrations during an oral glucose tolerance test (OGTT). The 1979 NDDG classification further included the category of impaired glucose intolerance (IGT), marked by an OGTT response above normal but below the diabetes diagnostic criteria. (For historical purposes, the terms "type I" and "type II" replaced "juvenile onset" and "adult onset," respectively. One problem with the age-based descriptors is that the elderly may be diagnosed with type I diabetes, hence the elimination of terms referring to age.)

The classification of diabetes further evolved in 1997. The terms IDDM and NIDDM were eliminated and replaced with the terms type 1 and type 2, respectively (The Expert Committee on the Diagnosis and Classification of Diabetes Mellitus [ECDCDM], 1997). Arabic numbers (1 and 2) are used instead of roman numerals to avoid confusing II with 11. The new terms are used according to etiology: type 1 for diabetes resulting from beta cell destruction typically mediated by the immune system, and type 2 for diabetes resulting from defects in insulin resistance and/or insulin secretion. The classification terms "IGT" and "GDM" have been retained.

DIAGNOSTIC CRITERIA

In addition to a new nomenclature, the diagnostic criteria for diabetes have also been modified. A diagnosis of diabetes can be based on any of three criteria (ECDCDM, 1997): (a) a plasma glucose value ≥ 200 mg/dl (or mg%) at any time plus the presence of classic symptoms, for example, polyuria, polydipsia; (b) fasting plasma glucose (FPG) ≥ 126 mg/dl; or (c) elevated plasma glucose in response to an OGTT performed according to WHO guidelines ≥ 200 mg/dl at the 2-hour time period. Confirmation on a subsequent day of any of these three criteria is strongly recommended. In clinical practice, however, diagnostic confirmation on a subsequent day is rare if the person presents with values significantly above the minimum values.

PREVALENCE AND INCIDENCE

It is estimated that 16 million Americans, or approximately 6% of the U.S. population have diabetes (ADA, 1996). The number of persons with diabetes (and the corresponding prevalence rate) has increased steadily over the past several decades. This is caused in part by a decreased mortality rate in persons with diabetes, better and more widespread screening efforts, and a corresponding increase in associated risk factors such as obesity and sedentary lifestyle (Kenny, Aubert, & Geiss, 1995).

Approximately 120,000 individuals ≤ 19 years of age and 300,000–500,000 persons of all ages have type 1 diabetes. Consequently, type 1 diabetes accounts for a very small percentage of all cases of diabetes. Although studies vary in their estimates, it is generally accepted that 1.7 per 1,000 individuals have type 1, making this one of the most prevalent chronic diseases of childhood. Incidence estimates in the United States suggest a rate of 30,000 new cases per year (LaPorte, Matsushima, & Chang, 1995).

Type 2 is clearly the most pervasive form of diabetes in the United States, with an estimated 7.8 million diagnosed cases and an equal number of undiagnosed cases. Considering persons of all ages, type 2 constitutes 90% or more of all cases of diabetes; at age ≥ 45, this percentage is even greater. Type 2 has a prevalence rate of about 1.2% for persons between ages 18 and 44 but climbs to 10.3% for those 65 and older. The average annual incidence rate for all ages is approximately 625,000 cases, or more than one new case of type 2 diabetes diagnosed every 60 seconds (Kenny et al., 1995).

Gestational diabetes mellitus occurs in approximately 4% of all U.S. pregnancies (Cousins, 1995). Testing for GDM between weeks 24–28 of gestation is therefore an important part of obstetric care for women who are at increased risk, for example, those with above normal body weight or a family history of diabetes (ECDCDM, 1997). Identification of GDM is important in order to reduce the associated fetal morbidities and mortality complications.

Risk Factors for the Development of Diabetes

In general, the stress-diathesis model of illness applies to the development of both types of diabetes—a genetic predisposition interacts with one or more environmental factors, conferring the expression of diabetes. Many factors thought to increase the risk of diabetes have been studied, including demographic, genetic, environmental/lifestyle, and physiologic. Risk factors are very different for type 1 and type 2, reflecting the differences in etiology between the two forms of the disease. Type 1 is viewed as an autoimmune disease caused by a pathogen that results in the destruction of beta cells responsible for the production of insulin. Type 2 is understood as a problem in insulin action (decreased insulin sensitivity) and/or insulin secretion (in a relative rather than absolute manner). Whether intervening to reduce a given risk factor would prevent or delay the onset of diabetes in unknown. Diabetes prevention trials are currently under way for both type 1 and type 2, however.

Type 1 Risk Factors

Sex, age, race/ethnicity. Males and females have similar incidence rates, indicating that gender is not a risk factor for type 1 diabetes. The odds of developing type 1 is greatest at the age of puberty (age 10–14, depending on gender). This increased risk period is thought to be a result of hormonal changes or growth activity (Dorman, McCarthy, O'Leary, & Koehler, 1995). Whites are generally more susceptible to type 1, with the countries of Finland and Sweden having the highest prevalence of the disease (Dorman et al., 1995). LaPorte et al. (1995) examined racial differences in type 1 incidence across several studies and found a significantly higher rate in Whites compared to either Blacks, Hispanics, or Asians.

Genetic. Only 20% of new cases of type 1 diabetes are linked to a family history of the disease. The risk of diabetes before age 30 for those with siblings, parents, or offspring with type 1 is 1%–15% compared to < 1% for those without a family history of the disease (Dorman et al., 1995). The concordance rate for identical twins is 25%–50% compared to 10% for a sibling of a person with diabetes (ADA, 1996). The identical-twin concordance rates reflect the importance of environmental factors.

Deoxyribose nucleic acid (DNA) research has implicated the human lymphocyte antigen (HLA) region of chromosome 6 in type 1 diabetes. Class II antigens include the DR locus antigens, and roughly 95% of individuals with type 1 have the DR3 and/or the DR4 antigen (Dorman et al., 1995). Persons with both antigens are extremely likely to develop type 1 diabetes.

Environmental/lifestyle. There is a seasonal tendency toward greater type 1 diagnosis during winter months. Because flu strains are more common in winter, this lends evidence to a viral agent or other pathogen as a contributing factor. Coxsackie B viruses (B2, B3, B4 and B5) and cytomegalovirus have been implicated in type 1 onset, but their potential contribution is not well understood (Dorman et al., 1995).

Nutrition may play a part in the onset of type 1 diabetes, for example, consumption of cow's milk. The putative mechanism is a link between bovine serum albumin (BSA) antibodies and diabetes. (BSA may trigger an autoimmune response involving the beta cells of the pancreas.) Scott, Norris, and Kolb (1996) examined animal and human dietary evidence and suggest that there are at least three type 1 diabetogenic foods—wheat, soy, and cow's milk. More research is needed to better understand the potential contribution of nutritional factors in the onset of type 1 diabetes.

Physiologic. Compared to people without diabetes, individuals with type 1 are much more likely to exhibit islet cell cytoplasmic antibodies (ICAs), antibodies to insulin, and/or antibodies to the enzyme glutamic acid decarboxylase (GAD) (Dorman et al., 1995). It is not known if these antibodies are directly or indirectly involved in the pathophysiology of type 1.

Type 2 Risk Factors

Sex, age, race/ethnicity. Although some studies suggest a greater prevalence of type 2 in women than men (ADA, 1996), such observations can be attributable to other risk factors rather than gender per se. When variables such as obesity and greater use of health care services are considered (both more common in women), the female:male ratio approaches 1 (Pareschi & Tomasi, 1989). Regarding age, the onset of type 2 is rare before age 30. After 30, age is directly and strongly related to the development of type 2 in most populations (Rewers & Hamman, 1995). Reaven and Reaven (1985) suggest much of the association can be attributed to age-related variables such as obesity and physical inactivity (discussed in the "Environmental/lifestyle" section that follows).

Prevalence rates of type 2 vary markedly depending on race and ethnic group. The highest rates are found in the American Pima Indians (50%), compared to the near zero prevalence rate in traditional societies such as the Mapuche Indians in Chile (Rewers & Hamman, 1995). U.S. data indicate African Americans and Hispanics have rates nearly twice that of non-Hispanic Whites (ADA, 1996).

Genetic. There is an 11% chance of developing type 2 diabetes by age 70 with no family history of the disease (ADA, 1996). This increases to 45% if both parents have type 2 diabetes. In reviewing studies assessing both monozygotic (MZ) and dizygotic (DZ) twin data, Rewers and Hamman (1995) noted at least a doubling of the concordance rate for MZ versus DZ twin pairs. The MZ concordance rates ranged from 34%–80% in these reports, with the mean rate substantially lower than 100%. Thus, environmental factors are important in the onset of type 2 diabetes.

Racial admixture data also reflect the (indirect) influence of genetic predisposition toward type 2. The percentage of Native American admixture across different groups (e.g., Pima Indians 100%, Barrio Mexican Indians 46%, mid-income Mexican Americans 27%) is strongly related to the prevalence rate of type 2 in each group (ADA, 1996). Potential group differences in environmental/lifestyle factors may also play a role in developing the disease.

More than 50 studies have investigated candidate genes for type 2 diabetes (Rewers & Hamman, 1995). Given the methodological challenges involved in this kind of research, how type 2 diabetes is inherited remains unclear. Overall, the data indicate polygenic influences rather than a single major locus influence.

Environmental/lifestyle. The question of whether specific dietary components (e.g., high sugar, high fat, low fiber) are diabetogenic has generated much research. Interpretation of such studies is difficult because of methodological concerns. Perhaps the biggest concern is that few dietary components appear to promote diabetes independent of obesity. An exception is a prospective study by Marshall and Hamman (1988), who reported a sevenfold increased risk for a 40 g/day higher fat intake controlling for obesity and other factors. Overall, however, the available longitudinal (prospective) data do not support the hypothesis that dietary composition per se promotes the onset of type 2 diabetes (e.g., Bennett, Knowler, Baird, Butler, & Reid 1984).

Physical inactivity may be a risk factor for type 2 diabetes. Research using a prospective epidemiological design has found that increased caloric expenditure is significantly related to a decreased risk of type 2 diabetes (Helmrich, Ragland, Leung, & Paffenbarger, 1991; Manson et al., 1992). Acute exercise enhances insulin sensitivity, but insulin sensitivity benefits diminish or disappear after only 3 days of inactivity (Schneider, Amorosa, Khachadurian, & Ruderman, 1984). Such evidence suggests adopting a lifestyle of physical activity (e.g., every 2–3 days) for both preventing and controlling type 2 diabetes.

Obesity is a strong risk factor for type 2 diabetes. This is a very robust finding and has been observed in many populations worldwide. Prospective epidemiologic research has documented the following: (a) the risk of developing type 2 diabetes is significantly related to being overweight, (b) increased risk occurs at even relatively low levels of obesity, and (c) statistically controlling for other assumed risk factors (e.g., age, blood glucose, family history of diabetes) indicates obesity is an independent predictor of type 2 onset (Ohlson et al., 1988; Westlund & Nicolaysen, 1972). It is important to note, however, that most overweight individuals do not develop diabetes, and conversely, nonobese persons are diagnosed with type 2.

The distribution of a person's adipose (fat) tissue has been repeatedly shown to predict the presence of diabetes. A common index of body-fat distribution is the waist-to-hip ratio (WHR), obtained by dividing the circumference of the waist by the circumference of the hip. WHR is a significant predictor of type 2 diabetes (Vague, DeCastro, & Vague 1986). Intraabdominal fat assessed by computer tomography (CT) scans has also been shown to predict the onset of type 2 (Bergstrom et al., 1990).

Physiologic. Between 1%–5% of persons with impaired glucose tolerance develop type 2 each year (ADA, 1996). Thus, although the majority of patients with IGT either remain so or revert to normal glucose tolerance, elevated blood or plasma glucose is a risk factor for diabetes. Insulin levels have been studied as impairment of insulin secretion/usage is considered a primary metabolic abnormality in these patients. Both reduced insulin secretion (Kadowaki et al., 1984) and hyperinsulinemia (Haffner & Stern, 1989) have been found to predict diabetes development.

FUNCTIONAL PRESENTATION OF DIABETES

Type 1: At Onset

The onset of symptoms for a person with type 1 diabetes is acute. Classic symptoms include polyuria (frequent urination), polydipsia (frequent drinking), polyphagia (frequent eating), and weight loss. Because the beta cells in the pancreas are no longer producing insulin, the body is unable to transfer glucose from the bloodstream into the organs, muscles, and so on. Although there is plenty of fuel (glucose) available in the blood, it cannot reach the target tissues without insulin. The result is often referred to as "starving in the midst of plenty."

Unable to effectively use and store food intake, the individual is caught in a vicious cycle. The sensation of hunger promotes polyphagia. Because of polyphagia and lack of insulin, the high concentration of glucose circulates through the kidneys. At or above concentrations of 160–180 mg/dl (the renal threshold), the overload of glucose is excreted in the urine (glycosuria). The body's drive to eliminate excessive glucose promotes polyuria. In turn, the person experiences dehydration, which promotes polydipsia. Caloric loss via glycosuria can be substantial and promote weight loss. In addition, because circulating glucose cannot be used as energy, the body begins to break down fat stores (lipolysis) as an energy source, further promoting weight loss. Lipolysis causes an increase in the blood level of free fatty acids and ketone bodies. Depending on the severity of symptoms, a person may reach a state of diabetic ketoacidosis (DKA), which reflects a dangerously high level of acid in the bloodstream. Although DKA is preventable and treatable, coma and possibly death may result if diagnosis and treatment are delayed.

Type 2: At Onset

The onset of symptoms for a person with type 2 diabetes is much more insidious. This explains in part the large number of undiagnosed cases in the United States. Because increasing age is associated with type 2 diabetes, many individuals perceive the slow onset of symptoms such as loss of energy, getting up at night to urinate, vision difficulties, and so on, as signs of aging. Individuals with type 2 rarely experience DKA because they do not suffer from absolute insulin deficiency. Given the insidious development of type 2, the discrepancy for some patients between meeting the diagnostic criteria for diabetes and actual diagnosis can be years.

Type 1 and 2: Acute Complications

There are several acute complications associated with the disease. Individuals with poorly controlled type 1 diabetes are at risk for DKA, a very serious (but preventable and correctable) metabolic problem. Hospital discharge records note DKA on 3%–4% of all diabetes admissions (ADA, 1996). Hypoglycemic episodes are fairly common in persons with type 1 (also called "insulin reactions"), but individuals with type 2 taking insulin or oral medication may also experience hypoglycemia. Two acute though rather rare metabolic conditions associated with type 2 are hyperosmolar hyperglycemic nonketotic syndrome (HHNS) and lactic acidosis (LA). In addition, people with diabetes are at greater risk for various forms of infections.

Type 1 and 2: Long-Term Complications

Microvascular Complications

There are a number of morbidities associated with diabetes that typically take years to develop. Patients with diabetes are very susceptible to microvascular disease, which can result in damage to the eye (retinopathy), kidney (nephropathy) and nerve functioning (neuropathy). Compared to nondiabetics, individuals with diabetes are 25 times more likely to become blind, 17 times more likely to develop renal disease, and 20 times more likely to develop gangrene (Davidson, 1986). It is believed that chronically elevated glucose levels (duration of diabetes interacting with degree of hyperglycemia) are primarily responsible for these problems (The DCCT Research Group, 1993).

Regarding retinopathy, diabetes is a leading cause of new cases of blindness in adults (12% of all new cases) (ADA, 1996). Klein and Klein (1995) reported 97% of insulin-taking and 80% of noninsulin-taking persons who have had diabetes for 15 or more years suffer some form of retinopathy. Bernbaum and Albert (1996) note that many diabetes patients with proliferative retinopathy are not referred for vision-related rehabilitation services by their ophthalmologist or diabetes care provider. There is a strong need to improve referrals to such services.

Nephropathy and renal disease are a common complication of diabetes. Diabetic nephropathy is defined as protein in the urine at a concentration > 30 mg/dl. Approximately 10%–21% of persons with diabetes have nephropathy. Progression of nephropathy can lead to end-stage renal disease (ESRD). Diabetes is the primary cause of ESRD and is responsible for approximately one third of new cases. Individuals with type 2 diabetes constitute the majority of new ESRD cases that are related to diabetes. From 1982 to 1991, the percentage of ESRD cases attributable to diabetes increased from 23% to 36%. In a parallel fashion, the mortality rate for diabetes-related renal disease doubled between 1979 and 1990. ESRD is usually seen ≥ 25 years duration and requires dialysis or a kidney transplant for survival (ADA, 1996).

The general definition of neuropathy refers to nerve damage, and there are many forms of diabetic neuropathy. Approximately 60%–70% of individuals with type 1 and type 2 diabetes suffer from subclinical or clinical neuropathy (Eastman, 1995). The various neuropathic conditions can have pervasive effects throughout the body. The most common form is peripheral sensory neuropathy, affecting the hands, feet, and legs. Fifty-four percent of individuals with type 1 and 45% of those with type 2 have this form. Carpal tunnel syndrome affects one third of persons with diabetes. Impotence, delayed gastric emptying, and bladder and bowel dysfunction are examples of autonomic neuropathy. Increased risk of silent myocardial infarction and sudden death in patients with diabetes is caused in part by autonomic neuropathy (ADA, 1996).

Macrovascular Complications

Persons with type 2 diabetes are at increased risk for large blood vessel disease, the leading cause of mortality in this population. Individuals with diabetes are 2 to 12 times more likely to suffer from cardiovascular disease and 2 to 4 times more likely to die from heart disease compared to those without diabetes (ADA, 1996). Peripheral vascular disease (PVD) affects about 10% of all patients with diabetes, but the rate is much higher with a disease duration > 20 years. PVD interferes with blood and oxygen flow to the lower extremities. PVD in concert with peripheral sensory neuropathy can lead to foot ulcerations, gangrene, and amputation. Approximately half of all nontraumatic amputations in the United States occur in patients with diabetes (ADA, 1996; Palumbo & Melton, 1995). In addition, stroke is 2 to 4 times more common, making cerebrovascular disease another significant morbidity associated with diabetes.

Mortality

Portuese and Orchard's (1995) review indicates > 15% of persons diagnosed with type 1 in childhood will be dead by the age of 40, reflecting a mortality rate some 20 times that seen in the general population. Mortality in type 2 individuals is also elevated compared to the general U.S. population but to a lesser degree. When type 2 onset occurs in middle age, these persons are observed to lose about 5 to 10 years of life expectancy. The onset of type 2 in people ≥ 70 years of age has negligible effects on life expectancy (Geiss, Herman, & Smith, 1995).

Economic Costs of Diabetes

Given the extensive morbidity and mortality problems related to diabetes, estimates of the direct and indirect costs attributable to the disease in 1997 totaled $98 billion (ADA, 1998a). The following is based on the results of this ADA study. In descending order of attributable cost, direct medical expenditures ($44.1

billion) were due to (a) excess prevalence of general medical conditions (e.g., flu), (b) excess prevalence of chronic complications, and (c) acute glycemic care. Indirect costs ($54.1 billion) were caused by disability ($37.1 billion) with the remainder a result of premature mortality. The average per capita cost of caring for a person with and without diabetes was $10,071 and $2,669, respectively, a nearly fourfold difference.

Reducing/Preventing Long-Term Complications

Until recently, it was not known if improving glycemic control would prevent or delay the progression of long-term complications associated with diabetes. This was the impetus for the Diabetes Control and Complications Trial (DCCT) (The DCCT Research Group, 1993). The main purpose of the DCCT was to determine if intensive treatment of patients with type 1 diabetes would decrease the likelihood of the three main microvascular complications, particularly retinopathy. Two cohorts were recruited: those with and without retinopathy. Patients without retinopathy allowed for the assessment of prevention, whereas the other cohort allowed for the assessment of progression. Patients within each cohort were randomly assigned to either intensive therapy (IT) or conventional therapy (CT). The former condition was designed to achieve optimal glycemic control, and used intensive self-monitoring of blood glucose (SMBG), frequent treatment contact, and either multiple daily injections (MDI; defined as ≥ 3/day) or an insulin pump. The CT group was treated with one or two daily insulin injections with a lower frequency of SMBG and treatment contact.

Compared to the CT condition, IT demonstrated a 76% reduction in risk of developing retinopathy (primary-prevention cohort). The progression of retinopathy was slowed by 54% in the secondary-intervention cohort. Both cohorts combined showed that IT provided (a) a 39% mean reduction in the occurrence of microalbuminuria (nephropathy indication), and (b) a 60% mean reduction in clinical neuropathy. There were no significant differences between the two treatment conditions in neuropsychological functioning or quality of life. Risks associated with IT included a threefold increase in severe hypoglycemia and a greater likelihood of becoming overweight. In sum, IT was extremely successful in preventing/managing long-term complications. The associated risks may interfere with the adoption of such treatment in certain patients, however (e.g., persons with difficulty detecting hypoglycemia, young women who are more concerned about weight gain than glycemic control).

Treatment of Diabetes

Although diabetes is a medical problem, effective management relies heavily on the patient to perform the appropriate self-care behaviors. Given the complexity and chronicity of diabetes self-management, coupled with the lack of an effective health care model for managing diabetes (Etzwiler, 1997), most patients with diabetes do not achieve proper glycemic control.

Treatment Goals

Type 1 and type 2 diabetes are characteristically different in terms of age at onset (and hence developmental challenges), level of obesity, lipid abnormalities, and other factors. Consequently, the focus of treatment is not identical for both forms of the disease.

The primary goals of treatment for type 1 diabetes are to (a) establish and maintain medical and psychological well-being; (b) avoid severe and frequent episodes of hypoglycemia, symptomatic hyperglycemia, and DKA; and (c) promote proper growth and development in children and adolescents (ADA, 1994a). A secondary goal is to provide the individual/family with the resources required to achieve optimal glycemic control in order to prevent/delay the diabetes-related micro- and macrovascular complications. The primary goals are viewed as very reasonable; the secondary goal requires much more effort and resources to achieve, though also providing greater benefits.

Primary treatment goals for patients with type 2 diabetes are to (a) promote normal metabolism (glucose and lipid), and (b) prevent or minimize micro- and macrovascular complications (ADA, 1994b). Because the majority of patients with type 2 diabetes are obese, normalizing lipid levels, blood pressure, and body weight are important for managing potential macrovascular complications.

Treatment Components

There are four basic components to the treatment of diabetes: medication (insulin, oral hypoglycemic agents), nutrition therapy, exercise, and self-monitoring of blood glucose (SMBG). Each component must be individualized for the patient. Medication, food intake, and exercise must be carefully balanced so the person maintains desirable glucose levels and avoids hypo- and hyperglycemia. SMBG is used as feedback to determine which aspects of the treatment regimen need adjustment.

Medication. For type 1 diabetes, all patients must take exogenous insulin to survive as they have an absolute or near-absolute deficiency in endogenous insulin production. The optimal goal of insulin administration is to mimic normal insulin secretion. This requires multiple daily injections (≥ 3/day) or use of an insulin infusion pump, however. Many type 1 patients do not want such an intensive regimen and opt for a twice-daily regimen, mixing both short-term and long-term insulins in each injection. In general, a twice-daily regimen yields poorer glycemic control compared to an MDI or pump approach (ADA, 1994a). The diabetes health care team and the patient must work together to determine an insulin administration plan that is acceptable to both parties while achieving the best possible glycemic control.

Medication for patients with type 2 include oral agents and insulin. Some type 2 patients are able to control their blood glucose with diet and exercise and do not need medication. This is a small minority, however. When diet alone is not successful, oral agents and possibly insulin are typically introduced in a stepped care approach.

Medical Nutrition Therapy. Regarding type 1 diabetes, current guidelines for macronutrient intake suggest calories be distributed as follows: protein—10%–20%; fat— < 10% from saturated fat, ≤ 10% from polyunsaturated fat; this leaves the remaining 60%–70% to come from carbohydrate and monounsaturated fat (ADA, 1998b). These guidelines are much more flexible than those used in the past. Consequently, terms such as "medical nutrition therapy" (MNT) or "meal planning" are used to better convey the current approach of determining proper caloric intake according to a set of nutrition-related goals. The primary aim of MNT is to promote proper glucose metabolism. Additional MNT goals for type 1 include healthy lipid levels, distribution of calories and types of foods to promote normal growth and development in children and adolescents, and prevention/treatment of hypoglycemic episodes (ADA, 1998b). All of these goals are developed with the individual while considering the person's health status, eating habits, cultural food preferences, and exercise habits.

MNT goals for persons with type 2 diabetes emphasize problems commonly seen in this population, for example, obesity, hypertension, and elevated lipid levels. Thus, in addition to normalizing glucose levels, primary goals for type 2 include modifying the quantity and quality of food intake to reduce weight, blood pressure and blood lipids.

Exercise. Exercise is recommended for individuals with diabetes. The potential benefits may include (a) decreased risk of cardiovascular disease via reducing obesity, blood pressure and elevated lipid levels, and by increasing HDL levels; (b) increased insulin sensitivity, which may enhance glycemic control and decrease dosage of antidiabetic medication; (c) improvements in mood and self-esteem; (d) enhancing quality of life and activities of daily living by improving muscle strength and joint flexibility; and (e) promoting weight reduction and maintenance of weight loss (ADA, 1994a, 1994b).

Potential risks associated with exercise for patients with diabetes are also numerous. These may include (a) cardiovascular effects such arrhythmias caused by ischemic heart disease, significant increases in blood pressure, and orthostatic hypotension following exercise; (b) microvascular problems such as retinal hemorrhage and increased proteinuria in patients with such preexisting problems; (c) metabolic decompensation such as promoting hyperglycemia caused by too little insulin when exercise is started, or hypoglycemia if too much insulin is present; and (d) musculoskeletal and related problems such as aggravating preexisting joint disease, and orthopedic injury and foot ulcers related to neuropathy (ADA, 1994a, 1994b). The benefit:risk ratio can be maximized by careful planning (with appropriate diabetes care providers) and tailoring physical activities to the person.

SMBG. Self-monitoring of blood glucose provides feedback regarding the effects of recent behavior (medication use, food intake, exercise) on blood glucose control. When used appropriately (i.e., accurate measurement and results properly used to modify regimen behavior), SMBG can be a powerful tool in optimizing glycemic control (The DCCT Research Group, 1993). However, SMBG performance and/or use of the results to guide eating or insulin adjustments are used by a minority of type 1 patients seen in an outpatient clinic setting (Fekete, Guare, Marrero, & Orr, 1997). Thus, SMBG is best viewed as a self-management tool, and there is no reason to believe it will enhance glycemic control unless it is used properly.

PSYCHOLOGICAL AND VOCATIONAL IMPLICATIONS

There are a number of psychological/behavioral and vocational issues relevant to diabetes. This section addresses adherence, stress, depression, eating disorders, insulin manipulation for weight control, sexual dysfunction, and adjustment to disability. These topics are representative of the psychosocial concerns in the diabetes literature and should not be construed as exhaustive.

Adherence

Given the multiple health behaviors involved in the self-management of diabetes, adherence should not be viewed as a unitary construct. Research has shown that an individual may adhere well to one behavior (e.g., SMBG) but not another (e.g., meal plan) (Johnson, 1994). Consequently, attempts to measure diabetes adherence behavior should be domain specific.

Partial or inconsistent adherence to one's diabetes treatment regimen is common (Kovacs, Goldston, Obrosky, & Iyengar, 1992). Patients often report the greatest difficulty following the meal-plan component (Ary, Toobert, Wilson, & Glasgow, 1986). Recent research indicates that an average of 16% (range 0%–50%) of the foods patients report consuming in a typical week would promote hyperglycemia (Fekete et al., 1997). The least difficult aspect of the regimen involves taking medication. Though most patients take their medication, however, many do not wait the appropriate amount of time between insulin administration and eating (Johnson, 1994).

Stress

Psychological stress has been thought to promote hyperglycemia and thus worsen glycemic control. Two mechanisms have been proposed to account for this hypothesis. Stress may indirectly affect blood glucose by interfering with one's behavior, for example, eating, exercise, and so on, which in turn promotes hyperglycemia. Another possibility is that glucose metabolism may be directly compromised by the neuroendocrine effects associated with stress, for example, increased catecholamine and/or cortisol levels.

Overall, the evidence that stress promotes metabolic decompensation in persons with diabetes is equivocal. The hypothesis that stress interferes with adherence to the type 1 regimen and consequently raises blood glucose has received mixed support (Hanson, Henggeler, & Burghen, 1987; Schafer, Glasgow, McCaul, & Dreher, 1983). Correlational studies have found that increased levels of stressful life events or daily hassles are significantly related to poorer glycemic control in persons with type 1 (Cox, Taylor, Nowacek, Holley-Wilcox, & Pohl, 1984) and type 2 diabetes (Aikens & Mayes, 1997). Conversely, lack of stressed-induced hyperglycemia has been reported in laboratory research manipulating acute stressors in type 1 (Kemmer et al., 1986) and type 2 diabetes (Bruce, Chisholm, Storlien, Kraegen, & Smythe, 1992). Stabler, Morris, Litton, Feinglos, and Surwit (1986) reported a greater blood glucose elevation in response to a competitive video task in Type-A-behavior vs. Type-B-behavior children with diabetes. Thus, the need to account for individual differences in response to stress is important.

Depression

Individuals with diabetes have to cope with the demands of managing an incurable disease, possibly putting them at risk for certain psychological problems. Depression has received the most attention in the area of diabetes. The finding that depression is more common in individuals with diabetes than healthy persons is well established. Gavard, Lustman, and Clouse (1993) conducted a systematic review of the depression and diabetes prevalence literature (20 studies). They concluded that approximately 15%–20% of persons with type 1 or 2 diabetes experience major depression at some point during their lifetime, a rate several times that of the general population. It is unclear whether persons with diabetes are more likely to experience depression compared to persons with other chronic medical conditions, however. Thus, the question remains if the increased risk is the result of having a chronic disease or diabetes per se.

Griffith and Lustman (1997) note the limited data addressing gender suggest depression in diabetes seem to follow the 2:1 female-to-male ratio seen in the general population. Given the recurring nature of depressive episodes and their significant impact on the person, diagnosing and treating depression in patients with diabetes should be an integral part of diabetes care. This is especially true for women.

Eating Disorders

There is substantial pressure on women in our society to be thin. Successful management of diabetes requires close attention to food intake. It has been hypothesized that young women with diabetes are at increased risk of eating disorders, especially bulimia nervosa. Initial research using self-report measures of eating-disordered behavior seems to support this hypothesis; however, two problems exist with self-report measures (Wing, Nowalk, Marcus, Koeske, & Finegold, 1986). One, although such measures are informative, they cannot be used to make a diagnosis of eating disorders. Two, persons with diabetes often endorse items that are appropriate for diabetes management, resulting in an artificially inflated score, for example, "I pay close attention to the food I eat."

Recent research using a structured-interview format and appropriate comparison subjects indicates the prevalence of eating disorders is relatively low in women with diabetes and comparable to that of their nondiabetic peers (Peveler, Boller, Fairburn, & Dunger, 1992). Subclinical eating-disordered behavior is a substantial problem, however. For example, scores on the Bulimia test-revised (BULIT-R) were a significant and independent predictor of glycemic control in adolescents and young adult females with diabetes (Guare et al., 1997a).

Insulin Manipulation for Weight Control

Adolescent females with diabetes are significantly more dissatisfied with their weight/body shape than their male counterparts, and such attitude differences diverge even more so as adolescence progresses (Guare & Orr, 1995). Individuals with type 1 diabetes can reduce/omit their insulin dose, which will promote loss of calories via glycosuria. Recent research indicates type 1 females aged 14–24 both decrease and skip their insulin dose specifically for weight-control purposes significantly more often than type 1 males (Guare et al., 1997b). Screening for weight dissatisfaction and possible insulin manipulation should be considered in type 1 females in this age category.

Sexual Dysfunction

Erectile dysfunction or impotence is reported by 50% of men with diabetes (Waxman, 1980). Both physiologic and psychologic factors may contribute to this problem. Women with type 2 (but not type 1) diabetes also report greater disturbance in sexual functioning compared to healthy women without diabetes in areas of sexual desire, orgasmic capacity, and lubrication (Schreiner-Engel, Schiavi, Vietorisz, & Smith, 1987). Research addressing sexual dysfunction in women with diabetes is relatively new and has produced mixed results, however. It is also not clear if diabetes has an organic contribution to sexual problems in women as it does in men. Future sexual-dysfunction research should stress the importance of assessing psychological and physiological factors and emphasize the study of women.

Disability and Employment

The following is based on a review of disability and diabetes by Songer (1995). Between 20%–50% of persons with diabetes report some form of disability, rates substantially higher than the general population. Activity limitations as well as restricted-activity days are reported 2 to 3 times more often by patients with diabetes. Increasing age and minority-group status are associated with greater impairment in activity and/or work. Reported activity limitations affect persons with type 2 (50.2%) more so than type 1 (42.3%), and are especially high for type 2 individuals taking insulin (63.5%). Long-term complications are a primary cause of disability.

Individuals with type 1 who are also disabled have higher rates of unemployment (49%) compared to nondisabled persons (12%). The same pattern holds true for absenteeism, 13.8 vs. 3.0/days per year. The average number of physician visits per year is double that for disabled persons with diabetes compared to those without disability. Activities of daily living (ADLs) are more likely to be limited by persons with diabetes (type 1: 8.8%; type 2: 4.9%) than without (2.3%).

SUMMARY AND FUTURE DIRECTIONS

Diabetes is a serious medical disorder that places significant demands on the person and the health care system. Substantial progress has been made in the field of diabetes care, however. Pharmaceutical companies have developed new antidiabetic medications (both oral and insulin) whose effects on long-term glycemic control are promising but as yet undetermined. Nompharmacologic efforts such as behavioral weight-loss interventions for overweight patients with type 2 diabetes have demonstrated improved glucose metabolism (Williams, Kelley, Mullen, & Wing, 1998). In addition, the ongoing development of minimally invasive and noninvasive blood-glucose meters for daily patient use will, we hope, improve diabetes self-care behavior. Perhaps most important, intensive management of type 1 diabetes significantly reduces the risk of diabetes-related sequalae. Whether the health care system will support and patients choose an intensive treatment approach to reduce long-term complications and disability remains to be seen.

REFERENCES

Aikens, J. E., & Mayes, R. (1997). Elevated glycosylated albumin in NIDDM is a function of recent everyday environmental stress. *Diabetes Care, 20,* 1111–1113.

American Diabetes Association. (1994a). *Medical management of insulin dependent (type II) diabetes* (2nd ed.). New York: American Diabetes Association.

American Diabetes Association. (1994b). *Medical management of non-insulin dependent (type II) diabetes* (3rd ed.). New York: American Diabetes Association.

American Diabetes Association. (1996). *Diabetes vital statistics.* New York: American Diabetes Association.

American Diabetes Association. (1998a). Economic consequences of diabetes mellitus in the U.S. in 1997. *Diabetes Care, 21,* 296–309.

American Diabetes Association. (1998b). Nutritional recommendations and principles for people with diabetes mellitus. *Diabetes Care, 21*(Suppl. 1), S32–S35.

Ary, D. V., Toobert, D., Wilson, W., & Glasgow, R. E. (1986). Patient perspective on factors related to non-adherence to diabetes regimen. *Diabetes Care, 9,* 168–172.

Bennett, P. H., Knowler, W. C., Baird, H. R., Butler, D. J., & Reid, J. M. (1984). Diet and development of noninsulin-dependent diabetes mellitus: An epidemiological perspective. In G. Pozza, P. Micossi, A. L. Catapano, & R. Pauletti (Eds.), *Diet, diabetes and atherosclerosis* (pp. 109–119). New York: Raven Press.

Bergstrom, R. W., Newell-Morris, L. L., Leonetti, D. L., Shuman, W. P., Wahl, W. P., & Fujimoto, W. Y. (1990). The association of elevated C-peptide level and increased intra-abdominal, fat distribution with development of NIDDM in Japanese-American men. *Diabetes, 39,* 104–111.

Bernbaum, M., & Albert, S. G.(1996). Referring patients with diabetes and vision loss for rehabilitation: Who is responsible? *Diabetes Care, 19,* 175–177.

Bruce, D. G., Chisholm, D. J., Storlien, L. H., Kraegen, E. W., & Smythe, G. A. (1992). The effects of sympathetic nervous system activation and psychological stress on glucose metabolism and blood pressure in subjects with type II non-insulin dependent diabetes mellitus. *Diabetologia, 35,* 835–843.

Cousins, L. (1995). *Obstetric complications. Diabetes mellitus and pregnancy: Principles and practice* (2nd ed.). New York: Churchill Livingstone.

Devlin, J. T., Hirshman, M., Hurton, E. D., & Horton, E. S. (1987). Enhanced peripheral and splanchnic insulin sensitivity in NIDDM men after single bout of exercise. *Diabetes, 36,* 434–439.

Cox, D. J., Taylor, A. G., Nowacek, G., Holley-Wilcox, P., & Pohl, S. (1984). The relationship between psychological stress and insulin-dependent diabetic blood glucose control: Preliminary investigations. *Health Psychology, 3*(1), 63–75.

Davidson, M. B. (1986). *Diabetes mellitus: Diagnosis and treatment.* New York: Wiley.

The Diabetes Control and Complications Trial Research Control Group. (1993). The effect of intensive treatment of diabetes on the development and progression of long-term complications in insulin dependent diabetes mellitus. *New England Journal of Medicine, 329,* 977–986.

Dorman, J. S., McCarthy, B. J., O'Leary, L. A., & Koehler, A. (1995). Risk factors for insulin dependent diabetes. *Diabetes in America* (2nd ed.) [NIH publication No. 95-1468]. Bethesda, MD: U.S. Government Printing Office.

Eastman, R. C. (1995). Neuropathy in diabetes. *Diabetes in America* (2nd ed.) [NIH publication No. 95-1468]. Bethesda, MD: U.S. Government Printing Office.

Etzwiler, D. D. (1997). Chronic care: A need in search of a system. *Diabetes Educator, 23,* 569–573.

The Expert Committee on the Diagnosis and Classification of Diabetes Mellitus. (1997). Report of the expert committee on the diagnosis and classification of diabetes mellitus. *Diabetes Care, 20,* 1183–1197.

Fekete, D., Guare, G., Marrero, D., & Orr, D. (1997). Self-management of "off-diet" food intake by adolescents and young adults with insulin-dependent diabetes mellitus. *Diabetes, 46,* 265A.

Garvard, J. A., Lustman, P. J., & Clouse, R. E. (1993). Prevalence of depression in adults with diabetes: An epidemiological evaluation. *Diabetes Care, 16,* 1167–1178.

Geiss, L. S., Herman, W. H., & Smith, P. J. (1995). Mortality in non-insulin dependent diabetes. *Diabetes in America* (2nd ed.) [NIH publication No. 95-1468]. Bethesda, MD: U.S. Government Printing Office.

Griffith, L. S., & Lustman, P. J. (1997). Depression in women with diabetes. *Diabetes Spectrum, 10,* 216–223.

Guare, J. C., Marrero, D., Orr, D., Kakos-Kraft, Fineberg, N., & Friedenberg, G. (1997a). Predictors of diabetic control in male and female adolescents and young adults with IDDM. *Diabetes, 46,* 266A.

Guare, J. C., Marrero, D., Orr, D., Kakos-Kraft, Fineberg, N., & Friedenberg, G. (1997b). Bulimia symptomatology and insulin manipulation in males and females with IDDM. *Diabetes, 46,* 265A.

Guare, J. C., & Orr, D. P. (1995). Changes in weight-related attitudes over a 2-year period in male and female adolescents with IDDM. *Diabetes, 44,* 97A.

Haffner, S. M., & Stern, M. P. (1989). Hyperinsulinemia is associated with 8-year incidence of NIDDM in Mexican Americans. *Diabetes, 38*(Suppl. 1), 92A.

Hanson, C. L., Henggeler, S. W., & Burghen, G. A. (1987). Model of associations between psychosocial variable and health-outcome measures of adolescents with IDDM. *Diabetes Care, 10,* 752–758.

Helmrich, S. P., Ragland, D. R., Leung, R. W., & Paffenbarger, R. S. (1991). Physical activity and reduced occurrence of non-insulin-dependent diabetes mellitus. *New England Journal of Medicine, 325,* 147–152.

Johnson, S. B. (1994). Methodological issues in diabetes research: measuring adherence. *Diabetes Care, 15,* 1658–1667.

Kadowaki, T., Miyake, Y., Hayura, R., Akanuma, Y., Kajinuma, H., Kuznya, N., Takahu, F., & Kokasa, K. (1984). Risk factors for worsening diabetes in subjects with impaired glucose tolerance. *Diabetologia, 26,* 44–49.

Kemmer, F. W., Bisping, R., Steingruber, H. J., Baar, H., Hardtmann, F., Schlaghecke, R., & Berger, M. (1986). Psychological stress and metabolic control in patients with type I diabetes. *New England Journal of Medicine, 314,* 1078–1084.

Kenny, S. J., Aubert, R. E., & Geiss, L. S. (1995). Prevalence and incidence of non-insulin-dependent diabetes. *Diabetes in America* (2nd ed.) [NIH publication No. 95-1468]. Bethesda, MD: U.S. Government Printing Office.

Klein, R., & Klein, B. E. K. (1995). Vision disorders in diabetes. *Diabetes in America* (2nd ed.) [NIH publication No. 95-1468]. Bethesda, MD: U.S. Government Printing Office.

Kovacs, M., Goldston, D., Obrosky, D. S., & Iyengar, S. (1992). Prevalence and predictors of pervasive non-compliance with the medical treatment among youths with insulin-dependent diabetes mellitus. *Journal of the American Academy of Child and Adolescent Psychiatry, 31,* 1112–1119.

Laporte, R. E., Matsushima, M., & Chang, Y. (1995). *Diabetes in America* (2nd ed.) [NIH publication No. 95-1468]. Bethesda, MD: U.S. Government Printing Office.

Manson, J. E., Nathan, D. M., Krowleski, A. S., Stampfer, M. J., Coldlitz, G. A., Willett, W. C., & Hennekens, C. H. (1992). A prospective study of exercise and incidence of diabetes among U.S. male physicians. *Journal of the American Medical Association, 268,* 63–67.

Marshall, J. A., & Hamman, R. F. (1988). Low carbohydrate, high fat diet, and the incidence of non-insulin-dependent diabetes mellitus. *Diabetes, 37,* 115A.

National Diabetes Data Group. (1979). Classification and diagnosis of diabetes mellitus and other categories of glucose intolerance. *Diabetes, 28,* 1039–1057.

National Institutes of Health. (1995). *Diabetes statistics* (NIH Publication No. 96-3926). Washington, DC: U.S. Government Printing Office.

Ohlson, L.-O., Larsson, B., Bjorntorp, P., Eriksson, H., Svardsudd, K., Welin, L., Tibblin, G., & Wilhelmsen, L. (1988). Risk factors for type II (non-insulin-dependent) diabetes mellitus. Thirteen and one-half years of follow-up of the participants in a study of Swedish men born in 1913. *Diabetalogia, 31*, 798–805.

Palumbo, P. J., & Melton, L. J. III (1995). *Diabetes in America* (2nd ed.) [NIH publication No. 95-1468]. Bethesda, MD: U.S. Government Printing Office.

Pareschi, P. L., & Tomasi, F. (1989). Epidemiology of diabetes mellitus. In M. Morsiani (Ed.), *Epidemiology and screening of diabetes* (pp. 77–113). Boca Raton, FL: CRC Press.

Peveler, R. C., Boller, I., Fairburn, C. G., & Dunger, D. (1992). Eating disorders in adolescents with IDDM. *Diabetes Care, 15,* 1356–1368.

Portuese, E., & Orchard, T. (1995). Mortality in insulin-dependent diabetes. *Diabetes in America* (2nd ed.) [NIH publication No. 95-1468]. Bethesda, MD: U.S. Government Printing Office.

Reaven, G. M., & Reaven, E. P. (1985). Age, glucose intolerance, and non-insulin-dependent diabetes mellitus. *Journal of the American Geriatrics Society, 33,* 286–290.

Rewers, M., & Hamman, R. F. (1995). Risk factors for non-insulin-dependent diabetes. *Diabetes in America* (2nd ed.) [NIH publication No. 95-1468]. Bethesda, MD: U.S. Government Printing Office.

Schafer, L. C., Glasgow, R. E., McCaul, K. D., & Dreher, M. (1983). Adherence to IDDM regimens: Relationship to psychological variables and metabolic control. *Diabetes Care, 6,* 493–498.

Schneider, S. N., Amorosa, L. F., Khachadurian, A. K., & Ruderman, N. B. (1984). Studies on the mechanism of improved glucose control during regular exercise in type II (non-insulin-dependent) diabetes. *Diabetologia, 26,* 355–360.

Schreiner-Engel, P., Schiavi, R. C., Vietorisz, D., & Smith, H. (1987). The differential impact of diabetes type on female sexuality. *Journal of Psychosomatic Research, 31,* 23–33.

Scott, F. W., Norris, J. M., & Kolb, H. (1996). Milk and type I diabetes: Examining the evidence and broadening the focus. *Diabetes Care, 19,* 379–383.

Songer, T. J. (1995). *Diabetes in America* (2nd ed.) [NIH publication No. 95-1468]. Bethesda, MD: U.S. Government Printing Office.

Stabler, B., Morris, M. A., Litton, J., Feinglos, M. N., & Surwit, R. S. (1986). Differential glycemic distress in type A and type B individuals with IDDM. *Diabetes Care, 9,* 550–552.

Vague, P., DeCastro, J. V., & Vague, J. (1986). The role of adipose tissue distribution in the pathogenesis of type II diabetes. In M. Serarano-Rios & P. J. Lefebvre (Eds.), *Diabetes 1985* (pp. 524–528). New York: Elsevier.

Waxman, S. G. (1980). Pathophysiology of nerve condition: Relation to diabetic neuropathy. *Annals of Internal Medicine, 92,* 297–201.

Westlund, K., & Nicolaysen, R. (1972). Ten-year mortality and morbidity related to serum cholesterol. *Scandinavian Journal of Laboratory and Clinical Investigation, 30*(Suppl. 127), 3–24.

Williams, K. V., Kelley, D. E., Mullen, M. L., & Wing, R. R. (1998). The effect of short periods of caloric restriction on weight loss and glycemic control in type 2 diabetes. *Diabetes Care, 21,* 2–8.

Wing, R. R., Nowalk, M. P., Marcus, M. D., Koeske, R., & Finegold (1986). Subclinical eating disorders and glycemic control in adolescents with type I diabetes. *Diabetes Care, 9,* 162–167.

World Health Organization. (1980). Report of the expert committee on diabetes [*WHO Technical Report Series*, no. 646]. Geneva, Switzerland: Author.

Chapter 11

Epilepsy

Robert T. Fraser

Epilepsy is the most common of the chronic neurological disorders. The term *epilepsy* derives from the Greek word for "to be seized." A seizure involves a disruption of the normal activity of the brain through neuronal instability. Neurons become unstable and fire in an abnormally rapid manner, and the excessive electrical discharging results in a seizure. A seizure may be confined to one area of the brain (a partial seizure) or may take place throughout the entire brain (a generalized seizure).

Seizures differ in their presentation, depending on the discharge focus within the brain. For some individuals, therefore, the focus of the electrical discharging can be in the motor cortex and simply involve some muscle twitching in a hand (simple partial seizure), whereas for others it involves most of the brain and results in a severe generalized tonic-clonic (formerly called grand mal) seizure. These seizures involve the whole body in convulsions and result in loss of consciousness.

Causes of epilepsy include traumatic brain injury, birth trauma, anoxia, brain tumors, infectious diseases in the mother, parasitic infections (e.g., meningitis), vascular diseases affecting the brain's blood vessels, and high concentrations of alcohol or street drugs. Only a small portion of patients with epilepsy (1%–2%) will have a diagnosable genetic etiology for their seizure occurrences (Anderson, 1988), whereas the general incidence of epilepsy is between 1% and 4%, varying with age groupings. In the Rochester studies (Hauser, Annegers, & Kurland, 1993), the cumulative risk for having epilepsy by age 80 was 4%, with the risk for having a single unprovoked seizure being 5%. Risk factors include alcohol abuse, hypertension, lower socioeconomic status, and depressive illness (Hauser, 1997). It should be underscored that epilepsy involves the occurrence of two or more seizures; the occurrence of one seizure is insufficient to make a diagnosis of epilepsy.

SEIZURE CLASSIFICATION

Seizures are generally classified by assessing clinical symptoms, supplemented by wake and/or sleep electroencephalograms (EEGs) and sometimes by more sophisticated procedures, such as 24-hour EEG-video monitoring. Seizures are generally categorized according to two types: generalized seizures, which affect both cerebral hemispheres, and partial seizures, which affect a specific part of the cerebral hemisphere. Partial seizures are further divided into simple partial seizures, in which consciousness is maintained, and complex partial seizures, which involve more than one symptom and in which consciousness is impaired. It is important to note that many partial seizures may secondarily evolve into generalized seizures. The classification proposed by the International League Against Epilepsy (ILAE) Commission on Classification and Terminology was published in 1981 and is provided in Table 11.1. This table provides the reader with a basic overview of the different types of seizure conditions in the generalized and partial categorizations. This classification schema is currently undergoing revision by the ILAE.

FUNCTIONAL PRESENTATION OF EPILEPSY

Generalized Seizures

Generalized seizures tend to involve both cerebral hemispheres and several areas of the brain (cerebral cortex, thalamus, brain stem structures, etc.) and are subcategorized into a number of specific types. The individual loses consciousness with each type. The most common form of generalized seizure is the tonic-clonic convulsion that occurs in 10% or less of epilepsy cases (Penry, 1986). This type of seizure involves two stages: the tonic stage, in which the body becomes rigid for a period of seconds, and the clonic stage, in which the person experiences a series of convulsive and jerky movements. The entire seizure generally lasts about 2 to 3 minutes. It is this type of seizure that tends to be remembered by the general public.

TABLE 11.1 An Abbreviated Classification of Epileptic Seizures

Generalized Seizures of Nonfocal Origin

Tonic-clonic
Tonic
Clonic
Absence
Atonic/akinetic
Myoclonic

Partial (Focal) Seizures

Simple partial seizures with elementary symptomatology(consciousness is not impaired)

a. With motor symptoms (including Jacksonisn, versive, and postural)
b. With sensory symptoms (including visual, somatosensory, auditory, olfactory, gustatory, and vertiginous)
c. With autonomic symptoms
d. With psychic symptoms (including dysphasia, dysmnesic, hallucinatory, and affective changes)
e. Compound (i.e., mixed) forms

Complex partial seizures with complex symptomatology (consciousness is impaired)

a. Simple partial seizures followed by loss of consciousness
b. With impairment of consciousness at the outset
c. With automatisms

Partial seizures evolving to secondarily generalized seizures

Unclassified Seizures

Reprinted with permission of the Epilepsy Foundation of America as Found in Pedlev and Hauser (1988, p. 3).

Tonic-clonic seizures should be timed. If the actual seizure activity exceeds 5 to 10 minutes, patients may enter an emergency state called status epilepticus, in which they suffer a continuing, prolonged seizure or experience recurring seizures within a brief period. This is an emergency situation and requires immediate hospital care. During the tonic-clonic seizure, it is best to discourage a crowd from gathering and to refrain from sticking anything into the person's mouth. It can be helpful to turn a person on one side and put a soft article of clothing under the head.

The other commonly known type of generalized seizure is the simple absence seizure (traditionally known as petit mal seizure). It takes only a few seconds, with a brief disruption of consciousness (less than 20 seconds) and autonomic symptoms such as pupil dilation and mild rhythmic movements of the eyelids. Simple absence seizures are distinguished by the three-per-second spike-and-wave tracings on the EEG. Most patients with this type of epilepsy begin having such seizures before age 12. Although they involve less than 5% of epilepsy cases (Penry, 1986), it is important to intervene medically, because not only can seizures affect a child's learning and influence behavior, they can also change into generalized tonic-clonic or more severe generalized seizures as the child approaches adolescence.

A number of adults still believe that they have these "petit mal" seizures because they had them as children, and they appear more benign in presentation than other seizure types. Often they simply do not know their precise seizure type, which may be partial-complex. On a vocational outreach grant at our center, between 25% and 30% of adults entering the study described their seizures as petit mal, which was generally not the case (Fraser & Clemmons, 1989). If patients do not know their seizure type, they may also be on an inappropriate medication.

Other types of seizures include tonic or clonic seizures, which are actually limited tonic-clonic seizures; atonic seizures, or brief drop attacks, which tend to affect children under 5 years of age; and generalized myoclonic jerks in adults, which are brief shocklike contractions affecting the entire body or segmented to a part of the body.

Partial Seizures

Partial seizures, as described in Table 11.1, can be divided into three categories: simple partial seizures with elementary symptoms, complex partial seizures with diverse symptoms, and partial seizures evolving into secondarily generalized seizures. Simple partial seizures may be motor, sensory, or autonomic, or they may involve some combination of symptoms without impaired consciousness. Many individuals can function quite well with simple partial seizures that are only of a few seconds duration and do not impair consciousness (e.g., the person may pull over to the side of the road when driving).

Complex partial seizures or partial seizures with complex symptoms, however, present a significant problem. First, consciousness is impaired. These seizures are also known for having an associated aura, or warning, which can involve a strange odor, aphasia, dizziness, nausea, headache, unusual stomach sensations, or a déjà vu experience. Common events include repetitive motor movements, fumbling with hands or clothing, lip smacking, and wandering. Partial-complex seizures without motor components are less common, but they can involve rapid emotional or sensory changes.

Approximately 60% of those with epilepsy have seizures classified in the partial seizure category (Pedley & Hauser, 1988). These patients are often not appropriately treated for their partial seizure but only for a later observed generalized (tonic-clonic) seizure into which the partial seizure has spread. Because of the impaired consciousness and strange characteristics of partial-complex seizures (clutching clothing, lip smacking, etc.), clients with partial-complex seizures are sometimes mistaken for psychiatric patients. This seizure type is often not appropriately identified in unsophisticated assessments. Accurate diagnosis is critical to appropriate medication treatment (e.g., from a clinical perspective an absence seizure and a partial-complex seizure may look the same—a brief period of unawareness and lack of response).

It should be noted that a subgroup of people initially diagnosed with chronic epilepsy are later determined to have "psychogenic" or "pseudo" seizures, which are nonepileptic events mimicking seizure activity. Kloster (1993) estimates this subgroup as between 10% and 20% of those initially diagnosed with syncope, hyperventilation, panic attacks, conversion disorders, dissociative events, and the like. Diagnosis can often be clarified by recording serum prolactin levels, which should be dramatically elevated 20–30 minutes postseizure (Betts, 1997), without more costly EEG and neuroimaging work confounding the situation. About 5% of those with established seizures also have nonepileptic seizures (Betts, 1997). Martin et al. (1997) utilized a Minnesota Multiphasic Personality Inventory–2 (MMPI–2) stepwise discrimination function to successfully classify 81% of patients with and without epilepsy. Obviously, other clinical information must be considered.

TREATMENT AND PROGNOSIS

Following an initial seizure, specifically a generalized tonic-clonic seizure, many individuals are briefly hospitalized or receive an initial outpatient evaluation. The physician may begin a medical treatment program or refer the individual to a general neurologist. If seizure control is not secured within 3 months, a neurological referral is recommended (National Association of Epilepsy Centers, 1990).

Neurological consultation includes physical examination and history taking, metabolic studies, and other evaluations, including routine EEG testing. Both awake and sleep EEGs provide the physician with a clearer definition of the nature of the abnormal neuronal discharging and have often confirmed a seizure diagnosis. When the diagnosis remains unclear in partial epilepsy, even when using two EEGs (approximately 25% of cases), other more specialized neuroradiological noninvasive techniques may be used to scan the brain and identify small focal lesions that may be the cause of partial seizures. Magnetic resonance imaging (MRI) is generally superior to CT scanning because of its definitiveness and sensitivity in clarifying small lesions or cerebral cortex abnormalities; but in an acute situation, if MRI is not available or there are other technical difficulties, a CT scan may be used (International League Against Epilepsy, 1997). Although the EEG is the only indicator of an actual abnormal brain state, MRI, CT, and single photon emission computed tomography (SPECT) or positive emission tomography (PET) clarify issues related to structural lesions. Multichannel magnetoencephalography (MEG) is a newer technique for measuring magnetic fields and appears to be more definitive in isolating sources of epileptiform discharges.

If seizure control is not achieved by the general neurologist within 9 months, a referral to a tertiary- or fourth-level epilepsy center should be made (National Association of Epilepsy Centers, 1990). These centers have neurologists and allied health teams that specialize in epilepsy, and they address such areas as pharmacological problems; possible psychogenic or pseudoseizures; the potential for epilepsy surgery; the need for invasive, intracranial video/EEG recording; and the need for complementary psychological or psychiatric expertise. It is important to acknowledge that antiepileptic medications are selectively effective for one or more different types of seizures (Wannamaker, Booker, Dreifuss, & Willmore, 1984). The neurologist matches the appropriate drug to the specific type. Table 11.2 presents an overview of the primary and secondary drugs that are most common for various seizure categories.

To achieve optimal daily life functioning for a patient (most effective treatment, fewer side effects), the normal course of treatment is the maximum tolerable dosage of one medication. A dosage should be established that maintains an appropriate concentration within the bloodstream throughout the day. Therapeutic ranges and toxicity levels have been established for the major recommended drugs. Table 11.3 shows pharmacological data on the major antiepileptic drugs.

Inappropriate or random taking of medications does not result in a steady state or maintenance of an appropriate level of the medication in the bloodstream. Excessive concentrations of medication (toxic ranges) can result in double vision, lethargy, impaired mental alertness/attention, coordination difficulties, weight gain, and other significant medical complications. Medication levels require periodic laboratory monitoring for assessing appropriate ranges. Even within appropriate ranges, drug side effects (such as facial hair on women or gum disease associated with phenytoin (Dilantin) may require intervention.

Antiepileptic medications first came on the market in the United States in the 1970s, and the 1980s were a period of further research. In the 1990s we have a number of new compounds (viz., gabapenten, felbamate, lamotrigine, tiagabine, topiramate, and vigabatrin), which have chiefly been tested as "add on," or adjunctive, drugs. All have shown effectiveness against complex partial and secondarily generalized seizures, but their spectrum of activity and dosages, possible (although chiefly subtle) side effects, and value as monotherapeutic agents against a broader range of seizures require further definition (Marson, Kadir, Hutton, & Chadwick, 1997; Porter & Meldrum, 1997).

Other treatment options, such as vagal nerve stimulation, which is receiving an increasing amount of research interest and compares favorably with the effectiveness of new antiepileptic drugs, are increasing in popularity. The ketogenic diet for children is receiving more recent attention because new long-term studies

TABLE 11.2 Seizure Types and Indicated Antiepileptic Drugs

Seizure type	Effective antiepileptic drugs (listed alphabetically)
Simple partial or complex partial	*Primary drugs*
	Carbamazepine (Tegretol)
	Phenobarbital (Lumanil)
	Phenytoin (Dilantin)
	Primidone (Mysoline)
	Secondary drugs
	Clonazepam (Klonopin)
	Methsuximide (Celontin)
	Valproic acid (Depakene)
Generalized tonic-clonic (primary or secondary generalized)	*Primary drugs*
	Carbamazopine
	Phenobarbital
	Phenytoin
	Valproic acid
	Secondary drugs
	Primidone (Mysoline)
Generalized absence	*Primary drugs*
	Ethosuximide (Zarontin)
	Valproic acid
	Secondary drugs
	Acetazolamide (Diamox)
	Trimethadione (Tridione)
Myoclonic	Clonazopam
	Valproic acid

Reprinted with permission of the Epilepsy Foundation of America as found in Leppik (1988, p. 13).

indicate > 50% seizure reduction for 40%–50% of the children treated (Gaillard, Shields, Stafstrom, & Vining, 1997). The vagal nerve stimulator is particularly exciting because seizure reduction persists and increases over time, compared to anticonvulsants' lesser effectiveness over time (Wilder, 1997). Much research, however, must be conducted in relation to these options, blended options, and behavioral or cognitive-behavioral training approaches (e.g., relaxation).

Medical Prognosis for Patients with Epilepsy

A review of seizure relapse studies would suggest that patients treated with medication generally achieve a 65% to 80% seizure-free status (Hauser & Hes-

TABLE 11.3 Common Anticonvulsant Properties

Drug	Therapeutic range (ug/ml)	Time to reach steady state (days)
Carbamazepine	0–12	3–4
Clonazepam	0.025–0.075	
Ethosuximide	40–100	7–10
Phenobarbital	15–30	14–21
Phenytoin	10–20	7–28
Valproic acid	50–100	1–2

Note: This information is current at the time of publication (1998). Guidelines for optimal therapeutic ranges can fluctuate with medical advances. The reader is encouraged to contact the Epilepsy Foundation of America, Landover, Maryland for the most current information.

dorffer, 1990). Annegers (1988) indicates that 10 years after epilepsy diagnosis, 65% of patients seen are in seizure remission; at 20 years, 76%. Although the probability of achieving remission after 10 years exceeds 60%, the probability of achieving remission during the next 10 years for those patients not having seizure control at 5 years from diagnosis was only 33%. The most important prognostic indicator for the eventual control of seizures is the duration of seizure occurrences. Other factors include seizure cause, seizure type, and age of onset (Annegers, 1988).

For patients with medically intractable seizures, surgical intervention can be a consideration after 1–2 years. This will principally be a consideration for the 10% to 25% of patients with partial epilepsy, primarily partial complex epilepsy (Hauser & Hesdorffer, 1990). Surgery is occasionally a consideration for management of intractable seizure conditions without a focus, but this is infrequent. A series of diagnostic tests, including neuropsychological and continuous EEG/video monitoring are conducted, in addition to utilization of the previously mentioned neuroimaging techniques, so that medical staff and patients have a clear understanding of surgery's viability as specific to the situation. If surface EEG and neuroimaging techniques are unclear in relation to seizure focus, depth electrodes, subdural grids, and direct intraoperative recording may be utilized (Hauser & Hesdorffer, 1990). In general, patients are chosen carefully for the operation and tend to have insignificant cognitive problems after surgery; they may actually perform better neuropsychologically after the operation. Neuropsychological data, however, are reviewed very carefully, specifically in relation to memory and language functions. For some individuals, however, stopping the seizures is paramount.

There are two different approaches to the surgeries. As described by Schaul (1987), these include a standard temporal lobectomy and a Penfield technique, in which the surgical procedure is tailored to the individual patient's seizure focus. As identification of patients with surgically treatable epilepsy becomes easier with neuroimaging and other approaches, 80% of those undergoing surgery can become seizure-free through more cost-effective approaches (Engel, Wieser, & Spencer, 1997). To some degree, surgical outcome is not completely clear because of different means of establishing outcome across surgical centers. For example, warning auras (the beginning warning component of a seizure) may be counted at some centers and not at others. In Schaul's (1987) review, it is estimated that there may be up to 120,000 surgical candidates within the United States who could profit from this type of surgery. For those with successful, seizure-free outcomes, medications are generally tapered off over 2–5 years; obviously, this involves significant discussion between patient, significant others, and the allied health team.

Neuropsychological Assessment

At the Epilepsy Center of Michigan, over a 5-year period, Rodin, Shapiro, and Lenox (1977) found that only 23% of their medical referrals had epilepsy only; among the remainder, brain impairment was the largest presenting difficulty across other psychosocial adjustment issues. In establishing functional abilities, this can be an important area to assess. Approximately 40% of those applying to the University of Washington's Regional Epilepsy Center Vocational Services indicated on their program application form that they had had a head injury. Additional research has shown that if individuals have more than 75 lifetime generalized tonic-clonic seizures or have an incidence of status epilepticus involving extended continuous seizure activity, their neuropsychological performance decreases (Dodrill, 1986).

It is reasonable to assume that those seeking vocational rehabilitation services would have diverse patterns of brain impairment that present more barriers to employment than would be common among a mainstream general or medical population. Rausch, Le, and Langfett (1997) indicate that common cognitive concerns for individuals with epilepsy include attention, speed of mental processing, memory and learning, and cognitive flexibility. A neuropsychologist can be helpful in providing brain-related information relative to these deficits and also in identifying assets on which the vocational rehabilitation program can be established—assets often being most important. The neuropsychological evaluation moves beyond basic intellectual assessment to look at the more subtle aspects of problem solving, motor performance, sensory perceptual abilities, memory capacities, attentional capacities, language skills, visual/spatial abilities, and other self-regulating activity.

Commonly used neuropsychological batteries include the Halstead-Reitan Neuropsychological Battery (Reitan & Wolfson, 1985) and the Luria-Nebraska Neuropsychological Battery (Goldin, Hammeke, & Parisch, 1980). Dodrill (1978) has established a comprehensive battery of 16 discriminative measures more sensitive to brain impairment and epilepsy. This battery includes Halstead's Neuropsychological Battery for Adults; the Aphasia Screening Test; the Trail Making Test; the Logical Memory and Visual Reproduction parts of the Wechsler Memory Scale, Form I; the Sensory-Perceptual Examination; the Stroop Test; and the Seashore Tonal Memory Test. Dodrill has also developed an abbreviated form of his battery that can be used as a screening instrument; and although not allowing detailed neuropsychological analysis, it is no less sensitive than the full battery in identifying brain impairment and providing a general indication of its overall extent. Neuropsychological testing is important both pre– and post–epilepsy surgery, particularly to assess surgical impact on memory and language functioning. The testing also can be helpful in clarifying epileptic foci.

It is important to emphasize that, among studies conducted at the University of Washington (Fraser, Clemmons, Dodrill, Trejo, & Freelove, 1986) with clients actively engaged in vocational rehabilitation services, it was aspects of brain impairment that discriminated between those who were able to go to work and maintain a job for 1 year and those who could not secure a job through our program (i.e., they tried to secure work through the program but were unsuccessful). Specifically, the impairments were visual/spatial problem solving and motor deficits. Most of these clients had job experience that was congruent with unskilled or semiskilled work, and the brain impairments were affecting their employability. These clients require longer training or coached work experience relative to accuracy and speed of functioning if they are to be able to secure and maintain a competitive job placement. They will also have to learn to use compensatory strategies to cope with their difficulties. For clients with a long history of generalized tonic-clonic seizures, neuropsychological test results can be very illuminating relative to rehabilitation planning.

Psychosocial Assessment

In assessing the psychosocial functioning of clients with epilepsy, measures traditionally used in clinical environments certainly have their place and are useful in the assessment process. These assessment measures include MMPI, 1 and 2, the Millon Clinical Multiaxial Inventory (MCMI) II or III, computerized psychiatric diagnostic interviews (SCID-II, DSR, etc.); and structured clinical interviews. For purposes of clinical interview, the reader might review the next section, on psychosocial adjustment, to identify risk factors to maladjustment that deserve attention in the interview.

It can be of particular benefit to use the Washington Psychosocial Seizure Inventory (WPSI) in assessing the psychosocial concerns of clients with epilepsy. This inventory, developed by Dodrill, Batzel, Queisser, and Temkin (1980) is helpful in identifying these concerns. It is an MMPI-like instrument in its development but has only 132 items, requiring 20 to 30 minutes for completion. Psychosocial concerns are identified across eight scales: family background, emotional, interpersonal, vocational, financial, adjustment to seizures, medicine and medical management, and overall psychosocial functioning. Other quality-of-life instruments have been developed more recently (e.g., Liverpool Quality of Life Battery, QOLIE-89 item, QOLIE-10 item), but these are more useful as outcome measures of medication changes or surgery outcome and are less helpful in guiding interventions.

PSYCHOLOGICAL AND VOCATIONAL IMPLICATIONS

Incidence of Psychosocial Maladjustment

In discussing the psychological and social adjustment issues of those with epilepsy, it is helpful to review findings using the WPSI. Trostle (1988) has found that most studies using the WPSI have identified 50% of the cases as having definite or severe problems on most of the WPSI scales. This author further indicates that maladjustment may approximate 50% to 60% of those sent for evaluation at a special epilepsy center, whereas overall psychosocial adjustment difficulties were identified for only 19% of a sample from Rochester, Minnesota (Trostle, Hauser, & Sharbrough, 1986). In general, it seems that referrals from private physicians have fewer adjustment difficulties than do clients referred from a medical center specializing in epilepsy treatment. The former may have less involved seizure conditions and simply not be as much at risk psychosocially.

The WPSI is basically a screening instrument and can be helpful in initial planning. If there appear to be more significant psychiatric concerns, a referral for a structured psychiatric interview and the use of inventories normed on psychiatric populations (MMPI–1 and -2, MCMI, II or III, etc.) can be more assistive.

Factors Influencing Psychosocial Adjustment

Hermann (1988) has synthesized the work of previous investigators in suggesting that four general forces affect adjustment among clients with epilepsy. These major influencing factors include biological, psychosocial, medication, and demographic factors. In Table 11.4, this multietiological model is presented with some additional factors identified by Fraser and Clemmons (1989). These factors cover most of those identified in the research literature as influencing the community adjustment of those with the disability. In the neurological category, items such as early age of onset, additional disabilities, associated neuropsychological impairment, type of seizure activity, and the like have been found to be important variables. Under the psychosocial category, a number of variables are identified, including perceived stigma and limitations, adjustment to seizures, vocational status, financial status, parental fears, limited socialization and recreation, divisive or dysfunctional parenting styles, and poor relationships with parents, siblings, and intrusive grandparents.

Other, more immediate issues, such as considerable life event changes, availability of social support, and perceived locus of control, seem to affect

TABLE 11.4 Multietiological Predictor Variables

Neurological	Psychosocial	
Age at onset	Perceived stigma	Parental fears
Duration of epilepsy	Perceived limitations	Divisive/dysfunctional parenting styles
Seizure type	Adjustment to seizures	
Associated neuropsychological impairment	Vocational adjustment	Limited socialization/ recreation
Laterality of lesion	Financial status	Poor relationships with sibling, parents, or grandparents
Presence/absence of multiple seizure types	Special education tracking	
Etiology	Locus of control	Social support
	Life event changes	
Medications	Demographics	
Monotherapy vs. polytherapy	Age	
Presence of barbiturate medications	Gender	
Serum levels of medications	Education	
	IQ	

Reprinted with modifications with permission from the Epilepsy Foundation of America as found in Hermann (1988, p. 30).

adjustment. Basic demographic issues such as age, gender, education, and intelligence also should be reviewed. Some older clients adapt well to the seizure condition because of positive prior life experiences and an integrated self-concept. For other individuals, despite their age, the onset of a seizure condition can be very unsettling. Young males tend to have more difficulties in adjusting than do females. It is of interest that the vocational interests and academic orientation of young males with more severe, early-onset seizures appear to be affected, compared to a norm group (Fraser, Trejo, Temkin, Clemmons, & Dodrill, 1985), but this is not true for young females. Special education tracking seems to relate to psychosocial maladjustment—this may be a masking variable for neuropsychological impairment (Goldin, Perry, Margolin, Stotsky, & Foster, 1977). In the medication category, the number of medications an individual takes and the appropriateness of medication levels also can affect community adjustment.

As emphasized by Hermann (1988), this type of model simply increases the reader's awareness of the range of factors that can influence a client's mental health. When emotional difficulties occur, depression and anxiety appear to be among the most frequent. There also is a significant rate of sexual dysfunction, particularly among males, with a propensity toward those having complex-partial or temporal lobe seizures (Hermann, 1988).

Work at the University of Washington Regional Epilepsy Center has demonstrated that early vocational rehabilitation program dropouts can be discriminated from those who have successfully become employed on a number of specific items from the WPSI (Fraser, Trejo, Clemmons, & Freelove, 1987). These items identified increased depression and anxiety, financial difficulties, and lack of adjustment to one's seizure condition as being more prominent among program dropouts. New 12-hour interventions were tested at our center as precursors to vocational programming in order to stabilize dropouts (Fraser et al., 1990) but were insufficient to render a difference.

VOCATIONAL IMPLICATIONS

In epilepsy rehabilitation it is very important to maintain an individualized approach to vocational evaluation and goal planning. Issues tend to arise around the seizure condition itself, associated disabilities, medication concerns, and seizure disclosure. Each of these salient issue categories is reviewed in the following section.

Clarification of Seizure Status

It is very important that the counselor have a clear understanding of the client's seizure status. If a seizure status remains unclear, it is important that the client be referred to a major epilepsy center (to which one can be directed by the Epilepsy Foundation of America) so that sophisticated testing and/or 24-hour EEG-video monitoring can be conducted. Some individuals will have pseudoseizures, which are emotionally rooted and require a different course of treatment. Some will have both real seizures, involving electrical discharges within the brain, and pseudoseizures. This also deserves clarification because the pseudoseizures can be brought under control in many cases more quickly than the organically based seizure activity. In each case the counselor must understand the following:

1. The specific type of seizure the client currently has, with a clear description of what occurs during a seizure. Of particular importance is establishing whether there is a loss of consciousness.

2. What type of seizure control has the client achieved? If the seizures are not controlled, it is important to understand whether there is any pattern to their occurrence. Many individuals will have seizures only early in the morning, while sleeping, or when taking a break from the day's work activities. For some clients, certain precipitants seem to trigger the seizures. These can include fatigue, having flu or other illness, flickering lights or screens, certain levels of stress in the work environment (which certainly vary for each client), and other events or health-related issues.

3. Does the client have a specific warning or aura (actually the initial part of the seizure) before the occurrence of a full seizure? A warning can be a feeling of lightheadedness, an uneasy sick feeling, other strange sensations, or déjà vu experiences. A consistent aura is very helpful in that it allows an individual to take safety precautions (e.g., sitting down, lying down, or otherwise removing oneself to a safe area before the seizure is in full progress).

4. What is involved in the recovery period? Some individuals can go directly back to work, others will require a brief nap, and some will have to take a sick day and spend the better part of the day recovering.

5. Has the client ever been otherwise injured as a result of a seizure? If not, this is very comforting for the employer.

6. Does the client have any other disabilities? In a recent study at our center (Fraser, Clemmons, Andrechak, & Dodrill, 1991), 89% of the clients served had one or more additional disabilities. It is particularly important to note whether there has been an additional head injury that precipitated the seizures or whether a head injury came about as a result of seizure activity (e.g., due to a fall). The additional or associated disabilities will often require specific assessment (e.g., neuropsychological).

7. What type of medication is the client taking, is it appropriate, and is he or she complying with the recommended medication and dosages? Might the

client with a clear focus and intractable seizures be a surgical candidate? Is the medication evaluation recent?

If counselors can answer the above questions, they are in a better situation to serve the client more appropriately. For example, recently at our center, as the result of a misunderstanding on the part of a counselor about a seizure type (which he believed to be a minor partial type), an individual was placed in a loading dock position in which he fell during a seizure, breaking his nose and sustaining a significant number of facial contusions and lacerations. In fact, he had had relatively frequent generalized tonic-clonic seizures that resulted in loss of consciousness and falling. In consideration of the heavy physical work he had been assigned and the potential for falling from the dock, the job assignment was inappropriate. It is a good standing policy to confirm the seizure description with a family member or significant other. As discussed earlier, many clients do not understand their seizure type and may provide inaccurate information. Many of them have never even witnessed a seizure and do not understand what occurs. A recent report (Bryant-Comstock, Hogan, Shumaker, & Tennis, 1997) indicates that a client's own perception of seizure severity, using the Liverpool Seizure Severity Scale, may be a better discriminator of employability than other seizure variables (e.g., seizure frequency).

Additional Disabilities

As discussed earlier, a majority of clients with epilepsy coming for rehabilitation services will have an additional disability. This is most commonly some type of neuropsychological impairment that has to be clarified. In early work at our center, we would miss detailed information about head injuries and other brain-related difficulties, which would result in mismatching individuals in the job placement process. An example would be an individual who had significant memory deficits and was placed in a locksmith job-training program, requiring him to remember a large number of different key molds. Clarification of some of these issues earlier would have redirected the placement effort, or the effort would have begun with more compensatory strategies being utilized. As discussed previously, clients who drop out of our rehabilitation program tend to do so because of emotional difficulties, such as depression, anxiety, financial fears, and so on. Individuals who are placed through the program but lose jobs after they are hired tend to do so because of cognitive or neuropsychological deficits.

To clarify these issues, the neuropsychological or epilepsy battery (Dodrill, 1978) that includes the Halstead-Reitan battery and other specialized measures is utilized to identify brain impairment issues. The WPSI is given to all clients in screening for emotional and psychosocial adjustment difficulties. Although neuropsychological issues and emotional concerns are more common, additional physical disabilities, mental retardation, cerebral palsy, and other medical concerns will be found in a subgroup of referrals. In review of some of these concerns, it becomes apparent that a number of clients will learn better in actual on-the-job training programs versus formal academic vocational/technical school training. Given specific cognitive deficits, it can be much easier to learn and retain the work tasks and requirements by training on the job site. This will be a counseling issue with clients who seek college training.

Medication Issues

The area of medication management deserves significant attention. A number of clients are simply on the wrong medication when they come for vocational rehabilitation or are receiving too many medications, which results in poorly managed seizures and negative side effects. Common side effects can include double vision, blurred vision, balance difficulties, lethargy, behavioral changes, gingival growth, nausea, weight gain, and liver enzyme elevations. As discussed earlier, if a client is not achieving good seizure control and has not been evaluated at an epilepsy center or by a neurological group that specializes in epilepsy, it can be appropriate to make a referral for current medication evaluation. A number of clients referred to our center may still be receiving Dilantin and phenobarbital, prescribed by a general practitioner to manage their seizures, which is inappropriate. These instances occur more frequently in rural areas.

It is also very common that clients do not take their medication as prescribed and do not understand that it can take days (depending upon their medication) to achieve a steady state of the anticonvulsant within their bloodstream. Consequently, a number of them take medication infrequently or in larger doses that result in toxicity and other side effects. They must be cautioned that it is necessary to take their medication consistently. This situation can be improved by taking the medication at a specific time or by using a pill counter or a medication box that has an alarm to remind patients when to take the medications.

Disclosure of Seizure Status

Disclosure of a seizure condition is a very individual consideration. For most people, we recommend that seizures be clearly discussed if they could affect work performance, preferably at the end of the interview, after they have had the opportunity to discuss their work-related background and skills. Consequently, they generally do not mention epilepsy on the application, but they have the interviewer note it at the time of their actual meeting with the employer. There can be a number of different approaches to disclosing. Because they do not lose consciousness, only have a seizure while sleeping, or have some other mitigating circumstance, some do not really have to discuss the issue with an employer or co-worker. They may prefer to tell an employer or co-worker that they have a seizure condition after they have been on the job some time and have established credibility as a worker. Under the new Americans with Disabilities Act, which was implemented in 1992, reasonable accommodation for many private-sector employers could involve minor modifications to the work site (layer of padding on a concrete floor or reassignment of work tasks (e.g., having a co-worker do some minimal driving that is required on the job if the client lacks a driver's license because of epilepsy).

In general, most studies show that the attendance and performance records for people with epilepsy are equal to or better than those of the general working population (McLellan, 1987). Risch (1968) demonstrated that time lost as a result of seizures was approximately 1 hour for every 1,000 hours worked by individuals with active seizure conditions. A study by Sands (1961) indicated that, over a 13-year period in the state of New York, there were more accidents in the workplace caused by sneezing or coughing on the job than related to seizures. Hiring people with epilepsy does not increase industrial insurance. In addition, second injury funds in most states protect an employer from bearing responsibility for total disability if the client has a seizure on the job that results in inability to work again. Working around machinery is generally not a problem of any significant measure in today's society. Most machinery has plastic guards and other safety features. Even equipment such as farm tractors has been modified with toggle switches to kill the engine when an individual experiences seizure activity while driving. For some individuals with active seizure conditions, however, working around heights may not be a reasonable idea, and in some cases working around boiling or molten materials can also present certain concerns. In the latter case, however, flame-resistant or -retardant clothing materials may still enable an individual to perform the job. On issues of accommodation, the Job Accommodation Network (JAN) at West Virginia University or the university rehabilitation research and training centers (identified through the U.S. Office of Special Education and Rehabilitative Services in Washington, DC) can be contacted for accommodation or ideas specific to individual seizure-related concerns.

CONCLUSIONS

This chapter has reviewed medical, psychosocial, and vocational implications of epilepsy as a disability. Within the past two decades, major strides have been made by the Epilepsy Foundation of America across the country in developing specialized vocational programs for adults and teens with epilepsy. These programs typically involve active job development, job-seeking skill training, job-related counseling, weekly job club activities, and the like. To assist the client with seizure status to obtain competitive work, there are 17 Epilepsy Foundation–administered employment programs, supported by Department of Labor funding. In addition, there are an increasing number of locally funded epilepsy programs based on the same Training and Placement Services (TAPS) employment preparation model as is funded by Department of Labor. The program has as good a success rate, approaching 75% of those served. With greater understanding of third-generation anticonvulsants' benefits, people with epilepsy should be more employable.

It is hoped that, by attention to a number of the concerns presented in this chapter, many state agency and other vocational rehabilitation counselors can be successful in working with the client with a seizure condition. In our experience, with good medical and psychosocial/vocational assessment, the seizure condition itself and associated disabilities can be worked with and around, resulting in a successful job match. It is hoped that with continued emphasis on training specific to this disability, local epilepsy association vocational rehabilitation programs and the efforts of vocational rehabilitation counselors nationally will continue to meet with increasing success.

ACKNOWLEDGMENT

The preparation of this chapter and a portion of the research reported therein were supported by grants NS 24823 and NS 17111 awarded by the National Institute of Neurological Disorders and Stroke, PHS/ DHHS, USA.

REFERENCES

Anderson, V. E. (1988). Genetics of the epilepsies. In W. A. Hauser (Ed.), *Current trends in epilepsy: A self-study course for physicians* (Unit 3). Landover, MD: Epilepsy Foundation of America.

Annegers, J. F. (1988). The natural history and prognosis of patients with seizures and epilepsy. In W. A. Hauser (Ed.), *Current trends in epilepsy: A self-study course for physicians* (Unit 1). Landover, MD: Epilepsy Foundation of America.

Betts, T. (1997). Psychiatric aspects of nonepileptics seizures. In J. Engel & T. A. Bedley (Eds.), *Epilepsy* (pp. 2101–2116). Philadelphia: Lippincott-Raven.

Bryant-Comstock, L., Hogan, P., Shumaker, S., & Tennis, P. (1997). Relation of seizure severity to employment status and education [Abstract]. *Epilepsia, 38*(Suppl.), 135.

Dodrill, C. B. (1978). A neuropsychological battery for epilepsy. *Epilepsia, 19,* 611–623.

Dodrill, C. B. (1986). Correlates of tonic-clonic seizures with intellectual, neuropsychological, emotional, and social functions in patients with epilepsy. *Epilepsia, 27,* 399–411.

Dodrill, C. B., Batzel, L. W., Queisser, H. R., & Temkin, N. R. (1980). An objective method for the assessment of psychological and social problems among epileptics. *Epilepsia, 21,* 123–135.

Engel, J., Wieser, H. G., & Spencer, D. (1997). Overview: Surgical therapy. In J. Engel & T. A. Bedley (Eds.), *Epilepsy* (pp. 1673–1676). Philadelphia: Lippincott-Raven.

Fraser, R. T., & Clemmons, D. C. (1989). Vocational and psychosocial interventions for youth with seizure disorders. In B. Hermann & M. Siedenberg (Eds.), *Childhood epilepsies: Neuropsychological, psychosocial, and intervention aspects* (pp. 201–220). Chichester, England: John Wiley & Sons.

Fraser, R. T., Clemmons, D. C., Andrechak, N., Dodrill, C. B., & Temkin, N. (1991, December). *Pre-vocational intervention in epilepsy rehabilitation: Outcome and pre/postintervention employability correlates.* Paper presented at the American Epilepsy Society Meeting, Seattle, WA.

Fraser, R. T., Clemmons, D. C., Dodrill, C. B., Trejo, W., & Freelove, C. (1986). The difficult to employ in epilepsy rehabilitation: Predictors of response to an intensive intervention. *Epilepsia, 27,* 220–224.

Fraser, R. T., Clemmons, D. C., Prince, S., Dodrill, C., Nelson, H., & Lucas, L. (1990, November). *Preliminary report of an intensive intervention in epilepsy rehabilitation.* Paper presented at the American Epilepsy Society annual meeting, San Diego, CA.

Fraser, R. T., Trejo, W., Clemmons, D. C., & Freelove, C. (1987, November). *Psychosocial adjustment of early dropouts compared to competitive placements.* Paper presented at the annual meeting of the American Epilepsy Society, San Francisco.

Fraser, R. T., Trejo, W., Temkin, N. R., Clemmons, D. C., & Dodrill, C. B. (1985). Assessing the vocational interests of those with epilepsy. *Rehabilitation Psychology, 30,* 29–33.

Gaillard, W., Shields, W. D., Stafstrom, C., & Vining, E. P. G. (1997). Ketogenic diet: What is the evidence that it works clinically and how to study it mechanically [Abstract]. *Epilepsia, 38*(Suppl.), 2.

Goldin, C. J., Hammek, T. A., & Parisch, A. D. (1980). *The Luria-Nebraska Neuropsychological Battery*: Manual. Los Angeles: Western Psychological Services.

Goldin, C. J., Perry, S. L., Margolin, R. F., Stotsky, B. A., & Foster, J. C. (1967). *Rehabilitation of the young epileptic.* Lexington, MA: D. C. Heath.

Hauser, W. A. (1997). Incidence and prevalence. In J. Engel & T. A. Bedley (Eds.), *Epilepsy* (pp. 47–58). Philadelphia: Lippincott-Raven.

Hauser, W. A., Annegers, J. F., & Kurland, L. T. (1993). The incidence of epilepsy and unprovoked seizures in Rochester, Minnesota, 1935–1984. *Epilepsia, 34,* 453–468.

Hauser, W. A., & Hesdorffer, D. C. (1990). *Epilepsy: Frequency, causes, and consequences.* New York: Demos.

Hermann, B. P. (1988). Interictal psychotherapy in patients with epilepsy. In W. A. Hauser (Ed.), *Current trends in epilepsy: A self-study course for physicians* (Unit 1). Landover, MD: Epilepsy Foundation of America.

International League Against Epilepsy (Neuroimaging Commission). (1997). Recommendations for neuroimaging of patients with epilepsy. *Epilepsia, 38*(Suppl. 10), 1–2.

Kloster, R. (1993). Pseudo-epileptic versus epileptic seizures: A comparison. In L. Gram, S. Johannessen, P. Osterman, & M. Sillanpas (Eds.), *Pseudoepileptic seizures* (pp. 3–16). Petersfield, UK: Wrightson Biomedical.

Leppik, I. (1988). Drug treatment of epilepsy. In W. A. Hauser (Ed.), *Current trends in epilepsy: A self-study for physicians* (Unit 3). Landover, MD: Epilepsy Foundation of America.

Marson, A. G., Kadir, Z. A., Hutton, J. L., & Chadwick, D. W. (1997). The new antiepileptic drugs: A systematic review of their efficacy and tolerability. *Epilepsia, 38,* 859–880.

Martin, R., Snyder, P., Gilliam, F., Roth, D., Fraught, E., & Kuzniecky, R. (1997). Classification accuracy of the MMPI-2 in the identification of patients with frontal lobe epilepsy and non-epileptic seizures [Abstract]. *Epilepsia, 38*(Suppl.), 159.

McLellan, D. L. (1987). Epilepsy and employment. *Journal of Social and Occupational Medicine, 3,* 94–99.

National Association of Epilepsy Centers. (1990). Recommended guidelines for diagnosis and treatment in specialized epilepsy centers. *Epilepsia, 32*(Suppl. 1), 1–12.

Pedley, T. A., & Hauser, W. A. (1988). Classification and differential diagnosis of seizures and of epilepsy. In W. A. Hauser (Ed.), *Current trends in epilepsy: A self-study course for physicians* (Unit 1). Landover, MD: Epilepsy Foundation of America.

Penry, J. K. (Ed.). (1986). *Epilepsy: Diagnosis, management, and quality of life*. New York: Raven Press.

Porter, R. J., & Meldrum, R. J. (1997). Overview: Antiepileptic drugs. In J. Engel & T. A. Bedley (Eds.), *Epilepsy* (pp. 1381–1382). Philadelphia: Lippincott-Raven.

Rausch, R., Le, M. T., & Langfett, J. L. (1997). Neuropsychological evaluation: Adults. In J. Engel & T. A. Bedley (Eds.), *Epilepsy*. Philadelphia: Lippincott-Raven.

Reitan, R. M., & Wolfson, D. (1985). *The Halstead-Reitan Test Battery: Theory and clinical interpretations*. Tucson, AZ: Neuropsychology Press.

Risch, F. (1968). We lost every game . . . but. *Rehabilitation Record, 9,* 16–18.

Rodin, E. A., Shapiro, H. L., & Lennox, K. (1977). Epilepsy and life performance. *Rehabilitation Literature, 38,* 34–38.

Sands, H. (1961). Report of a study undertaken for the committee on neurological disorders in industry. *Epilepsy News, 7,* 1.

Schaul, N. (1987). Epilepsy surgery. *New York Journal of Epilepsy, 5,* 14–15.

Trostle, J. A. (1988). Social aspects of epilepsy. In W. A. Hauser (Ed.), *Current trends in epilepsy: A self-study course for physicians* (Unit 1). Landover, MD: Epilepsy Foundation of America.

Trostle, J. A., Hauser, W. A., & Sharbrough, F. W. (1986). Self-regulation of medical regimens among adults with epilepsy in Rochester, MN. *Epilepsia, 27,* 640.

Wannamaker, B. B., Booker, H. E., Dreifuss, F. E., & Willmore, L. J. (1984). *The comprehensive clinical management of the epilepsies*. Landover, MD: Epilepsy Foundation of America.

Wilder, B. J. (1997). Vagal nerve stimulation. In J. Engel & T. A. Bedley (Eds.), *Epilepsy* (pp. 1353–1358). Philadelphia: Lippincott-Raven.

Chapter 12

Speech, Language, Hearing, and Swallowing Disorders

Patricia Kerman Lerner and Kimberly Hauck

The ability to share experiences, emotions, needs, and thoughts is a basic component of daily interactions between individuals and a cornerstone to social structure. Indeed "the need for socialization is the core of human existence and the desire to communicate with others is the essence of that socialization" (Chapey, 1994). Therefore, impairment in the ability to communicate disrupts all aspects of the human experience: establishment and maintenance of relationships, participation in educational programs, pursuit and retention of employment, and the fulfillment of self-actualization and independence.

The ability to communicate is a complete and unique behavior that is influenced by interacting biological, psychological, and environmental factors. Communication requires adequate speech, language, and hearing, working in an integrated manner to produce an effective exchange of information. Unfortunately, many individuals have impaired communication systems. It is conservatively estimated that nearly 23 million individuals in the United States have some form of communication impairment (Adams & Benson, 1990). Speech, language, and hearing disorders can impede economic self-sufficiency, academic performance, and employment opportunities.

In recent years, swallowing impairments, often coexisting with a communication disorder, have been identified, diagnosed, and remediated. The swallowing disorder often encompasses the same oral, pharyngeal, and laryngeal structures that are involved in the production of speech and language. Disorders of swallow function can be uncomfortable, embarrassing at times, and even life threatening. According to a major study (Simmons, 1986), difficulty in swallowing affects more than 10 million Americans.

Disorders of communication and swallowing can impose social isolation and personal suffering on an affected individual and may place an enormous emotional and economic burden on the individuals's family and on society. Maximizing the ability of a person to communicate is integral to his or her education, vocational plans, and social interactions. Maintaining a person's ability to swallow foods and liquids is essential for his or her health, nutrition, and emotional well-being.

Communication and swallowing deficits may be seen throughout the age spectrum. Discussion of all possible communication and swallowing disorders, including those that are congenital or acquired, functionally or organically based, is beyond the scope of this chapter. Therefore, only those impairments with a medical etiology that are frequently encountered by the rehabilitation specialist are reviewed. This chapter provides the reader with a description of the major communication and swallowing disabilities and their medical correlates, the treatment and prognosis for these disorders, and the subsequent psychological and vocational ramifications.

SPEECH AND LANGUAGE DISORDERS

Aphasia and Apraxia of Speech

According to the National Institutes of Health at least 500,000 people are victims of a cerebral vascular accident, or stroke, each year, and it is the third leading cause of death in the United States (NINDS, 1990). Of this population, approximately two thirds are believed to have the concomitant language deficit, aphasia. Aphasia is defined as an inability to express and/or comprehend language as a result of organic damage to the brain, usually in the left cerebral cortex. The person with aphasia demonstrates dysfunction in language content or meaning, language form or structure, and language usage or function, along with the underlying cognitive processes such as memory, reasoning, and recognition (Chapey, 1994). This dysfunction disrupts the individual's ability to listen and understand, read, speak, and write in varying degrees and is not attributable to confusion, hearing loss or motor impairment.

Aphasia can also result from other neurological insults including, but not limited to, brain tumor, head trauma, subcortical infarcts, and infectious diseases. Infrequently, aphasia occurs following right hemisphere damage, especially in left-handed individuals, and as the result of focal subcortical lesions.

An elderly man who once delighted in reading now struggles to make sense of the morning headlines; the newsprint is clear, but the words appear to him like random squiggles on the page. A middle-aged woman speaks haltingly, groping for words that once flowed with ease. Thousands of alert, intelligent individuals find themselves suddenly plunged into a world of jumbled communication because damage to the brain has left them with aphasia. Aphasic symptoms are usually not restricted to deficits in one language modality. The aphasic individual has reduced abilities in all language areas, including oral expression, auditory comprehension, reading, writing, and even use and understanding of meaningful gestures. Generally, persons with aphasia have impairments of differing severity in both the expressive and receptive components of language.

Difficulty with verbal output and writing is often commonly termed expressive aphasia; difficulty with comprehension of what is heard and/or read is often described as receptive aphasia. The specific pattern of exhibited linguistic deficits forms the basis for classifying people with aphasia. Central to a description and classification of aphasia is the ability to view verbal output as either fluent or nonfluent. Fluent forms of aphasia are marked by effortless speech, with ease in articulation and the production of long strings of words in a variety of grammatical contexts. Normal speech rhythm and melody are usually preserved. Word-finding difficulty, often termed anomia, is evidenced, however, for substantive nouns and picturable action words. Words devoid of content, nonspecific words, and circumlocutions frequently occur. At times, meaningless jargon is used.

In contrast, in the nonfluent aphasia, the flow of speech is impaired. The speech uttered is usually limited in quantity, is spoken slowly and with great effort, and is frequently poorly articulated. The language may be telegraphic, containing only the information words and excluding the grammatical words such as verb tenses and prepositions. The nonfluent aphasic knows what he wants to say but cannot find the words he needs; he has thoughts but cannot access or organize the language to express them (Kerman-Lerner, 1988).

Occasionally, individuals show a severe impairment of communicative ability across all language modalities, resulting in little or no understanding or ability to communicate. This is termed global aphasia. It usually results from extensive damage to the language areas of the left hemisphere or occasionally from a subcortical lesion.

One widely used descriptive system to classify aphasic speakers is the Boston classification schema by Goodglass and Kaplan (1983) based on the speech output of the individual. Subtypes of aphasia in the Boston system include the more common Broca's aphasia, Wernicke's aphasia, and global aphasia, as well as the less common transcortical types.

Not all aphasias fit neatly into a single classification schema nor a specific aphasia syndrome. Variations of these syndromes occur not only because lesions differ in location and extent but because the response to the same injury is not fixed among individuals (Goodglass & Kaplan, 1983). In addition, the symptoms and configuration of the aphasia may change as the time from onset increases and the severity decreases. Initially, the individual's language may have been diagnosed as a global aphasia yet may resolve toward a nonfluent aphasia with slow, labored, one- or two-word utterances during the acute stage. Following a period of therapeutic intervention, auditory comprehension and verbal expression may improve, approaching the cluster of symptoms seen in anomic aphasia.

A disorder that often coexists with aphasia is apraxia of speech. Apraxia was defined by Darley, Aronson, and Brown (1965) as a neurogenic speech disorder resulting from impairment of the capacity to program sensorimotor commands for the positioning and movement of muscles for volitional production of speech. It can occur without significant weakness or neuromuscular slowness and in the absence of disturbances of conscious thought or language. This definition has stood the test of time and is consistent with those currently used by leaders in the field of motor speech (Duffy, 1995).

The person with apraxia can hear and comprehend a requested task and can perform a movement or series of movements reflexively. But when he attempts voluntary performance of a speech task, he cannot sequence and execute the movements. The speech pattern of the person with apraxia is usually slow and labored, with numerous vowel and consonant articulatory errors. The speaker is often aware of his errors but is unable to modify or correct them.

Management Considerations. Language rehabilitation must be individualized to meet the communication needs of the client while being specific to the language deficits requiring remediation. The goal of aphasia treatment is to maximize the functional communication abilities of the person in daily living situations. Treatment tasks and goals depend on the nature and severity of the aphasia.

Remediation targets the achievement of a set of language skills and the generalization of these skills to the daily communication environment of the aphasic. Therapeutic approaches are derived from a theoretical framework based on a variety of linguistic models. Holistic paradigms address the communication abilities of the individual as a whole. Deficit-specific approaches focus on remediation of the impaired language behaviors, whereas functional approaches focus on maximizing communication effectiveness, using any and all language modalities. Technology, such as the use of microcomputers with language-enhancing software, often furthers or supplements the treatment delivered (Duffy, 1995).

The prognosis for recovery from aphasia depends on many factors, including the location, extent, and type of cerebral damage; the severity of language symptoms; and any additional associated impairments, such as apraxia. The time from onset of the brain damage also affects outcome predictions. Prognosis is generally more positive if the onset of aphasia has been recent. Behavioral factors, including motivation for recovery, error awareness, and ability to self-correct errors, all affect the ability of the individual to benefit from treatment.

Dysarthria

A major communication disorder that is often confused with aphasia is the motor-speech impairment known as dysarthria. Dysarthria is manifested as a disruption in oral communication caused by paralysis, weakness, abnormal tone, or incoordination of the muscles used in speech. It encompasses disorders of respiration, phonation, resonation, articulation, and prosody. Dysarthria does not refer to the symbolic language impairments that result from aphasia; rather, the person with dysarthria has retained the language symbols necessary for communication but speaks unclearly. Speech production may sound distorted, unintelligible, or bizarre. In addition to the speech symptomatology, difficulty in mastication, swallowing, and controlling salivation are frequently observed.

The functional speech intelligibility of the client depends on the degree of neuromuscular impairment. Some individuals have only slightly distorted speech; they can communicate most needs verbally but may have to repeat an utterance or overarticulate for clarity. Others have a more marked impairment, with involved speech systems interacting inefficiently. Their speech sounds slow and labored, with imprecise consonant production and decreased control of vocal pitch and volume. In other situations, some persons have speech systems that are severely impaired; they can generate only minimal intelligible speech production, even at the single-word level. In its most severe form the individual cannot produce any intelligible words or even sounds, an impairment termed anarthria (Rosenbek & LaPointe, 1982).

Dysarthria results from a lesion or impairment of the central or peripheral nervous system, or both, including the cerebrum, cerebellum, brain stem, and cranial nerves. The neuromotor effects may include spasticity, flaccidity, ataxia, tremor, rigidity, and chorea. Some neurogenic disorders causing dysarthria are stable, whereas others are degenerative in nature. Speech characteristics will vary according to the site of neurological lesion and the severity of the physiological impairment. A useful classification schema has been developed by Darley, Aronson, and Brown (1975), describing six major types of dysarthria associated with specific neuromuscular deficits and disordered speech subsystems, each having a unique cluster of deviant speech dimensions.

Management Considerations. When a person with dysarthria attempts to communicate, success will depend on overall speech intelligibility and the naturalness of speech production. The successful therapeutic management of the person with dysarthria focuses on increasing effective communication either through speech or through alternative and augmentative systems. Specific techniques for improving speech intelligibility often encompass the use of behavioral, instrumental, and prosthetic treatments. The goals of treatment vary with the severity of the disability and with the progression of the disorder.

For the mildly involved dysarthric speaker, whose speech is fairly intelligible in certain situations, treatment includes enhancing communication efficiency while maintaining clarity and speech naturalness. For those moderately involved dysarthric speakers who are able to communicate with speech but who are not completely intelligible, the primary goal of treatment is to maximize their speech intelligibility. Traditional behavioral methods have focused on improving the strength and coordination of the speech musculature. New technology, encompassing the use of microcomputers and instrumental biofeedback, has facilitated the modification of acoustic parameters in speech performance. In some instances, however, these methods produce only limited changes in functional production. Compensatory techniques to enhance speech intelligibility may also be employed, along with prosthetic intervention to aid vocal intensity and/or resonance (e.g., palatal lift).

For the severely involved dysarthric speaker who has poor or nonfunctional speech intelligibility, as well as severe physical disabilities, treatment may include augmentative communication intervention. This population has little or no verbal, written, or gestural communication. The selection of an appropriate augmentative system depends on the communication needs as well as the physical and cognitive abilities of the person. Systems range from simple letter and word boards (communication boards) to computer-based systems that provide synthesized speech, printed output, and memory (Yorkston, Beukelman, & Bell, 1988).

The prognosis for recovery from dysarthria depends on many factors, including whether the underlying neuropathology is stable or degenerative. With a stable neurological situation, functional gains may be realized; with a degenerative disorder, maintaining the current status and preparing for further decline is viewed as a favorable outcome. Other factors affecting prognosis include extent and type of neurological damage; additional impairments, such as aphasia or cognitive deficits; the ability of the individual to correct his errors; and the individual's motivation.

Right Hemisphere Dysfunction

Individuals with right hemisphere dysfunction, in contrast to those with aphasia, demonstrate cognitive and extralinguistic impairments as their primary communication disorder. Deficits include disturbances in attention, initiation, perception, visual memory, and the social use of language (e.g., humor). Paucity of facial expression while speaking, poor eye contact, failure to use gesture, and a lack of vocal inflection all characterize the interaction style. Right hemisphere–impaired individuals are often labeled "difficult personalities." Problems with social interactions may develop. These individuals often become isolated, with limited vocational options and family support.

Management Considerations. Extralinguistic and cognitive factors within a communicative context are the primary focus of therapeutic intervention for the person with right hemisphere impairment. Remediation of attention, recall, and initiation of conversation are three areas frequently addressed. Individuals often show a lack of awareness of communication style and of the resulting impact upon others. Therefore, activities that involve both clinician and peer feedback, role playing, and social interaction in group communication are valuable therapeutic tools.

Traumatic Brain Injury

Traumatic brain injury is the leading cause of death and disability for individuals under 40 years of age, with a mortality rate of approximately 56,000 deaths per year. For those who survive, 500,000 require hospitalization, with an estimated cost to society of $25 billion each year (Adamovich, 1997; Kraus & McArthur, 1996). Individuals who suffer traumatic brain injury will present with communication disorders subsequent to impairment of both cognitive and linguistic skills. Unlike cerebrovascular accidents, damage to the cortex is often diffuse, affecting a variety of perceptual and linguistic behaviors. As a result, language is impaired as part of a complex constellation of memory and cognitive deficits rather than as the isolated disorder noted in aphasia. Characteristics of the disorder often include impaired attention, perception, auditory comprehension, and recall. The individual may exhibit disorientation and confusion in verbal output, along with anomia (word-finding deficit). Difficulty in integrating, analyzing, and synthesizing information affect abstract reasoning and problem-solving abilities. Subsequent to such impairments, almost all aspects of daily living and communication may be compromised. Functional disability ranges in severity from a comatose state, with little or no response to the environment, to mild brain injury or postconcussive syndrome, which results in subtle manifestation of deficits (Ylvisaker & Szekeres, 1994).

Management Considerations. Prognosis for recovery from traumatic brain injury depends on the nature and extent of cortical damage, the time from onset of injury, the length of coma, and the nature of intact abilities. Significant restoration of function is frequently noted early in the process as a result of spontaneous recovery. Improvement in cognitive and linguistic function may be realized secondary to rehabilitation; in most cases some form of residual cognitive dysfunction will persist over the long term. A 7-year follow-up study of 190 brain injury survivors conducted by Tennant, Macdermott, and Neary (1995) revealed 7.4% had died postdischarge, 17% had not achieved a good recovery, and 36% were failing to occupy their time in a meaningful way.

The majority of brain-injured victims are under the age of 30, with concomitant physical disabilities. As a result, treatment must be designed to address their current communication needs and to anticipate the cognitive demands of future educational and vocational endeavors. The direction of treatment is continually modified during the recovery process. Early intervention methods focus on remediation of deficit areas and instructional techniques aimed at restoration of skills. As recovery in function begins to plateau, efforts target implementation and training of compensatory strategies. The culmination of rehabilitation is directed toward carryover of skills and strategies into the everyday life of the client.

Dementia

Dementia is viewed as a progressive diffuse pathology that results in chronic deterioration of intellect, memory, and communication function. The cluster of cognitive deficits most often associated with dementia include disorientation, impaired memory, emotional lability, and poor learning. Dementia not only affects the overall mental functioning of an individual but also the ability to use language to interact with caregivers and the environment.

Dementia may result from a variety of progressive neuropathological conditions, including Alzheimer's disease, Pick's disease, Parkinson's disease, multiinfarct dementia, Huntington's chorea, acquired immune deficiency syndrome (AIDS), and multiple sclerosis. Deterioration of language function in dementia may be correlated with the progression of the disease (Bayles, Tomoeda, & Trosset, 1992).

Management Considerations. Treatment for dementia is directed toward compensation for lost skills, support of the remaining functional abilities, structure or control of the environment, and education of caregivers and families in effective communication techniques. Application of compensatory strategies in the environment facilitates enhancement of orientation, memory, and comprehension skills. Interactions are structured to be within the cognitive and linguistic abilities of the individual in order to reduce frustration and increase communication effectiveness. Within this context, nonverbal communication, such as touch, facial expression, eye contact, and gesture, can enhance communication effectiveness and foster interactions with patients who no longer respond to verbal stimuli (Bayles, 1994; Hoffman, Platt, & Barry, 1988).

AIDS

AIDS has rapidly become a major health crisis in our time, with devastating repercussions. Along with the significant medical complications accompanying the progression of the disease, there are associated impairments of neurological, cognitive, and communicative functions. Disorders involving language, speech, cognition, and swallowing may occur. In accordance with the progressive course of the disease, these deficits will frequently increase in severity as the individual advances through the early, middle, and late stages of AIDS.

Manifestation of communication and cognitive deficits during the AIDS disease process ranges from minimal impairments that are almost undetectable to severe dementia and mutism. In the early stages of AIDS, speech and language skills appear to be primarily intact, yet mild cognitive deficits begin to emerge. Difficulty in recalling recent events and in sustaining attention, as well as slowing of mental processes, is observed. As the disease progresses, the person may have difficulty responding to complex questions and organizing his thoughts. Aphasic-type deficits can appear, reading may become difficult, and writing may be affected by motor retardation. Dysarthria of speech also may become evident.

Degeneration of function will advance to include global cognitive impairments, slowed motor responses, swallowing impairments, and impoverished verbal expression. In the late stage, the individual with AIDS often becomes mute and demonstrates little or no response to his environment (Navia, Jordan, & Price, 1986).

Management Considerations. Because of the progressive nature of AIDS and the association with chronic morbidity, remediation efforts are best directed toward maximizing the use of existing skills. Modification of the environment to enhance function, as well as education and counseling of the AIDS patient, are important components of remediation. Dysarthric speech may benefit from short-term speech treatment to teach strategies that maximize intelligibility, or augmentative communication methods may be required. Swallowing techniques and posture and diet modifications are effective in delaying the necessity of nonoral feeding methods and in reducing the risk of aspiration pneumonia. Most important, educating the patient regarding the nature of his deficits and future expectations is an important factor in the management of the frustrations, concerns, and anxieties that accompany AIDS.

Voice Disorders

Phonation, or voice, is a complex neuromotor activity that requires coordination of respiration, laryngeal function, and resonance. Disruption of any one of these processes can result in a disordered voice, termed dysphonia. Such conditions may result from pathological, neurological, traumatic, or behavioral conditions. This discussion is confined to those conditions that relate to a medical or neurological etiology.

Vocal fold pathologies disrupt the biomechanics of laryngeal function, thereby causing a phonatory disturbance. Vocal nodules, vocal polyps, contact ulcers, and laryngitis are the most prevalent benign conditions. Vocal fold pathologies are usually characterized by hoarse, breathy, strained, or harsh vocal quality and, at times, low vocal intensity. In addition, neurological or traumatic insult to the central nervous system or the larynx may result in vocal cord paralysis, resulting in a breathy voice of low intensity or, in more severe eases, a total lack of phonation, which is termed aphonia. Laryngeal tumors, of which approximately 80% are malignant, also may exist (English, 1976). Tumors are often indicated by a prolonged hoarse vocal quality combined with complaints of pain. Depending on the extent of surgical remediation for the tumor, the individual can be rendered dysphonic or even aphonic.

A common medical procedure that produces an aphonia is a tracheotomy. When the upper airway is compromised, an artificial airway, or tracheostomy, is surgically created below the cricoid cartilage of the larynx. Inhalation and exhalation take place below the larynx, precluding the passage of air through the vocal folds to produce voice. Individuals may undergo tracheostomy for a variety of medical conditions, including chronic obstructive pulmonary disease, laryngeal trauma, and progressive neurological diseases such as amyotrophic lateral sclerosis or myasthenia gravis.

Management Considerations. Management of voice disorders requires the coordinated efforts of a speech-language pathologist and various medical specialists. Treatment of noncancerous vocal fold pathologies often includes medical intervention (e.g., surgical resection) along with a period of vocal rest. When vocal abuse or misuse is identified as a cause of the pathology, voice therapy is recommended. The goal is the elimination of vocal abuse behaviors and the promotion of good vocal hygiene.

In the case of vocal fold paralysis, remediation focuses on improving vocal fold approximation to produce speech. Surgical interventions, such as silastic tube implantation, thyroplasty, Teflon injections, and vocal cord repositioning, are used to aid vocal cord closure. Voice therapy for this condition is usually employed to facilitate maximum gains. More recently, botulin toxin injections have been used experimentally to facilitate increased vocal fold function in specific phonatory disorders, such as spasmodic dysphonia.

Treatment for malignant vocal fold pathologies incorporates surgical resection, radiation or chemotherapy, and voice strengthening or restoration. A total laryngectomy, for example, requires the excision of the entire larynx, from the trachea to the base of the tongue. The laryngectomy renders the patient aphonic, and respiration takes place via a surgically created airway in the neck, the stoma. Restoration of speech is usually accomplished by the use of an artificial larynx, esophageal speech, or a tracheoesophageal puncture.

For the tracheotomized individual with an intact larynx, voice restoration is the primary goal. Finger occlusion or capping of the tracheostomy tube is often adequate to redirect exhaled air through the vocal folds so that normal phonation is produced. Additionally, the use of prosthetic speaking valves or a talking tracheostomy tube will facilitate the return of voice.

Prognosis for successful intervention depends on the etiology of the disorder, the severity of the dysphonia, and the regeneration of the vocal physiology. Of course, behavioral factors, including motivation and willingness to accept a modified but functional voice, are also important components. A summary of the functional presentation of speech and language disorders is provided in Table 12.1.

SWALLOWING DISORDERS

The ability to swallow is a basic function essential to our health and well-being, affording us both pleasure and nutrition. The act of swallowing encompasses the interaction of a complex anatomical and physiological system. Even small alterations in the events, structures, or physiology involved in swallowing can have a profound influence on the process and significantly alter a person's quality of life.

Difficulty in swallowing, or dysphagia, affects people throughout the age spectrum with a wide range of medical etiologies. A person with dysphagia may have an unsafe swallow, causing food or saliva to enter his airway, termed aspiration. Or a person may have a weak and slow swallow, resulting in difficulty in taking in adequate food and liquids to ensure proper nutrition. Mastication (chewing) may be impaired, and some people may experience drooling. Other people may have difficulty in propelling food through their pharynx and into the esophagus. These deficits create serious problems in sustaining a healthy and satisfying quality of life. Furthermore, profound changes in nutritional status may be seen. Consequences of dysphagia range from discomfort (e.g., throat pain) to coughing and choking or even life-threatening illness. Serious sequelae include silent aspiration, aspiration pneumonia, dehydration, and malnutrition.

Swallowing disorders are found in both the pediatric and adult population. Problems can arise from various causes, including neurological involvement; degenerative diseases; alteration of the anatomy and physiology following surgery, trauma, or radiation therapy; cardiovascular and other systematic diseases; developmental disabilities; congenital defects; and failure to thrive.

Millions of Americans suffer from some type of swallowing disorder caused by a wide range of medical problems. Up to 50% of persons with head trauma (Lazarus & Logemann, 1987), 30% of patients who have suffered a cerebrovascular accident (CVA) (Groher & Bukatman, 1986; Veis & Logemann, 1985), 20%

TABLE 12.1 Summary of Functional Presentation

Disorder	Verbal expression	Writing	Auditory comprehension	Reading
Expressive aphasia	Impaired production of connected speech; may be able to produce greetings, yet has difficulty producing names and single words	Impaired production of single words or sentences; may be able to write name and numbers	Usually impaired, yet better than expressive language	Impairment is similar to that of auditory comprehension
Receptive aphasia	Verbal expression usually impaired due to comprehension deficits	May be impaired but often better than receptive language	Impairment in auditory comprehension, increasing with length and complexity; difficulties more pronounced with abstract or ambiguous language	Usually marked impairment, severity similar to that of auditory comprehension deficits
Global aphasia	Severely impaired expression; not able to produce single words or connected speech	Severely impaired writing; unable to write name, words, or numbers	Severely impaired auditory comprehension; difficulty with basic commands and questions	Severely impaired reading comprehension; unable to read single words
Right hemisphere syndrome	Basic language skills are intact; however, pragmatic language and initiation of verbal expression are often impaired	Intact	May present comprehension deficits due to cognitive impairment; difficulty understanding abstract language	Reading comprehension may be impaired
Head trauma	Expressive aphasia may be present with deficits in word retrieval, discourse cohesion and coherence, and pragmatic language	Difficulty with spelling, grammar, and paragraph formation may exist	Auditory attention and processing impairments often impact on comprehension; difficulty with abstract ideas, complex syntax, and humor	Same as receptive language; visual perceptual deficits may limit acuity and scanning of written material

of Speech and Language Disorders

Cognition	Motor speech	Voice	Swallowing
Intact	May present with apraxia or dysarthria of speech	Usually intact	Usually intact
Intact	May present with apraxia or dysarthria of speech	Usually intact	Usually intact
Cognitive impairment may coexist; unable to determine parameters due to severe language deficits	May present with apraxia or dysarthria of speech	Usually intact	Swallowing disorder may be present
Impairments in attention, initiation, memory, and abstract reasoning may be present; visual perceptual deficits often coexist	May have concomitant dysarthria ranging from mild to severe	Usually intact	Usually intact, although may be impaired especially when dysarthria coexists
Significant cognitive impairment affecting attention, memory, information processing, problem solving, organization, and abstract reasoning; difficulty with self-monitoring and awareness; may significantly impact on behavior	Apraxia or dysarthria of speech may coexist	Traumatic vocal fold damage or vocal cord paralysis may occur; aphonia due to tracheostomy may be present	Swallowing disorder may be present

(continued)

TABLE 12.1 *(continued)*

Disorder	Verbal expression	Writing	Auditory comprehension	Reading
Dementia, Alzheimer's disease, Organic brain syndrome	Reduction in verbal output and syntactic complexity; word-finding difficulties evident; deficits increase in severity over time leading to scarce or no verbal output	Similar to verbal expression; writing difficulties increase over time to eventual loss of written expression	Comprehension deficits progressive in nature; initial difficulty understanding complex paragraphs progressing to difficulty understanding basic commands and questions	Same as receptive language; reading comprehension ability lessons over time
Parkinson's disease	Intact language skills; see Motor Speech	May be limited due to impairment of motor skills	Intact	May be limited by visual perceptual deficits
Other progressive neurological diseases	Intact language skills; see Motor Speech	Writing skills will progressively degenerate, with impairment of motor skills	Intact	Intact
Head and neck cancer	Intact language skills	Intact	Intact	Intact

TABLE 12.1 *(continued)*

Cognition	Motor speech	Voice	Swallowing
Progressive deficits in memory, orientation, problem solving, and learning new material; advances to global cognitive impairment over time	Intact	Intact	Swallowing physiology may be intact, yet oral feeding may be compromised by cognitive status
In later stages mild–moderate overall cognitive dysfunction may occur; cognition may also be reduced by side effects of medications	Speech becomes distorted with reduced articulatory precision, poor coordination with respiration and rushes of unintelligible speech	Progressive loss of vocal intensity and vocal inflection pattern	Swallowing impairment often results as disease progresses; diet modifications or nonoral feedings may be needed in later stages
Intact in amyotrophic lateral sclerosis; may have impairments in multiple sclerosis and Huntington's chorea, especially in later stages	Dysarthria progressing from mild to severe disability; speech will become unintelligible in late stages of disease and may evolve to anarthria	Volume and vocal quality may be reduced; strained erratic voicing pattern noted	Progressive degeneration of swallowing requiring diet modification; in later stages may require nonoral feeding
Intact	Resection of tongue, mandible, or other portions of the oral cavity may reduce intelligibility of speech depending on the extent of surgical excision	In cancer of the larynx, voicing may be moderately impaired (hemilaryngectomy), or absent (total laryngectomy); voice restoration may be possible via puncture or esophageal speech	Oral, pharyngeal, or laryngeal swallowing impairment may occur

of patients with pneumonia, and 30% of patients with head and neck resections (Echelard, Thoppil, & Melvin, 1984) show a swallowing impairment. Research indicates that 12% to 15% of patients in acute care hospitals exhibit swallowing impairments (Groher & Bukatman, 1986). Thirty-five percent of patients in rehabilitation settings (Gordon, Hewer, & Wade, 1987) and up to 50% of individuals in nursing homes (Feinberg, Ekberg, Segall, & Tully, 1992; Jones & Donner, 1988) have difficulty with swallowing.

Swallowing Stages

Swallowing is a complex series of events involving the cerebral cortex, brain stem, six cranial nerves, and over 25 different facial and oral muscles, working together to initiate the swallowing process. Normal swallowing is a rapid, safe, and efficient process taking less than 2 seconds to move foods or liquids from the mouth, through the pharynx, and into the esophagus (Logemann, 1998). Swallowing occurs in three stages: oral (preparatory and oral transit), pharyngeal, and esophageal. The first stage is voluntary and is controlled by cortical centers located in the brain. The next two stages are involuntary and are coordinated by brain stem centers.

In the oral preparatory stage, food is mixed with saliva and chewed to an appropriate size and consistency. Oral transit follows as the material is propelled toward the back of the mouth and then enters the pharynx. When material is in the pharynx, several processes occur simultaneously to halt respiration, protect the airway, and transport the material being swallowed into the esophagus and stomach.

After the pharyngeal swallow reflex is initiated, a series of events is set into motion to safely move the material through the pharynx. Simultaneously, the airway entrance is closed to prevent aspiration, and pressure is applied to the food by the base of tongue and the pharyngeal walls to propel it through the pharynx and into the esophagus. Material must be efficiently transported in order to prevent delayed aspiration of foodstuffs into the airway and to assure adequate nutrition. The speed of the swallow is defined by combining the oral and pharyngeal transit times, which in normal swallowing is 2 seconds or less. If the combined transit times are more than 10 seconds for all types of food swallowed, it is unlikely that the patient will be able to take in sufficient nutrition by mouth to maintain good health.

The final stage of swallowing, the esophageal stage, begins with the initiation of the esophageal swallow. The peristaltic wave carries the swallowed material through the length of the esophagus until the material passes through the gastroesophageal junction into the stomach. The esophageal stage normally takes 3–10 seconds.

Management Considerations

In recent years, with technology-enhanced diagnostics and physiology-based treatment techniques, health care professionals have discovered that active intervention with the swallowing-impaired individual often aids in the person's return to normal feeding and swallowing (Groher, 1997). Treatment is designed to reestablish or increase oral intake, maintain adequate nutrition, improve the safety of the swallow, and eliminate aspiration. Therapy is usually directed at specific anatomical or physiological deficiencies detected from clinical and instrumental assessments. Intervention can include swallow rehabilitation and, if needed, specific medical/surgical techniques.

Remediation involves identifying problems and selecting correct swallowing techniques to address these problems. Through exercises and management strategies many individuals will eventually show improvement in swallowing function. Treatment can be divided into three types: (1) management of the impaired swallow by changing the types and consistencies of foods and liquids to aid intake and reduce risk of aspiration; (2) compensatory strategies to eliminate the symptoms of the swallowing problem while not necessarily changing the swallow physiology; and (3) specific therapy techniques, designed to change swallow physiology. A recent study has shown that rehabilitation can be successful in returning over 80% of individuals with dysphagia to oral intake (Rademaker et al., 1993).

Compensatory strategies such as postural changes and diet restrictions alter the way food flows through the oral cavity and pharynx, permitting a person to eat by mouth. The correct positioning of food in the mouth during eating and alternating solids and liquids to wash residue from the mouth or pharynx are examples of compensatory techniques. The advantage of compensatory strategies is that they can be put into effect quickly, enabling many people to immediately improve swallow function. In contrast there are a number of direct rehabilitation techniques designed to change the swallow physiology. They may include (1) exercise programs to improve muscle strength, range of motion, and muscle coordination; (2) sensory input treatment to improve the awareness of food in the mouth or the speed at which the pharyngeal swallow is triggered; and (3) specific maneuvers, designed to change selected aspects of the pharyngeal swallow.

In many cases the individual is best managed when both compensatory and direct treatment techniques are used simultaneously. That is, the patient is given a compensatory technique that enables him to eat by mouth while swallow treatment is initiated. The direct treatment will eventually improve oropharyngeal muscle function and enable the patient to eat without compensatory postures.

If swallowing therapy does not prove effective, there are limited prosthetic and surgical options that focus on the elimination of aspiration and may be appropriate for selected patients. To illustrate, a palatal lift elevates the soft palate to achieve separation between the oral and nasal cavity, thus preventing regurgitation of food through the nose. In the case of vocal cord paralysis, injection of the vocal cord with Teflon or other substance to increase vocal cord closure may decrease the chance of aspiration. A cricopharyngeal myotomy is performed to allow greater opening into the upper cervical esophagus. A tracheostomy with a plastic tracheotomy tube and inflatable cuff may be the only option for some patients with intractable aspiration. Once in place, it provides a separate entrance for the airway and decreases the risk of aspiration. This procedure, however, deprives the patient of the ability to speak by diverting air from the vocal cords.

A multidisciplinary team approach enhances the diagnosis and treatment of a swallowing disability. Using the expertise of rehabilitation specialists and, when indicated, medical specialists such as a neurologist, gastroenterologist, pulmonologist, otolaryngologist, and radiologist affords the individual a comprehensive approach to a multifaceted disorder.

HEARING

Hearing requires the detection, transmission, analysis, and integration of sound into meaningful symbols. The act of hearing is an integral component of communication. Unfortunately, more than 20 million Americans are believed to have a significant hearing impairment (Adams & Benson, 1990). This estimate includes over 2 million who have a profound hearing loss with little or no speech discrimination ability. These people are considered deaf. According to the National Institute on Deafness and Other Communication Disorders (1990), such numbers are expected to increase substantially in the next few decades because of increase in longevity and consequent overall aging of the population. The U.S. Office of Technology Assessment has designated hearing impairment as the third most prevalent chronic condition among the elderly in the United States (National Institute on Deafness and Other Communication Disorders, 1990).

Hearing impairments are classified on the basis of site of lesion in the auditory system. This provides information leading to appropriate diagnosis, prognosis, and aural rehabilitation for the hearing-impaired individual. Within this scheme there are three types of organic hearing loss: conductive, sensorineural, and mixed. The site of lesion indicated in conductive hearing loss is in the outer or middle ear or both. A sensorineural hearing loss results from lesions to the cochlea and/or auditory nerve. The presence of sensorineural loss accompanied by conductive hearing loss in the same ear is referred to as mixed hearing loss. In some cases, hearing loss is present with no organic pathology in the auditory system to validate the loss. The term *functional hearing loss* is applied in such cases.

Conductive Hearing Loss

Pathological conditions of the outer and middle ear may produce a barrier to sound transmission, resulting in conductive hearing loss. In this instance sound energy is attenuated and not efficiently transferred to the inner ear. As a result, the individual perceives sound as muffled and of insufficient intensity. Speech sounds are not distorted; the individual is usually able to understand speech when it is increased in intensity.

Abnormalities of the outer ear tend to produce hearing loss of varying degrees. Outer ear pathologies include malformations of the auricle or absence of the external auditory canal (meatus), which may be a hereditary condition, such as Treacher Collins syndrome, or the result of traumatic injury. Otitis externa (swimmer's ear) results in a conductive hearing loss caused by swelling of the skin lining in the external auditory canal. Tumors (both malignant and benign) and cerumen (ear wax) interfere with sound transmission when they completely obstruct the ear canal and eardrum.

As in the outer ear, any barrier or abnormality of the middle-ear system often produces a conductive hearing loss. The most common condition arises from otitis media, an inflammation of the middle ear. In chronic cases, fluid accumulation in the middle ear dampens the sound signal and can rupture the tympanic membrane (eardrum). Often, individuals with middle-ear fluid report a "plugged up" sensation in the affected ear accompanied by a decrease in hearing sensitivity.

Structural abnormalities of the middle ear, such as fusion or absence of the ossicles, result in an inability to transmit sound from the middle to the inner ear. Otosclerosis is a progressive structural condition that results in the formation of spongy bone over the stapedial footplate, causing fixation of the ossicles. The disease can be unilateral or bilateral and may affect the anatomy of the inner ear. An individual with otosclerosis speaks in a very soft voice because he or she perceives his or her own voice as louder than normal (Sataloff, 1966). Damage to the ossicles also occurs as a result of trauma or perforation of the ear drum from tumors that invade the middle ear.

Sensorineural Hearing Loss

Abnormalities or damage to the cochlea (sensory loss) or to the auditory nerve (neural loss) result in sensorineural hearing loss. Determining whether the site of lesion is in the cochlea or auditory nerve will affect the individual's ability to benefit from amplification and indicate whether further exploration of the medical condition is required. A sensorineural loss, especially a high-frequency loss, will produce diminished clarity for specific sounds, making it difficult to distinguish consonants in connected speech. Consequently, word intelligibility may be significantly compromised, especially in noisy environments that mask consonant sounds. Word intelligibility becomes further compromised as the hearing deficit advances in severity. An individual with sensorineural loss frequently complains that he or she can hear but finds it difficult to understand speech even when the intensity of the speech is increased.

A sensorineural loss can result from a congenital condition or an acquired disorder. A congenital hearing loss results from either genetic factors (35%–50% of the cases) or prenatal or perinatal conditions (English, 1976). Prenatal conditions that result in hearing loss include rubella, RH incompatibility, anoxia, viruses, and the use of ototoxic drugs during the birth process. Genetic conditions that may result in hearing loss at birth or later in life (perinatal) include Warrdenburg's syndrome, Crouzon's disease, and Pierre Robin syndrome.

An acquired hearing loss can be caused by various conditions, including viruses, degenerative diseases, tumor, ototoxic drugs, or noise exposure. Common viruses that may produce a sensorineural hearing loss are measles, mumps and meningitis. Degenerative changes to the auditory system associated with the aging process result in a progressive sensorineural hearing loss called presbycusis. Lesions of the auditory nerve (acoustic neuromas) are additional causes of acquired hearing loss. Lastly, prolonged and excessive use of well-known drugs such as aspirin, quinine, and antibiotics may produce temporary or permanent hearing loss (Martin, 1986).

Noise-induced sensorineural hearing loss usually results from excessive exposure to industrial or environmental noise. The severity is dependent on the intensity and duration of the noise exposure. Hearing loss resulting from noise may be temporary, as with brief exposure to high levels of intensity, or permanent if the exposure is repetitive over long periods (Martin, 1986). Noise exposure can worsen hearing loss in individuals taking toxic drugs.

One disease often seen clinically is Ménière's disease. Ménière's disease is characterized by fluctuating sensorineural hearing loss, accompanied by vertigo, vomiting, tinnitus, and fullness in the affected ear. The site of lesion is cochlear; however, there is no definitive cause for this disease. In the course of Ménière's disease, either cochlear hearing loss or vestibular symptoms may be present but usually will not co-occur. Ménière's disease occurs at any age but is most prevalent in adults (Paparella, DaCosta, Fox, & Yoon, 1991).

Functional Hearing Loss

Occasionally, in daily practice, the professional evaluates a client whose hearing loss cannot be explained by organic pathology. The term "functional hearing loss" is frequently used to describe this behavior. A functional loss is also referred to as pseudohypoacusis, nonorganic hearing loss, psychogenic hearing loss, or hysterical deafness. The term "malingering" has been used and described in individuals who consciously falsify physical or psychological symptoms. The audiological evaluation may not be able to determine if a nonorganic hearing loss is the result of unconscious or conscious behavior. Financial gain, compensation, and psychological or emotional factors can contribute to this behavior. In fact, it is believed that some individuals with functional hearing loss have a nonorganic component superimposed on an organic loss (Katz, 1992).

Classification of Hearing Impairments

Classifying hearing impairments by the degree and type of loss is a convenient method of interpreting audiological results and aids in determining the effect of the hearing handicap on communication. Although inferences can be made from interpreting the test results, the degree of impairment is affected by a variety of other factors, including the type, degree, and configuration of hearing loss, age of onset, cognitive status, educational background, and the individual's personality.

The following classification schema, with functional manifestations and a rating of hearing handicap, may be assistive to the professional's understanding of the hearing-impaired individual.

Mild hearing loss: The individual often has difficulty with faint speech, distant speech, or understanding conversational speech in background noise; slight hearing handicap.

Moderate hearing loss: The individual has difficulty understanding conversational speech, especially in noisy environments, if the distance between the speaker and listener is more than 3 feet; mild handicap.

Moderately severe hearing loss: The individual requires speech to be loud and may have difficulty understanding speech in most listening situations, unable to hear conversational speech; marked hearing handicap.

Severe hearing loss: The individual hears loud speech approximately 1 foot from the speaker and is aware of some environmental noises; speech sounds in conversation will not be heard; severe hearing handicap.

Profound: The individual's understanding of speech is poor; conversational speech is not audible, but some loud sounds may be heard; unable to rely on hearing as the only modality in communication situations; extreme hearing handicap.

Management of Hearing Impairment

It is useful to view management for the hearing-impaired population as either medical or surgical intervention, followed by appropriate aural rehabilitation as needed. One or all of these treatment modalities may be required to maximize the individual's functional communication capability.Medical intervention is indicated once a conductive or mixed hearing loss is identified. Hearing sensitivity is often improved or restored through treatment with antibiotics when a middle-ear infection is present. Surgery is frequently the treatment of choice for structural or physiological etiologies. Outer-ear pathologies are addressed through plastic surgery to create an ear canal or a more normal pinna. Surgical options for middle-ear pathologies restore effective transmission of sound energy from the outer ear to the inner ear. The procedure implemented is dependent on the location of the middle-ear disruption and includes myringoplasty, tympanoplasty, stapedectomy, and insertion of myringotomy tubes (Miller, Groher, Yorkston, & Rees, 1988; Schein & Miller, 1990). Most sensorineural hearing losses are not amenable to medical or surgical intervention. A life-threatening tumor or disease associated with sensorineural hearing loss, however, can necessitate otologic surgery. Hearing preservation is not the primary concern in this situation.

Following the appropriate medical or surgical intervention, aural rehabilitation is initiated. Aural rehabilitation includes amplification, speechreading, and auditory training. The aim of aural rehabilitation is to maximize the use of residual hearing in order for the hearing-impaired individual to function in social, educational, and vocational roles. A secondary purpose is to educate the individual to manage his or her hearing aid, to optimize communication strategies, and to prevent the possibility of further hearing impairment.

Amplification is central to a treatment program of aural rehabilitation. Amplification includes hearing aids that intensify the speech signal to a comfortable listening level for the hearing-disordered person. Hearing aids are frequency-specific, allowing for amplification of those frequencies in which hearing loss is present (Hartford, 1988). The three most common types of hearing aids are behind the ear, in the ear, and in the canal.

In recent years, amplification has been improved, with advances in the micronization of hearing aid components. This has resulted in the miniaturization of hearing aids and has enabled greater frequency specificity. In addition, technology has allowed for the development of programmable or digital hearing aids. These have the capacity to be programmed to acoustically accommodate different listening environments. The digital hearing aid also can be programmed to more than one user-selected listening mode. For instance, in a noisy situation the hearing aid wearer can adjust the aid to reduce low-frequency input and reduce background noise (Sammeth, 1990).

When little or no benefit from conventional amplification is realized, the hearing-impaired individual may be a candidate for a cochlear implant. The device is surgically implanted into the mastoid area and the cochlea. Sounds are transformed into small electrical currents that stimulate auditory nerves found in the cochlea and produce hearing sensations. A cochlear implant is designed to amplify acoustically some of the speech spectrum information in an attempt to enhance lipreading ability (Boothroyd, Geers, & Moog, 1991; Staller, Dowel, Beiter, & Brimcombe, 1991).

In some situations, an individual can use not only a traditional hearing aid but also an assistive listening device. This device captures sound inches from the source and transmits it directly to the listener's ear without losing the sound intensity of the speech signal and without amplifying unwanted environmental sounds. For example, in a lecture hall, the lecturer wears a microphone inches from his or her mouth. The signal is transmitted through the air, by either infrared or FM waves, directly to the listener's hearing aid, a special FM unit or a special infrared unit. Other assistive listening devices available include a closed caption decoder for television, flashing smoke detectors, flashing alarm clocks, and vibrator alarm beds.

For severely hearing-impaired or deaf individuals, sign language may be the primary method of communication. The most commonly used form of sign in the United States is American Sign Language (ASL). Sign language may be implemented as the sole means of communication, or used in conjunction with any combination of the previously described management methods. An important piece of technology designed for this population is the telecommunication device for the deaf (TDD). The TDD allows direct interface with a phone line. The message is typed and either transmitted to a visual display screen or printed out at the receiver's TDD. Many phone companies provide toll-free numbers so that a hearing-impaired person using a TDD can communicate via telephone with a normal hearing person.

Finally, speechreading, traditionally called lipreading, consists of using visual cues for the recognition of speech sounds and incorporates the use of facial expressions, body movements, and gestures. Speechreading alone, however, is ineffective because only one-third of English speech sounds are visible. Auditory training, instructing the individual to maximize his residual hearing, in conjunction with speechreading, enables the person to use minimal auditory cues most effectively. The combination of speechreading, auditory training, and amplification offers the hearing-disordered individual enhanced comprehension of speech (Miller, Groher, Yorkston, & Rees, 1988).

PSYCHOLOGICAL AND VOCATIONAL IMPLICATIONS

As human communication is central to an individual's feelings of well-being, a disruption in this ability has a significant impact on daily living. Most obvious is the limitation imposed on the ability of a person to express his wants and needs and to hear and understand the messages of others. When these difficulties are compounded by a swallowing disorder or even when difficulty with swallowing occurs in isolation, an individual's feelings of well-being and the ability to participate in all the vocational, social, and family events that take place around the ingestion of foods and liquids are disturbed. Individuals recount experiences of social isolation. Body image and physical vulnerability take on new importance as swallowing, a function so basic to living, is now fraught with difficulties.

The emotional reactions to a communication and/or swallowing disability depend on a variety of factors, including its severity, its chronicity, and the extent of organic sequelae. Vocational expectations and pursuits may be jeopardized as a consequence of the disability. The personality style and coping patterns of the individual, as well as the acceptance and coping styles of significant others, will affect the psychological well-being of that individual.

A severe communication disability frequently produces a strong emotional response from the impaired individual. For example, in receptive aphasia with auditory comprehension deficits, paranoia may develop around the individual's lack of verbal understanding. On the other hand, expressive aphasia may be accompanied by an agitated depression punctuated by explosive outbursts. Often, persons with severe cognitive impairments will have difficulty in making sense of their environment, as well as of their disability and its impact on their lives. In addition, a severe dysarthric who is unable to produce even a single word yet has complete and accurate comprehension will experience a high degree of anxiety and anger. The swallowing-impaired individual may become withdrawn and depressed, refusing to attempt any nutrition by mouth when in the company of other people. At times, a catastrophic reaction to frustration and anger can be seen with any of these disabilities.

Depending on the rate and extent of recovery, emotional reactions may lessen with improvement or become more intense and culminate in a depressive state should gains not meet the expectations and needs of the individual. Attainment of a productive vocational role is highly integrated into the individual's perception of recovery. Many become depressed and discouraged when the reality of a slow, painstaking, and typically incomplete recovery has to be faced, along with the awareness that complete restoration of function may never occur.

Significant issues of loss and mourning are noted in individuals with communication deficits and swallowing impairment secondary to chronic degenerative conditions and other neurological impairments. These reactions can be exacerbated by lack of productive employment. In some cases the reactions of an individual to a stroke can be similar to that associated with bereavement or terminal illness, showing the stages of denial, anger, depression, and eventual acceptance.

In cases of head trauma, organically based psychological and behavioral deficits impact on one's ability to engage in interpersonal interaction and affect premorbid work and family roles. Posttraumatic psychosocial difficulties can represent a continuation or intensification of premorbid personality and behavioral patterns. Individuals who suffer head trauma report symptoms of slowness, forgetfulness, excessive irritability, lability, fatigue, hypersensitivity, reduced frustration tolerance, anxiety, and depression (Ponsford, 1990). Such behavioral changes have been identified as elements commonly responsible for job loss in this population. The marked and persistent cognitive deficits following head injury limit the individual's return to premorbid employment and ability to develop new work roles. As a result, many head-injured clients are in a double-bind situation: they are faced with long-term and frequently permanent stressors without adequate personal coping resources (Moore, Stambrook, & Peters, 1988; Myers, 1983).

The onset of a hearing loss forces an individual to make adjustments in interpersonal relationships, social activities, and vocational plans. Extra effort and an increase in visual awareness are required to follow a conversation. Anxiety results from a fear of misunderstanding what has been said. People with impaired hearing may also feel embarrassed by callous comments made by others. Hearing disability frequently becomes a factor affecting major life decisions concerning vocation, marriage, or retirement plans. Adults in the work force worry about the possibility of making costly errors, being unable to handle job demands, or meeting eligibility for career advancement. Employers may stereotype the hearing-impaired into work roles that are isolated and require minimal communication with others. Careful reevaluation of job tasks will frequently identify methods of modification that will compensate for the hearing loss (Schien, 1982).

The Americans with Disabilities Act (ADA) requires most employers to provide reasonable accommodations for the hearing-disabled person (e.g., devices such as the TDD, assistive listening devices, and amplifiers). Such adaptations, combined with consideration of the acoustic environment in the work setting, allows an individual to operate at his or her optimal potential.

The person who was born with or acquired a hearing loss prelingually may not feel the sense of loss as would a postlingually deafened adult, nor experience the major life changes of an acquired disorder and the related denial and grieving period. On the other hand, an adult who loses all usable hearing will feel a great sense of loss and will go through the stages of grief mentioned earlier. The severely hard-of-hearing or deaf person may become isolated from colleagues at work and from neighbors. Most social contacts depend on quick, easy exchanges. When conversations have to be repeated or written out, frustration prevails.

The ability to return to work will affect overall adjustment to the disability. Not only is vocational satisfaction highly integrated with issues of self-esteem, it also has significant economic ramifications. Vocational outcomes are influenced by the nature and severity of the disability, the cognitive and communicative requirements of the job tasks, the work environment, and the individual's vocational expectations. Identification of appropriate vocational pursuits requires careful analysis of job tasks, the work setting, and the communication demands. Does the job require speech? Is auditory or reading comprehension an integral component? Is normal hearing required for safety or co-worker interaction? Is the individual required to put thoughts into written or verbal expression? Is a high level of memory or problem solving required? Following such a task analysis, the client's deficits and strengths are compared with the demands of the job. When there is a conflict between work requirements and the individual's abilities, methods of compensation for communication or cognitive deficits are explored. It is important to consider not only the feasibility of such compensation but also the ability of the environment to accept such adaptation. The work setting might be required to support additional equipment (e.g., augmentative systems or TDD) or methods (e.g., structured work lists or supervision), as well as provide social and emotional acceptance of such adaptations.

The personality characteristics that a communicatively or swallowing-impaired individual brings to the disability will have a significant impact on the adjustment to the deficits and the subsequent life changes. Such life changes are highly integrated with the expectations of significant others and must be incorporated into the treatment process. Being able to modify expectations, develop new goals that incorporate the disability, alter family roles and vocational responsibilities, and apply socially acceptable defenses and behaviors are crucial components for a successful recovery from a speech, language, swallowing, or hearing disability.

REFERENCES

Adamovich, B. L. (1997). Traumatic brain injury. In L. LaPointe (Ed.), *Aphasia and related neurogenic language disorders* (2nd ed., pp. 226–237). New York: Thieme.

Adams, P. F., & Benson, V. (1990). Current estimates from the National Health Interview Survey, 1989. In *Vital and Health Statistics*, Series 10 (176). Washington, DC: National Center for Health Statistics.

Bayles, K. A. (1994). Management of neurogenic communication disorders associated with dementia. In R. Chapey (Ed.), *Language intervention strategies in adult aphasia* (3rd ed., pp. 540–543). Baltimore: Williams and Wilkins.

Bayles, K. A., Tomoeda, C. K., & Trosset, M. W. (1992). Relation of linguistic communication abilities of Alzheimer's patients to stage of disease. *Brain and Language, 42,* 454–472.

Boothroyd, A., Geers, A. E., & Moog, J. S. (1991). Practical implications of cochlear implants in children. *Ear and Hearing, 12*(Suppl. 290), 815–895.

Chapey, R. (1994). *Language intervention strategies in adult aphasia* (3rd ed.). Baltimore: Williams and Wilkins.

Darley, F., Aronson, A. W., & Brown, J. R. (1975). *Motor speech disorders.* Philadelphia: W. B. Saunders.

Duffy, J. R. (1995). *Motor speech disorders: Substrates, differential diagnosis, and management*. St. Louis: C. V. Mosby.

Echelard, P. D., Thoppil, E., & Melvin, J. (1984, October). *Rehabilitation of dysphagia*. Paper presented at the American Congress of Rehab Medicine, Boston.

English, G. M. (1976). *Otolaryngology*. New York: Harper & Row.

Fein, D. J. (1983). The prevalence of speech and language impairments. *American Speech and Hearing Association, 25*(2), 37.

Feinberg, M., Ekberg, O., Segall, L., & Tully, J. (1992). Deglution in elderly patients with dementia: Findings of videofluorographic evaluation and impact on staging and management. *Radiology, 183,* 811–814.

Goodglass, H., & Kaplan, E. (1983). *The assessment of aphasia and related disorders*. Philadelphia: Lea & Febiger.

Gordon, C., Hewer, R. L., & Wade, D. T. (1987). Dysphagia in acute stroke. *British Journal of Medicine, 295,* 411–414.

Groher, M. (1997). *Dysphagia: Diagnosis and management* (3rd ed.). Boston: Butterworth-Heinemann.

Groher, M. E., & Bukatman, R. (1986). The prevalence of swallowing disorders in two teaching hospitals. *Dysphagia, 1,* 3–6.

Hartford, E. R. (1988). Hearing aid selection for adults. In M. Pollack (Ed.), *Amplification for the hearing impaired* (3rd ed., pp. 175–210). Orlando, FL: Statton.

Hoffman, S., Platt, C. A., & Barry, K. E. (1988). Comforting the confused: The importance of non-verbal communication in the care of people with Alzheimer's disease. *American Journal of Alzheimer's Care and Related Disorders and Research, 3*(1), 25–30.

Jones, B., & Donner, M. (1988). Examination of the patient with dysphagia. *Radiology, 167,* 319–326.

Katz, J. (1992). *Handbook of clinical audiology* (4th ed.). Baltimore: Williams and Wilkins.

Kerman-Lerner, P. (1988). Communication disorders. In J. Goodgold (Ed.), *Rehabilitation medicine* (pp. 787–814). St. Louis: C. V. Mosby.

Kraus, J. F., & McArthur, D. L. (1996). Epidemiologic aspects of brain injury. *Neurologic Clinics, 14,* 435–450.

Lazarus, C., & Logemann, J. A. (1987). Swallowing disorders in closed head trauma patients. *Archives of Physical Medicine and Rehabilitation, 68,* 79–84.

Logemann, J. (1998). Evaluation and treatment of swallowing disorders (2nd ed.). Austin, TX: Pro-Ed.

Martin, F. N. (1986). *Introduction to audiology* (3rd ed.). Englewood Cliffs, NJ: Prentice-Hall.

Miller, R. M., Groher, M., Yorkston, K. M., & Rees, T. S. (1988). Speech, language, swallowing and auditory rehabilitation in rehabilitation medicine. In J. A. DeLisa (Ed.), *Principles and practice* (pp. 118–134). Philadelphia: J. B. Lippincott.

Moore, A. D., Stambrook, M., & Peters, L. C. (1988). Coping strategies and adjustment after closed-head injury: A cluster analytical approach. *Brain Injury, 3*(2), 171–175.

Myers, P. S. (1983). Right hemisphere communication disorder. In W. H. Perkins (Ed.), *Current therapy in communication disorders* (pp. 213–229). New York: Thieme-Stratton.

National Institute on Deafness and Other Communication Disorders Advisory Board. (1990). *Annual report*. Bethesda, MD: Author.

National Institute on Neurological Disorders and Stroke. (1990). *Aphasia: Hope through research* (Publication No. 90-391). Bethesda, MD: Author.

Navia, B. A., Jordan, B. D., & Price, R. W. (1986). The AIDS dementia complex: 1. Clinical features. *Annals of Neurology, 19,* 517–524.

Paparella, M., DaCosta, S., Fox, R., & Yoon, T. H. (1991). Ménière's disease and other labyrinthine diseases. In M. M. Paparella, D. A. Shumrick, J. C. Gluckman, & J. L. Meyerhoff (Eds.), *Otolaryngology* (3rd ed., 291–321). New York: W. B. Saunders.

Ponsford, J. L. (1990). Psychological sequelae of closed-head injury: Time to redress the imbalance. *Brain Injury, 4*(2), 111–114.

Rademaker, A. W., Logemann, J. A., Pauloski, B. R., Bowman, J., Lazarus, C., Sisson, G., Milianti, F., Graner, D., Cook, B., Collins, S., Stein, D., Berry, Q., Johnson, J., & Baker, T. (1993). Recovery of postoperative swallowing in patients undergoing partial laryngectomy. *Head and Neck, 15,* 325–334.

Rosenbek, J. C., & LaPointe, L. L. (1982). A physiological approach to the dysarthrias. *Journal of Speech and Hearing Disorders, 47,* 334.

Sammeth, C. A. (1990). Current availability of digital and hybrid hearing aids. *Seminars in Hearing, 11,* 91–100.

Sataloff, J. (1966). *Hearing loss.* Toronto: J. B. Lippincott.

Schein, J. D. (1982). Group techniques applied to deaf and hearing impaired persons. In M. Seligman (Ed.), *Group psychotherapy and counseling with special populations* (pp. 143–161). Baltimore: University Park Press.

Schein, J., & Miller, M. (1990). Diagnosis and rehabilitation of auditory disorders. In F. J. Kottke & J. F. Lehmann (Ed.), *Krusen's handbook of physical medicine and rehabilitation* (3rd ed., pp. 935–966). Philadelphia: W. B. Saunders.

Simmons, K. (1986). Multidisciplinary approach aids successful swallowing. *Journal of the American Medical Association, 255,* 3209–3212.

Staller, S. J., Dowell, R. C., Beiter, A. L., & Brimcombe, J. A. (1991). Perceptual abilities of children with the Nucleus 22-Channel Cochlear Implant. *Ear and Hearing, 12,* 345–475.

Tennant, A., Macdermott, N., & Neary, D. (1995). The long-term outcome of head injury: implications for service planning. *Brain Injury, 9,* 595–605.

Veis, S. L., & Logemann, J. A. (1985). Swallowing disorders in persons with cerebrovascular accident. *Archives of Physical Medicine and Rehabilitation, 66,* 372–375.

Ylvisaker, M. S., & Szekeres, S. F. (1994). Management of the patient with closed head injury. In R. Chapey (Ed.), *Language intervention strategies in adult aphasia* (pp. 546–567). Baltimore: Williams & Wilkins.

Yorkston, K. M., Beukelman, D., & Bell, K. (1988). *Clinical management of dysarthria speakers.* San Diego, CA: College Hill.

Chapter 13

Hematological Disorders

Bruce G. Raphael

Normal blood cells are produced in the bone marrow. A resting stem cell or progenitor cell will, under appropriate stimulus, divide and mature into the various blood cells. These include the red blood cells that carry oxygen to the tissues, the white blood cells that help fight infection, and the platelets, which are the blood-clotting cells. The white blood cells are further divided into a variety of cell types. The two most important white blood cell types are granulocytes, which fight bacterial infection, and lymphocytes, which make the antibodies, control the immune reactions, and help with viral infections. Cancers that develop because of abnormal proliferation of the white blood cells are called leukemia and lymphoma.

LYMPHOMA

Disease Description

Lymphomas are a malignant proliferation of one of the white blood cell types: lymphocytes, which are divided into B lymphocytes and T lymphocytes. B lymphocytes are cells that go through a complicated maturation process in which only a portion of the genetic material that codes for antibody production is activated, so each B cell produces a single antibody against a specific foreign protein. T lymphocytes go through similar maturation, with activation of other portions of genetic material. These cells then specialize in helping (helper cells) or suppressing (suppressor cells) the immune reaction. Once formed, these cells migrate to the lymph nodes, and when exposed to a foreign protein or infectious agent, those lymphocytes programmed to make the specific antibodies for the one specific agent will divide, enlarge, and multiply, producing large numbers of cells and antibodies to neutralize the invading organism. The T helper cells will aid this reaction; and when the organism is cleared, T suppressor cells will inhibit the immune reaction, and the swollen lymph gland will shrink back to the quiescent state (Skarin, 1989).

When one of the maturing and dividing lymphocytes undergoes malignant change and divides uncontrollably, an accumulation of these cells occurs as a tumor, called a lymphoma. The cause of this malignant change is unknown, but certain viruses (the Epstein-Barr virus and T cell lymphotrophic virus) have been implicated in a small number of B and T cell lymphomas, respectively. Additionally, chromosomal breaks that occur during the division and maturation of each individual lymphocyte can lead to mutations of genes involved in proliferation and to uncontrolled growth (Williams, Butler, Erslev, & Lichtman, 1990). Three percent of all cancers in the United States result from lymphomas, with 70%–80% of B-cell origin and the rest derived from T cells (Skarin, 1989). There is a rising incidence of aggressive lymphoma in acquired immune deficiency syndrome (AIDS) patients and in patients on immunosuppressive drugs (i.e., posttransplant state). The speculative cause of these lymphomas is excessive immune stimulation of B lymphocytes with chromosomal breaks and poor immune surveillance by the reduced T lymphocytes, which are destroyed by the AIDS virus (Raphael & Knowles, 1990).

Pathology

The lymphomas are all classified by the appearance of malignant lymphocytes on biopsy of the tumor. As stated earlier, normal lymphocytes go through various stages of maturation. A lymphoma is an accumulation of malignant lymphocytes that are arrested at one stage of maturation. Clinical behavior of the tumor is often correlated with the level of maturation of abnormal lymphocyte. Hence, a recent classification of lymphomas is divided into three categories: (a) low, (b) intermediate, and (c) high grade (Rosenberg, 1982) (see Table 13.1). Low-grade lymphomas contain cells that are smaller, slower growing, and often asymptomatic. Intermediate-grade lymphomas have cells that are larger and faster growing. High-grade lymphomas are very fast growing, immature lymphocytes, which often present in extranodal as well as nodal tissues. Additionally, the tumor can present in a nodular (follicular) pattern or diffusely, replacing the architecture

TABLE 13.1 Classifications of Lymphoma

Low grade
Malignant lymphoma, small lymphocytic
Malignant lymphoma, follicular, predominantly small cleaved cell
Malignant lymphoma, follicular, mixed small and large cell
Intermediate grade
Malignant lymphoma, follicular, predominantly large cell
Malignant lymphoma, diffuse, mixed small and large cell
Malignant lymphoma, diffuse large cell cleaved
High grade
Diffuse large cell, immunoblastic
Malignant lymphoma, lymphoblastic
Malignant lymphoma, small noncleaved cell

of the lymph node. Slower growth is associated with the former pattern, and more aggressive behavior is related to the latter (Rosenberg, 1982).

Functional Presentation

Patients present with swollen, growing lymph glands (nodal disease) or tumors in other organs (extranodal disease). Patients can be asymptomatic (A) or have one or more of the B symptoms, which include fever, drenching night sweats, loss of 10% of body weight, and pruritus. A staging evaluation is done to determine the extent of disease. This includes a proper physical examination to determine any lymph node group that is enlarged or any abnormal organ enlargement. Additionally, CT scans of chest, abdomen, and pelvis are done to determine internal organ and nodal involvement. A bone marrow biopsy is used to examine for bone marrow involvement by lymphoma. In the high-grade lymphomas, the central nervous system is more often involved, and spinal fluid analysis is required. The stage of disease is then determined by the number of lymph nodes involved and presence of disease in other organs (Table 13.2). Once the type of lymphoma is known and patient stage and clinical presentation are determined, a decision on treatment can be made.

Treatment and Prognosis

The vast majority of lymphomas present in multiple areas of the body, Stage 3 or 4, as the abnormal lymphocytes are free to travel to other areas of the body

TABLE 13.2 Staging of Lymphoma

Stage	Characteristics
I	Involvement of a single lymph node region or single extra nodal organ or site
II	Involvement limited to one side of the diaphragm with two or more lymph node regions
III	Involvement of lymph node regions on both sides of the diaphragm
IV	Diffuse or disseminated involvement of one or more extralymphatic organs

through the blood. Hence localized treatment with surgery or radiation are rarely curative (Ruthoven, 1987; Skarin, 1989). Treatment is, therefore, primarily chemotherapy, in which chemicals are used to poison the growing malignant cells. Lymphomas are very sensitive to chemotherapy, but no drug is specific for only the tumor cell. This leads to the side effects of chemotherapy: normal-growing cells are affected as well as specific organs that are sensitive to the toxic effects of these agents. Some of the disability that patients experience may be due to the presence of the tumor in a disease site, and some may be related to the side effects of the chemotherapy. Prognosis is dependent on the grade and stage of the lymphoma. The earlier the stage, the more curable the lymphoma.

Additionally, other prognostic variables have been determined, including bulky disease of greater than 10-cm mass; performance status, which refers to degree of debilitation and symptoms; bone marrow and central nervous system involvement; and high level of lactic dehydrogenase, which is an enzyme correlated with rapid growth. Low-grade lymphomas can be controlled for many years, with average survival of 7 years, but are rarely curable (Skarin, 1989). The intermediate lymphomas now have a 50%–70% cure rate, depending on stage, using combinations of multiple chemotherapy agents (Skarin, 1989; Williams et al., 1990). High-grade lymphomas are treated with high, intensive doses of chemotherapy, leading to a 30% cure rate but often to rapid death within a year for those who relapse (Skarin, 1989).

For patients who do not respond to primary treatment, bone marrow transplantation is increasingly used. High-dose chemotherapy is used to kill the lymphoma that was resistant to conventional treatment. The bone marrow from the patient (autologous transplant) or from a tissue-matched relative (allogeneic transplant) is stored away before the procedure and given back to rescue the patient from the lethal effects on the bone marrow of high-dose chemotherapy. Other organs are damaged during the intensive therapy, infections are frequent, and immune suppressive drugs are sometimes needed. The result is a prolonged hospital stay with multiple complications and a lengthy recovery period requiring rehabilitation. Biological agents, such as antibodies that attack the tumor cells directly, as well as vaccine therapy that induces the body to make an immune reaction against the tumor cells, are now being tested as additional therapy to rid the body of residual tumor (Hsu et al., 1997).

LEUKEMIA

Disease Description

Acute leukemia is characterized by an abnormal proliferation of immature white blood cells. As stated earlier, lymphoma represents an accumulation of lymphocytes arrested at one stage of maturation; leukemia is the accumulation of the earliest white blood cells, called blasts or progenitor cells. These cells normally divide and mature into the normal white cells that help fight infections, and they are continually renewed. Hence, the effect of lack of maturation is the presence of large numbers of these young cells in the bone marrow and lack of normal bone marrow cells. Patients then present with signs and symptoms of low red blood cell count (anemia), decreased white blood cells (granulocytopenia) with infection and fever, and a low platelet count (thrombocytopenia) with bleeding. Additionally, infiltration of various organs by these tumor cells can lead to enlargement of liver, spleen, and lymph nodes, as well as to gum hypertrophy and skin nodules.

The incidence of acute leukemia is 9 cases per 100,000 population, and the incidence rises with age (DeVita, Hellman, & Rosenberg, 1989). Unlike some other tumors, however, acute leukemia occurs in childhood and is the most common childhood malignancy. There are two main forms of acute leukemia: acute lymphoblastic leukemia (ALL) is a cancer of the earliest stages of lymphocyte maturation, and acute nonlymphoblastic leukemia (ANLL) usually is a malignancy of the progenitor of the granulocyte series called the myeloblast. ALL occurs more often in the young; ANLL is more common with adults. Cytogenetic studies show a variety of chromosomal breaks associated with various types of leukemia. The proteins encoded by these mutated genes cause dysregulation of division and maturation and hence accumulation of myeloblasts or lymphoblasts (Berman, 1997).

Pathology

Patients' routine blood tests show low blood counts (pancytopenia) and/or early white cell forms (blasts). Bone marrow analysis shows a hypercellular specimen with almost complete replacement by early white cell forms. Only a few remaining normally maturing blood cells can be found. The cells are analyzed by morphology, staining characteristics, biochemistry, and immunological typing to differentiate between ANLL or ALL. Additionally, infiltration by leukemic cells may be detected in a variety of sites, such as gums, skin, lymph nodes, liver, and lungs.

Functional Presentation

Patients with acute leukemia usually present critically, with signs and symptoms of lack of normal blood elements. If they present late in the course of the disease, the white blood cell counts are high because the leukemic cells have multiplied and spilled into the blood, or there is organ dysfunction due to infiltration by the leukemic cells. Patients are admitted immediately and stabilized by correcting the anemia with red blood cell transfusions, treating any uncontrolled infection resulting from lack of mature white blood cells, stopping any bleeding with platelet transfusion, and starting chemotherapy to kill the leukemia cells. Although treatment for ANLL differs from treatment for ALL, the principle is the same. Induction therapy involves large doses of chemotherapy to poison the tumor cells (Gale & Foon, 1987; Hoelzer & Gale, 1987). However, these drugs are toxic to all blood cells, resulting in the death of the few remaining normal bone marrow cells and the development of aplasia in the bone marrow. Once chemotherapy stops, tumor cells die, the normal stem cells in the marrow that are resistant to chemotherapy divide, and their progeny cells mature and repopulate the marrow over the next 3 weeks. Until sufficient cells grow to produce the necessary mature, functioning peripheral blood cells, the patient is very sick and must receive antibiotics, fluids, and transfusions on a daily basis. Remissions occur in up to 80% of cases, but relapses are the rule, and additional consolidation chemotherapy is given after recovery to prevent recurrence (Gale & Foon, 1987; Hoelzer & Gale, 1987). This further slows recovery, adds days of admissions to the hospital, and results in more disability.

Furthermore, the chemotherapy drugs are toxic to other organs as well as bone marrow. Myopathy caused by steroids and neurotoxicity from the drug vincristine are common in the treatment of ALL. Heart damage from anthracycline chemotherapy drugs and fluid overload due to multiple intravenous fluids and transfusions are common to all patients. Finally, nausea, mouth sores, and gastric irritation are typical with this type of chemotherapy, making adequate nutritional intake difficult and further adding to the general level of debilitation. In cases of relapse, as well as in some experimental protocols for patients in remission, bone marrow transplantation is offered as a way of using very high doses of chemotherapy to rid the body of any remaining leukemia cells and to prevent any further relapses (Williams et al., 1990). The physical problems secondary to this intensive therapy are multiplied, compared to conventional therapy. Hence, patients with leukemia face months of treatment and weeks of hospitalization with each treatment. The resulting physical, psychological, and financial toll is substantial.

Psychological and Vocational Implications

A further discussion of the relationship of cancer and psychosocial adaptation will be found in another chapter in this book. However, several points that are unique to lymphoma and leukemia will be discussed here.

As stated earlier, lymphoma and leukemia affect a wider age range than do most cancers, and the psychosocial implications will vary with age. Younger adults, ages 18 to 36, with leukemia and lymphoma were surveyed by Daiter et al. (Daiter, Larson, Weddington, & Ultmann, 1988). As might be expected, patients with less favorable prognoses experienced more stress but also significant personal growth and maturation. Additionally, family and friends who provided social support reported more stress with less favorable prognoses but also sometimes expressed more prolonged anxiety after treatment was completed than did the patient. Psychological stress has been reported to be lower for leukemia than for breast cancer.

Older patients have additional concerns about financial matters, how their spouses and children are coping and functioning, and interpersonal relationships at work. Depression, sleep disorder, and anxiety over personal appearance are common. Long-term survivors also have persistent problems; one study reported 73% of patients with Hodgkin's disease having at least one of five problems including decreased energy level, negative body image, depression, employment problems, and marital problems (Fobair et al., 1986).

Finally, because bone marrow transplantation has become a common therapy for refractory lymphoma and leukemia, studies of the psychosocial morbidity of these procedures have been done. Jenkins, Linington, and Whittaker (1991) report a 40% prevalence of depression with impaired function, but most cases were temporary and resolved with resumption of normal activities and return to work. Wolcott, Wellisch, Fawzy, and Landsverk (1986) also reported that 15%–20% of bone marrow transplant recipients have a degree of psychological distress that would benefit from intervention. Somerfield et al. (Somerfield, Wingard, Baker, & Fogarty, 1996) noted a list of most frequently endorsed fears of transplant patients, which included increased vulnerability to illness, uncertain future, reduced energy, and inability to have children. Additionally heightened concern over somatic symptoms leads to panic attacks that the cancer is returning. In particular, patients with continuing medical problems were more likely to need help. In addition to routine physical therapy, aerobic training has been tested in patients after high-dose chemotherapy and it reduced fatigue and enhanced physical performance (Dimeo et al., 1997).

In summary, patients with leukemia and lymphoma require intensive chemotherapy and, in some cases, repeated hospitalizations, which can lead to a host of psychological and vocational difficulties. Remarkably, most patients adapt well, but significant numbers may benefit from at least temporary counseling and rehabilitation services.

DISORDERS OF HEMOSTASIS

Hemostasis is the process by which blood clots in response to injury to the vessels. When a vessel is cut, it may constrict, reducing blood flow and bleeding. Platelets, the blood-clotting cells, then adhere to the open wound and clump together to form a plug. Coagulation factors are activated from an inactive proenzyme form, sequentially activating larger and larger numbers of other coagulation proteins until conversion of fibrinogen (Factor I) to fibrin occurs. Fibrin strands mesh with platelets, forming a stable clot that will not break down until the vessel repairs itself. Abnormal bleeding may occur when there is a defect in the number or function of the platelets or any of the 13 coagulation factors. Hemophilia A and B are the most common congenital deficiencies of these plasma proteins, and we will discuss them in more detail as prototypes of a chronic bleeding disorder.

Hemophilia

Disease Description

As stated previously, there are 13 coagulation factors. Factor XII is activated first, and then a series of factors are converted to their active form. This cascade of activation will be stopped or slowed if there is a deficiency of any one factor required to convert the next factor. Factor VIII is the most common congenital deficiency, accounting for 75% of hemophilias. It is a rare disease, however, with an incidence of 1 in 10,000 male births (Williams et al., 1990). The protein is encoded by a gene on the X chromosome; hence, males need inherit only one defective gene from the mother to be affected. Females, who have two X chromosomes, are rarely affected.

Hemophilia B, a deficiency of Factor IX, is also an X-linked recessive hemorrhagic disease. It occurs in 1 of 75,000 male births and clinically is indistinguishable from hemophilia A (Williams et al., 1990). The diagnosis of both of these disorders is made by functionally assaying the plasma for the level of either protein compared to normal plasma.

Functional Presentation

The genes controlling production of either Factor VIII or Factor IX may have one of many mutations. This can lead to no production, decreased production, or production of a defective protein. Hence, the patient can present with mild, moderate, or severe hemorrhagic disease, depending on the amount of active protein produced. Activity of the protein is measured in a timed clotting assay and compared to normal plasma. Mothers of hemophilia patients are obligate carriers and have 50% or greater activity. Mild hemophiliacs have 6%–50% activity, rarely bleed spontaneously, and usually are discovered after excessive bleeding secondary to trauma or surgery. Moderately affected individuals have 1%–5% levels of the active protein and have rare episodes of spontaneous bleeding but can hemorrhage with any trauma. Finally, patients with less than a 1% level have severe disease, with frequent spontaneous hemorrhage from early childhood (Williams et al., 1990). Patients can bleed anywhere, but bleeding into joints (hemarthrosis), soft tissue (such as muscle), urine (hematuria), and the brain are common. Chronic bleeding into joints or an acute bleed into the brain or spinal canal can lead to chronic disabilities, both functional and psychological.

Treatment and Prognosis

The general principle of treatment of hemophilia is, first, to avoid drugs that can interfere with clotting, particularly aspirin and other nonsteroidal antiinflammatory agents that inhibit platelet function (Williams et al., 1990). Second, early recognition of bleeding episodes or potential trauma and treatment with replacement Factor VIII or IX is imperative. Concentrates of these factors from normal plasma are commercially available. The number of units of coagulation protein infused depends on the initial level of the factor in the patient's plasma and the level of factor desired. Minor trauma or bleeding may require factor levels of only 20% of normal to stop bleeding, whereas major hemorrhage, especially intracranial, will require larger doses to raise levels of the factor to greater than 50% of normal (Kasper & Dietrich, 1985; Williams et al., 1990). If surgery is required, factors VIII and IX must be raised before the operation. Because Factor VIII is degraded in the plasma, half the dose is gone in 8–12 hours; treatment is given every 12 hours for several days to allow healing and prevent late hemorrhage. Factor IX has a longer half-life, 18–24 hours, and reinfusion can take place less often.

Prognosis improved with the advent of factor concentrate treatment in the 1960s, with fewer severe bleeds, less crippling arthritis from hemarthrosis, and less intracranial bleeding. Complications of multiple transfusions, such as hepatitis and, more recently, AIDS, have greatly influenced the prognosis, however. Although new preparation techniques have eliminated the hepatitis and human immunodeficiency virus (HIV), many hemophiliacs, particularly those who are severely affected and who have had many transfusions, are infected by HIV and will ultimately die of AIDS. Additionally, because therapy has allowed normal growth and development, adult hemophiliacs are sexually active, and the risk of sexually transmitting the AIDS virus is problematic. New patients appear safe from transmission of these viruses because of the new concentrates, but it will be many years before the problem of transfusion-related viral infections in the older patients will disappear.

Psychological and Vocational Implications

The medical advancement of efficient factor replacement has led to a great improvement in the psychosocial aspect of caring for hemophilia patients. A study from the Netherlands (Rosendall et al., 1990) showed that most patients consider their health and quality of life no different from that of the general population. Additionally, those who were employed had positions consistent with their education. In the older patient, however, joint damage correlated with increased disability and decrease in marriage and having children. Twenty-two percent of patients were unemployed and receiving some disability compensation. Vocational training should stress jobs that limit potentially hazardous situations. Patients who are on effective replacement therapy can compete equally for most jobs. It is clear that programs like home therapy slow the rate of progression of arthropathy, and most young hemophiliacs who are under appropriate medical care can and should be fully employed and leading normal lives.

However, the patients who were infected with the AIDS virus during therapy from 1980 to 1985 will require special psychological help and will experience greater disability. Social counseling for sexual partners is imperative. The impact of this tragic complication should be temporary as future patients are protected by the newer generation of coagulation factor replacement products.

Sickle Cell Disease

Disease Description

Normal red blood cells have a biconcave shape with a pliable cell membrane and cytoplasm in the center filled with a protein called hemoglobin. This protein is a combination of two alpha-globin chains and two beta-globin chains, forming a complex molecule that binds a heme molecule in the center, which allows the protein to bind oxygen. Hemoglobin is soluble in the cytoplasm, so the red cell shape can change and thereby squeeze through small vessels to deliver the oxygen to the tissues. Sickle cell disease occurs when the beta chain has one amino acid changed from a glutamic acid to valine in the sixth position of a 146-amino acid chain that makes up the beta globin protein molecule (Williams et al., 1990). The substitution of one amino acid for another allows bonding to occur between adjacent hemoglobin molecules, forming a tubular insoluble structure and causing the red cell to assume a nonpliable sickle shape. This process occurs only when the hemoglobin molecule has lost the oxygen molecule at the level of the tissue, and it can be reversed by reoxygenating the hemoglobin in the lungs as the blood returns to the left side of the heart. However, permanent membrane change occurs after several cycles of sickling and unsickling, resulting in an irreversibly sickled cell. The resultant cellular defect leads to the main manifestations of disease, which include (a) premature death of the cells, called hemolytic anemia; (b) vascular occlusion of vessels (due to plugging of vessels by sickle cells that cannot pass through the small capillaries) and subsequent tissue infarction; and (c) increased susceptibility to infection.

Sickle cell disease patients are homozygous for the abnormal gene controlling beta-chain production. Hence, both parents must be heterozygous for the abnormal gene. The frequency of one abnormal gene in the Black population of America is 1 in 12, and the incidence of sickle cell anemia is 1 in 650 in American Blacks (Williams et al., 1990). Milder forms of this disease can be seen with one sickle cell beta gene and either deletion of the other beta gene (thalassemia) or occurrence of a second type of sickle gene, called sickle C. The latter results from replacement of the glutamic acid by lysine at the sixth position on the beta chain (Williams et al., 1990).

Functional Presentation

Patients usually present in the first decade of life with complications of the three main characteristics of sickle cell disorder. As stated earlier, anemia results from hemolysis secondary to irreversible shape change and the quick breakdown of blood cells, with large amounts of hemoglobin being released into the blood, converted into bilirubin, and secreted into the bile. Bile stones develop early, and the clinical picture is that of a patient with anemia, jaundice, and gallstone attacks. Also, the bone marrow expands, producing extra red blood cells to make up for the anemia, causing bone deformity. This hypercellular marrow is susceptible to vitamin deficiency and viral infection, leading to an abrupt decrease in production, a condition called aplastic crisis.

The second set of clinical symptoms results from the plugging of small blood vessels by the nonpliable sickle cells. Infarction of any organ or, particularly, bone results in a painful crisis. Additionally, strokes and cardiac and pulmonary infarction are major complications of the vascular occlusive disease. Leg ulcers develop for the same reason, heal poorly because of poor tissue perfusion, and can cause physical disability. Finally, the spleen, an organ that helps clear certain infectious agents from the blood, shrinks and is nonfunctional as a result of many infarctions in early childhood. The result is a susceptibility to infections, particularly pneumococcal pneumonia. Another infectious complication results from the combination of devitalized bone and a propensity for salmonella to lodge in the diseased gallbladder, leading to seeding of the bone and salmonella osteomyelitis.

Treatment and Prognosis

There is no specific treatment for sickle cell disease; hence, most therapy is supportive in treatment of the complications. Painful crises are treated with fluids, pain medication, and careful search for causes, such as an infection (Charache, 1974). Early recognition of infection, administration of prophylactic antibiotics, and vaccination may forestall or prevent other complications (Scott, 1985). If painful crisis persists or there is infection of a major organ (brain, lung, or heart), exchange transfusion is performed to remove some of the sickle red cells. Normal red cells are transfused to lower the concentration of sickle hemoglobin to 50% (Charache, 1974). At this level no significant sludging, further thromobosis, or complications will occur. This effect is temporary, however, as the transfused red cells die and new sickle cells are produced. Additionally, transfusion carries risks of infection, allergy, and sensitization to donor blood. Hence, this mode of treatment is used only for severe cases. Investigational approaches to therapy include inhibition of hemoglobin S polymerization, reduction of the intracellular hemoglobin concentration, and pharmacologic induction of hemoglobin F as a substitute for hemoglobin S (Bunn, 1997). Bone marrow transplantation and possible gene therapy, in which the normal beta-globin gene is placed in the patient's stem cell, hold hope for the future, but many technical hurdles still remain. Prognosis has improved with good supportive care, and many patients survive into middle age. However, frequent admissions for painful crisis, the complication of sickle cell disease, narcotic use and abuse due to chronic pain, and absence from school and work lead to significant psychological and vocational problems.

Psychological and Vocational Implications

The psychological impact of a chronic, painful disease has been documented by several authors (Barrett et al., 1988; Damlous, Kevess-Cohen, Charache, Georgopoulos, & Folstein, 1982). In one paper the findings suggested that a relationship between the chronicity and dependence on the medical care system was the best predictor of psychosocial functioning (Damlous et al., 1982). Others have shown links between medical complications and psychopathology (Barrett et al., 1988). The psychological impact can include drug addiction, hysterical conversion reaction, and malingering, as well as low self-esteem, dependency, and depression (Barrett et al., 1988).

Adolescents with sickle cell disease must deal with defining their personal identity along with their chronic illness. Delays in sexual maturation and adolescent growth spurt contribute to poor self-image. Physical limitations, particularly in sports, also lead to low self-esteem. Fifteen percent of patients between the ages of 13 and 40 have been reported to be depressed (Kinney & Ware, 1996).

Physical limitations stemming from stroke in childhood, along with decreased IQ (Hariman, Griffith, Hartig, & Keehn, 1991) and medical complications, may contribute to both psychosocial and vocational limitations. The greatest dysfunction was found in areas of employment, finances, sleep habits, and performance of daily activities (Barrett et al., 1988). Hence, the implications of these findings suggest a strong need for vocational rehabilitation services, training in areas of communication and self-esteem (Barrett et al., 1988), medical treatment, and psychological help for depression and drug dependence. A national sickle cell disease program with 10 regional centers has been set up to provide the comprehensive care required, but many patients and families still have difficulty in obtaining the help they need (Scott, 1985). The centers provide cost-effective day treatment to handle the majority of patient complaints that are neither emergent nor life-threatening. Additionally, the psychological, rehabilitation, and vocational services can be provided in a family setting for the patient (Koshy & Dorn, 1996).

REFERENCES

Barrett, D. H., Wisotzek, I. E., Abel, G. G., Rouleu, J. L., Platt, A. F., Pollard, W. G., & Echman, J. R. (1988). Assessment of psychosocial functioning of patients with sickle cell disease. *Southern Medical Journal, 81,* 745–750.

Berman E. (1997). Recent advances in the treatment of acute leukemia. *Current Opinion in Hematology, 4,* 256–260.

Bunn, H. F. (1997). Pathogenesis and treatment of sickle cell disease. *New England Journal of Medicine, 337,* 762–769.

Charache, S. (1974). The treatment of sickle cell anemia. *Archives of Internal Medicine, 133,* 698–705.

Daiter, S., Larson, R. A., Weddington, W. W., & Ultmann, J. E. (1988). Psychosocial symptomatology, personal growth and development among young adult patients following the diagnosis of leukemia or lymphoma. *Journal of Clinical Oncology, 6,* 613–617.

Damlous, N. F., Kevess-Cohen, R., Charache, S., Georgopoulos, A., & Folstein, M. F. (1982). Social disability and psychiatric morbidity in sickle cell anemia and diabetes patients. *Psychosomatics, 23,* 925–931.

DeVita, V. T., Hellman, S., & Rosenberg, S. A. (Eds.). (1989). *Cancer: Principles and practice of oncology* (3rd ed.). Philadelphia: J. B. Lippincott.

Dimeo, F. C., Tilmann, M. H., Bertz, H., Kanz, L., et al. (1997). Aerobic exercise in the rehabilitation of cancer patients after high dose chemotherapy and autologous peripheral stem cell transplantation. *Cancer, 79,* 1717–1722.

Fobair, P., Hoppe, R. T., Bloom, J., Cox, R., Varghese, A., & Spiegle, D. (1986). Problems in Hodgkin's disease survivors. *Journal of Clinical Oncology, 4,* 805–813.

Gale, R. P., & Foon, K. A. (1987). Therapy of acute myologenous leukemia. *Seminars in Hematology, 24,* 40–54.

Hariman, L. M. P., Griffith, E. R., Hartig, A. L., & Keehn, M. T. (1991). Functional outcomes of children with sickle cell disease affected by stroke. *Archives of Physical Medicine and Rehabilitation, 12,* 498–502.

Hoelzer, D., & Gale, R. P. (1987). Acute lymphoblastic leukemia in adults: Recent progress, future directions. *Seminars in Hematology, 24,* 27–39.

Hsu, F. J., Caspor, C. B., Czerwinski, D., Kwak, L. W., Liles, T. M., Syrengelas, A., Taidi-Laskowski, B., & Levy, R. (1997). Tumor-specific idiotype vaccines in the treatment of patients with B-cell lymphoma: Long term results of a clinical trial. *Blood, 89,* 3129–3135.

Jenkins, P. L., Linington, A., & Whittaker, I. A. (1991). A retrospective study of psychosocial morbidity in bone marrow transplant recipients. *Psychosomatics, 32,* 65–71.

Kasper, C. K., & Dietrich, S. L. (1985). Comprehensive management of hemophilia. *Clinics in Haematology, 14,* 489–512.

Kinney, T. R., & Ware, R. E., (1996). The adolescent with sickle cell anemia. *Hematology-Oncology Clinics of North America, 10,* 1255–1264.

Koshy, M., & Dorn, L. (1996). Continuing care for adult patients with sickle cell disease [Review]. *Hematology-Oncology Clinics of North America, 10,* 1265–1273.

Raphael, B. G., & Knowles, D. M. (1990). Acquired immunodeficiency syndrome: Associated non-Hodgkin's lymphoma. *Seminars in Oncology, 17,* 361–366.

Rosenberg, S. A. (Chairman). (1982). National Cancer Institute sponsored study of classifications of non-Hodgkin's lymphomas: Summary and description of a working formulation for clinical usage. *Cancer, 49,* 2112–2135.

Rosendall, F. R., Smit, C., Varekamp, L., Brockervrunos, A. H. J. T., Van Dijck, J., Saurmeijer, T. P. B. M., Vanderbrouckes, J. P., & Breit, E. (1990). Modern hemophilia treatment: Medical improvements and quality of life. *Internal Medicine, 282,* 633–640.

Ruthoven, J. J. (1987). Current approaches to the treatment of advanced-stage non-Hodgkins lymphoma. *Canadian Medical Association Journal, 136,* 29–36.

Scott, R. B. (1985). Advances in the treatment of sickle cell disease in children. *American Journal of Diseases of Children, 139,* 1219–1222.

Skarin, A. T. (1989). Non-Hodgkin's lymphoma. *Archives of Internal Medicine, 34,* 209–242.

Somerfield, M. R., Curbow, B., Wingard, J. R., Baker, F., & Fogarty, L. A. (1996). Coping with the physical and psychosocial sequelae of bone marrow transplantation among long-term survivors. *Journal of Behavioral Medicine, 19*(2), 163–184.

Williams, W. J., Butler, E., Erslev, A. J., & Lichtman, M. A. (Eds.). (1990). *Hematology* (4th ed.). New York: McGraw-Hill.

Wolcott, D. L., Wellisch, D. K., Fawzy, F. I., & Landsverk, J. (1986). Adaptation of adult bone marrow transplant recipient long term survivors. *Transplantation, 41,* 478–484.

Chapter 14

Developmental Disabilities

Richard J. Morris and Yvonne P. Morris

Developmental disability can be traced to the work of Jean Itard, a French physician, and his attempts, beginning in 1799, to educate Victor, the Wild Boy of Aveyron (Itard, 1962). According to Humphrey (1962), Itard believed that Victor's condition could be cured because he felt that the reason for Victor's "apparent subnormality" was his lack of typical language experiences and social interactions that form an integral part of the development of a "normal civilized person." Itard placed Victor under his care for 5 years at the Paris institution where he worked. Although Victor improved over this period, he did not achieve Itard's initial expectations and predictions of becoming "normal."

Itard's work influenced the writings, research, and treatment practices of a number of early workers in the field of developmental disabilities, notably, Edouard Seguin. Their writings, in turn, led directly, in the United States, to the building of residential schools and facilities for mentally retarded and other developmentally disabled persons. The first facility was established in Watertown, Massachusetts, in 1848 as part of the Perkins Institution for the Blind (MacMillan, 1982), and the second was built in Syracuse, New York, in 1851, as an independent facility for mentally retarded and other developmentally disabled persons. Although the primary residents of these facilities were children, adults and adolescents were placed in the same institutions. These persons were generally referred to as "feebleminded" or, more specifically, as either "idiots," "imbeciles," or "morons"—"moron" being applied to those people who were in the highest-functioning category of feeblemindedness, followed by "imbeciles," who were in the middle range of functioning, and "idiots," who were in the lowest-functioning category (Kanner, 1948).

Seguin and others (e.g., Samuel Howe) intended these facilities to be established on an experimental basis as educational institutions rather than as custodial asylums. The hypothesis underlying this form of intervention was that after mentally retarded or other developmentally disabled people received training, education, or other forms of treatment to help them in their functioning in society, they would then be returned to their natural homes within the community. The hypothesis, however, was not supported by empirical data (Baumeister, 1970). In fact, few persons who entered these institutions ever returned to society, and by the beginning of the 20th century, the state educational schools became the state custodial institutions (Baumeister, 1970; Blatt, 1984; Brown et al., 1986; Kanner, 1964; Morris & Kratochwill, 1998; Wolfensberger, 1972). This custodial emphasis began to change in the late 1960s and early 1970s, with the introduction of behavior modification treatment (e.g., Ayllon & Azrin, 1968; Baer, Wolf, & Risley, 1968; Gardner, 1970; Lovaas & Bucher, 1974; Morris & McReynolds, 1986; Thompson & Grabowski, 1972), the deinstitutionalization and normalization movements (e.g., Blatt, 1968, 1984; Blatt & Kaplan, 1966; Nirje, 1969; Wolfensberger, 1969, 1972), and legal advocacy for the mentally retarded (e.g., Friedman, 1975; *Halderman v. Pennhurst*, 1977; *New York State Association for Retarded Children v. Rockefeller*, 1973; *Pennsylvania Association for Retarded Children v. Commonwealth of Pennsylvania*, 1971; *Wyatt v. Stickney*, 1971).

DESCRIPTION OF DISABILITY

Developmental disability encompasses a wide range of diagnostic conditions and behaviors (e.g., Blackman, 1983; Wright, 1987) and typically refers to those chronic or lifelong mental and/or physical conditions that develop prior to 18 years of age and require specific forms of agency services and intervention strategies that may occur over an extended duration (Ehlers, Prothero, & Langone, 1982; Scheerenberger, 1987). In addition, social adaptability and competence enter into the specific definition of one of these disabilities, mental retardation (American Association on Mental Retardation, 1992; Leland, 1991; Scheerenberger, 1987).

The major forms of developmental disability are mental retardation, cerebral palsy, epilepsy and other types of seizure disorder, and autism (pervasive developmental disorder). Some of the common characteristics that are often found in developmentally disabled persons are functional limitations in some or most of the following areas: self-care and self-help skills, receptive and/or expressive language, cognition and learning ability, mobility, self-direction, economic independence, and the ability to live on their own without assistance (see, e.g.,

American Psychiatric Association, 1994; Cole & Gardner, 1993; Developmental Disabilities Act, 1984). In addition, these persons are often characterized as scoring in the subaverage range on individually administered standardized tests of intelligence. Two types of developmental disability will be emphasized in this chapter: mental retardation and autism.

FUNCTIONAL PRESENTATION

Mental Retardation

In 1959, the American Association of Mental Deficiency (AAMD)—now called the American Association on Mental Retardation (AMMR)— defined mental retardation in terms of a person's level of intellectual ability and level of adaptive behavior. This statement was revised over the years; the current definition is as follows:

> Mental retardation refers to substantial limitations in present functioning. It is characterized by significantly subaverage intellectual functioning, existing concurrently with related limitations in two or more of the following applicable adaptive skill areas: communication, self-care, home living, social skills, community use, self-direction, health and safety, functional academics, leisure, and work. Mental retardation manifests before age 18. (AAMR, 1992, p. 5)

"Substantial limitations in present functioning" refers to difficulty in the learning and performance of particular daily skills and manifests itself in a "substantial limitation" in a person's cognitive, social, and practical intelligence (AAMR, 1992). "Significantly subaverage intellectual functioning" is defined by AAMR as an approximate IQ of 70 to 75 or below based on an individually administered general intelligence test. In addition, the subaverage intellectual functioning must occur concurrently with the person's limitations in adaptive skills, and such limitations should be related to the intellectual functioning versus those resulting from cultural or linguistic diversity or sensory limitations (AAMR, 1992). Moreover, the limitations in adaptive skills must be assessed in relation to the person's age, with such an assessment and the subaverage intellectual functioning taking place before the person's 18th birthday. This definition must also take place under the following assumptions:

1. Valid assessment considers cultural and linguistic diversity as well as differences in communication and behavioral factors.

2. The existence of limitations in adaptive skills occurs within the context of community environments typical of the individual's age peers and is indexed to the person's individualized needs for support.
3. Specific adaptive limitations often coexist with strengths in other adaptive skills or other personal capabilities.
4. With appropriate supports over a sustained period, the life functioning of the person with mental retardation will generally improve. (AAMR, 1992, pp. 6–7)

The revised AAMR definition has not been completely endorsed by the American Psychiatric Association's (APA) *Diagnostic and Statistical Manual of Mental Disorders*, fourth edition (DSM-IV; APA, 1994). For example, the APA definition indicates that the person should have an IQ "about 70 or below" instead of the AAMR's view that the IQ should be "70–75 or below." In addition, the APA includes the phrase "accompanied by significant limitations in adaptive functioning in at least two of the following skill areas" (p. 39) when referring to what AAMR states as "related limitations in two or more . . . applicable adaptive skill areas" (AAMR, 1992, p. 5).

Unlike previous descriptions, in which the AAMR identified different levels of mental retardation—such as mild, moderate, severe, and profound mental retardation—the current AAMR categorization system identifies "intensities of supports" that typically parallel the person's limitations. These levels of needed support are listed in Table 14.1. To determine a person's support level, the AAMR recommends that the person's interdisciplinary team take into consideration (a) the person's cognitive functioning and adaptive skills level; (b) the emotional and other psychological issues being presented; (c) physical, health, and etiological issues; and (d) environmental concerns (AAMR, 1992).

According to AAMR (1992), this new diagnostic and support level system "reflects the contemporary perspective regarding the expectation for growth and potential of people; focus on personal choice, opportunity, and autonomy; and the need for people to be both in and of the community" (p. 34). This new conceptualization could lead a clinician and/or team to the following type of diagnosis: "Mental retardation with limited supports needed in communication skills, self-direction, and social skills." This type of diagnostic system, however, is inconsistent with the APA's DSM-IV degree-of-severity categories, in which support levels are not addressed. Instead, the DSM-IV lists severity levels that reflect a person's degree of cognitive or intellectual impairment, such as (a) mild mental retardation, which encompasses the IQ range of 50–55 to approximately 70; (b) moderate mental retardation, which encompasses an IQ range of 35–40 to 50–55; (c) severe mental retardation, which encompasses an IQ range of 20–25 to 35–40; and (d) profound mental retardation, which encompasses an IQ range below 20 or 25 (APA, 1994). The DSM-IV also provides for another severity

TABLE 14.1 Definition and Examples of Intensities of Supports

Intermittent Supports on an "as needed basis." Characterized by episodic nature, person not always needing the support(s), or short-term supports needed during life-span transitions (e.g., job loss or acute medical crisis). Intermittent supports may be high or low intensity when provided
Limited An intensity of supports characterized by consistency over time, time-limited but not of an intermittent nature; may require fewer staff members and cost less than more intense levels of support (e.g., time-limited employment training or transitional supports during the school-to-adult provided period)
Extensive Supports characterized by regular involvement (e.g., daily) in at least some environments (such as work or home) and not time-limited (e.g., long-term support and long-term home living support)
Pervasive Supports characterized by their constancy and high intensity; provided across environments; potentially life-sustaining in nature. Pervasive supports typically involve more staff members and intrusiveness than do extensive or time-limited supports

Note: From American Association of Mental Retardation. *Mental Retardation. Definition, Classification, and Systems of Support* (9th ed.). Washington, DC: American Association of Mental Retardation. Copyright 1992 by the American Association of Mental Retardation. Reprinted with permission.

category, "Mental retardation: Severity unspecified," in which the clinician and/or team concludes that "there is a strong presumption of mental retardation but the person's intelligence is untestable by standard tests" (APA, 1994, p. 46). The AAMR does not recognize an "unspecified" category.

A number of concerns have been raised about the new AAMR definition and its inconsistency with the DSM-IV as well as with many state and federal statutes pertaining to mental retardation, each of which contain wording that is similar to the DSM-IV's severity levels and is consistent with Grossman's (1983) and AAMR's earlier conceptualization of mental retardation (see, e.g., Gresham, MacMillan, & Siperstein, 1995; Hodapp, 1995; MacMillan, Gresham, & Siperstein, 1993; Matson, 1995). The implementation of the AAMR's new diagnostic and support-level system may therefore be problematic for many clinicians, schools, state and locally funded community service agencies, and residential treatment centers.

With regard to prevalence data, using Grossman's (1983) and AAMR's pre-1992 definition, it has been estimated that between 5% and 6% of all school-age children are typically diagnosed as having mental retardation, whereas approximately 1% of all individuals over 18 years of age receive this diagnosis. The apparent discrepancy between these two estimates appears to be related to the acquisition of adaptive skills as people grow older. As these skills are developed and maintained over time, many adults who were diagnosed as mentally retarded in school no longer appear to meet the criteria for the diagnosis because, as adults, they manifest sufficiently high levels of adaptive behavior skills to offset any cognitive abilities limitations. Thus, even though a person may still score below 70 or 75 on an IQ test, if he or she does not demonstrate any significant deficits in adaptive skills (i.e., communication, self-care, home living, social skills, community use, self-direction, health and safety, functional academics, leisure, and work), then the person can not be classified as having mental retardation.

An appreciable amount of research has been devoted to determining the causes of mental retardation, as well as to developing techniques and strategies for the treatment and prevention of this disorder (see, e.g., Aman & Singh, 1991; Berg, 1975; Cole & Gardner, 1993; Coutler, 1991; Gullone, King, & Cummins, 1996; Matson & Coe, 1992; Matson, Appelgate, Smirdo, & Stallings, 1998; Peterson & Martens, 1995; Williams, Kirkpatrick-Sanchez, & Crocker, 1994; Zigler & Hodapp, 1986). It is estimated that certain known physical conditions (e.g., metabolic disorders, chromosomal abnormalities, maternal infections, alcoholism or drug abuse, and birth trauma) account for less than 25% of those persons who have been diagnosed as having mental retardation (APA, 1994; Grossman, 1983). These factors also tend to be associated with the presence of sensory, motor, metabolic, anatomical, and/or emotional abnormalities. Most of the physical causes are also associated with moderate, severe, or profound forms of mental retardation, not mild mental retardation. Table 14.2 lists some of the physical conditions associated with mental retardation. For the other 75% of the individuals, whose mental retardation is not accounted for by these conditions, the etiology is largely unknown, although social deprivation and the associated inadequate level of environmental stimulation is considered to be a primary factor (Matson et al., 1998).

Autism

More than 50 years ago, Leo Kanner (1943) described a group of 11 children who displayed a similar pattern of specific symptoms that were significantly different from those of other childhood behavior disorders. Kanner called this form of childhood psychopathology "early infantile autism" and noted that among its characteristics were marked withdrawal; dislike of being held; unresponsiveness to people as well as to the environment; manipulation of objects in a

TABLE 14.2 Some Conditions or Events Associated with Mental Retardation

Period of development	Type of condition or event	Examples
Pre- and periconceptual	Metabolic disorders	Mucopolysaccharidoses Tay-Sachs disease
	Brain malformation	Encephalocele Hydranencephaly
	Neurocutaneous syndromes	Tuberous sclerosis Neurofibromatosis
	Chromosomal abnormalities	Down's syndrome Cri du chat syndrome
Prenatal	Teratogens	Chemicals Radiation Alcohol
	Infection	Rubella Cytomegalovirus
	Fetal malnutrition	Mother with high blood pressure or kidney disease
Perinatal	Prematurity	Complications such as poor oxygenation of the brain and intracranial hemorrhage
	Metabolic abnormalities	Asphyxia at birth Hypoglycemia
	Trauma	Misapplication of forceps
	Infection	Herpes simplex encephalitis
Postnatal	Infection	Meningitis
	Trauma	Automobile accident Child abuse
	Lack of oxygen	Near drowning Strangulation
	Severe nutritional deficiency	Kwashiorkor
	Environmental toxins	Lead
	Environmental and social problems	Psychosocial deprivation Parental psychiatric disorders

From: Blackman, J. A. (Ed.). (1983). *Medical aspects of developmental disabilities in children birth to three*. Iowa City, IA: University of Iowa Press. Reprinted with permission.

rigid, stereotyped manner; lack of appropriate play; failure to acquire normal speech; echolalia and difficulties with pronoun use; anxious insistence on sameness in the environment; excellent rote memories; normal physical appearance; and good cognitive potential.

Currently, autism is characterized by the following: (a) qualitative impairment in reciprocal social interaction; (b) qualitative impairment in verbal and nonverbal communication, as well as in imaginative activity; (c) restricted and stereotyped patterns of behavior, interests, and activities; (d) delays or abnormal functioning in at least one of these areas, with onset prior to 3 years of age; and (e) the disturbance is not better accounted for by Rett's disorder or childhood disintegrative disorder (pervasive developmental disorders in which there is a period of normal functioning after birth, followed by the development of multiple specific deficits or marked regression in multiple areas of functioning) (APA, 1994). Charlop-Christy, Schreibman, Pierce, and Kurtz (1998) have noted that the significant characteristics of autistic children include profound deficits in social behavior (including failure to develop relationships with people); problems in understanding the intentions, motivations, and beliefs of others or of themselves (i.e., an impaired "theory of mind"); problems in the development of speech and language (e.g., echolalia, pronominal reversal, failure to acquire functional speech) that affect the child's ability to learn, communicate, and develop relationships with others; ritualistic behavior and the insistence on sameness; abnormalities in response to the physical environment; self-stimulatory behavior; self-injurious behavior; and limited intellectual functioning.

According to Ritvo and Freeman (1978), the majority of autistic children are functioning in the mentally retarded range; the majority having IQs below 70. Accurate assessment of intellectual functioning of children with autism may be difficult, however, as inappropriate behaviors may interfere with test taking, they may not be motivated to do well on IQ tests, and individuals with language impairment tend to perform poorly on tests of abstract reasoning and symbolic logic (L. K. Koegel, R. L. Koegel, & Smith, 1997; Schreibman & Charlop, 1987). Nevertheless, IQ scores of children with autism are generally stable and tend to be predictive of educational performance (Rutter, 1978; Rutter & Bartak, 1973).

TREATMENT AND PROGNOSIS

The modern approach to treating developmentally disabled persons began in the late 1960s and early 1970s. Previously, treatment was typically limited to custodial care within institutional settings, education in private or church-related schools for those who were functioning in the severe and profound range of mental retardation, segregated classroom education (i.e., classrooms for the trainable and educable) for mildly retarded and higher-functioning children and youth, and sheltered workshop activities both within and outside the custodial institution for older youths and adults who were high-functioning. Although psychotherapy and counseling services were available, they were very limited prior to the 1970s (e.g., Cowen, 1963; Stacey & DeMartino, 1957). It was not until the behavior modification treatment research of the early to mid-1960s became more widely disseminated in the late 1960s and early 1970s that the treatment emphasis with mentally retarded and autistic persons began to change (see, e.g., Ayllon & Azrin, 1968; Gardner, 1971; Matson & McCartney, 1981; Morris, 1976; Thompson & Grabowski, 1972; Ullmann & Krasner, 1965).

Mental Retardation

So much has been written about the relative effectiveness of behavior modification procedures with people who have mental retardation that few writers today would question its utility and the role that these procedures have played in assisting people to live more comfortable and humane lives, independent of their level of mental retardation (see, e.g., Brown et al., 1986; Cole & Gardner, 1993; Matson et al., 1998; Matson & Schaughency, 1988; Wacker & Berg, 1988).

Reinforcement Procedures

Reinforcement is typically defined as an event that immediately follows a specific behavior that has been designated for change (called the target behavior) and that results in an increase in the frequency of occurrence of that behavior (e.g., Skinner, 1938, 1953). Because reinforcement is defined for our purposes in terms of its effects on the person, something that might be reinforcing to one person may not be reinforcing to another person. It is therefore very important when using reinforcement procedures to make sure that the clinician, teacher, or other care provider knows what is a reinforcer for the person with whom she or he is working.

There are typically five categories of *positive reinforcement*: social praise ("Very Good," "That's right," "Fine," "You're terrific," etc.), nonverbal messages (smiling, tickling, hugging, kissing, etc.), edibles (small amounts of the person's favorite foods or snacks or favorite drinks), objects (pencil, paper, book, coupons, toys, cosmetics, etc.), and activities (playing catch, playing video games or other electronic games, going to the county fair, going to a shopping mall or park, etc.) (Morris, 1985). The positive reinforcers used by the clinician, teacher, or other care provider should be appropriate for the person's age, and if possible, the clinician or other behavior modifier should avoid the use of edibles or liquids. Use of edibles and liquids is usually reserved for clients who are severely to profoundly handicapped. The most commonly used method for distributing positive reinforcers is through the use of a conditioned reinforcer, called a token, within a *token economy program* (see, e.g., Ayllon & Azrin, 1968; Kazdin, 1994; Morris, 1985). A token is an object (such as a metal washer, poker chip, "credit card" receipt, or check mark on a personalized identity card) that can be earned by the client each time he or she engages in the target behavior and that has a quantitative relationship to the obtainment (i.e., "purchasing") of particular positive reinforcers such as those listed above.

Positive reinforcement can be applied on a continuous or intermittent basis but, whenever possible, should be applied on an intermittent basis. In addition, reinforcement can be applied when the client performs the target behavior or, in the case of *differential reinforcement of other behavior* (DRO) or *differential reinforcement of incompatible behavior* (DRI), when the client engages, respectively, in a behavior(s) other than the target behavior (DRO) or a behavior(s) that is incompatible with the target behavior (DRI). Another procedure, *shaping*, is used when the clinician or other behavior modifier wants to teach a complex target behavior to the client in successive steps, with each step gradually leading to an approximation of the desired behavior. For example, instead of attempting to teach a severely handicapped client a whole complex behavior pattern, the behavior modifier would break up the behavior into its component parts and teach each component in successive steps that lead eventually to the performance of the complex behavior pattern (Morris, 1985).

Each of these reinforcement procedures has been used successfully with persons with mental retardation to teach them a variety of target behaviors, such as self-help/self-care skills, social skills, reading, math, writing, job interview skills, job-finding skills, independent living skills, assertiveness, speech and sign language, and vocational/prevocational skills (see, e.g., Cole & Gardner, 1993; Matson et al., 1998; Matson & McCartney, 1981; Morris & McReynolds, 1986).

Behavior-Reduction Procedures

Behavior-reduction procedures involve the introduction of a dissatisfying or unpleasant event immediately following a person's performance of the target behavior that results in a decrease in the probability that the target behavior will occur again the next time that the same antecedent or situational stimuli are present (Skinner, 1938, 1953). The most commonly used behavior-reduction procedures are extinction, time-out from positive reinforcement, response cost, and overcorrection (Morris, 1985). *Extinction* refers to the removal of the reinforcing consequences that normally follow a particular target behavior (Skinner, 1953). To use this procedure, the clinician, teacher or other care provider must be able to (a) identify those consequences that are reinforcing or maintaining the client's undesirable behavior, (b) determine whether those consequences will follow the client's behavior each time the behavior is performed, (c) control the occurrence of those consequences, and (d) be consistent in the use of the procedure each time the target behavior is performed (Morris, 1985). If these conditions cannot be met, another behavior-reduction procedure should be used.

Time-out from positive reinforcement involves removing the person from an attractive and positively reinforcing situation (or withdrawing a positive reinforcing activity) for a particular period of time immediately following the client's performance of the undesirable target behavior. The type of time-out setting in which the client is placed is very important and should contain fewer positive aspects than the positive reinforcing area. Three types of time-out procedures have been applied with persons with mental retardation. "Contingent observation" involves having the client who performs the undesirable target behavior step away from the reinforcing setting (e.g., small group discussion, athletic event, group vocational activity) for a specified period and watch the other people in the setting perform appropriate behaviors and receive positive reinforcement from the clinician or other behavior modifier. The client then rejoins the group after a specific time has elapsed. A second time-out method is called "exclusion time-out." In this method, the person is removed from the reinforcing setting for a specific time and placed in a situation that has a lower reinforcement value to the client each time he or she performs the undesirable target behavior. Typically, the client is not removed to another room or environment with this procedure; rather, he or she is placed in an isolated area in the same room with his or her back to the group activity.

A third procedure is "seclusion time-out," in which the client is removed from the reinforcing situation for a specific period and placed in a supervised isolated area (e.g., vacant room, cubicle) that is separate from the reinforcing setting. The isolated area must be well ventilated, well lighted, and unlocked, and the person must be monitored on a regular basis (Kazdin, 1994; Morris, 1985).

Another behavior reduction procedure is *response cost.* This procedure is typically combined with a token-economy positive reinforcement method and involves placing a cost on a client's performance of a specific undesirable target behavior. Thus, this procedure consists of the removal or withdrawal of a particular quantity of reinforcers (tokens) from the person each time he or she performs the target behavior. *Overcorrection* is a procedure that includes both an educational and a response-suppression component (Foxx & Azrin, 1972). These components are "restitution" (the person corrects the environmental effects of the impact of his or her undesirable behavior to a vastly improved state) and "positive practice" (the person is required to intensely practice appropriate types of behavior in the environmental setting in which he or she performed the undesirable behavior).

These methods have been used effectively to decrease the frequency or eliminate the occurrence of a wide variety of target behaviors, including physical aggression, verbal aggression, disruptive behaviors, property destruction, stealing, noncompliance, head banging and other self-injurious behavior (SIB), and self-stimulation. However, they should be used only in conjunction with positive reinforcement procedures to teach alternative desirable target behaviors to clients (Kazdin, 1994; Morris, 1985).

Modeling/Imitation Learning Procedures

Behavior change that results from the observation of another person has been typically referred to as *modeling* (Bandura, 1969; Bandura & Walters, 1963). The modeling procedure consists of an individual called the model (e.g., therapist, teacher, parent, aide) and a person called the observer (e.g., the client). The observer typically observes the model performing the desirable target behavior in a familiar setting, where the model experiences reinforcement for engaging in the behavior. Another approach to modeling follows Skinner's (1938, 1953) position, in which the clinician, teacher, or other care provider first demonstrates the target behavior and then reinforces the person for successfully imitating the target behavior of the therapist. Modeling or imitation learning often reduces the amount of time that a person needs to learn a particular behavior.

Although modeling and imitation learning have been found effective in teaching persons with mental retardation, there are certain preconditions that must be met for it to be helpful. First, the person should be able to attend to the various aspects of the modeling situation. Second, the person should be able to reproduce motorically the modeled behavior. Third, the person should be motivated to perform the target behavior that she or he has observed (Bandura, 1969; Rimm & Masters, 1979). If any of these factors is absent, the clinician should consider using another behavior modification procedure to teach the target behavior. Modeling has been used effectively to teach such behaviors as social skills, speech and related conversational skills, and recreational activities.

Self-Management Procedures

Self-management refers to a group of procedures in which the person becomes the primary agent directing and controlling his or her behavior to lead to preplanned and specific behavior changes and/or consequences (e.g., Goldfried & Merbaum, 1973; Kanfer, 1980; Karoly & Kanfer, 1982; Lloyd, Hallahan, Kauffman, & Keller, 1998; Matson et al., 1998). Self-management methods have the following as their common base: (a) the recognition of the contribution of cognitive processes to behavior change and (b) the view that individuals can regulate their own behavior. A third common base involves the presence of a clinician, teacher, or other care provider to motivate the person to begin the self-management plan and to teach him or her how, when, and where to use it (Kanfer, 1980).

The essence of a self-management approach involves the following general steps: (a) having the mentally retarded person discuss with the clinician or teacher the negative thinking styles that may be preventing the person from working effectively or that may lead him or her to become emotionally upset; (b) developing with the person specific self-statements, rules, or strategies that can be used to assist him or her in performing the appropriate target behavior, educational task, or work activity; and (c) providing the person with positive reinforcement and feedback for his or her use of the self-management procedure (e.g., Meichenbaum & Genest, 1980).

Self-management procedures represent a potentially effective approach for changing the behaviors of mentally retarded people (Ferretti, Cavalier, Murphy, & Murphy, 1993). The relative effectiveness of this approach, however, is tied not only to the level of structuring provided by the clinician but also to the receptiveness, interest, and motivational level of the client in implementing the procedure. Moreover, in some cases, if the level of cognitive functioning in the client is quite low, the procedures may be contraindicated—although there is research literature to suggest that they can also be used effectively with severely handicapped clients (e.g., Ferretti et al., 1993; Rusch, McKee, Chadsey-Rusch, & Renzaglia, 1988; Shapiro, 1981, 1986). Self-management has been used effectively with teaching such behaviors as on-task activity, exercise skills, chores, and social skills.

Autism

Until the mid-1960s the most widely used therapeutic approach with people who had autism was psychoanalytically based treatment. It was assumed that the basis for autism was a pathological parent-infant relationship (see, e.g., Bettelheim, 1950, 1967, 1974; Kanner, 1943, 1948). By the mid-1960s alternative approaches to the understanding and treatment of autism began to appear in the research and practice literature (Harris, 1988). An early alternative approach was associated with the organic theory of autism as proposed by Rimland (1964). After thoroughly reviewing the literature on autism, Rimland concluded that the disorder had a biological basis. His book stimulated a great deal of interest in the biological bases of autism, and treatment programs based on his assumption of a neurological or a biochemical dysfunction were developed (see, e.g., Perry & Meiselas, 1988; Schopler, 1965; Schopler & Reichler, 1971).

More recent research on the biochemical basis of autism has focused on the role of the neurotransmitter serotonin, which is involved in the body's arousal system. Altered serotonergic function in individuals with autism has been reported by Freeman and Ritvo (1984), who note that 30% to 40% of autistic individuals maintain an elevated level of blood serotonin throughout their lifetime rather than demonstrating the expected decrease in serotonin level with maturation. Some studies on pharmacological treatment to reduce blood serotonin levels (e.g., with fenfluramine) have reported improved eye contact, social awareness, attention, IQ scores, and sleep patterns, as well as decreased hyperactivity and repetitive behavior (e.g., August, Raz, & Baird, 1985; Ritvo et al., 1984). However, other studies have failed to demonstrate behavioral or other improvements as a result of pharmacological treatment to decrease blood serotonin level (e.g., Duker et al., 1991; Ekman, Miranda-Linne, Gilberg, & Garle, 1989). Charlop-Christy et al. (1998) have noted that, in general, pharmacological treatment of children with autism has had limited success, with most drug treatments focusing on the reduction or alleviation of disruptive symptoms.

In addition to studies on the biochemical basis of autism, other recent studies have focused on abnormal neuronal organization and brain development in individuals with autism (e.g., Waterhouse, Fein, & Mohdahl, 1996). Neuroimaging studies using MRIs and CT scans, as well as postmortem examinations, have revealed a higher incidence of structural brain defects, particularly in the cerebellum, in autistic than in normal individuals (e.g., Courchesne, 1989; Courchesne et al., 1994; Haas et al., 1996; Rapin & Katzman, 1998). The cerebellum is involved in the regulation of incoming sensation, and it has been suggested that decreased cerebellar volume in autistic individuals contributes to difficulties in coordinating and shifting attention (i.e., problems in "joint attention" and in shifting attention between people and between people and objects). It should also be noted that studies on the heritability of autism have found a high concordance rate in monozygotic but not dizygotic twins, suggesting that autism is an autosomal recessive genetic disorder (e.g., Ritvo, Freeman, Mason-Brothers, Mo, & Ritvo, 1985; Ritvo, Spence, et al., 1985). No genetically based treatment programs have been developed, but information on the heritability of autism may be of use in genetic counseling.

Most contemporary intervention programs for the treatment of autism are based on the use of *behavior modification procedures*, and the behavioral approach is reported to be the major treatment model that has been empirically demonstrated to be effective in treating autistic children (Charlop-Christy et al., 1998). One of the earliest behavioral programs was proposed by Lovaas and his associates (e.g., Lovaas, 1977; Lovaas, Berberich, Perloff, & Schaeffer, 1966). They used behavior modification techniques to modify many of the behavioral characteristics associated with autism, including increasing the frequency of eye contact, developing functional speech and social skills, and reducing self-injurious and stereotypic behaviors. More recently, Lovaas (1987) reported on the results of a treatment study in which preschool children with autism received intensive behavioral treatment (i.e., more than 40 hours per week of intensive one-to-one behavioral intervention), while similar children in a control group received less intensive treatment (i.e., 10 hours per week of behavioral treatment). Results indicated that 47% of the children in the intensive treatment group, compared to 2% of the children in the control group, achieved normal intellectual functioning and were placed in the regular first-grade education program.

A review of behavioral treatment programs for individuals with autism suggests that most studies have focused on the use of procedures to reduce or eliminate behavior problems (e.g., tantrums, aggression, SIB, self-stimulation) and to develop and strengthen communication and social skills. Programs for treating behavior problems have typically used extinction, as well as such positive reinforcement techniques as DRO and DRI. In addition, many of the programs have included a functional analysis of the problem behavior prior to the start of treatment so that an appropriate replacement behavior, such as tapping the teacher rather than yelling, could be identified (e.g., Durand & Carr, 1991; Horner & Day, 1991). One of the problems in initiating behavioral treatment programs with individuals who have autism is that they tend to have a pervasive lack of motivation to learn (Charlop-Christy et al., 1998) which, in turn, may cause difficulty in identifying salient reinforcers for them—or any reinforcers other than food, liquids, and the avoidance of pain. Some researchers, however, have utilized internal reinforcers (e.g., opportunities to engage in self-stimulatory behaviors) in teaching them new skills (e.g., Charlop, Kurtz, & Casey, 1990).

It has been estimated that approximately 50% of children with autism are functionally mute, many of them having problems with receptive and expressive language (Rimland, 1964). Behavioral programs for teaching language to these children have included both verbal language and sign language training (e.g., Carr, 1979; Carr, Kologinsky, & Leff-Simon, 1987; Fay & Schuler, 1980; Lovaas, 1977). Most such programs focus primarily on the development of functional language, using positive reinforcement and shaping procedures for imitating the clinician's vocalizations. Language enhancement programs, such as Natural Language Programming (NLP), also have been developed to teach nonverbal autistic children to talk (see, e.g., R. L. Koegel, O'Dell, & Koegel, 1987). In NLP, language training through modeling and imitation takes place in a naturalistic setting, with the autistic children imitating the speech of the teacher/model as they play with high-interest toys or engage in high-interest activities. R. L. Koegel et al. (1987) have reported higher rates of imitated verbalization, as well as greater generalization of verbalizations to other settings, with the use of NLP than with the more traditional forms of functional language training.

Behavioral programs focusing on the development of social skills in individuals with autism also have utilized modeling and imitation learning. For example, Strain and his associates (e.g., Odom, Hoyson, Jamieson, & Strain, 1985; Odom & Strain, 1984; Strain, Kerr, & Ragland, 1979) integrated autistic and nonautistic peers in a naturalistic setting, with the socially competent children acting as peer models in initiating and carrying out social interactions. Other social skills studies have used adults to model social interactions, utilized verbal prompts to initiate social interaction patterns, and used self-management and self-reinforcement procedures for developing social interaction (e.g., R. L. Koegel & Frea, 1993; Krantz, MacDuff, & McClannahan, 1993).

In addition to behavior modification procedures, reference to two other treatment procedures for individuals with autism have been reported in the literature, namely, the use of facilitated communication and auditory integration training. *Facilitated communication* was introduced in the United States in the early 1990s (see, e.g., Biklin, 1990, 1992; Biklin & Schubert, 1991; Crossley, 1988) and was hailed as a communication breakthrough for individuals with autism or other expressive language problems (e.g., Makarushka, 1991). In facilitated communication a "facilitator" helps the person with a communication difficulty to express thoughts by supporting his or her arm or shoulder and assisting in pointing or pressing the keys of a typing or other communication device. Unfortunately, several research studies have failed to document the validity of this technique and suggest either conscious or unconscious facilitator influence (see, e.g., Jacobson, Mulik, & Schwartz, 1995; Szempruch & Jacobson, 1993; Wheeler, Jacobson, Paglieri, & Schwartz, 1993). The use of this procedure has therefore been called into question by such professional associations as the American Psychological Association (1994) and the American Academy of Child and Adolescent Psychiatry, the AAMR, and the APA (Autism Society of America, 1996).

A second treatment program, *auditory integration training* (AIT), also was introduced into the United States in the late 1980s. AIT is based on the premise that some characteristics of autism occur because of auditory sensory dysfunction. The two main AIT programs used in the United States are the Berard method (Berard, 1993) and the Tomatis method, with most studies using the Berard method. Both programs were developed by European physicians, and both involve the use of auditory training to treat auditory system problems, including hypersensitivity to certain sound frequencies and problems in sound discrimination as a result of asymmetrical hearing, as well as to regulate the vestibular system through reprogramming of the inner ear. Only limited research on AIT is available (e.g., Bettison, 1996; Madell & Rose, 1994; Rimland & Edelson, 1994, 1995), and its efficacy in treating autism has not yet been established. It seems important to conduct research in this area because, as O'Neill and Jones (1997) have noted, there are many published firsthand accounts and published findings detailing the hyper- and hyposensitivity, sensory distortion, and multichannel receptivity and processing difficulties of people with autism (e.g., Grandin, 1986; Stehi, 1992; Williams, 1992).

PSYCHOLOGICAL AND VOCATIONAL IMPLICATIONS

As a result of the deinstitutionalization and normalization movements that began in the late 1960s and early 1970s, as well as the research advances in behavior modification treatment, more developmentally disabled persons are living in group homes, semiindependent apartment/homes, or independent living residences than ever before in the history of the treatment and care of these persons. Although this situation certainly reflects the advances that have taken place in developmental disabilities over the past 20–25 years, it is not without its problems (see, e.g., Brown et al., 1986; Cole & Gardner, 1993; Lovaas & Buch, 1992; Matson et al., 1998; Smith, Parker, Taubman, & Lovaas, 1992). One of the major problems that researchers are currently experiencing is how treatment gains can be maximized by (1) generalizing the behaviors that have been modified or successfully developed in persons with developmental disabilities in their natural environment (stimulus generalization) and (2) maintaining these treatment gains over time in the person's natural environment (temporal generalization).

The issue of generalization and transfer of training has major implications for the psychological and vocational aspects of a person's treatment and habilitation process. Several writers have made suggestions in regard to this issue (see, e.g., Luce, Christian, Anderson, Troy, & Larsson, 1992; Matson & Coe, 1992; Matson et al., 1998; Perel, 1992; Wacker & Berg, 1988; Wetzel, 1992; Wetzel & Hoschouer, 1984), but more systematic research in this area is needed before any definitive statements can be made regarding how this issue can be rectified. In addition, little is known at present regarding how we as a society and knowledgeable professionals can make the adult life of developmentally disabled persons more meaningful and fulfilled so that these persons can live productive and rewarding lives as well as being gainfully employed (Patton, 1988).

NOTES

Portions of this chapter are based on the work of R. J. Morris (1985). For discussions regarding other possible forms of developmental disability, depending on the age of onset in the person, see chapters 8, "Cardiovascular Disorders"; 11, "Epilepsy"; 13, "Speech, Language, Hearing and Swallowing Disorders"; 15, "Neuromuscular Disorders"; 21, "Pulmonary Disorders"; and 27, "Visual Impairments" in this volume.

REFERENCES

Aman, M. G., & Singh, N. N. (1991). Pharmacological intervention. In J. L. Matson & J. A. Mulick (Eds.), *Handbook of mental retardation* (2nd ed., pp. 347–372). New York: Pergamon Press.

American Association on Mental Retardation. (1992). *Mental retardation: Definition, classification, and systems of supports* (9th ed.). Washington, DC: Author.

American Psychiatric Association. (1994). *Diagnostic and statistical manual of mental disorders* (4th ed.). Washington, DC: Author.

American Psychological Association. (1994, August). *Resolution on facilitated communication by the Council of Representatives of the American Psychological Association.* Los Angeles, CA: Author.

August, G. J., Raz, N., & Baird, T. D. (1985). Brief report: Effects of fenfluramine on behavioral, cognitive, and affective disturbances in autistic children. *Journal of Autism and Developmental Disorders, 15,* 97–107.

Autism Society of America. (1996). *Autism Society facilitated communication info . . . : Statements from professional organizations* [On-line]. Available: http://www.autism-society.org/

Ayllon, T., & Azrin, N. H. (1968). *The token economy: A motivational system for therapy and rehabilitation.* New York: Appleton-Century-Crofts.

Baer, D. M., Wolf, M., & Risley, T. R. (1968). Some current dimensions of applied behavior analysis. *Journal of Applied Behavior Analysis, 1,* 91–97.

Bandura, A. (1969). *Principles of behavior modification.* New York: Holt.

Bandura, A., & Walters, R. H. (1963). *Social learning and personality development.* New York: Holt.

Baumeister, A. A. (1970). The American residential institution: Its history and character. In A. A. Baumeister & E. Butterfield (Eds.), *Residential facilities for the mentally retarded* (pp. 1–28). Chicago: Aldine.

Berard, G. (1993). *Hearing equals behavior.* New Caanan, CT: Keats Publishing.

Berg, I. M. (1975). Aetiological aspects of mental subnormality: Pathological factors. In A. M. Clark & A. D. B. Clarke (Eds.), *Mental deficiency: The changing outlook* (pp. 81–117). New York: Free Press.

Bettelheim, B. (1950). *Love is not enough.* Glencoe, IL: Free Press.

Bettelheim, B. (1967). *The empty fortress.* New York: Free Press.

Bettelheim, B. (1974). *A home for the heart.* New York: Knopf.

Bettison, S. (1996). The long-term effects of auditory training on children with autism. *Journal of Autism and Developmental Disorders, 26,* 361–374.

Biklin, D. (1990). Communication unbound: Autism and praxis. *Harvard Educational Review, 60,* 291–314.

Biklin, D. (1992). Typing to talk: Facilitated communication. *American Journal of Speech Language Pathology, 1,* 15–17.

Biklin, D., & Schubert, A. (1991). New words: The communication of students with autism. *Remedial and Special Education, 12,* 46–47.

Blackman, J. A. (Ed.). (1983). *Medical aspects of developmental disabilities in children birth to three.* Iowa City: University of Iowa.

Blatt, B. (1968). The dark side of the mirror. *Mental Retardation, 6,* 42–44.

Blatt, B. (1984). Biography in autobiography. In B. Blatt & R. J. Morris (Eds.), *Perspectives in special education: Personal orientations* (pp. 263–307). Glenview, IL: Scott, Foresman.

Blatt, B., & Kaplan, F. (1966). *Christmas in purgatory: A photographic essay on mental retardation.* Boston: Allyn & Bacon.

Brown, L., Shiraga, B., Ford, J. R., Nisbet, J., VanDeventer, P., Sweet, M., York, J., & Loomis, R. (1986). Teaching severely handicapped students to perform meaningful work in nonsheltered vocational environments. In R. J. Morris & B. Blatt (Eds.), *Special education: Research and trends* (pp. 131–189). New York: Pergamon Press.

Carr, E. G. (1979). Teaching autistic children to use sign language: Some research issues. *Journal of Autism and Developmental Disorders, 9,* 345–359.

Carr, E. G., Kologinsky, E., & Leff-Simon, S. (1987). Acquisition of sign language by autistic children: 3. Generalized descriptive phases. *Journal of Autism and Developmental Disorders, 17,* 217–229.

Charlop, M. H., Kurtz, P. F., & Casey, F. G. (1990). Using aberrant behaviors as reinforcers for autistic children. *Journal of Applied Behavior Analysis, 22,* 275–285.

Charlop-Christy, M. H., Schreibman, L., Pierce, K., & Kurtz, P. (1998). Childhood autism. In R. J. Morris & T. R. Kratochwill (Eds.), *The practice of child therapy* (3rd ed., pp. 271–302). Needham Heights, MA: Allyn & Bacon.

Cole, C. L., & Gardner, W. I. (1993). Psychotherapy with developmentally delayed children. In T. R. Kratochwill & R. J. Morris (Eds.), *Handbook of psychotherapy with children and adolescents* (pp. 426–471). Boston: Allyn & Bacon.

Coulter, D. L. (1991). Theoretical basis of the definition. In R. Luckasson (Ed.), *Classification in mental retardation: Draft—1991.* Washington, DC: American Association on Mental Retardation.

Courchesne, E. (1989). Neuroanatomical systems involved in infantile autism: The implications of cerebellar abnormalities. In G. Dawson (Ed.), *Autism: New perspectives on diagnosis, nature, and treatment* (pp. 119–143). New York: Guilford Press.

Courchesne, E., Saitho, O., Yeung-Courchesne, R., Press, G. A., Lincoln, A. J., Haas, R. H., & Schreibman, L. (1994). Abnormality of cerebellar vermian lobules VI and VII in patients with infantile autism: Identification of hypoplastic and hyperplastic subgroups by MR imaging. *American Journal of Roentgenology, 162,* 123–130.

Cowen, E. (1963). Psychotherapy and play techniques with the exceptional child and youth. In W. M. Cruickshank (Ed.), *Psychology of exceptional children and youth* (2nd ed., pp. 526–592). Englewood Cliffs, NJ: Prentice-Hall.

Crossley, R. (1988). *Unexpected communication attainments by persons diagnosed as autistic and intellectually impaired.* Paper presented at International Society for Augmentative and Alternative Communication, Los Angeles.

Developmental Disabilities Act. (1984). Washington, DC: U.S. Government Printing Office.

Dickerson, M. U. (1988). Adulthood and maturity. In E. E. Lynch & R. B. Lewis (Eds.), *Exceptional children and adults* (pp. 619–647). Glenview, IL: Scott, Foresman.

Duker, P. C., Welles, K., Seys, D., Rensen, H., Vis, A., & van der Berg, G. (1991). Brief report: Effects of fenfluramine on communicative, stereotypic and inappropriate behaviors of autistic-type mentally handicapped individuals. *Journal of Autism and Developmental Disorders, 21,* 355–363.

Durand, V. M., & Carr, E. G. (1991). Functional communication training to reduce challenging behavior: Maintenance and application in new settings. *Journal of Applied Behavior Analysis, 25,* 251–264.

Ehlers, W. H., Prothero, J. C., & Langone, J. (1982). *Mental retardation and other developmental disabilities* (3rd ed.). Columbus, OH: Merrill.

Ekman, G., Miranda-Linne, F., Gillberg, C., & Garle, M. (1989). Fenfluramine treatment of 20 children with autism. *Journal of Autism and Developmental Disabilities, 19,* 511–532.

Fay, W. H., & Schuler, A. L. (1980). *Emerging language in autistic children.* Baltimore: University Park Press.

Fereitti, R. P., Cavalier, A. R., Murphy, M. J., & Murphy, R. (1993). The self-management of skills by persons with mental retardation. *Research in Developmental Disabilities, 14*, 189–206.

Foxx, R. M., & Azrin, N. H. (1972). Restitution: A method of eliminating aggressive-disruptive behavior of retarded and brain-damaged patients. *Behaviour, Research, and Therapy, 13*, 15–28.

Freeman, B. J., & Ritvo, E. R. (1984). The syndrome of autism: Establishing the diagnosis and principles of management. *Pediatric Analysis, 13,* 284–305.

Friedman, P. (1975). *The rights of the mentally retarded.* New York: Avon.

Gardner, W. I. (1970). *Behavior modification in mental retardation.* Chicago: Aldine.

Gardner, W. I. (1971). *Behavior modification: Applications in mental retardation.*Chicago: Aldine.

Goldfried, M. R., & Merbaum, M. A. (1973). A perspective on self-control. In M. R. Goldfried & M. Merbaum (Eds.), *Behavior change through self-control* (pp. 127–143). New York: Holt.

Grandin, T. (1986). *Emergence: Labeled autistic.* Novato, CA: Academic Therapy Publications.

Gresham, F. M., MacMillan, D. L., & Siperstein, G. N. (1995). Critical analysis of the 1992 AAMR definition: Implications for school psychology. *School Psychology Review, 10,* 1–19.

Grossman, H. J. (Ed.). (1983). *Classification in mental retardation.* Washington, DC: American Association on Mental Deficiency.

Gullone, E., King, N. J., & Cummins, R. A. (1996). Fears of youth with mental retardation: Psychometric evaluation of the Fear Survey Schedule for Children—II (FSSC-II). *Research in Developmental Disabilities, 17*, 269–284.

Haas, R. H., Townsend, J., Courchesne, E., Lincoln, A. J., Schreibman, L., & Yeung-Courchesne, R. (1996). Neurologic abnormalities in infantile autism. *Journal of Child Neurology, 11,* 84–92.

Halderman v. Pennhurst, 446 F. Supp. 1295 (1977).

Harris, S. L. (1988). Autism and schizophrenia: Psychological therapies. In J. L. Matson (Ed.), *Handbook of treatment approaches in childhood psychopathology* (pp. 289–300). New York: Plenum.

Hodapp, R. M. (1995). Definitions in mental retardation: Effects on research, practice, and perceptions. *School Psychology Review, 10*, 24–28.

Horner, R. H., & Day, H. M. (1991). The effects of response efficiency on functionally equivalent competing behaviors. *Journal of Applied Behavior Analysis, 24,* 719–732.

Humphrey, G. (1962). Introduction. In J. M. C. Itard, *The wild boy of Aveyron* (G. Humphrey & H. Humphrey, Trans.). New York: Appleton-Century-Crofts.

Itard, J. M. C. (1962). *The wild boy of Aveyron* (G. Humphrey & H. Humphrey, Trans.). New York: Appleton-Century-Crofts.

Jacobson, J. W., Mulick, J. A., & Schwartz, A. A. (1995). A history of facilitated communication: Science, pseudoscience, and antiscience. *American Psychologist, 50,* 750–765.

Kanfer, F. H. (1980). Self-management methods. In F. H. Kanfer & A. P. Goldstein (Eds.), *Helping people change* (2nd ed., pp. 334–389). New York: Pergamon Press.

Kanner, L. (1943). Autistic disturbances of affective contact. *Nervous Child, 2*, 217–250.

Kanner, L. (1948). *Child psychiatry*. Springfield, IL: Charles C Thomas.

Kanner, L. (1964). *A history of the care and study of the mentally retarded*. Springfield, IL: Charles C Thomas.

Karoly, P., & Kanfer, F. H. (Eds.). (1982). *Self-management and behavior change: From theory to practice*. New York: Pergamon Press.

Kazdin, A. E. (1994). *Behavior modification in applied settings* (5th ed.). Homewood, IL: Dorsey.

Koegel, L. K., Koegel, R. L., & Smith, A. (1997). Variables related to differences in standardized tests outcomes for children with autism. *Journal of Autism and Developmental Disorders, 27,* 233–243.

Koegel, R. L., & Frea, W. D. (1993). Treatment of social behavior in autism through the modification of pivotal skills. *Journal of Applied Behavior Analysis, 26,* 369–377.

Koegel, R. L., O'Dell, M. C., & Koegel, L. K. (1987). A natural language teaching package for nonverbal autistic children. *Journal of Autism and Developmental Disorders, 17,* 187–200.

Krantz, P. J., MacDuff, M. T., & Mc Clannahan, L. E. (1993). Teaching children with autism to initiate to peers: Effects of a script fading procedure. *Journal of Applied Behavior Analysis, 26,* 121–132.

Leland, H. (1991). Adaptive behavior scales. In J. L. Matson & J. A. Mulick (Eds.), *Handbook of mental retardation* (pp. 234–251). New York: Pergamon Press.

Lloyd, K. W., Hallahan, D. P., Kauffman, J. M., & Keller, C. E. (1998). Academic problems. In R. J. Morris & T. R. Kratochwill (Eds.), *The practice of child therapy* (3rd ed., pp. 167–198). Needham Heights, MA: Allyn & Bacon.

Lovaas, O. I. (1977). *The autistic child.* New York: Irvington Publishers.

Lovaas, O. I. (1987). Behavioral treatment and normal education and intellectual functioning in young autistic children. *Journal of Consulting and Clinical Psychology, 55*, 3–9.

Lovaas, O. I., Berberich, J. P., Perloff, B. F., & Schaeffer, B. (1966). Acquisition of imitative speech by schizophrenic children. *Science, 151*, 705–707.

Lovaas, O. I., & Buch, G. (1992). Editor's introduction. *Research in Developmental Disabilities, 13*, 1–8.

Lovaas, O. I., & Bucher, B. D. (Eds.). (1974). *Perspectives in behavior modification with deviant children.* Englewood Cliffs, NJ: Prentice-Hall.

Luce, S. C., Christian, W. P., Anderson, S. R., Troy, P. J., & Larsson, E. V. (1992). Development of a continuum of services for children and adults with autism and other severe behavior disorders. *Research in Developmental Disabilities, 13,* 9–25.

MacMillan, D. L. (1982). *Mental retardation in school and society*. Boston: Little, Brown.

MacMillan, D. L., Gresham, F. M., & Siperstein, G. N. (1993). Conceptual and psychometric concerns about the 1992 AAMR definition of mental retardation. *American Journal on Mental Retardation, 98*, 325–335.

Madell, J. R., & Rose, D. E. (1994, March). Auditory integration training. *American Journal of Audiology,* pp. 14–18.

Makarushka, M. (1991, October 6). The words they can't say. *New York Times Magazine*, pp. 32–33, 36, 70.

Matson, J. L. (1995). Comments on Gresham, MacMillan, and Siperstein's paper "Critical Analysis of the 1992 AAMR Definition: Implications for School Psychology." *School Psychology Review, 10*, 20–23.

Matson, J. L., Appelgate, H., Smirdo, B., & Stallings, S. (1998). Mentally retarded children. In R. J. Morris & T.R. Kratochwill (Eds.), *The practice of child therapy* (3rd ed., pp. 303–324). Needham Heights, MA: Allyn & Bacon.

Matson, J. L., & Coe, D. A. (1992). Applied behavior analysis: Its impact on the treatment of mentally retarded emotionally disturbed people. *Research in Developmental Disabilities, 13*, 171–187.

Matson, J. L., & McCartney, J. R. (Eds.). (1981). *Handbook of behavior modification with the mental retarded.* New York: Plenum.

Matson, J. L., & Schaughency, E. A. (1988). Mild and moderate mental retardation. In J. C. Witt, S. N. Elliott, & F. M. Gresham (Eds.), *Handbook of behavior therapy in education* (pp. 631–652). New York: Plenum.

Meichenbaum, D., & Genest, M. (1980). Cognitive behavior modification: An integration of cognitive and behavioral methods. In F. H. Kanfer & A. P. Goldstein (Eds.), *Helping people change* (2nd ed., pp. 390–422). New York: Pergamon Press.

Morris, R. J. (1976). *Behavior modification with children: A systematic guide*. Cambridge, MA: Winthrop Publishers.

Morris, R. J. (1985). *Behavior modification with exceptional children: Principles and practices*. Glenview, IL: Scott-Foresman.

Morris, R. J., & Kratochwill, T. R. (1998). Historical context of child therapy. In R. J. Morris & T. R. Kratochwill (Eds.), *The practice of child therapy* (3rd ed., pp. 1–4). Needham Heights, MA: Allyn & Bacon.

Morris, R. J., & McReynolds, R. A. (1986). Behavior modification with special needs children: A review. In R. J. Morris & B. Blatt (Eds.), *Special education: Research and trends* (pp. 66–130). New York: Pergamon Press.

New York State Association for Retarded Children v. Rockefeller, 357 F. Supp. 752 (1973).

Nirje, B. (1969). The normalization principle and its human management implications. In R. B. Kugel & W. Wolfensberaer (Eds.), *Changing patterns in residential services for the mentally retarded* (pp. 179–195). Washington, DC: President's Commission on Mental Retardation.

Odom, S. L., Hoyson, M., Jamieson, B., & Strain, P. S. (1985). Increasing handicapped preschoolers' peer social interactions: Cross-setting and component analysis. *Journal of Applied Behavior Analysis, 18,* 3–16.

Odom, S. L., & Strain, P. S. (1984). Classroom based social skills instruction for severely handicapped preschool children. *Topics in Early Childhood Special Education, 4,* 97–116.

O'Neill, M., & Jones, R. S. (1997). Sensory-perceptual abnormalities in autism: A case for more research? *Journal of Autism and Developmental Disorders, 27,* 283–293.

Oppenheim, R. (1974). *Effective teaching methods for autistic children.* Springfield, IL: Charles C Thomas.

Patton, P. (1988). Preparation for adulthood. In E. E. Lynch & R. B. Lewis (Eds.), *Exceptional children and adults* (pp. 588–618). Glenview, IL: Scott, Foresman.

Pennsylvania Association for Retarded Children v. Commonwealth of Pennsylvania, 334 F. Supp. 1257 (1971).

Perel, I. (1992). Deinstitutionalization at a large facility: A focus on treatment. *Research in Developmental Disabilities, 13,* 81–86.

Perry, R., & Meiselas, K. (1988). Autism and schizophrenia: Pharmacotherapies. In J. L. Matson (Ed.), *Handbook of treatment approaches in childhood psychopathology* (pp. 301–325). New York: Plenum.

Peterson, F. M., & Martens, B. K. (1995). A comparison of behavioral interventions reported in treatment studies and programs for adults with developmental disabilities. *Research in Developmental Disabilities, 16*, 27–42.

Rapin, I., & Katzman, R. (1998). Neurobiology of autism. *Annals of Neurology, 43,* 7–14.

Rimland, B. (1964). *Infantile autism.* New York: Appleton-Century-Crofts.

Rimland, B., & Edelson, S. M. (1994). The effects of auditory integration training in autism. *American Journal of Speech-Language Pathology, 5,* 16–24.

Rimland, B., & Edelson, S. M. (1995). Auditory integration training: A pilot study. *Journal of Autism and Developmental Disorders, 25,* 61–70.

Rimm, D. C., & Masters, J. C. (1979). *Behavior therapy: Techniques and empirical findings.* New York: Academic Press.

Ritvo, E. R., & Freeman, B. J. (1978). National Society for Autistic Children definition of the syndrome of autism. *Journal of Autism and Childhood Schizophrenia, 8*, 162–167.

Ritvo, E. R., Freeman, B. J., Mason-Brothers, A., Mo, A., & Ritvo, A. (1985). Concordance for one syndrome autism in 40 pairs of affected twins. *American Journal of Psychiatry, 142,* 74–77.

Ritvo, E. R., Freeman, B. J., Yuwieler, A., Geiler, E., Yokota, A., Schroth, P., & Novak, P. (1984). Study of fenfluramine in outpatients with the syndrome of autism. *Journal of Pediatrics, 105,* 823–828.

Ritvo, E. R., Spence, M. A., Freeman, B. J., Mason-Brothers, A., Mo, A., & Marzarita, M. L. (1985). Evidence of autosomal recessive inheritance in 46 families of multiple incidences of autism. *American Journal of Psychiatry, 142,* 187–182.

Rusch, F. R., McKee, M., Chadsey-Rausch, J., & Renzaglia, A. (1988). Teaching a student with severe handicaps to self-instruct: A brief report. *Education and Training of the Mentally Retarded, 23,* 51–58.

Rutter, M. (1978). Diagnosis and definition of childhood autism. *Journal of Autism and Childhood Schizophrenia, 8,* 139–161.

Rutter, M., & Bartak, L. (1973). Special education treatment of autistic children: A comparative study. II. Follow-up of findings and implications for services. *Journal of Child Psychology and Psychiatry, 14,* 241–270.

Scheerenberger, R. C. (1987). *A history of mental retardation*. Baltimore: Brookes Publishing.

Schopler, E. (1965). Early infantile autism and receptor processes. *Archives of General Psychiatry, 13*, 327–335.

Schopler, E., & Reichler, R. J., (1971). Psychobiological referents for the treatment of autism. In D. W. Churchill, G. P. Alpern, & M. K. DeMyer (Eds.), *Infantile autism* (pp. 327–335). Springfield, IL: Charles C Thomas.

Schreibman, L., & Charlop, M. H. (1987). Autism. In V. B. Van Hasselt & M. Hersen (Eds.), *Psychological evaluation of the developmentally and physically disabled* (pp. 155–177). New York: Plenum Press.

Shapiro, E. (1981). Self-control procedures with the mentally retarded. In M. Hersen, R. M. Eisler, & P. M. Miller (Eds.), *Progress in behavior modification* (Vol. 12, pp. 265–297). New York: Academic Press.

Shapiro, E. S. (1986). Behavior modification: Self-control and cognitive procedures. In R. P. Barrett (Ed.), *Severe behavior disorders in the mentally retarded* (pp. 259–276). New York: Plenum.

Skinner, B. F. (1938). *The behavior of organisms*. New York: Appleton-Century-Crofts.

Skinner, B. F. (1953). *Science and human behavior*. New York: Macmillan.

Smith, T., Parker, T., Taubman, M., & Lovaas, O. I. (1992). Transfer of staff retraining from workshops to group homes: A failure to generalize across settings. *Research in Developmental Disabilities, 13*, 57–71.

Stacey, C. L., & DeMartino, M. F. (Eds.). (1957). *Counseling and psychotherapy with the mentally retarded*. Glencoe, IL: Free Press.

Stehli, A. (1992). *Sound of a miracle: A child's triumph over autism.* Roxbury, CT: Georgiana Organization.

Strain, P. S., Kerr, M. M., & Ragland, E. U. (1979). Effects of peer-mediated social initiations and prompting/reinforcement procedures on the social behavior of autistic children. *Journal of Autism and Developmental Disorders, 9,* 41–54.

Szempruch, J., & Jacobson, J. W. (1993). Evaluation facilitated communications of people with developmental disabilities. *Research in Developmental Disabilities, 14,* 253–264.

Thompson, T., & Grabowski, J. (Eds.). (1972). *Behavior modification of the mentally retarded*. New York: Oxford University Press.

Ullmann, L., & Krasner, L. (Eds.). (1965). *Case studies in behavior modification.* New York: Holt.

Wacker, D. P., & Berg, W. K. (1988). Behavioral habilitation of students with severe handicaps. In J. C. Witt, S. N. Elliott, & F. M. Gresham (Eds.), *Handbook of behavior therapy in education* (pp. 719–737). New York: Plenum.

Waterhouse, L., Fein, D., & Mohdahl, C. (1996). Neurofunctional mechanisms in autism. *Psychological Review, 103,* 457–489.

Wetzel, R. J. (1992). Behavior analysis of residential program development. *Research in Developmental Disabilities, 13*, 73–80.

Wetzel, R. J., & Hoschouer, R. (1984). *Residential teaching communities*. Glenview, IL: Scott, Foresman.

Wheeler, D. L., Jacobson, J. W., Paglieri, R. A., & Schwartz, A. A. (1993). An experimental assessment of facilitated communication. *Mental Retardation, 31,* 49–60.

Williams, D. (1992). *Nobody, nowhere: The extraordinary life of an autistic.* New York: Times Books.

Williams, D. E., Kirkpatrick-Sanchez, S., & Crocker, W. T. (1994). A long-term follow-up of treatment for severe self-injury. *Research in Developmental Disabilities, 15,* 487–501.

Wolf, M. M., Risley, T. R., & Mees, H. (1964). Application of operant conditioning procedures to the behavior problems of an autistic child. *Behavior Research and Therapy, 1*, 305–312.

Wolfensberger, W. (1969). The origin and nature of our institutional models. In R. B. Kugel & W. Wolfensberger (Eds.), *Changing patterns in residential services for the mentally retarded* (pp. 59–171). Washington, DC: President's Commission on Mental Retardation.

Wolfensberger, W. (1972). *The principle of normalization in human services*. Washington, DC: National Institute on Mental Retardation.

Wright, E. B. (1987). Developmental disabilities. In C. R. Reynolds & L. Mann (Eds.), *Encyclopedia of special education* (Vol. 1, pp. 486–488). New York: Wiley Interscience.

Wyatt v. Stickney, 325 F. Supp. 781 (1971).

Zigler, E., & Hodapp, R. M. (1986). *Understanding mental retardation.* New York: Cambridge University Press.

Chapter 15

Neuromuscular Disorders

Hana Ilan

The following is an attempt to familiarize the rehabilitation professional with some of the neuromuscular conditions most commonly encountered in the rehabilitation clinic. This by no means is an exhaustive list. The intention is to review representative causes of two major physical deficiencies and to demonstrate that, in spite of apparently similar outcomes, these diseases differ not only in anatomical site of pathology but also in course of progression, functional disability, and implications for rehabilitation. The two physical deficiency categories are muscle weakness and movement disorders. Of the conditions covered, five fall under either category, and one is best represented by both, as shown in the following list:

- Combined muscle weakness and movement disorder
  - Multiple sclerosis
- Muscle weakness
  - Amyotrophic lateral sclerosis
  - Muscular dystrophy
    - Duchenne muscular dystrophy
    - Facioscapulohumeral muscular dystrophy
    - Myotonic dystrophy
  - Charcot-Marie-Tooth syndrome (hereditary motor and sensory

neuropathy Type 1)

Movement disorders

Parkinson's disease

Friedreich's ataxia (hereditary spinocerebellar ataxia)

It is hoped that, upon reviewing this chapter, the reader will have gained an understanding of the following: Rehabilitation goals, including vocational and psychological implications, must be established on the basis of an accurate diagnosis of a neuromuscular disorder, the natural course of the disease, and its functional ramifications. The rehabilitation professional has a responsibility to build on this information and develop a realistic and rational treatment program.

MULTIPLE SCLEROSIS

Multiple sclerosis (MS) is a nonhereditary chronic disease of the central nervous system, with onset mostly in young adult life. It is characterized by exacerbations and remissions of a multitude of signs and symptoms indicative of damage to several areas of the brain and spinal cord. In most cases, symptoms begin between ages 20 and 40, although onset before age 10 and after 60 has been reported. MS is rare in some parts of the world and more common in others. It increases in frequency with latitude in both northern and southern directions. Thus, it is nonexistent near the equator, as in parts of Africa. In most of northern Europe, northern United States, and southern Australia, it occurs with a prevalence of 60/100,000 population; in the Shetland and Orkney islands off the coast of Scotland, the prevalence is 150/100,000 population. It is rare in Asia and most of South America. There seems to be a genetic predisposition to the disease that is modified by some environmental influence. It has been shown that individuals emigrating to another country before the age of 15 years will have the same risk of acquiring MS as the native-born residents of that country. Additionally, although MS is rare among African Blacks, the incidence among U.S. Blacks is only slightly lower than that of U.S. Whites (Merritt, 1989).

The exact cause is unknown, but the most widely held theory today is that MS occurs in persons who have a genetically determined (i.e., born with a predisposition to) increased immune response to viral infections and that some part of the immune response "attacks" the myelin sheath covering the different components of the central nervous system. The resulting pathological picture is that of scattered areas of demyelination, or plaques, in the brain and spinal cord (Merritt, 1989).

The clinical course of MS is chronic, lasting for several decades. The onset of exacerbations is acute, and remission can occur within days. The first exacerbation is almost always followed by complete recovery, and subsequent attacks are gradually less completely resolved. With each subsequent attack, there may be a recurrence of old symptoms and some additional ones. The signs and symptoms vary in nature and severity, depending on the area of injury in the central nervous system and the chronicity of the illness. The most common are muscle weakness and spasticity, impaired sensation and coordination, unexplained pain, visual disturbances, gait abnormalities, urinary difficulties, and mental status changes. Among the mental symptoms, euphoria and depression are common. A tendency to extend symptoms beyond the actual basic organic deficit is well known. There are also subtle cognitive deficits, such as aphasia and memory disturbances. Because some of the visual and sensory symptoms can be as short-lived as several seconds, patients are described as hysterical. A typical characteristic of MS is that all of its symptoms tend to vary in both nature and severity with time.

MS can be described according to increasing chronicity. At one end of the spectrum are the cases that remain clinically silent for life and are incidentally discovered at autopsy. At the other end are the cases that progress to death within a few weeks of onset. The more common cases fall into the following recently standardized four categories:

1. Relapsing-remitting (about 2/3 of cases at onset); characterized by acute exacerbations, with complete or close to complete recovery and a stable disease level between exacerbations
2. Primary-progressive; characterized by a continuous disease progression, with minor improvements or plateaus and with no acute exacerbations
3. Secondary-progressive; characterized by an initial relapsing-remitting course, followed by continuous disease progression, with or without further episodes of exacerbation
4. Progressive-relapsing; characterized by a continuous disease progression, with episodes of near acute exacerbations, with complete or incomplete recovery, and with continuous disease progression between exacerbations (Lublin & Reingold, 1996)

Functional Disability

All aspects of function can be affected by disability, including ambulation, transfers, activities of daily living (ADL), vision, hearing, and mental status. Gait difficulties are the most common. They can include spasticity, ataxia, loss of position sense, weakness, and various combinations thereof. They can vary functionally from a need for assistive devices (orthoses) to an inability to ambulate and need for a wheelchair because of paralysis, severe spasticity and contractures, or a severe balance disorder. Arm and hand function can be similarly affected, and there is often an intention tremor, which further makes self-care activities difficult or impossible (Jette, Branch, & Berlin, 1990). Bladder functions are affected, and management includes intermittent self-catheterization. In a patient with impaired hand function this requires dependence on a caretaker. As paralysis or spasticity becomes severe, functional independence is further compromised. Deteriorating vision, hearing, and speech, along with mental depression or unrealistic euphoria, progressively impair independent social interaction and communication.

Treatment and Prognosis

Medical management in MS is twofold. One is the use of medication to arrest exacerbations and possibly delay or moderate recurrent symptoms. The second is the maintenance of function and prevention of physical and functional deterioration, using a multidisciplinary rehabilitation team approach.

Current medical therapy of acute exacerbations in MS involves the oral or intravenous administration of corticosteriods. The latter appears to speed recovery, moderately lengthen remission, and cause less severe steroid side effects (Ebers, 1994). There has been extensive recent research involving the use of pharmacological agents that will modify the immune response and thus more permanently limit the frequency and intensity of exacerbations. Interferon-β 1-b, Interferon-β 1-a, and copolymer-1 are thought to reduce inflammation and demyelination. Protein growth factor is believed to enhance remyelination, and potassium channel blockers (4-aminopyridine) may improve conduction through demyelinated fibers (Miller, 1997).

Although these recent drugs are bringing some hope of reduced relapse rate, there has been no adequate demonstration of reduction in disability. Most MS patients become progressively disabled (Freeman, Langdon, Hobart, & Thompson, 1997). A comprehensive rehabilitation program, introduced at the time of diagnosis, remains a major factor in improving function and reducing disability (Mertin, 1994). The rehabilitation of MS patients includes management of pain, weakness, and spasticity via the following: neurophysiological physical therapy techniques; physical agents and medications; prescription of needed orthotics, shoes, and assistive devices to help various gait disorders; occupational therapy to manage ADL, adaptive equipment, splinting, transfer training, and eventually wheelchair needs; management of neurogenic bladder with various medications, intermittent self-catheterization, follow-up tests, and behavioral techniques (Anderson & Goodkin, 1996).

Spasticity remains the major source of disability in MS, leading to weakness, pain, loss of motor function, and eventually the consequences of inactivity. In addition to the well-established oral medications, various injectable local anesthetics, and several neurosurgical techniques, recent early clinical trials have reported that the use of intramuscular injection of botulinum toxin (BTX) has reduced lower extremity spasticity in MS patients (Simpson, 1997).

During the advanced stage of the disease, physical and occupational therapy are still useful in preventing flexion contractures and decubitus ulcers, and nursing care is essential to prevent bladder and renal infection and to maintain proper nutrition and hydration. The average survival of MS patients is 35 years. Death is usually secondary to respiratory, renal, or decubitus ulcer infections (Merritt, 1989).

Psychological and Vocational Implications

Patient and family must be informed of the diagnosis, given a realistic prognosis, and offered supportive psychological and vocational services (Critchley & Mitchell, 1987). The rehabilitation psychologist can help the patient moderate the mood swings, deal with the anxiety generated by the bizarre symptoms that may label the patient hysterical, and teach the patient and family to live with a chronic progressive illness and to obtain the proper treatment and rehabilitation required to prevent rapid deterioration toward severe complications. A periodic neuropsychological evaluation is desirable to determine the presence and extent of cognitive impairment and to offer the patient a guide to modifications in the functional and work environment.

Patients who fall into the first two diagnostic categories of MS (relapsing-remitting and primary-progressive) can be expected to work for 25 years past onset or longer. As they begin to use orthotics, assistive devices for ambulation, hearing aids, eyeglasses, and upper extremity splints, modifications in their work environment may be needed. Those with vocations requiring heightened physical activity, such as walking, prolonged standing, and exertion of physical force, will benefit from vocational retraining early on in the disease. Vocational counselors can intervene on behalf of the patient in the workplace, where employers may not be responsive to accommodating the worker with physical and functional modifications. Counselors can also assist patients in locating and dealing with the appropriate agencies that offer allied health and social services.

AMYOTROPHIC LATERAL SCLEROSIS

Amyotrophic lateral sclerosis (ALS) is a chronic disease of middle to late adult life, affecting the voluntary motor pathways of the central nervous system. It is hereditary in 10% of cases and is characterized by muscle weakness and fasciculations. Symptoms usually begin after age 40, with rare exceptions occurring earlier.

There are four widely accepted subgroups of ALS: familial, Guamanian, secondary, and sporadic. The sporadic type is the most commonly seen worldwide, affecting all sexes and races, with a prevalence rate of 4–6/100,000 population (Merritt, 1989). On Guam, ALS occurs at rates 50 to 100 times greater. The familial type of ALS is transmitted from parent to offspring in an autosomal dominant or recessive fashion. The exact cause is unknown. Several hypotheses have been examined, including a slow viral infection and an autoimmune problem, but none has been proved. An aging DNA repair mechanism is presently being considered. On the island of Guam, exposure to a toxin from the cycad nut is thought to be the agent causing the disease. In the secondary subgroup, ALS-like symptoms have been associated with syphilis, hypoglycemia, and plasma cell disorders, such as multiple myeloma (Merritt, 1989).

The defect responsible for the symptoms of ALS includes degeneration of different nerves and nerve nuclei along the voluntary motor system within the brain and spinal cord (affecting mostly the brain stem and anterior horn cells). The clinical course is rapidly progressive, beginning with muscle atrophy and loss of power and fasciculations in the extremities and face and progressing to muscle spasticity and severe weakness. Symptoms therefore include gait abnormalities, arm function deficits, and impaired speech and swallowing mechanisms. Respiratory muscle weakness may occur at any time during the course of the disease and may be rapidly progressive. Intellectual functions are not affected in ALS.

Functional Disability

Gait difficulties, loss of arm muscle power, and fatigue are common early complaints, requiring a variety of assistive devices, including lower extremity braces and upper extremity splints to maintain posture and assist in function. As symptoms progress, trunk and neck braces and specialized feeding devices are needed. The patient rapidly becomes dependent on a caretaker, progressing to complete loss of functional independence. Impaired feeding mechanism leads to weight loss and increasing debility, and a need for some form of tube feeding arises. Loss of speech function, combined with an inability to write and eventually to use a computerized communication aid, leads to physical and mental isolation in spite of intact intellect and mental status.

Treatment and Prognosis

In spite of trials with different agents, there is no specific drug treatment for ALS. The most recent trial involved the administration of oral branched-chain amino acids to ALS patients in an attempt to slow disease progression. A double-blind placebo-controlled treatment trial failed to demonstrate any beneficial effect of this treatment (Tandan et al., 1996). Other attempts at treatment—with recombinant growth-hormone (Smith et al., 1993) and with high-dose intravenous immunoglobulin (Dalakas et al., 1994)—also have failed to demonstrate any reduction in motor unit loss or slowing of disease progression. Cell and gene transfer therapy are considered promising future treatments (Hugon, 1996).

Spasticity of extremity muscles and those involved in chewing and swallowing is reduced with medication. Physical and occupational therapy are necessary from the onset to aid in ADL and to maintain muscle range and power. Training in the use of splints, orthotics, and assistive devices is also essential. Speech therapy for improved food intake and swallowing, as well as training in alternative modes of communication are essential early on (Critchley & Mitchell, 1987). Eventually, the placement of a feeding tube, via a gastrostomy or esophagostomy, must be addressed by the patient and the family. Death usually occurs within 5 years of onset, from respiratory failure, aspiration of oral contents, or infection. The consequences of respiratory failure can be delayed by the timely use of assisted ventilation and a tracheostomy.

Psychological and Vocational Implications

For the younger patient, not yet near retirement age, a vocational counselor ideally should intervene with the employer to keep the patient on the job while accommodating his or her special needs, such as rest periods and the increased use of computerized tools. Heavy physical labor could not be sustained by an ALS patient, and attempts at retraining should be made. Because intellectual capacity is preserved, the patient should be supported by the rehabilitation team and encouraged to remain a productive member of society for as long as possible. Once dependence on assisted ventilation and alternative feeding methods ensues, the patient requires full-time care. Psychological support is essential for both patient and family, to help them through the devastating progression of this disease (Critchley & Mitchell, 1987).

MUSCULAR DYSTROPHY

The muscular dystrophies are a group of progressive hereditary diseases characterized by muscle weakness, muscle loss, joint contractures, and deformity. They differ by mode of inheritance, age of onset, and clinical features. The three major types of muscular dystrophy are Duchenne, facioscapulohumeral (FSH), and myotonic muscular dystrophy.

Duchenne muscular dystrophy is an X-linked hereditary disorder occurring in males only, although some atypical females are affected by a Duchenne-like form. The prevalence rate is 1.9–3.4/100,000 population worldwide (Swash & Oxburg, 1991). Symptoms first appear in early childhood, before age 3, and are characterized by a "waddling gait" and difficulties in climbing and running. Rising from a chair or from a supine position requires a maneuver of "climbing" up one's body (known as Gowers' sign) or the support of nearby objects. The calves and upper arm muscles are overdeveloped, a condition known as pseudohypertrophy. As muscle weakness and wasting progress, a characteristic posture of toe walking, with bent knees and an increased lumbar lordosis, is assumed. A progressive scoliosis of the thoracic and lumbar spine occurs in many cases. Mild to moderate mental retardation is common. If the ability to ambulate is maintained beyond age 12, the condition is Becker's muscular dystrophy, a more slowly progressive form of the disease.

FSH muscular dystrophy is a group of syndromes inherited in an autosomal dominant fashion and differing from each other in extent of clinical expression. Prevalence is 0.2–0.5/100,000 population (Swash & Oxburg, 1991). Onset of symptoms occurs during adolescence and includes upper arm and shoulder girdle weakness, impaired eye and lip closure, and eventually footdrop. Muscles involved in eye movement and the chewing mechanism are spared. There is no intellectual deficit. Muscles of the pelvic girdle are affected later on, but their involvement is mild.

Myotonic muscular dystrophy is an autosomal dominant hereditary disorder with varied clinical expression, affecting males more than females, with a prevalence of 5/100,000 population (Mumenthaler, 1990). Symptoms include an inability of the muscles to relax after a forced contraction (myotonia); loss of muscle power and bulk in the face and neck, leading to poor head control; a flat facial expression; swallowing difficulties; and weakness of the distal extremities. Eyes are affected by cataracts, and there are cardiac arrhythmias and gastrointestinal motility problems. Mild mental retardation and personality disorders have been noted, although a tendency toward depression has been found to be caused by the progressive nature of the disease and not a characteristic of it (Duveneck, Portwood, Wicks, & Lieberman, 1986). Onset of symptoms is in the early adult years, between ages 20 and 30, with facial, hand, and foot weakness appearing first. Myotonia, however, may be present in infancy.

In Duchenne muscular dystrophy, a defect in the gene coding for a particular muscle protein has been identified. In myotonic dystrophy, the location of the disease marker has been identified. In all three disorders, the production of muscle fibers is impaired (Merritt, 1989). The clinical course of Duchenne muscular dystrophy is rapidly progressive. Most patients are unable to walk or care for themselves as a result of severe muscle weakness by early adolescence. Death from respiratory failure usually occurs toward the end of the second decade.

FSH patients have a near-normal life expectancy because of the chronic, slowly progressive disease course, and ambulation is often preserved. Myotonic dystrophy is slowly progressive; patients with mild muscle involvement may not become disabled, and they have a normal life expectancy. If muscle weakness is severe, the patient will become incapacitated in the fourth to fifth decade of life (Merritt, 1989).

Functional Disability

In all three forms, muscle weakness and wasting lead to impaired ambulation, arm function, and general mobility. Young Duchenne patients present initially with gait difficulties and need training to prevent untimely loss of power. They progress to require lower extremity and trunk orthoses, as well as assistive devices, and eventually need assistance with arm function and general mobility. Once they are wheelchair-bound, a motorized wheelchair and dynamic upper extremity orthoses are useful in prolonging their functional independence. When muscles of respiration become involved, patients can be placed on ventilatory support via tracheostomy and may continue to live at home using portable ventilation units.

FSH patients require prevention of rapid muscle power loss and contractures. Assistance with self-care activities and feeding will allow them functional independence. Gait difficulties are mild and can usually be corrected by the use of orthoses, shoes, and assistive devices.

Myotonic dystrophy patients may be disabled by the myotonia or may be only mildly affected. Facial muscle weakness and involvement of the smooth muscles of the gastrointestinal tract may present feeding and speech difficulties. Weakness of the neck, hands, and feet requires special orthoses for support and prevention of contractures. Patients often maintain functional independence within a sheltered environment. In the rapidly progressive cases, confinement to a wheelchair or bed, with total supervision, may be required.

Treatment and Prognosis

There is no specific drug treatment for the muscular dystrophies. Several recent studies have repeatedly demonstrated that administration of low-dose prednisone to Duchenne muscular dystrophy patients improves muscle force, or slows muscle deterioration, thus improving function (Backman & Henriksson, 1995). This treatment has recently been offered to Duchenne muscular dystrophy patients who are still ambulatory, just before they become wheelchair-dependent. Treatment benefits must be weighed against steroid side effects, which may have a deleterious effect on the disease course (Fenichel et al., 1991). Physical therapy is essential early on in Duchenne muscular dystrophy to prevent joint contractures and maintain muscle power (Russman, 1990). Orthopedic management of contractures via tendon lengthening and transfer procedures is advisable and should be followed by appropriate splint and physical therapy prescriptions. As weakness increases, the patient should be fitted with the proper extremity and spinal orthoses. Occupational therapy is essential to provide assistance with activities of daily living, home equipment, and wheelchair fitting, including specialized seating arrangements, and the accommodation of a portable ventilator unit. In myotonic dystrophy, speech therapy can offer maintenance of the muscles of mastication and deglutition, as well as alternative modes of communication when speech is no longer possible.

Death in Duchenne muscular dystrophy usually occurs in the middle to late second decade of life and is secondary to respiratory failure or aspiration. FSH and myotonic dystrophy patients can have a normal life expectancy, or they may die of the complications of severe deconditioning (Merritt, 1989).

Psychological and Vocational Implications

If the diagnosis of Duchenne muscular dystrophy is confirmed, vocational training is not feasible because of rapid disease progression. Patients in the second decade of life who are still partially independent functionally should continue to attend school and may be guided into light part-time employment (Jamero & Dundore, 1982). Vocational retraining is appropriate in Becker's muscular dystrophy, keeping in mind the chronic yet slow progression toward muscle weakness. FSH and myotonic dystrophy patients may be able to sustain their chosen vocations or, if more severely affected, may need job retraining that accommodates future upper-body and upper-extremity weakness. About 30% of Duchenne muscular dystrophy patients are mentally retarded (Jamero & Dundore, 1982) and, because of their very dependent lifestyle, may be socially immature. Social skills training is useful as an integral part of a comprehensive specialized educational program. Psychological guidance for patient and family in dealing with the consequences of rapid disease progression, as well as the difficult issue of accepting artificial ventilatory support, is crucial.

CHARCOT-MARIE-TOOTH SYNDROME

Charcot-Marie-Tooth syndrome (hereditary motor and sensory neuropathy Type I; peroneal muscular atrophy) is a slowly progressive hereditary disease of the peripheral nervous system, characterized by muscle weakness and deformity of the feet and hands. Symptoms are usually noted late in the first decade or early in the second decade of life. It is mostly transmitted in an autosomal dominant fashion and occasionally is autosomal recessive or x-linked. The prevalence is 2–5/100,000 population.

The disease is caused by a peripheral nervous system defect—a loss of the myelin "covering" of those nerves, with damage to the exposed nerves and replacement of all by scarlike tissue. The cause of this damage is unknown. Congenital foot deformities may be the only symptoms in some families. In others, loss of leg muscle bulk, footdrop, and a "stocking and glove" loss of sensation occur early. Hand deformity caused by loss of the small muscles occurs later on. Spinal deformities and a tremor may be seen in some patients. The combination of Charcot-Marie-Tooth symptoms, in conjunction with a tremor, is also known as Roussy-Lévy syndrome. Cognitive and mental functions are not affected.

Functional Disability

Congenital foot deformities may be mild and not interfere with the development of ambulation. The more severe deformities and those progressing to bilateral foot weakness create difficulty in walking. The use of a variety of shoe orthoses, braces, and assistive devices is indicated. Eventual loss of hand muscle power will cause difficulties with daily living and work activities and necessitate functional retraining and the use of splints.

Treatment and Prognosis

There is no known drug treatment. Physical therapy is necessary as soon as orthoses and assistive devices are introduced. The goal is to retain ambulation and preserve joint range of motion, as well as to protect the sound joints from damage and deformity. Occupational therapy is important in preventing hand and arm deformity and in retraining function. Life expectancy is normal, and most patients remain ambulatory until old age (Swaiman, 1989).

Psychology and Vocational Implications

Because onset generally occurs before the age of vocational training, the rehabilitation counselor should be instrumental in planning for a vocation that does not require extensive ambulation or generalized physical exertion and can be carried out in spite of eventual hand weakness and deformities. In more advanced cases, supportive psychotherapy is indicated, to help the individual deal with the physical deformities and with depression due to nearly complete functional dependency.

PARKINSON'S DISEASE

Parkinson's disease (paralysis agitans) is the major cause of neurological disability in people over 60 years of age. It is a nonhereditary chronic disease of the brain, characterized by abnormal movement and posture. Symptoms usually begin between the ages of 50 and 65, although rare cases of childhood onset are known. It affects both sexes and all races equally. Prevalence throughout the world is 100–150/100,000 population.

The underlying brain dysfunction responsible for the disease symptoms is loss of dopamine, a chemical neurotransmitting substance from the basal ganglia, as well as destruction of another deep-seated brain structure, the substantia nigra (Chusid, 1985). The cause of this deficiency is unknown. Among the possibilities being considered today are infection with a viral or subviral agent causing a defect in the production of some neural structures, an inherent abnormality in DNA repair, and exposure to an external toxin, such as an environmental pollutant. The clinical course of Parkinson's disease is progressive, leading to a steady decline in function after the first 3 years (Merritt, 1989). The characteristic symptoms include a tremor described as "pill rolling," muscle rigidity described as "cog wheeling," motor slowness, and a tendency to be suddenly "frozen" in one position. There are changes in body posture affecting the trunk, hands, and feet. The gait is characterized by small, rapid, shuffling steps known as a festinating gait. Functions controlled by the autonomic nervous system are affected, resulting in poor temperature control, leading to profuse sweating; episodes of hypotension and syncope; and inadequate bowel and bladder emptying. Psychological disturbances range from cognitive, perceptual, and memory deficits to frank dementia.

Functional Disability

In 70% of cases, tremors is the initial complaint (Merritt, 1989). It is often preceded by a decrease in facial and eye movements and a tendency to remain in one postural position for a long time. Although an annoyance, these may not affect highly skilled movements. With the onset of muscle rigidity and slowness, the patient rapidly deteriorates to a state of total dependency on a caretaker. All self-care tasks may require 10 times the normal duration, and no assistive devices can alleviate loss of arm swing, muscle stiffness, pain, and fatigue. Walking is so slow and laborious, interrupted by periods of "freezing" in place, that an assistive device and close supervision are necessary. Voice volume and speech production are affected, and with the earlier loss of writing ability, communication is severely challenged. Drooling and swallowing difficulties affect eating and lead to weight loss and further debility. The eventual deterioration of intellectual function, affecting memory and cognition and in some cases leading to dementia, requires confinement to the home under constant supervision.

Treatment and Prognosis

The medical treatment of Parkinson's disease consists of lifelong administration of certain medications, rehabilitation, and psychotherapeutic support. The drug of choice functions to replenish dopamine in the brain. In high doses and after prolonged use, involuntary dystonic body movements may appear (Merritt, 1989). For patients in the early stages of the disease, stereotactic brain surgery has been used to control one-sided arm tremor and rigidity. The most recent drug-management protocol is close control of motor fluctuations and neurological and psychological side effects. This approach can give patients increased symptomatic relief and longer functional independence. Options available are alterations in dosing frequency of levodopa, use of controlled-release and liquid levodopa, and the use of various neuroprotective agents (Stern, 1997; Waters, 1997). In some patients who no longer respond to symptomatic drug management, pallidotomy has been effective in reducing dyskinesia. Neural transplants of fetal or genetically engineered cells into the patient's substantia nigra remain in the research stage (Stern, 1997).

The rehabilitation team is involved in increasing mobility via use of assistive devices, prescribing supportive home equipment, providing training in self-care activities, preventing and managing joint flexion contractures and decubitus ulcers, and prolonging communication. The patient should be trained to carry out a daily home therapeutic exercise program (Liang, Gall, Partridge, & Eaton, 1983). Prior to the use of medication, 25% of Parkinson's disease patients died within 5 years of onset, and 80% of the survivors died within 15 years. Levodopa has reduced the mortality rate by 50% and has increased survival by several years. Levodopa is most effective in the first 3 years of treatment, but other medications used today help to control and prevent symptoms and postpone the onset of severe disability (Merritt, 1989).

Psychological and Vocational Implications

Through psychological counseling, the patient should be helped to deal with the anxiety and depression that occur from the time of initial diagnosis and are exacerbated with progression of symptoms. Fears of disability, dependency, and dementia cause Parkinson's disease patients to withdraw from interpersonal relations. Families should be taught the symptoms of Parkinson's disease as well as the treatments and their side effects so that they can better help the patient remain in the mainstream of society. Support groups and individual counseling are effective. With early diagnosis and administration of medication, symptom progression may be slowed down or delayed considerably. Patients will be able to continue working in most vocations that are not extremely demanding physically, for example, sedentary white-collar jobs not requiring manual dexterity and most professional occupations. As the disease progresses, there is a tendency to decrease public contact and to work more in isolation. Occupations that involve heavy manual labor or shifts in posture and position should be changed if onset is in the early 50s and the patient is not near retirement. Additionally, the rehabilitation vocational counselor can coordinate psychological, family, and vocational services.

FRIEDREICH'S ATAXIA

Friedreich's ataxia is a common, rapidly progressive hereditary disease of the brain and spinal cord, characterized by loss of coordination in the voluntary muscles of the extremities, trunk, and speech apparatus. Symptoms begin during the first decade or early second decade of life, between ages 7 and 13, but may be present in infancy. The disease is passed from parent to offspring in an autosomal recessive manner; it is commonly seen in families, but some patients are unable to identify family members with the disease. It occurs worldwide, in all races, and is more common in males. The prevalence in Europe and North America is 1–2/100,000 population (Asbury, McKhann, & McDonald, 1986).

The brain defect leading to the disease symptoms is replacement by scar tissue of the various corticospinal and spinocerebellar tracts, including some deep-seated structures of the cerebellum and the posterior horns and dorsal roots of the spinal cord. The cause is unknown, although a defective gene is thought to be located on chromosomes 9 and 11 (Merritt, 1989).

The course of Friedreich's ataxia is rapidly progressive, except in a few cases in which early symptoms are arrested and no new ones develop. The first symptom to occur is usually loss of coordination in the legs, known as gait ataxia. This is followed by hand or body tremors, known as titubations, and a speech disturbance described as "scanning speech." Leg muscle weakness leading to paralysis and muscle atrophy occur later. Loss of position sense and other sensations in the legs and trunk make it difficult for the patient to stand, walk, and sit. The rate of seizures is higher than that in the general population. In most cases, intelligence is normal to high, but mental retardation and dementia have been noted in some.

Almost 75% of Friedreich's ataxia patients are born with clubfoot, and 80% are born with scoliosis and kyphosis of the upper spine. Cardiac abnormalities, such as an enlarged heart or myocardial fibrosis, are common. In most cases, complete loss of independent function occurs 10 to 15 years after onset. Death may be sudden, secondary to a cardiac complication, or may result from an infection following complete physical deterioration.

Functional Disability

Walking is usually affected from the start. In the few cases that do not progress beyond foot and skeletal deformities, special shoe modifications may suffice. For the more chronic cases, the need for foot orthoses and ambulation aids progresses to dependence on a wheelchair with special supports. Advanced ataxia, paralysis, and loss of speech necessitate total dependence on a caretaker.

Treatment and Prognosis

There is no known drug for the treatment of Friedreich's ataxia. During the early phase and in the more chronic, less rapidly progressive cases, physical therapy is indicated for maintenance of muscle range and strength. Various orthopedic surgical procedures are helpful in correcting foot deformities and require follow-up prescription or orthoses and assistive devices, as well as physical therapy.

Psychological and Vocational Implications

Because the onset of Friedreich's ataxia occurs before the age at which vocational choices are made, the need for retraining is low. In some of the less progressive cases that do not require total dependency on a caretaker, vocational/educational guidance is indicated. The goal is to help the patient to choose a vocation that is intellectually appropriate yet not demanding in terms of physical strength and coordination. Psychological support to patient and family in dealing with the diagnosis, the poor prognosis, and physical deformities, as well as the stresses of social interaction, is a requirement.

REFERENCES

Anderson, P. B., & Goulkin, D. E. (1996). Current pharmacologic treatment of multiple sclerosis symptoms. *Western Journal of Medicine, 165,* 313–317.

Asbury, A. K., McKhann, G. M., & McDonald, W. I. (1986). *Diseases of the nervous system: Clinical neurobiology.* Philadelphia: W. B. Saunders.

Backman, E., & Henriksson, K. G. (1995). Low-dose prednisolone treatment in Duchenne and Becker muscular dystrophy. *Neuromuscular Disorders, 5,* 233–241.

Brod, S. A., Lindsey, W., & Wolinsky, J. S. (1996). Multiple sclerosis: Clinical presentation, diagnosis and treatment. *American Family Physician, 54,* 1301–1307.

Chusid, J. G. (1985). *Correlative neuroanatomy and functional neurology* (9th ed.). Los Altos, CA: Lange.

Critchley, E. M. R., & Mitchell, J. (1987). Explanation and management of neurological disability. *Medical Practice, 204,* 1203–1205.

Dalakas, M. C., Stein, D. P., Otero, C., Sekul, E., Cupler, E. J., & McCrosky, S. (1994). Effect of high-dose intravenous immunoglobulin on amyotrophic lateral sclerosis and multifocal motor neuropathy. *Archives of Neurology, 51,* 861–864.

Duveneck, M. J., Portwood, M. M., Wicks, J. J., & Lieberman, J. S. (1986). Depression in myotonic muscular dystrophy. *Archives of Physical Medicine and Rehabilitation, 67,* 875–877.

Ebers, G. C. (1994). Treatment of multiple sclerosis. *Lancet, 343,* 275–279.

Fenichel, G. M., Florence, J. M., Pestronk, A., Mendell, J. R., Moxley, R. T., III, Griggs, R. C., Brooke, M. H., Miller, J. P., Roibison, J., King, W., et al. (1991). Long-term benefit from prednisone therapy in Duchenne muscular dystrophy. *Neurology, 41,* 1874–1877.

Freeman, J. A., Langdon, D. W., Hobart, J. C., & Thompson, A. J. (1997). The impact of inpatient rehabilitation on progressive multiple sclerosis. *Annals of Neurology, 42,* 236–244.

Hugon, J. (1996). ALS therapy: Targets for the future. *Neurology, 47,* 5251–5253.

Jamero, P., & Dundore, D. (1982). Three common neuromuscular diseases: Considerations for vocational rehabilitation counselors. *Journal of Rehabilitation, 48,* 43–48.

Jette, A. M., Branch, L. G., & Berlin, J. (1990). Musculoskeletal impairments and physical disablement among the aged. *Journal of Gerontology: Medical Sciences, 45*(6), 203–208.

Liang, M. H., Gall, V., Partridge, A., & Eaton, H. (1983). Management of functional disability in homebound patients. *Journal of Family Practice, 17,* 429–435.

Lublin, F. D., & Reingold, S. C. (1996). Defining the clinical course of multiple sclerosis: Results of an international survey. *Neurology, 46,* 907–911.

Mertin, J. (1994). Rehabilitation in multiple sclerosis. *Annals of Neurology, 36,* 5130–5133.

Merritt, H. (1989). *A textbook of neurology* (8th ed.). Philadelphia: Lea & Febiger.

Miller, A. (1997). Current and investigational therapies used to alter the course of disease in multiple sclerosis. *Southern Medical Journal, 90,* 367–374.

Mumenthaler, M. (1990). *Neurology* (3rd ed.). New York: Thieme.

Russman, B. S. (1990). Rehabilitation of the pediatric patient with a neuromuscular disease. *Neurologic Clinics, 8,* 727–740.

Simpson, D. (1997). Clinical trials in the treatment of spasticity. *Muscle and Nerve, 6,* 5169–5173.

Smith, R. A., Melmel, S., Sherman, B., Frane, J., Munsat, T. L., & Festoff, B. W. (1993). Recombinant growth hormone treatment of amyotrophic lateral sclerosis. *Muscle and Nerve, 16,* 624–633.

Stern, M. (1997). Contemporary approaches to the pharmacotherapeutic management of Parkinson's disease: An overview. *Neurology, 49*(Suppl. 1), 52–59.

Swaiman, K. F. (1989). *Pediatric neurology.* St. Louis: C. V. Mosby.

Swash, M., & Oxburg, J. (1991). *Clinical neurology.* New York: Churchill Livingstone.

Tandan, R., et al. (1996). A controlled trial of amino acid therapy in amyotrophic lateral sclerosis. *Neurology, 47,* 1220–1226.

Waters, C. H. (1997). Managing the late complications of Parkinson's disease. *Neurology, 49*(Suppl. 1), 549–557.

Chapter 16

Orthopedic Impairments

Edwin F. Richter III

Orthopedic impairments are almost inevitable developments for most individuals. Routine activities of daily living stress the musculoskeletal system. Degenerative changes accumulate in joints over time. Environmental and lifestyle factors may influence this process. In the geriatric population, osteoporotic weakening of bones becomes increasingly evident. These forces may affect even the healthiest members of the adult population.

Acute traumatic events can suddenly create an orthopedic problem. Premorbid characteristics play major roles in shaping responses to such developments. Psychological factors influence response to the acute trauma, the medical treatment, and the rehabilitation process. Other medical illnesses may limit treatment options or interfere with recovery. Economic forces may act on patients, families, health care providers, employers, and other institutions. Social support systems are challenged when orthopedic impairments lead to disability.

FUNCTIONAL PRESENTATION

Many common orthopedic impairments develop gradually and often cause only limited disability in early stages. Osteoarthritis, a degenerative change seen in joints, is commonly associated with frequent and vigorous activity. Bearing the weight of the human body is a substantial stress over time. Even relatively light individuals load their body weight on and off their lower extremities each time they take a normal step. Running, carrying extra weight, exposure to hard surfaces, choice of footwear, and variations in anatomy may increase the stresses across the joints. Long-term use of crutches by active persons with gait disorders may lead to similar effects on the shoulders. The affected joints may initially be painful intermittently. Over time the severity, frequency, and duration of painful episodes typically escalate, sometimes leading to persistent pain even when the joint is at rest.

Concurrent loss of range of motion may occur in osteoarthritis and other joint pain syndromes. This may limit functional use of the joint, depending on which joint is involved and the number of degrees lost in a particular plane of motion, as well as the specific tasks that the person needs to do (Triffit, 1998). Loss of mobility at a given joint may be the result of contracture of the soft tissues around the joint, fusion of bony structures, or mechanical blockage (such as by a loose piece of cartilage blocking the swinging of the knee joint's hinge mechanism). Pain may also prompt a functional restriction of movement, which may take place without conscious effort. "Guarding" may also reflect apprehension or quests for secondary gain.

Other joints may be able to compensate for loss of normal motion at a site of pathology. This strategy is not without risk. Normal body mechanics can be altered to such a degree that other structures may be harmed. A more subtle but quite serious problem occurs when the energy efficiency of an important activity is impaired. Normal gait involves strategic movements at several joints to lower metabolic costs (Winter, 1983). Interference with this process may stress cardiovascular and pulmonary systems. Speed and endurance would be jeopardized.

Low back pain deserves special attention when considering orthopedic impairments. The overall incidence of back pain is high. At least one debilitating episode affects 80% of Americans by age 55 (Frymoyer, 1988). Fortunately, most episodes resolve with conservative management. The cost of this condition, however, remains quite high. The direct expense has been estimated to be from $20 to $50 billion in the United States (Nachemson, 1992). This has raised concerns among health care providers, insurers, employers, and government agencies.

Many potential risk factors for back pain have been reviewed. Increasing age has some association with increasing likelihood of episodes. There is interest in anthropometric factors (Battie, Bigos, & Fisher, 1990), but the predictive value of height and weight is limited. Abdominal and lumbar muscle strength have been studied (Gardner-Morse & Stokes, 1998), but biomechanical models do not always correspond well with clinical realities.

Much attention has been paid to risk factors related to the workplace. Direct trauma, overexertion, or repetitive stresses can cause injuries, whereas postural factors may be more relevant to those with sedentary occupations (Bendix & Biering-Sorensen, 1983). Attributing an individual worker's pain to a specific ergonomic problem is often a challenge. Psychosocial factors have been implicated. Occupational factors, including an injured employee's prior attitudes toward his work, must be considered (Battie, Bigos, & Fisher, 1989).

Problems in the clinical evaluation of back pain complicate the situation. Gross assessment of lumbar movement may be hindered by hip joint factors (such as tight hamstring muscles) or voluntary guarding. Physical examination maneuvers such as straight leg raising (Lasègue's test) to look for nerve root involvement rely on the patient's verbal response, as well as the examiner's assessment of facial expression and body language. Subtle abnormalities on neurological testing of sensory and motor function or reflex activity are difficult to quantify.

Differences of opinion between practitioners are common when evaluating and treating back pain. The Agency for Health Care Policy and Research (AHCPR) has promoted practice guidelines (Bigos, Bowyer, & Braen, 1994), but on surveys of practicing physicians from eight specialties that commonly treat such patients there was little consensus on selection of diagnostic tests (Cherkin, Deyo, Wheeler, & Ciol, 1994). Patients do not limit themselves to seeking care from allopathic physicians, thereby introducing further potential controversies. One third of patients in a study conducted in North Carolina reported seeking care initially from a chiropractor (Carey et al., 1996).

Different anatomical structures may be involved in low back pain. Acute muscle strains may be accompanied by significant spasm and local tenderness. Most cases respond well to oral analgesics and possibly muscle relaxants, which may work primarily as central sedatives (Robinson & Brown, 1991), brief periods of rest, and limited physical therapy interventions.

Degenerative changes may affect the spine as well. Osteophytes (bone spurs) may compress critical structures, such as nerve roots. Many of these spurs, however, may look impressive on an x-ray without causing any clinical problem. Facet joint arthritis has been implicated as a source of pain, which may radiate down the lower extremities. An injection with local anesthetic may temporarily relieve such pain, helping to make this diagnosis (Gamburd, 1991). Some physicians would then treat the condition with radio frequency ablation of the local nerve supply.

An acute disk herniation may cause compression of the spinal cord or nerve roots. The size and location of the protruding disk material are essential factors. The size of the spinal canal is also important, as this determines how much extra room is available to accommodate any invading structure. Computerized tomography (CT) and magnetic resonance imaging (MRI) have represented major advances over plain radiographs and traditional myelograms (x-rays done after injection of dye) (Herzog, 1991). Abnormal findings on imaging studies of asymptomatic individuals remind us that such tests do not obviate the need for clinical judgment (Frymoyer & Haldeman, 1991). Electrodiagnostic testing yields physiological rather than anatomical data but can be painful. It can also be difficult to distinguish between new and chronic abnormalities.

Many competing theories have been advanced in the debate over treatment of herniated disks and other lumbar pathologies. At least a brief period of rest may be beneficial, but prolonged bed rest has risks that may outweigh its benefits. Trunk muscle weakness may follow such inactivity. As little as 2 days of bed rest may be appropriate (Deyo, Diehl, & Rosenthal, 1986). Similar concerns have been raised about prolonged use of corsets. The efficacy of traction has been challenged, as considerable forces are required to provide distraction of the lumbar spine before any reduction of pressure within a disk can be achieved. Suspending as little as 5 or 10 pounds from the apparatus is at best only a means of enforcing bed rest.

Therapeutic exercises are also the subject of different schools of thought. Some clinicians advocate strengthening flexor muscles or extensors; others recommend both approaches. Hyperextended postures are used in some methods, such as the McKenzie technique, whereas body mechanics are stressed in the "back school" approach (Sinaki & Mokri, 1996). Programs aimed at dynamic lumbar muscular stabilization have been reported to be quite successful (Saal & Saal, 1991). That approach seeks a "neutral" position of the lumbar spine, which its adherents favor over the extreme positions of hyperextension programs. Analysis of this controversy is beyond the scope of this chapter, but it is safe to assume that some patients are perplexed by the conflicting advice they receive.

Another area of conflict is the role and timing of surgery. Patients with progressive neurological dysfunction, especially involving bowel or bladder control, require acute attention. Some physicians will try high-dose steroid treatment in such scenarios before moving to surgical options, but great caution is required. Patients with less dramatic deficits are more likely to receive longer courses of conservative management before having invasive procedures.

Communication with patients involves selection of medical terms. Use of terms like "herniated," "ruptured," or "bulging" disks may be interpreted in various ways. Assuming that a patient understands the clinical significance of such words is inappropriate.

Acute back pain may result from osteoporotic vertebral body compression fractures. This situation initially warrants short periods of rest, analgesics, and efforts to prevent constipation. Spinal supports may help to maintain posture and reduce uneven distribution of forces on the vertebral body (Sinaki, 1995). During ambulation, some patients experience less pain when using a rolling walker to place more weight on their upper extremities, reducing the forces across the fracture site.

Fracture management must consider the location and severity of the injury. Fortunately at least some fractures are relatively stable and can be treated symptomatically. Uncomplicated fractures of ribs or distal phalanges of the toes are often in this category. Other fractures are moderately unstable. Manipulation of the bone fragments may yield adequate positioning. (When done without surgery, this is a closed reduction.) Maintaining alignment may require controlling the joint above and below the site (Zuckerman & Newport, 1988). Traditional plaster casting techniques have been augmented by use of fiberglass material.

The use of special braces for fracture care allows faster mobilization in some cases. This approach invokes the importance of mechanical forces across the fracture site. Control of surrounding soft tissues allows a limited degree of movement at the fracture, which facilitates the healing process (Kumar, 1995). Weight bearing causes small local electric fields, which may enhance new bone formation. Braces may also be used to limit weight bearing by shifting weight to appropriate structures. The ischial bone of the pelvis and the patellar tendon below the kneecap are capable of supporting weight through braces in selected cases. Orthotic designs utilizing plastic and metal components can be strong but light. They are often more comfortable than a cast and can be removed for inspection and hygiene, but noncompliant patients find them easier to remove.

Some fractures will be quite unstable without operative intervention (Zuckerman & Newport, 1988). Open reduction and internal fixation (ORIF) allows direct access to the site. Various types of hardware have been developed, such as screws, nails, and pins to directly secure fragments of bone. These are also used to anchor metallic plates, spanning a fracture site, to healthy areas of bone. Rods may also be placed inside a long bone to span a fracture site.

An alternative method of using external fixation was pioneered by Ilizarov in the Soviet Union. This approach came into worldwide use during the 1980s (Bianchi, 1997). Pins can be placed above and below a fracture site and attached to a strong external apparatus. The sites where the pins puncture the skin must be carefully cleaned and monitored. The appearance of the device may be disconcerting to some patients, but it can facilitate early mobilization.

There are several acute medical issues potentially associated with fractures (Duong, 1995). Infection may delay healing or even lead to amputation or death. Bleeding may be dramatic or gradual. Pressure from a collection of blood (hematoma) or watery fluid (edema) may compress nerves or blood vessels or may hinder wound healing. Inflammatory responses may be dramatic. These factors may all subsequently decrease adjacent joint mobility, even if the joints were not directly injured. Contractures are of great concern in this setting. A patient may be disabled long after a fracture heals if nearby joints never regain adequate range of motion.

Chronic pain may follow orthopedic injury via a number of mechanisms. Direct nerve injury or indirect compression may lead to chronic burning pain or hypersensitivity in the sensory territory of that nerve. Reflex sympathetic dystrophy is a more complicated syndrome, involving pain and vasomotor instability. Skin changes, soft tissue atrophy, and osteoporotic changes may be seen (Subbarao & Blair, 1995). There are many controversies surrounding this subject, but early mobilization is suggested as a preventive measure.

Hip fractures are particularly associated with problematic complications. These fractures typically affect geriatric patients. Osteoporosis and increased risk of falling are the main risk factors. Bone mineral density below the fracture threshold level puts patients at risk from relatively low impact falls from seated or standing positions (Goh, Bose, & Das, 1996). Mortality rates have been measured at 20% at 1 year and 33% at 2 years after injury (Emerson & Andersson, 1988). The mortality rate has been linked with poorly controlled systemic disease, cognitive disorders, and surgery before medical stabilization (Lyons, 1997).

Deep vein thrombosis (DVT) is a special concern after hip fracture. Decreased mobility and perhaps slowing of venous return past the site of injury are implicated in the increased risk of blood clot formation. Estimates of incidence are as high as 70% (Cifu, 1995), although clinically significant cases are clearly somewhat less common. The main concern is that thrombotic material may break loose, reaching the vascular supply to the lungs. This can cause a potentially fatal pulmonary embolus. Patients with atrial septal defects have a hole between the upper chambers of the heart, which could allow an embolic stroke to occur.

Pharmacological prophylaxis is the primary method of prevention (Agnelli & Sonaglia, 1997). Oral anticoagulation with warfarin is effective but requires frequent blood tests and increases risk of bleeding. Subcutaneous injection of low-molecular-weight heparin also has been used effectively. It does not require monitoring with blood tests. This medication also increases bleeding complications (Greaves, 1997). Injections are not always feasible in home settings after discharge. Some patients are treated prophylactically with aspirin, despite a lack of compelling evidence in medical literature. Patients who are at very high risk of clot formation can have a filter placed in the vena cava to block access to vital organs.

Hip fracture patients who avoid major medical complications must confront problems with mobility and self-care performance. The amount of weight they can bear on the affected extremity is determined by the orthopedic surgeon. The type of fracture and the hardware used to repair it influence this decision. Quality of bone at the fracture site is also important. Complete avoidance of weight bearing is very difficult or impossible for some elderly patients. Even toe touching for balance requires that almost all body weight be supported through the arms to advance the uninvolved leg. A walker is required in this situation, unless the patient has adequate coordination to utilize bilateral crutches. Climbing stairs is very difficult unless at least partial weight bearing is allowed.

Compliance with precautions is important. Excessive weight bearing increases risk of failure of the repair. Refusing to use adequate assistive devices increases risk of another fall and further injury.

Mobility and self-care skills may never recover after hip fracture. In one study, 1 year after hip fracture 40% of patients could not walk independently, 60% had difficulty with one or more activity of daily living, and 27% had entered nursing homes for the first time (Cooper, 1997). Premorbid dementia and postoperative confusional states decrease the likelihood of recovering walking ability (Lyons, 1997).

Rehabilitation efforts should begin as soon as possible. Reimbursement policies discourage lengthy stays in acute care hospitals. Patients who are not ready to go home directly and who can benefit from an active program typically have gone to acute rehabilitation services. Patients with limited endurance can receive less vigorous regimens at subacute programs, typically at skilled nursing facilities. Further restrictions on reimbursement for traditional inpatient rehabilitation programs may shift greater numbers of orthopedic patients to subacute care or day programs. Providers will likely seek outcome data to justify support for their form of care.

Patients who undergo elective hip replacement face some of the same challenges as hip fracture patients. (Some hip fracture patients receive joint replacement hardware if the injury is near the head of the femur and extensive degenerative changes are present.) The majority of the patients facing hip arthroplasty demonstrate very advanced joint disease. Osteoarthritis and rheumatoid arthritis are typical etiologies. Many patients are elderly and have some other chronic conditions, although very frail or medically unstable patients should be discouraged from having this procedure. Arthritic involvement of the upper extremities may hinder use of walkers or canes. Prior limitation of activity because of pain may have decreased exercise tolerance. Abnormal gait patterns may have developed.

Total hip replacement has become a popular procedure. Approximately 120,000 were performed annually in the early 1990s (Harris & Sledge, 1990; Poss, 1993), and interest has remained strong. Restoring ability to ambulate without pain is the usual goal.

Deep venous thrombosis is a potential major complication (Brandes, Stulberg, & Chang, 1994). Pneumatic compression boots can be used postoperatively, and elastic compression stockings are commonly used subsequently. The medications usually prescribed to prevent clots are the same as those used after hip fracture.

Anticoagulation increases the risk of major bleeding at the operative site. Bleeding into the thigh may cause significant pain and swelling, which may cause nerve compression, possibly leading to muscle weakness. Major blood loss may require treatment with transfusions. Some patients will donate their own blood preoperatively in anticipation of postoperative anemia.

Heterotopic ossification may occur after any hip surgery but is most likely to be seen after arthroplasty. Calcification within muscle tissue can lead to a serious loss of range of motion. Severe cases may require surgical resection, followed by prophylactic radiation therapy or medication, such as indomethacin or etidronate, to prevent recurrence. These medications may have gastrointestinal side effects.

The implanted hardware includes a ball-and-socket joint that mimics the function of the original joint. Preventing dislocation of the prosthetic joint is critical. Standard instructions after a posterolateral approach include avoiding hip flexion past 90 degrees and hip adduction or internal rotation past neutral. Triangular pillows can be placed between the legs to encourage compliance. High chairs and raised toilet seats reduce the need to flex the hips while sitting. Long-handled shoe horns, sock pullers, and reachers are useful devices that facilitate safe dressing. Patients may require substantial reinforcement to use them correctly. Eventually, the healing of soft tissues around the hip reduces the risk of dislocation. Patients who dislocate may need to be brought back to the operating room. Subsequent care may include a brace that holds the hip in abduction and limits flexion. Patients tend to find such devices uncomfortable.

Weight-bearing limitations depend on several factors. Use of cement to help bind the femoral component to the bone immediately may increase the amount of weight bearing that the surgeon allows. Weight bearing as tolerated may be ordered, with a walker being used for a standard period of time before advancing to less restrictive devices as the patient's comfort level permits. The faster mobilization in this scenario may be offset by earlier loosening of the bond between hardware and bone in later years. Noncemented prostheses may have better long-term fitting of hardware to bone. Initial restrictions on bearing weight are usually more conservative, although substantial variations are noted, depending on the individual orthopedist's protocol. If the greater trochanter of the femur was cut as part of the surgical approach, which may be done for a revision, then active hip exercises may be restricted further (Brandes et al., 1994).

The durability of the replacement may depend on the activity level of the patient. Vigorous sports or active manual labor may hasten failure of the interface between hardware components and bone. Traditional concerns about variable levels of activity in patient populations have been supported by current research. Joint replacement patients less than 60 years old walked 30% more on average than those over 60 (Schmalzried et al., 1998). The plastic lining of the acetabular cup may wear. The metal elements are unlikely to break, because they are stronger than the surrounding bone.

Total knee replacements are also commonly performed at many centers. Postoperative swelling and pain may respond well to cold modalities. Wounds are monitored closely for signs of infection. Initial ambulation orders may specify partial weight bearing. Adaptive equipment may facilitate activities of daily living. Dislocation is not a concern after this procedure, in contrast to hip replacement cases. Failure to achieve adequate range of motion is a major issue. Inpatient goals on acute rehabilitation services may include attaining 90 degrees of active knee flexion while lacking no more than 5 degrees of extension. This allows normal sitting posture and adequate ambulation for most patients. Reaching full extension and over 100 degrees of flexion will help performance on stairs, ramps, and curbs.

Given the importance of range of motion (ROM) goals, there has been great interest in continuous passive motion (CPM) machines. There is controversy over whether the reported initial benefits will lead to improved long-term outcomes (Naftulin & Niergarth, 1995). With ongoing interest in developing standard clinical pathways, it is likely that future use of these devices will hinge on resolution of this debate.

Prophylaxis of deep vein blood clots is again an important issue. Risks of major bleeding events, especially at the surgical site, must be weighed against potential mortality from pulmonary emboli.

Successful outcomes are common after this procedure. Ability to walk more than 1 mile is usually anticipated. There is about a 1% annual failure rate (Insall, 1993).

Replacement of other joints is much less common. Most of the patients who undergo those procedures have severe inflammatory arthritis involving multiple joints. Rehabilitation efforts must consider their overall condition in detail, rather than concentrating exclusively on the recent surgery.

Psychological and Vocational Implications

Individuals with similar orthopedic impairments may have very different levels of physical disability. In some cases, this is easily predicted. A well-conditioned athlete should be able to move relatively well on crutches even if an injured leg can't bear weight. Cardiopulmonary disorders might prevent other patients with similar fractures from meeting the substantial energy demands of this abnormal way of walking. Coordination, strength of uninjured limbs, and body weight can also be critical.

Disability evaluations should take into account appropriate goals for each person. Vocational and avocational interests, family supports, social roles, and environmental factors must be noted. The athlete or manual laborer who can ambulate well with crutches may be unable to return to his usual work. Ability to care for a child may be compromised. Favorite recreational activities may be curtailed. Other people with severe physical problems may be able to continue their work effectively. Key factors include ability to travel, accessibility of the work site, specific tasks performed, and need to attend medical appointments.

Rehabilitation programs should assess travel needs. Training in car transfers or use of public transportation can be addressed, and telecommuting options can be explored.

Architectural barriers may hinder access to a building or movement once inside. Creative advice from rehabilitation professionals should include the most efficient and practical approaches to modification. Arranging access to a service entrance may be much faster than initiating construction projects. Advocacy with employers or landlords may be required.

On the macroeconomic level, the impact of orthopedic impairments is impressive. Low back pain care alone is a multibillion dollar industry in the United States, and indirect costs are estimated to double the expense (Andersson, 1997). Employers face substantial compensation claims. Additional personal injury litigation may add to total expenses. Action may be taken against equipment manufacturers, landlords, or other parties not covered under compensation insurance.

At the individual level the potential for lost income is obvious. Coverage for professional health care varies significantly. Patients who require care from an attendant at home after discharge may face major out-of-pocket expenses. (Opening the home to strangers, even under the supervision of a home care agency, is also a source of anxiety to some frail individuals.) Relatives who take on direct care responsibilities also may lose income opportunities.

It is harder to quantify the social stresses that result from these conditions. Valued leadership roles in the family or community may be lost by the patient. Parents may become dependent on children. Sexuality may be affected by pain, mobility, apprehension, and altered body image. Barriers to communication about sexual issues have been noted (Gilbert, 1996), and many rehabilitation professionals are aware of this. Alteration of traditional gender roles may also be of special concern to patients and their families. Sensitivity to diverse cultural backgrounds will enhance care providers' effectiveness.

Many of the psychosocial aspects of orthopedic impairment overlap with other disabling conditions. Pain issues are of special importance. An injury may directly limit function mechanically or overwhelm pain tolerance. Fear of exacerbating the condition or of causing recurrent injury may restrict activity after good physical recovery. Even after elective procedures, such as knee replacements, patients may fear the implications of pain. Understanding their specific concerns allows effective counseling. In some cases, rehabilitation emphasis is placed on functional restoration rather than pain reduction. Sustaining patient involvement requires acceptance of those priorities.

Orthopedic disorders may affect body image. Surgical scars are not the only concern for some patients. Reduced exercise tolerance may lead to weight gain or decreased muscle bulk. Some individuals who appear to be in very good physical condition will still express concerns over changes from their baseline. This may raise questions about whether they were in excellent condition before injury or are exaggerating their current deficits. Opportunities for secondary gain are often invoked as explanations, but many factors may be involved. Patients with extensive physical limitations may expect to achieve high levels of performance. Some cases clearly involve inappropriate levels of denial, whereas others reflect realistic determination.

Orthopedic impairments create challenges for patients, families, providers, insurers, employers, and other agencies. Rehabilitation teams can look beyond traditional medical issues to address psychosocial issues. Complex cases warrant interdisciplinary interventions, including concerted efforts at patient education and counseling.

REFERENCES

Agnelli, G., & Sonaglia, F. (1997). Prevention of venous thromboembolism in high-risk patients. *Haematologica, 82,* 496–502.

Andersson, G. B. J. (1997). Guest editorial. *Journal of Rehabilitation Research and Development, 34,* ix–x.

Battie, M. C., Bigos, S. J., & Fisher, L. (1989). Isometric lifting strength as a predictor of industrial back complaints. *Spine, 14*, 851–856.

Battie, M. C., Bigos, S. J., & Fisher, L. (1990). Anthropometric and clinical measures as predictors of back pain complaints in industry: A prospective study. *Journal of Spinal Disorders, 3,* 195–201.

Bendix, T., & Biering-Sorensen, F. (1983). Posture of the trunk when sitting on forward reclining seats. *Scandinavian Journal of Rehabilitation Medicine, 15*, 197–203.

Bianchi, M. A. (1997). Historical view of the method according to Ilizarov. *Bulletin of the Hospital for Joint Diseases, 56*(1), 16–18.

Bigos, S. J., Bowyer, O., & Braen, G. (1994). Acute low back problems in adults. In *Clinical practice guideline* (AHCPR Publication 95-0642). Rockville, MD: U.S. Department of Health and Human Services.

Brandes, V. A., Stulberg, D. S., & Chang, R. W. (1994). Rehabilitation following hip and knee arthroplasty. *Physical Medicine and Rehabilitation Clinics of North America, 5,* 815–836.

Carey, T. S., Evans, A. T., Hadler, N. M., Lieberman, G., Kalsbeek, W. D., Jackman, A. M., Fryer, J. G., & McNutt, R. A. (1996). Acute severe low back pain. *Spine, 21*, 339–344.

Cherkin, D. C., Deyo, R. A., Wheeler, K., & Ciol, M. A. (1994). Physician variation in diagnostic testing for low back pain. *Arthritis and Rheumatology, 37,* 15–22.

Cifu, D. X. (1995). Rehabilitation of fractures of the hip. *Physical Medicine and Rehabilitation: State of the Art Reviews, 9*(1), 125–140.

Cooper, C. (1997). The crippling consequences of fractures and their impact on quality of life. *American Journal of Medicine, 103*(2A), 12S–17S.

Deyo, R. A., Diehl, A. K., & Rosenthal, M. (1986). How many days of bedrest for acute low back pain? *New England Journal of Medicine, 315*, 1064–1070.

Duong, T. T. (1995). Complications of fractures. *Physical Medicine and Rehabilitation: State of the Art Reviews, 9*(1), 17–30.

Emerson, S., & Andersson, G. B. J. (1988). Ten year survival after fractures of the proximal end of the femur. *Gerontology, 34,* 186–191.

Frymoyer, J. W. (1988). Back pain and sciatica. *New England Journal of Medicine, 318,* 291–300.

Frymoyer, J. W., & Haldeman, S. (1991). Evaluation of the worker with low back pain. In M. H. Pope, G. B. J. Andersson, J. W. Frymoyer, & D. B. Chaffin (Eds.), *Occupational low back pain* (pp. 151–182). St. Louis: Mosby-Year Book.

Gamburd, R. S. (1991). The use of selective injections in the lumbar spine. *Physical Medicine and Rehabilitation Clinics of North America*, *2*(1), 79–96.

Gardner-Morse, M. G., & Stokes, I. A. F. (1998). The effects of abdominal muscle coactivation on lumbar spine stability. *Spine*, *23*, 86–90.

Gilbert, D. M. (1996). Sexuality issues in persons with disabilities. In R. L. Braddom (Ed.), *Physical medicine and rehabilitation* (pp. 605–629). Philadelphia: W. B. Saunders.

Goh, J. C., Bose, K., & Das, D. S. (1996). Pattern of fall and bone mineral density measurement in hip fractures. *Annals of the Academy of Medicine of Singapore, 6,* 820–823.

Greaves, J. D. (1997). Serious spinal cord injury due to haematomyelia caused by spinal anaesthesia in a patient treated with low dose heparin. *Anaesthesia*, *52*, 150–154.

Harris, W. H., & Sledge, C. B. (1990). Total hip and total knee replacement. *New England Journal of Medicine*, *323*, 725–731.

Herzog, R. J. (1991). Selection and utilization of imaging studies for disorders of the lumbar spine. *Physical Medicine and Rehabilitation Clinics of North America, 2*(1), 7–60.

Insall, J. N. (1993). *Surgery of the knee* (2nd ed.). New York: Churchill, Livingstone.

Kumar, V. N. (1995). Fracture bracing. *Physical Medicine and Rehabilitation: State of the Art Reviews, 9*(1), 11–16.

Lyons, A. R. (1997). Clinical outcomes and treatment of hip fractures. *American Journal of Medicine*, *103*(2A), 51S–63S.

Nachemson, A. L. (1992). Newest knowledge of low back pain: A critical look. *Clinical Orthopedics*, *279*, 8–20.

Naftulin, S., & Niergarth, S. (1995). Continuous passive motion. *Physical Medicine and Rehabilitation: State of the Art Reviews, 9*(1), 51–65.

Poss, R. (1993). Total joint replacement: Optimizing patient expectations. *Journal of the American Academy of Orthopedic Surgeons*, *1*, 18–23.

Robinson, J. P., & Brown, P. B. (1991). Medications in low back pain. *Physical Medicine and Rehabilitation Clinics of North America*, *2*(1), 97–126.

Saal, J. A., & Saal, J. S. (1991). Initial stage management of lumbar spine problems. *Physical Medicine and Rehabilitation Clinics of North America, 2*(1), 187–204.

Schmalzried, T. P., Szuszczewicz, E. S., Northfield, M. R., Akizuki, K. H., Frankel, R. E., Belcher, G., & Amstutz, H. C. (1998). Quantitative assessment of walking activity after total hip or knee replacement. *Journal of Bone and Joint Surgery*, *80-A*, 54–59.

Sinaki, M. (1995). Rehabilitation of osteoporotic fractures of the spine. *Physical Medicine and Rehabilitation: State of the Art Reviews*, *9*(1), 105–124.

Sinaki, M., & Mokri, B. (1996). Low back pain and disorders of the lumbar spine. In R. L. Braddom, *Physical medicine and rehabilitation* (pp. 813–850). Philadelphia: W. B. Saunders.

Subbarao, J. V., & Blair, S. J. (1995). Reflex sympathetic dystrophy syndrome. *Physical Medicine and Rehabilitation: State of the Art Reviews, 9*(1), 31–50.

Triffit, P. D. (1998). The relationship between motion of the shoulder and the stated ability to perform activities of daily living. *Journal of Bone and Joint Surgery, 80-A*, 41–46.

Winter, D. (1983). Energy generation and absorption at the ankle and knee during fast, natural, and slow cadences. *Clinical Orthopedics, 175*, 147–154.

Zuckerman, J. D., & Newport, M. L. (1988). Rehabilitation of fractures in adults. In J. Goodgold (Ed.), *Rehabilitation medicine* (pp. 441–456). St. Louis: C. V. Mosby.

Chapter 17

Ostomy Surgeries

Mary Ellen Olbrisch, Jolie Blankenship, Kathleen Hudson, and Elisabeth D. Sherwin

Numerous medical conditions, including congenital defects, trauma, inflammatory bowel disease (IBD), and bowel and bladder cancer can be treated by surgeries that close the normal route of elimination of bodily wastes and create a new opening. These various surgical procedures are collectively referred to as ostomies, and the abdominal openings created are called stomas. Understanding the reason for the ostomy surgery can be more important in understanding issues related to adjustment and rehabilitation than knowing the details of the specific surgery. Table 17.1 presents a summary of the indications for various types of ostomy surgery.

PEDIATRIC OSTOMIES

A number of conditions, many congenital, necessitate ostomy surgery for pediatric patients. Congenital anomalies associated with intestinal ostomies are imperforate anus, rectal atresia, spina bifida, myelomeningocele, Hirschspring's disease, and necrotizing enterocolitis (NEC). Conditions affecting the urinary tract primarily include posterior urethral valves, bladder exstrophy, spina bifida, and myelomeningocele. Intermittent catheterization is used more now than in previous years, eliminating the need for permanent urostomy. Occasionally, a child is born

TABLE 17.1 Indications for Ostomies

Large intestine

Disease
- Cancer (rectal most common)
- Crohn's
- Diverticular
- Neoplasms (lipomas, carcinoid)
- Tumors, leiomyomas
- Adenomas, familial polyposis

Diversion
- Trauma
- Fistula
- Obstruction
- Loss of sphincter control
- Abscess

Defect
- Rectal atresia[a]
- Volvulus
- Necrotizing enterocolitis (NEC)[a]
- Hirschspring's[a]
- Imperforate anus[a]
- Meconium ileus[a]

Small intestine

Disease
- Crohn's
- Ulcerative colitis
- Cancer
- Familial polyposis

Diversion
- Trauma
- Obstruction
- Toxic megacolon
- Vascular infarction (involving the large intestine)

Defect
- NEC[a]

Urinary system

Disease
- Cancer (bladder, urethra, cervix, rectum)

Diversion
- Trauma
- Neurogenic bladder
- Chronic cystitis/urinary tract infection
- Acquired spinal cord injury
- Incontinence
- Urethral stricture
- Recurrent reflux
- Radiation cystitis

Defect
- Megaureters
- Exstrophy[a]
- Obstructive
- Anomalies
- Spina bifida[a]
- Myelomeningocele[a]

[a]Indicates congenital anomalies.

with cloacal exstrophy, or prune belly syndrome, also known as Eagle-Barrett syndrome, that would manifest in deformities in both the intestinal and urinary tracts. Many of these conditions may necessitate ostomy surgery as a temporary measure, with restorative surgery performed at a later date. Prognosis for recovery is generally good. A few ostomies remain permanent. Children with NEC who have lost a significant portion of small intestine may face short- or long-term support with total parenteral nutrition.

Tumors in the pelvis are rare in children. Rhabdomyosarcoma can occur in the bladder as well as in the prostate, with an incidence of 0.5 to 0.7 cases per million children younger than 15 years. Generally, chemotherapy, radiation therapy, and surgery are required to control the tumor. Children who have no residual tumor after surgery have an excellent prognosis; those with microscopic residual disease generally can expect a relapse.

Preteens and teenagers with Crohn's disease or ulcerative colitis are grouped together as having IBD. Long-term steroid therapy, along with exacerbations of the disease, can have a negative effect on normal growth and development as well as on emotional development. Many young patients lose a great deal of time from school and work. Both ulcerative colitis and Crohn's disease are characterized by inflammation of the lining of the gastrointestinal (GI) tract, although in ulcerative colitis the inflammation is confined to the large intestine. In Crohn's disease, inflammation and granulomatous lesions can occur anywhere in the GI tract, beginning in the mouth and including the esophagus, stomach, small intestine, large intestine, and anus. Diarrhea, fatigue, and poor absorption of nutrients are among the most common problems for IBD patients. Because Crohn's disease can recur anywhere in the GI tract, surgery is almost never curative and is therefore reserved for patients for whom management with medications and bowel rest have failed. Ostomy surgery is usually performed for complications or if the disease affects the perianal area. The risk of colon cancer is particularly high in patients who have ulcerative colitis, doubling every 10 years that the patient lives with the disease. For this reason, most ulcerative colitis patients will eventually have surgery to remove the large bowel, as this is a curative procedure. Many will have a permanent ileostomy, although newer procedures may require only a temporary stoma or none at all.

ADULT OSTOMIES

Trauma, IBD, cancer, perforations, and diverticulitis are the most common reasons for ostomy surgery in adult patients. Colorectal cancer is one of the most common cancers affecting adults of both sexes. The disease is frequently asymptomatic; patients must prepare for colostomy surgery very soon after learning of a diagnosis of malignancy. Colostomy is indicated in those cases where the tumor cannot be resected, an obstruction is present, or the tumor is too low in the rectum to permit anastomosis of the remaining portions of large bowel. If the tumor has not metastasized, colostomy surgery can be curative. If the disease has spread beyond the large bowel, however, additional treatments such as chemotherapy and radiation may be necessary, and the prognosis is poorer.

Pelvic exenteration is a radical surgical procedure occasionally recommended for advanced rectal and gynecological malignancies. It has also been performed in some tumors involving the urinary tract if the tumor has spread to other organs within the pelvis. Generally, removal of the rectum, distal sigmoid colon, all reproductive organs, the urinary bladder, distal ureters, internal iliac vessels, and pelvic lymph nodes is performed. Some women may also require a partial or total removal of the vagina depending on the location of the tumor. When vaginal resection is necessary to ensure surgical margins that are free from tumor, reconstructive surgery can be performed. Vaginal reconstruction is accomplished by using portions of muscles from the thighs and skin grafts. This will allow for penile penetration (Piver, 1996). Pelvic exenteration surgery requires the patient to wear one external pouch to collect the stool and another to collect the urine. Some of the newer continent urinary diversions allow patients to eliminate the external pouch and just intubate the stoma to drain. Tumors involving the anterior pelvis may allow for sparing of bowel function. Those involving the posterior pelvis may allow for sparing the urinary tract, but nerves may be damaged, causing an alteration in bladder function. This surgery is approached as a curative measure and is therefore contraindicated for patients whose tumors have metastasized beyond the pelvis. Radiation therapy treatments may be a part of the preoperative regimen, particularly in gynecological tumors, and may lead to postoperative complications such as poor wound healing, intestinal obstruction, or fistula development.

TYPES OF OSTOMY SURGERIES

GI Stomas

Figure 17.1 shows the normal lower GI system. The following are types of GI stomas:

Jejunostomy is an opening into the jejunal portion of the small intestine. A stoma located in this portion of the bowel may be done to relieve obstruction or divert stool when a traumatic injury has occurred. Nutritional and fluid-absorptive capabilities are limited when the distal bowel is not functional. Nutritional supplements may be required to maintain appropriate body weight and physical well-being.

Ileostomy is an opening into the ileum, or terminal portion of the small intestine. It may be done for a variety of medical problems. Three common procedures are (1) an end, or Brooke, ileostomy (Figure 17.2), (2) a Kock pouch or internal reservoir, and (3) loop ileostomy. The effluent (discharge) is usually liquid to mushy and may be somewhat odorous. It contains intestinal enzymes that are irritating to the skin surrounding the stoma.

Cecostomy is indicated as a preliminary step in the presence of a large-bowel obstruction when old age or other conditions may make a patient a poor surgical

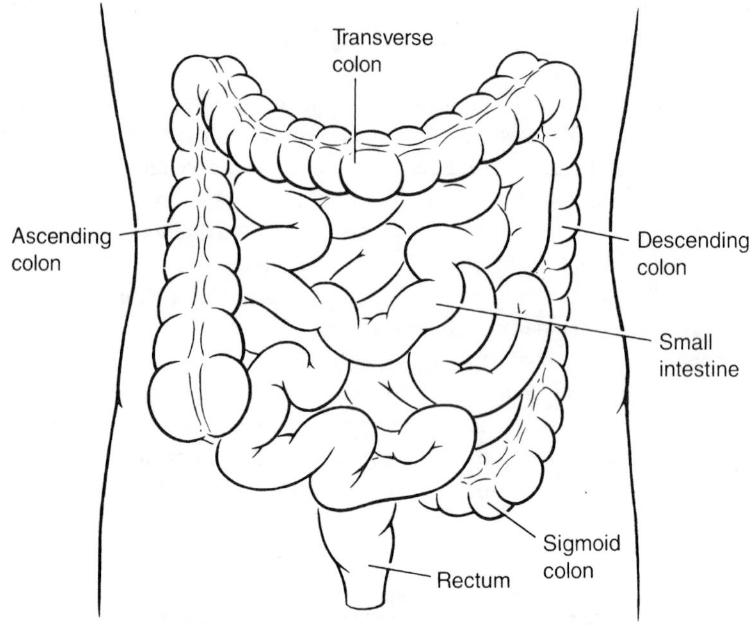

FIGURE 17.1 The normal gastrointestinal system. (Permission to use and/ or reproduce this copyrighted material has been granted by the owner, Hollister Incorporated.)

risk. The incision is located in the lower right quadrant. A tube may or may not be inserted.

Colostomy is an opening created anywhere in the large intestine. Fecal matter exits from that point through the stoma. Colostomies may be end, loop, or double-barreled. The location depends on the site of the disease. Colostomies may be created in the ascending, transverse, descending, or sigmoid colon. A transverse colostomy, occurring in the upper part of the large intestine, drains semiliquid to soft effluent. Output is usually odorous and can irritate peristomal skin. Double-barreled colostomies have two openings. Loop colostomies have one opening but two tracks, the active (proximal), which discharges fecal matter, and the inactive (distal), with a mucous discharge.

Descending or sigmoid colostomies (Figure 17.3) have semisolid to solid drainage. Discharge is malodorous and irritating to skin around the stoma. Frequency of output is unpredictable and varies with each patient. Routine colostomy

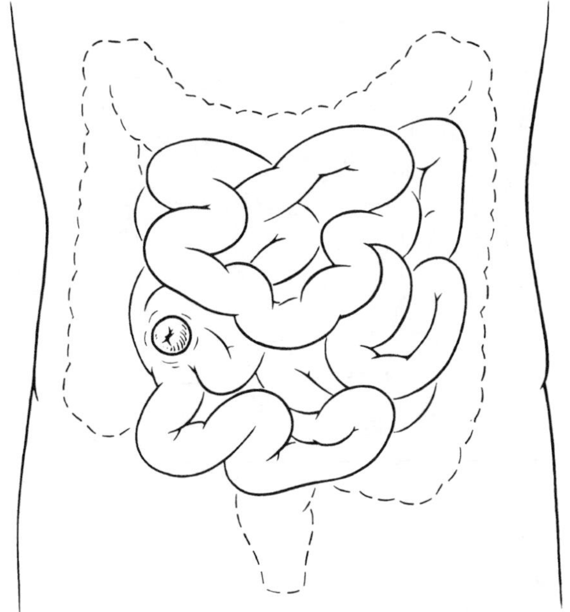

FIGURE 17.2 Ileostomy. The entire colon is removed and a stoma is created at the end of the small intestine. (Permission to use and/or reproduce this copyrighted material has been granted by the owner, Hollister Incorporated.)

irrigation is most effective for individuals who have a permanent or long-term descending or sigmoid colostomy. This procedure, essentially an enema through the stoma, allows many with colostomies the opportunity to control bowel movements and allow them to wear a much smaller security pouch or no pouch at all. Routine irrigation is not indicated in many patients with stomal complications or radiation enteritis or those with a poor prognosis (Hampton & Bryant, 1992).

Urinary Stoma

A urinary conduit (urinary diversion, ileal conduit, or urostomy) is a standard surgical procedure from a urological standpoint. The bladder may or may not be removed (cystectomy). A 20-cm segment from the small intestine (ileum) is removed, with the mesentery intact. The ureters are implanted into the segment

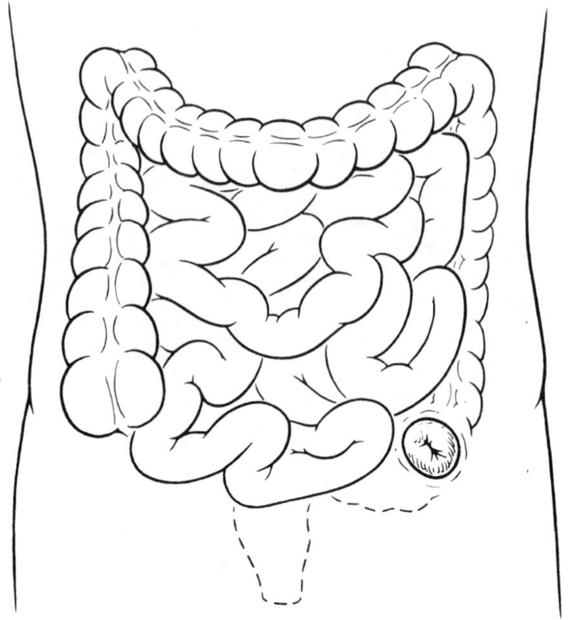

FIGURE 17.3 Sigmoid colostomy. The rectum and part of the sigmoid colon is removed, and a stoma is created in the sigmoid colon. (Permission to use and/or reproduce this copyrighted material has been granted by the owner, Hollister Incorporated.)

to create a passage for urine to be diverted. One end of the ileum is sutured closed; the other end is brought out to the skin to create a stoma (Figure 17.4). The bowel is sutured back together, and there are no changes in the digestive system. Urine output is constant, with mild odor. The urine is usually not irritating to the skin; however, if it is left to remain on the skin for an extended period, the skin will become macerated and problematic. Elderly patients with medical problems are ideal for this type of surgery.

ALTERNATIVE PROCEDURES

Ostomy surgery as described above is considered standard, and the majority of patients have success or minimal technical problems with their stomas. Currently, surgeons are creating alternatives to ostomy surgery and are attempting to create

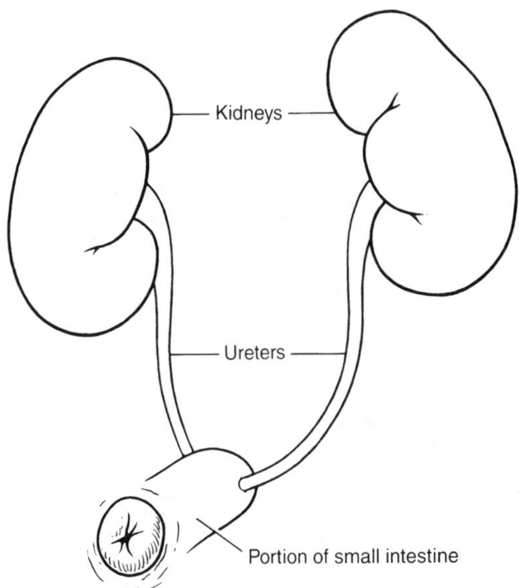

FIGURE 17.4 Ileal conduit. The bladder has been removed, and the ureters are connected to a portion of small bowel, which has been resected and used to create a small collection pouch. The small bowel is reconnected in the area of the resection to maintain normal fecal continence. (Permission to use and/or reproduce this copyrighted material has been granted by the owner, Hollister Incorporated.)

continence or establish other means to regulate the elimination process: allowing the patient to eliminate the ostomy pouch, allowing for continence to be reestablished, preserving normal fluid and electrolyte balance, avoiding metabolic abnormalities, or allowing the patient to manage a colostomy for social situations.

Continent ileostomy (Kock pouch) is a surgical technique developed in 1967 by a Swedish surgeon, Dr. Nils G. Kock, to improve continence for patients with ileostomies. A proctocolectomy (removal of the large intestine) is performed, with 15 cm of the ileum created into a cuplike structure. The flaps of tissue are brought together and sutured, creating an internal pouch structure. The nipple valve is formed by intussuscepting the ileum into the reservoir. A flush stoma (skin level) is sutured to the abdominal wall. The nipple valve operates like a mechanical valve, forcing the valve to close as stool and flatus enters the reservoir. Directing a catheter into the stoma permits the patient to drain the pouch on a schedule, therefore allowing flexibility and preventing leakage. Contraindications include Crohn's disease, age less than 18 years, morbid obesity, and emergency surgery. Patients must be monitored closely for teaching and follow-up in order to deal with unexpected complications and for assistance in dealing realistically with their high expectations for this procedure.

Ileoanal reservoir or anastomosis is a surgical procedure that may take from one to three stages to form the reservoir. Stages of healing vary from patient to patient, and factors such as steroids and anastomotic healing are taken into consideration. Patients on high-dose steroids at the time of operation may experience fewer complications if a two-stage procedure with fecal diversion is employed. The patient will undergo a proctocolectomy with a stump closure of the rectum along with a stripping of the rectal mucosa. A certain population of patients may be anastomosed at the same time (hence, a one-step procedure) according to the findings at the time of surgery. The rectal mucosa is not stripped in a one-stage procedure. Patients must have yearly proctoscopy to rule out recurrent disease in the remaining mucosa.

Other patients may receive loop ileostomy. The creation of the pouch reservoir (the distal ileum placed into the anorectal canal) can be precarious, depending on the medical history and current drug therapy. Therefore, the surgeon will allow the anastomosis and healing phase. The third stage of this procedure involves taking down the ileostomy and converting the newly created pouch to assume normal continence. The small intestine eventually will be able to take over the absorption and storage functions of the resected bowel. The pouch may resemble a *J* or an *S* in shape to take on a side-to-side anastomotic structure. Selection criteria for the procedure include motivation, disease process (Crohn's disease is contraindicated), physical status, and competent rectal sphincter.

Continent Urinary Diversions

Over the past decade, newer surgical options or techniques have become more advanced, with a favorable outlook for the patient. The practice of intermittent catheterizations has expanded the options for patients to retain their continence and eliminate the need for wearing an external pouch; hence, an individual can experience periods of dryness that would prove socially acceptable. It also reduced the costs of specific supplies and allows the individual to experience a positive outlook.

There are many factors that should be taken into consideration before this type of surgery is undertaken. A detailed explanation of the surgery must take place between the surgeon and the patient. What the operation will entail and what will occur over the following 6 weeks, as well as long term, should be discussed. A bowel prep is necessary when the bowel is involved. Also, antibiotics are considered important to reduce the infection rate.

Patients undergoing extended pelvic surgery are at high risk for development of deep vein thrombosis (DVT). Compression hose or wraps, along with low-dose heparin will assist to promote venous return. Smoking should be discouraged for at least 1 month prior to the surgery. Early ambulation and vigorous pulmonary toilet are fundamental to the success of the patient's postoperative recovery.

An enterostomal therapist (ET) nurse should mark the patient for a standard urinary diversion if the procedure is unable to be performed. An accessible area of the patient's abdomen can also be evaluated for the procedure. Psychological evaluation and counseling is an integral part of the patients total recovery in this type of surgery.

Patient selection is the most significant factor if the surgery is to be considered a true success. The following conditions must be met: a true understanding of the surgery, along with emotional maturity and manual dexterity. Indications for continent urinary diversions include primary bladder cancers, failed radiation treatments for prostate or bladder, neurogenic bladder, congenital abnormalities, interstitial cystitis, and the patient's choice for continence (Marshall, 1996). The surgery involves ensuring that adequate bowel with good blood supply can be obtained. The efferent end is identified in a mobilized area. The segments of the bowel reservoir are marked in centimeters for the arms of the reservoir (3–4 areas). The bowel is opened, and the nipple valves are created (afferent and efferent limbs). The loops of bowel are used to create the internal pouch and the GIA Stapler is used to take the place of sutures.

The success of this surgery is dependent on careful selection of the individual after physical and emotional stability has been established. Several other factors are also important: the clinical and surgical expertise of the physician, availability of necessary and particular equipment and supplies, and also access to other members of the surgical staff for assistance if necessary.

Neobladder

An anastomosis of the ureters to a segment of bowel allows micturition, which has been preferred in the male patient who has met all the standards. This surgical procedure is a prolonged operation, is technically challenging, and has a high complication rate. A detailed evaluation of the patient must be considered. Medical history must be carefully taken in to account and risk factors excluded. Contraindications for surgery exist in patients who are elderly, have an involved medical and/or surgical history (that includes bowel disease), are nutritionally compromised, have undergone radiation therapy, or have a decreased motivational level.

TABLE 17.2 Types of Continent Diversions

Name	Pouch
Mansson	Ascending and transverse colon
Kock	Ileum U-shaped
Mainz	Ileocecum sideways, S-shaped
Mitrofanoff	Any detubularized[a] reservoir or bladder
Indiana	Ascending colon
Hautmann neobladder	Ileum W-shaped
Studer neobladder	Ileum U-shaped
Hemi-Kock neobladder	Ileum U-shaped
Mainz neobladder	Ileocecal sideways, S-shaped

[a]Reestablishment of the bowel into a detubularized structure is the most important aspect to be maintained to result in a low pressure/high volume reservoir.

For several weeks after the surgery (4–6 weeks) the patient will have catheters and drainage tubes. Once they are removed, x-rays and blood tests are performed. Voiding must be relearned. By utilizing abdominal straining, the Valsalva maneuver, and certain relaxation methods, the patient is able to void with a stream. The neobladder gradually enlarges over 6 months. Follow-up with testing is very important to the patient's well-being.

FUNCTIONAL PRESENTATION OF OSTOMIES

Equipment for stoma care is one of the most important factors to consider. Selecting specific supplies should reflect their availability to the patient; cost; type of ostomy; characteristics of the patient's abdomen, including scars, skin folds, and creases; characteristics of the stoma (flush, retracted, or budded); the patient's capabilities and limitations; patient size; patient preference; and patient activity level. Postoperatively the incision, stoma size, drains, and tubes will affect selection of equipment.

Patient teaching should occur on a daily basis to aid the patient in learning to manage the ostomy, learning proper skin care, and becoming adept in the use of appropriate equipment. Shorter hospitalizations have necessitated continued teaching by home health nurses after discharge. An ostomy visitor who has undergone similar surgery is usually extremely helpful to the patient in providing role modeling, support, information, and encouragement. Besides direct care and management of the stoma and surrounding skin, the patient may have to make dietary adjustments to prevent blockages, to maintain a regular schedule for elimination, or to maintain optimal urinary pH to prevent infection. These adjustments do not generally require major lifestyle alterations.

TREATMENT AND PROGNOSIS

Ostomies themselves are not disabling, and the original reason for the surgery will probably say more about prognosis than the fact of ostomy surgery itself. Many ostomy surgeries are temporary, allowing healing time for damaged tissues. Reconnection will generally return the patient to normal elimination patterns. Permanent ostomies will, for some patients, represent cure of a disabling illness and removal of the threat of life-threatening disease, as is usually the case for ulcerative colitis. For patients with other diseases, the stoma may serve as a reminder of vulnerability to malignancy or other problems. Most patients can anticipate a reasonably active lifestyle, assuming that preexisting disease does not contribute to further deterioration.

PSYCHOLOGICAL AND VOCATIONAL IMPLICATIONS

There is little doubt that the creation of a stoma requires adjustment on the part of the patient: issues such as self-image, sexuality, interpersonal relationships, care of the stoma, and the economics associated with a chronic condition must all be faced. One of developmental tasks a child faces is the control and management of waste—mastering "toilet training." Accomplishing this task often elevates the toddler, at least in the eyes of the family, to that of a young child, a maturational stage. Moreover, in psychodynamic terms, anal function and anal products "are closely linked to issues of control [and] orderliness" (Gonsalves-Ebrahim, 1982, p. 1). Thus, the removal of a body part, the closure of a natural body orifice, and the creation of an external opening for the elimination of fecal material or urine can be expected to be a stressful physiological and psychological event.

Changes in Body Image

Much of the literature on adjustment to a stoma has focused on the expected psychological distress associated with a change to body and self-image (e.g., Mikolon, 1982b; Pieper & Mikols, 1996; Walsh, Grunert, Telford, & Otterson, 1995). However, such research has often suffered from methodological difficulties, ranging from the nature of retrospective data collection and lack of consistency in instruments used to measure unclearly defined concepts to subject biases (Tomaseli, Jenks, & Morin, 1991). Moreover, such research has often combined two polar populations: individuals who are undergoing an ostomy surgery for cancer and those who suffer from Crohn's disease and similar ailments.

In general, attention has focused on the interaction between the stress associated with the creation of the stoma and its implication, namely, that the stoma symbolizes lack of control over bodily excretions as well as the relocation of such functions to a less private site (e.g., Cohen, 1991; Gonsalves-Ebrahim, 1982; Kelman & Minkler, 1989; Quayle, 1994; Smith & Babaian, 1989; Tomaseli et al., 1991). In line with these concerns, Klopp (1990) reports that individuals with fecal stomas have a poorer body image than do individuals with urinary stomas: Moreover, body image appears particularly threatened by the sensory phenomena associated with a stoma: the effluence and the odor and sound of involuntary passage of flatus. These are aggravated by the constant fear of leakage that many persons with ostomies report (Goldberg, 1991). Patients with alternative procedures allowing continence express more satisfaction (Boys et al., 1987), although patient selection may be a more compelling factor. Emotions such as shame and embarrassment, feelings of being mutilated, fears of rejection and of being viewed as an invalid, and anxiety over role responsibility and ability to meet expectations are all associated with the stoma.

Psychosocial Issues

Uninformed patients may assume that they are unique and alone in their condition (Mikolon,1982b), whereas, in fact, in 1989 it was estimated that there were 1.5 million patients with some type of ostomy (Kelman & Minkler, 1989), and 100,000 such operations are performed annually in the United States (Klopp, 1990). Thus, it is not surprising that a "striking commonality among studies involving persons with stomas is the high incidence of depression" (Klopp, 1990, p. 104). Klopp reports a 70% incidence of depression among her subjects. This depression may be a reflection and an integral product of a grieving process that has been conceptualized as necessary in rehabilitation and readjustment. Sultenfuss (1982) delineates four stages for this process: shock and panic, defensive retreat, acknowledgment, and adaptation and resolution. Kelman and Minkler (1989) note that the third stage, acknowledgment, "occurs when the individual realizes that the stoma is real and begins to explore its meaning. This may be the most painful stage" (p. 5). In line with general research on bereavement, Kelman and Minkler note that an "inability to adapt after a one year period is a positive indication for psychiatric intervention" (p. 5). Adjustment to ostomy is not solely determined by the absence of depression, however, but also by the ability to engage in normal activities and overcome limitations (Burckhardt, 1990).

Yet the most powerful predictors of postoperative adjustment are the preoperative physical and emotional status (Follick, Smith, & Turk, 1984; Liss, 1982; Mikolon, 1982b). Variables as diverse as personality style, extent of social support, health, and nature of employment all affect the quality of postsurgery life and adjustment to the stoma. Mikolon (1982b) summarizes previous research by noting that "overall, the dependent individual who expresses a need to have support and interaction from other people, yet who has difficulty in expressing affection (or may indeed feel little affection), is apparently the type of individual who does not return to a satisfactory lifestyle" (p. 440). At the same time, she notes that "the response of close family members to the presence of an ostomy is a key factor in a person's adjustment to an ostomy" (p. 440).

Social support and understanding of those close to the ostomy patient have been significantly associated with better marital, family, and sexual adjustment (Follick et al., 1984; Oades-Souther & Olbrisch, 1984; Olbrisch, 1983; Rheaume & Gooding, 1991). Rheaume and Gooding (1991) note that there are self-help groups that exist to help the patients with an ostomy to adjust. These researchers approached members in two United Ostomy Association groups. The majority of their respondents had had ostomies for over 10 years. Rheaume and Gooding report that their subjects had high levels of perceived support, scored high on the Quality of Life Index, and used significantly more problem-oriented coping strategies as opposed to affective coping strategies. Problem-focused coping has been associated with better overall adjustment (Strentz & Auerbach, 1988).

On a more intimate level, Mikolon (1982b) stresses that "family members should be reminded that the patient will silently look to them in the beginning as an index of how the world at large will regard them" (p. 441). Unfortunately, the illness of a husband or wife may not necessarily elicit the desired support and comfort from the spouse (Mikolon, 1982b). The illness brings about a disequilibrium in the relationship. Reactions such as revulsion or rejection of their partners were more commonly expressed by wives than by husbands (Dyk & Sutherland, 1956). Nearly 40 years later, the response to the stoma has not changed; Liss (1982) reports the "during the convalescent period, almost 50% of patients concealed the colostomy from their spouses" (p. 434). Yet ultimately, it is the quality of the preoperative relationship that will largely determine the nature of postoperative support and intimacy (Gloeckner, 1991; Nagata, 1982).

The fear of rejection by one's spouse is closely associated with perceived changes in sexual attractiveness. However, 80% of those responding to Gloeckner's (1983) questionnaire indicated that their partners were comfortable with the physical changes resulting from the surgery. Nagata (1982) stresses that, to facilitate the resumption of normal healthy sexual relationships, sexual counseling is to begin early on, "before a person has adjusted by repression or suppression of sexuality" (p. 455). Future goals and expectations must be delineated and addressed, and Nagata endorses the PLISSIT model of counseling: permission, limited information, specific suggestions, and intensive therapy.

Simmons (1983), an ostomy patient herself, offers explicit and concrete guidelines to other women with ostomies. She suggests reformulating one's expectations and focusing initially on emotional intimacy rather than physical intercourse. Nagata (1982) offers similar suggestions: absence of sensation does not mean absence of feelings, inability to move does not mean inability to please, inability to perform does not mean inability to enjoy, and loss of genitals does not mean loss of sexuality.

In preparation for sexual intimacy, Nagata (1982) suggests the following:

1. Emptying the ostomy appliance before sexual activity and taping the appliance for added security.
2. Using a pouch deodorant or odor-proof pouches.
3. Maintaining body cleanliness and, if helpful, using desired colognes and perfumes.
4. Using boxer shorts (men) or panties with the crotch removed (women) for persons wishing to hide the stoma or pouch.
5. Using pouch covers, opaque pouches, or belts.
6. If a break in the pouch seal occurs, one may wish to bathe and continue sexual activities in the tub or shower. (p. 457)

Of special note are the sexual needs of the nontraditional patient, such as the adolescent and the homosexual adult. Both of these groups often fall between the cracks, as the health professional assumes there should be no sexual concerns (the adolescent) or an assumption of heterosexuality is made and the patient's specific needs are ignored. Etnyre (1988) notes that many of sexual concerns of the homosexual patient may be similar to those of the heterosexual. Yet some may perceive the stoma to be a form of punishment, and if these perceptions go unaddressed, this may result in depression. Etnyre suggests that the ET nurse be alert and make no assumptions regarding the patient's sexual orientation nor about the nature and meaning of the loss the patient is experiencing because of the stoma. A prerequisite to any discussion of sexuality with any patient is that the health care professional be familiar and comfortable with his or her own sexuality. Creating a climate for disclosure; building basic rapport; employing adaptable, inclusive language; initiating discussion about sexual concerns while employing a direct approach are all guidelines for effective communication regarding sex. Moreover, "in all cases the patient must be reassured that knowledge of his or her sexual orientation will be treated confidentially. . . . Under no circumstances should information about sexual orientation be placed in the chart" (p. 124).

When dealing with an adolescent, Landmann (1989) exhorts ET nurses to remember the unique developmental tasks and the body image issues confronting an adolescent. The adolescent, like any ostomy patient, requires "useful and factual information" about possible changes in dress style, dating, sexuality, peer relationships, diet, and activities such as sports and leisure activities. Time must be set aside to answer specific questions and concerns. Landmann stresses that "it is important to stress that the presence of a stoma and pouching system will not interfere with one's customary attire or physical activities" (p. 88). But the primary directive for a health professional dealing with an adolescent is to remember that "adolescents want the health care provider to show respect for them and to talk with them" (p. 88). Manworren (1996) notes that activity limitations are a major concern for teenage boys, although body image, independence, social relationships, and sexuality are also concerns.

Preoperative health status, or the reason for the ostomy, is a variable that often confounds the literature. As Oades-Souther and Olbrisch (1984), Liss (1982), and Follick, Smith, and Turk (1984) note, the two major groups undergoing ostomy surgery are cancer patients and those suffering from IBD. These two populations differ greatly from each other. Patients suffering from IBD, in contrast to cancer patients, usually have a long history of impairment resulting from their condition. It has often caused severe disruption in work and social functioning (Liss, 1982). In contrast, the cancer patient may be taken unaware by both the diagnosis and the need for an ostomy. The acuteness of the trauma associated with the cancer diagnosis often preempts preoperative explanations, preparation by the ET nurse, and visits from other patients with ostomies—all variables that have been significantly associated with better coping (Goldberg, 1991; Hedrick, 1987; Mikolon, 1982a, 1982b).

The cancer patient is often older than the chronic disease patient and often undergoes a colostomy rather than an ileostomy, a surgery more prevalent among IBD patients (Follick et al., 1984; Oades-Souther & Olbrisch, 1984). This procedural distinction is critical, as "a higher rate of sexual dysfunction seems to exist among males with colostomies than among males with ileostomies" (Oades-Souther & Olbrisch, 1984, p. 232). Ultimately, the differential recovery among these two groups appears to be associated with the intrinsic difference in the catalyst for surgery. Whereas "the colitis patient . . . soon realizes that the stoma means freedom to live an almost normal life . . . , the cancer patient will be more concerned with death and the chances of survival than with the care of the ostomy" (Liss, 1982, p. 433). Differences in perceived sexual attractiveness were also found between those who underwent surgery because of cancer and those suffering from inflammatory disease. Gloeckner (1984) reports that those with IBD perceived themselves as more attractive than those with cancer.

Economic and Vocational Issues

Mikolon (1982a) notes that "clearly, the economic costs of living with an ostomy can be considerable when complications from the stoma or disease process develop" (p. 460). Yet the cost in and of itself, she claims, should not be the primary influence in the choice of equipment. Rather, "obtaining a secure, odor-proof, comfortable seal is most important, followed by individual preference, ease of application and emptying, availability and appearance" (p. 460). Naturally, a return to employment is crucial in both defraying the cost of ostomy appliances and enhancing the ostomy patient's self-esteem (Kelman & Minkler, 1989). Ostomy surgery itself does not present obstacles to most vocational functioning. Nevertheless, underlying disease processes may influence patients' potential for return to work. Issues of eligibility for health insurance reimbursement and government-associated programs available to defray the cost of ostomy supplies are described in detail by Mikolon (1982a).

Interventions and Resources

The role of the ET nurse and the information and counseling he or she provides appears to have been underrated according to recent research (Follick et al., 1984; Kelman & Minkler, 1989). However, the significant contribution of ET nurses has been documented. Follick, Smith, and Turk (1984) note that technical difficulties were frequently and negatively correlated with psychosocial adjustment, and significant correlations were found between preparatory information and postsurgical adjustment. Kelman and Minkler (1989) noted that patients who received counseling intervention demonstrated positive alteration in self-concept and self-esteem. Righter (1995) emphasizes the authority and educational role of the ET nurse in helping patients derive meaning from the experience of illness and surgery.

Sultenfuss (1982) suggests that the more a therapist is aware and accepting of her or his own barriers to issues potentially precipitated by ostomy surgery, the more available she or he may be to the ostomy patient. The message an ET nurse should strive to relay is one of acceptance:

1. Whatever you communicate is normal and acceptable.
2. Whatever you communicate is not threatening or frightening to me.
3. You will not be rejected or isolated for whatever you communicate. (p. 443)

When working with the elderly, Kuhn and Flaherty McCrann (1990) suggest that ET nurses take the time to identify the strength of their patients, restore self-esteem, and use knowledge about the geriatric population—sensory changes, reaction time, memory and intellectual capacity, and motivation—while teaching. The meaning of ostomy surgery is likely to be different for elderly patients facing possible death and dependency than it is for younger patients (Mihalopoulos, Trunnell, Ball, & Moncor, 1994).

Alternative interventions are offered by individuals such as Trunnell (1996), Simmons (1983), and Frager and Griffis (1978) and through organizations such as the local chapters of the United Ostomy Association. Ostomy visitors from the United Ostomy Association are people who have had their ostomies for at least 1 year and are assessed by their physicians or ETs as coping well with the changes that have occurred. They are required to attend a training program, then are matched as closely as possible for age, sex, and type of ostomy. People who live in rural areas may not have access to this service. Information is still available to them in *Ostomy Quarterly*, a magazine that each member receives. It addresses pertinent issues of ostomy patients of all ages. Other support groups, like the Crohn's Colitis Foundation of America (formerly NFIC) and the Oley Foundation PEN (Parenteral and Enteral Nutrition), offer assistance to those with specific chronic or long-term illness. The American Cancer Society often will help the ostomy patient who is also combating cancer.

REFERENCES

Boys, S. D., Feinberg, S. M., Skinner, D. E., Lieskovsky, G., Baron, D., & Richardson, J. (1987). Quality of life survey of urinary diversion patients: Comparison of ileal conduits vs. Kock urinary reservoirs. *Journal of Urology, 138,* 1386–1389.

Burckhardt, C. S. (1990). The Ostomy Adjustment Scale: Further evidence of reliability and validity. *Rehabilitation Psychology, 35*, 149–155.

Cohen, A. (1991). Body image in the person with a stoma. *Journal of Enterostomal Therapy, 18,* 68–71.

Dyk, R. B., & Sutherland, A. (1956). Adaptation of the spouse and other family members to the colostomy patient. *Cancer, 9*, 123.

Etnyre, W. S. (1988). Meeting the psychosocial needs of the homosexual person with a stoma. *Journal of Enterostomal Therapy, 15,* 121–125.

Follick, M. J., Smith, T. W., & Turk, D. C. (1984). Psychosocial adjustment following ostomy. *Health Psychology, 3,* 505–517.

Frager, S. R., & Griffis, J. (1978, Spring). If you are an ostomate because of cancer you need to read this! *Ostomy Quarterly*, p. 43.

Gloeckner, M. R. (1983). Partner reaction following ostomy surgery. *Journal of Sex and Marital Therapy, 9,* 182–190.

Gloeckner, M. R. (1984). Perceptions of sexuality after ostomy surgery. *Journal of Enterostomal Therapy, 18,* 36–38.

Gloeckner, M. (1991). Perceptions of sexual attractiveness following ostomy surgery. *Research in Nursing and Health, 7,* 87–92.

Goldberg, M. T. (1991). Promoting positive self-concept in patients with stomas: Nursing interventions. *Progressions: Developments in Ostomy and Wound Care, 3,* 3–11.

Gonsalves-Ebrahim, L. (1982). *Psychological implications of temporary and permanent ostomies.* Unpublished manuscript.

Hampton, B., & Bryant, R. (1992). *Ostomies and continent diversions*. St. Louis: Mosby Year Book.

Hedrick, J. K. (1987). Effects of ET nursing intervention on adjustment following ostomy surgery. *Journal of Enterostomal Therapy, 14*, 229–239.

Kelman, G., & Minkler, P. (1989). An investigation of quality of life and self-esteem among individuals with ostomies. *Journal of Enterostomal Therapy, 16,* 4–11.

Klopp, A. L. (1990). Body image and self-concept among individuals with stomas. *Journal of Enterostomal Therapy, 17*, 98–105.

Kuhn, J. K., & Flaherty McCrann, M. J. (1990). Helping ostomy patients back to independence. *Journal of Gerontological Nursing, 16*, 27–30.

Landmann, L. A. (1989). When your ostomy patient is an adolescent. *Journal of Enterostomal Therapy, 16,* 87–88.

Liss, J. L. (1982). Psychiatric issues in ostomy management. In D. C. Broadwell & B. S. Jackson (Eds.), *Principles of ostomy care* (pp. 431–437). St. Louis: C. V. Mosby.

Manworeen, R. C. (1996). Development effects on the adolescent of a temporary ileostomy. *Journal of Wound Care, Ostomy and Continence Nursing, 23,* 210–217.

Marshall, F. F. (1996). Ileal conduit urinary diversion. In E. Shapiro (Ed.), *Textbook of operative urology, 54*, 438–444. Philadelphia: W. B. Saunders.

Mihalopoulos, W. C., Trunnell, E. P., Ball, K., & Moncor, C. (1994). The psychologic impact of ostomy surgery on persons 50 of age and older. *Journal of Wound Care, Ostomy and Continence Nursing, 21*, 149–155.

Mikolon, S. (1982a). Economic facilitators and barriers to living with an ostomy. In D. C. Broadwell & B. S. Jackson (Eds.), *Principles of ostomy care* (pp. 460–467). St. Louis: C. V. Mosby.

Mikolon, S. (1982b). Psychosocial issues in ostomy management. In D. C. Broadwell & B. S. Jackson (Eds.), *Principles of ostomy care* (pp. 438–442). St. Louis: C. V. Mosby.

Nagata, F. K. (1982). Human sexuality. In D. C. Broadwell & B. S. Jackson (Eds.), *Principles of ostomy care* (pp. 450–459). St. Louis: C. V. Mosby.

Oades-Souther, D., & Olbrisch, M. E. (1984). Psychological adjustment to ostomy surgery. *Rehabilitation Psychology, 4,* 221–237.

Olbrisch, M. E. (1983). Development and validation of the ostomy adjustment scale. *Rehabilitation Psychology, 28*, 3–12.

Pieper, B., & Mikols, C. (1996). Predischarge and postdischarge concerns of persons with an ostomy. *Journal of Wound Care, Ostomy and Continence Nursing, 23*, 105–109.

Piver, M. S. (Ed.). (1996). *Handbook of gynecologic oncology* (2nd ed., pp. 118–120). Boston: Little, Brown.

Quayle, B. K. (1994). Making positive choices: Body image and the new ostomy patient. *Ostomy/Wound Management, 40,* 16–21.

Rheaume, A. N., & Gooding, B. A. (1991). Social support, coping strategies, and long-term adaptation to ostomy among self-help group members. *Journal of Enterostomal Therapy, 18,* 11–15.

Righter, B. M. (1995). Uncertainty and the role of credible authority during the ostomy experience. *Journal of Wound Care, Ostomy and Continence Nursing, 22*, 100–104.

Simmons, K. N. (1983). Sexuality and the female ostomate: Patient-to-patient advice. *American Journal of Nursing, 83,* 409–411.

Smith, D. B., & Babaian, R. J. (1989). Patient adjustment to an ileal conduit after radical cystectomy. *Journal of Enterostomal Therapy, 16*, 244–246.

Strentz, T., & Auerbach, S. M. (1988). Adjustment to the stress of simulated captivity: Effects of emotion-focused versus problem-focused preparation on hostages differing in locus of control. *Journal of Personality and Social Psychology, 55,* 652–660.

Sultenfuss, S. R. (1982). Psychosocial issues and therapeutic intervention. In D. C. Broadwell & B. S. Jackson (Eds.), *Principles of ostomy care* (pp. 443–449). St. Louis: C. V. Mosby.

Tomaseli, N., Jenks, J., & Morin, K. H. (1991). Body image in patients with stomas: A critical review of the literature. *Journal of ET Nursing, 18,* 95–99.

Trunnell, E. P. (1996). Mindfulness and people with stomas. *Journal of Wound Care, Ostomy and Continence Nursing, 23,* 38–45.

Walsh, B. A., Grunert, B. K., Telford, G. L., & Otterson, M. F. (1995). Multidisciplinary management of altered body image in the patient with an ostomy. *Journal of Wound, Ostomy and Continence Nursing, 22,* 227–236.

Chapter 18

Pediatric Disorders: Cerebral Palsy and Spina Bifida

Joan T. Gold

Physically challenged children present with a variety of developmental and neuromuscular disabilities that are often difficult to diagnose, harder to remediate, and impossible to cure. The restrictions of such disability may not permit the patient the motoric control or experiences to acquire skills at the same rate as an unimpaired child, and secondary delays may occur (Missuna & Pollack, 1991). Social isolation, parental dependency, and financial burdens act as stressors for patients, parents, and siblings (Worley, Rosenfeld, & Liscomb, 1991).

It is the purpose of this chapter to discuss cerebral palsy and spina bifida, two of the more handicapping conditions of childhood, and the strategies that allow for appropriate medical treatment and habilitation. This information permits the health professional to serve as an advocate for optimization of care, prevention of complications, referral to early intervention programs, and placement in the least restrictive school setting. Additionally, potentially abusive and neglectful behaviors of parents and caretakers may be circumvented (Benedict, White, Wulff, & Hall, 1990).

CEREBRAL PALSY

Cerebral palsy denotes a group of static encephalopathies of diverse etiologies that result from nonprogressive lesions of the brain sustained in the pre-, peri-, or postnatal period. They are characterized by abnormalities of muscle tone, movement, and posture, of which spasticity is the most common. Secondary dysfunction and deformities occur but not the frank neurological regression seen with neurodegenerative disorders, such as the leukodystrophies. Other symptoms of cerebral dysfunction, such as learning disabilities, mental retardation, and seizures, may be seen, but it is the motoric dysfunction that is essential to its recognition (Ingram, 1955).

Incidence

The incidence of cerebral palsy over the past 20 years has remained at 2 cases per 1,000 births in the United States (Nelson & Ellenberg, 1986), with 400,000 patients currently being affected despite advances in intrapartum monitoring that can herald fetal distress and neonatal respiratory support (Grant, O'Brien, Joy, Hennessy, & MacDonald, 1989; Stanley & Blair, 1991). This implies that some low-birth-weight infants are surviving unscathed and that efforts expended at the time of delivery may be employed after the fact (Ford, Kitchen, Doyle, Richards, & Kelly, 1990). It is possible that incidence figures may gradually increase as more extremely low-birth-weight infants (less than 1,000 g) survive. From 44% to 56% of this group may require special education services, although a frank diagnosis of cerebral palsy is made in less than 25% of the cases (Vohr & Msall, 1997).

Etiology and Risk Factors

Cerebral palsy was first described by Little in 1843 in former premature infants who developed increased tone and incoordination primarily affecting the lower extremities (spastic diplegia). With changes in medical treatment, a reduced association with dystocia (difficult labor), erythroblastosis (Rh-negative blood incompatibility), and encephalitis and an increased association with multiple births, prematurity, acquired hydrocephalus (following intracranial bleeding), and trauma have been noted (Capute, Shapiro, & Palmer, 1981). Accordingly, fewer patients are affected with the writhing movement disorder of athetosis, seen with erythroblastosis and basal ganglia involvement, and more have diffuse cerebral dysfunction with spasticity and cognitive difficulties.

Etiology can be identified in up to 71% of quadriplegics (four-extremity involvement) and 40% of nonquadriplegics (Naeye & Peters, 1989). A gestational age of less than 32 of 40 weeks is the greatest predictor of cerebral palsy. Other risk factors, such as maternal mental retardation, birth weight of less than 2,001 g, the presence of congenital malformations, and symptomatic intoxications such as fetal alcohol syndrome, support a largely prenatal etiology (Coorsen, Msall, &

Duffy, 1991; Ellenberg & Nelson, 1981). Factors that result in chronic antenatal hypoxia with brain injury include maternal anemia, preeclampsia/gestational hypertension, a drop in third-trimester blood pressure, postterm delivery, and multiple births (Nelson, 1989). Premature delivery and findings associated with birth asphyxia, such as meconium staining, low Apgar scores at 10 minutes, apneic (breath-holding) spells, seizures, persistent neurological abnormalities, and slow head growth, may be manifestations of prior intrauterine events resulting in brain damage rather than its cause (Nelson, 1989); they have a high association with congenital malformations.

A prenatal etiology for cerebral palsy has been identified in up to 50%–60% of patients (Holm, 1982; Naeye & Peters, 1989), most presenting with hypotonia, ataxia, or hemiplegia. Thrombotic events in utero may explain many cases of cerebral palsy. Identification of a parental coagulopathy could potentially identify a population at risk and allow for development of preventative treatment protocol (Kraus, 1997). A perinatal etiology has been identified in 10%–30% of cases. True perinatal asphyxia may be related to obstetrical complications such as placental abruption, nuchal cord, or meconium aspiration and may affect heart and kidney function. Other perinatal etiologies include central nervous system bleeding (Williams, Lewandowski, Coplan, & D'Eugenio, 1987) and meningeal infections. Patients in this group are most likely to be spastic. A postnatal etiology occurs in about 10% of patients (Holm, 1982); factors include head trauma (often abuse-related), central nervous system infections, and cerebrovascular accidents. Such patients are likely to be hemiparetic (have unilateral limb involvement). A mixed etiology occurs in approximately 7% of the cases (Holm, 1982).

Neonatal indicators for development of static encephalopathy include intracranial hemorrhage, seizures, microcephaly (small head size), hyper- or hypotonia, abnormal suck/cry/grasp/reflexes, jitteriness, temperature instability, and feeding difficulties (Nelson & Ellenberg, 1979). Apgar scores that reflect immediate neonatal status are not as predictive as once thought (Nelson & Ellenberg, 1981). Periventricular hemorrhage in association with attenuation of the white matter around the ventricles (periventricular leukomalacia) and formation of cysts correlates with the development of cerebral palsy (Graham, Levene, & Trounce, 1987).

Delineation of etiology may imply a specific clinical presentation and prognosis that permits parents to be supplied with an overview of the child's potential outcome. Counseling parents that actions during the time of conception and pregnancy are most likely unrelated to the development of the cerebral palsy permits feelings of guilt to be assuaged and promotes better acceptance of the child.

Functional Presentation

Cerebral palsy is classified on the basis of etiology, tone, and anatomical distribution of neurological abnormalities (Perlstein, 1952). Pyramidal or spastic (clasp-knife) cerebral palsy is the most common, occurring in 65%–75% of all cases. Resistance is noted when muscles are stretched rapidly beyond a critical point. There is associated hyperreflexia and up-going plantar responses. Quadriplegia occurs in about 20% of these cases, with diffuse cortical involvement, and, in the most disabled, widespread atrophy with cavity formation and decreased white matter density. Hemiplegia occurs in about 30% and is associated with atrophy/gliosis of the contralateral cerebral hemisphere, likely caused by a vascular disturbance. Liquefaction necrosis may occur, resulting in a perencephalic cyst (Mannino & Traunor, 1983).

Diplegics, who comprise over 50% of this population, are generally, but not exclusively, premature infants who have undergone significant intraventricular hemorrhages (Blair & Stanley, 1990; Hagberg & Hagberg, 1989). The periventricular areas have cortical radiations to the lower extremities, which are more involved with spasticity than the upper extremities; this differentiates them from quadriplegics, in whom all extremities are involved to the same degree (Banker & Larroche, 1962). Diplegia and cerebral palsy in general in premature infants is most correlated with periventricular leukomalacia demonstrated on ultrasound and MRI studies. The severity of these findings seems to correlate with the degree of the child's sensorimotor involvement. Infants in this group who also demonstrate thalamic lesions are more likely to have more severe motor and cognitive dysfunction (Yokochi, 1997). Monoplegia and triplegia (affecting one and three limbs, respectively) are rare. Bilateral involvement is the most common presentation, occurring in 75% of preterm and 45% of term patients (Hagberg & Hagberg, 1996).

Extrapyramidal or nonspastic types of cerebral palsy are responsible for about 20% of cases. Patients who have athetosis or rigidity have basal ganglia dysfunction that accounts for their movement disorders. Ataxic patients have difficulties with balance and position sense resulting from cerebellar pathology. Diagnostic workup is most important with ataxias, as posterior fossa brain tumors and degenerative inherited diseases, such as ataxia telangiectasia and Friedrich's ataxia, may have similar presentations.

Hypotonic patients have widespread damage to cortical and subcortical areas, so spasticity cannot be mounted as a response, and they have the poorest prognosis for cognitive and motor function. Some hypotonic patients may become athetoid with time. The remainder of cases have mixed features (i.e., diffuse cerebral involvement and impaired motor function).

Differential Diagnosis

Up to 40% of patients with an initial diagnosis of cerebral palsy have been incorrectly diagnosed. Other disorders that present with gross motor delays, aberrant tone, and abnormal movement patterns include mental retardation, neurodegenerative disorders, hydrocephalus, subdural effusion, slowly growing brain tumors, spinal cord lesions, muscular dystrophy, spinal muscular atrophy, and congenital cerebellar ataxia. Obviously, prognosis, inheritance pattern, and treatment would differ widely (Molnar & Taft, 1977).

Investigations that may be helpful in substantiating or excluding the diagnosis of cerebral palsy include the following: CT or MRI scans to assess for structural lesions, ultrasound of the head to exclude the possibility of intraventricular hemorrhage, lumbar puncture to exclude the elevation in protein in the cerebrospinal fluid that is seen with neurodegenerative disorders, serum uric acid and blood and urine assays for amino and organic acids to exclude congenital metabolic disorders, viral and parasitic titers (TORCH) to exclude the possibility of intrauterine-acquired infections, and chromosomal studies to exclude such abnormalities, especially in dysmorphic children.

Associated Medical Problems

Mental retardation coexists in 50%–60% of patients with cerebral palsy; communication and learning disorders, in 40%–50%; visual problems, including strabismus and myopia, in 50%; deafness, in 6%–16%; seizure disorders, in 33%; and orthopedic deformities, in 50% (Robinson, 1973). Hemiplegics have the highest incidence of seizures because of their discrete lesions. Electroencephalograms and visual and auditory evoked potentials are helpful in delineation of such problems.

The parietal lobe syndrome is characterized by hemiplegia, limb length discrepancies (the upper extremity being more affected), and sensory deficits as manifested by reduced two-point discrimination, stereognosis, and graphesthesia (Staheli, Duncan, & Schafer, 1960). A less common triad, seen with erythroblastosis-related disease, includes kernicterus (bilirubin deposition from red blood cell breakdown in the basal ganglia) with resultant athetosis, hearing loss, and paralysis of upward gaze.

Oropharyngeal incoordination may result in poor oral intake, with failure to thrive, occasionally necessitating placement of a gastrostomy tube for caloric supplementation (Vaughn, Neilson, & O'Dwyer, 1988). Misdirected swallowing and gastroesophageal reflux may result in aspiration pneumonias (Drvaric, Roberts, Burke, King, & Falterman, 1987; Gisel & Patrick, 1988). Poor hand function, pooling of saliva, and abnormal muscle tone can result in poor dental hygiene and malocclusion (Rosenstein, 1982). Restrictive pulmonary disease may result from hypertonicity, and scoliosis may limit endurance (Rothman, 1978). Bladder spasticity and sphincteric incoordination, rather than cognitive limitations, may cause urinary incontinence and may be responsive to uropharmacological and behavioral management (Keating, McCarron, James, Gruenberg, & Lonczak, 1985; McNeal, Hawtrey, Wolraich, & Mapel, 1983). Orthopedic complications include the development of contractures and deformities, dislocations especially at the hips, and scoliosis due to prolonged muscle imbalance. All of these conditions may require surgical intervention, as discussed below. Fractures may occur in these patients as a result of osteopenia concomitant with spasm and secondary effects of anticonvulsant administration (Lingam & Joester, 1994).

Clinical Findings and Prognostic Indicators

Cerebral palsy may be difficult to identify at less than 1 year of age. Although gross motor milestones may be delayed, hypertonicity, movement disorders, and early hand dominance may have not yet occurred (Levine, 1980). The infant with spastic quadriplegia is generally identified by 5 months of age; diplegics are not identified until 12 months, on average, and hemiplegics at 21 months (Harris, 1989). Difficulty in diagnosis is compounded by the plasticity of the immature nervous system, with compensatory branching of corticospinal tract fibers (Farmer, Harrison, Ingram, & Stephens, 1991), allowing cerebral palsy to disappear in up to 55% of cases (Tardorf, 1986). Labeling an infant "high-risk" may result in overinterpretation of normal physical findings (Ashton, Piper, Warren, Stewin, & Byrne, 1991).

Motor development in the subtypes of cerebral palsy varies, but common denominators exist (Bobath & Bobath, 1975). Abnormal positioning of the hands, hypertonicity of the neck extensors, inability to isolate lower-extremity movements (i.e., an all-flexor or all-extensor pattern), difficulty in bringing the elbows across midline, poor head control, microcephaly, abnormal deep tendon reflexes, persistence of grasp reflexes, and up-going plantar responses beyond 12 months of age are suspect findings. Lack of symmetrical movements and of early onset of hand dominance is suggestive of hemiparesis. Not only may gross motor activities be delayed, but when they are performed, they may be carried out in an abnormal way. For example, a child may be unable to crawl in a reciprocal manner in quadruped but can creep on his abdomen, dragging his legs behind him.

Major support for the diagnosis of a static encephalopathy is given by the persistence of primitive reflexes. These subcortical reflexes are normally suppressed by 6 months. They can always be summoned but are modulated by more advanced learned motor activities. When these reflexes occur each time a child is placed in a position, they interfere with ability to change position and maintain antigravity posture. These reflexes include the symmetric and asymmetric (fencer response) tonic neck reflexes, the tonic labyrinthine response, positive support reaction, and the Moro (startle) response. Postural reactions such as head and neck righting responses may be delayed or absent. The persistence of more than one reflex beyond 2 years and the child's inability to sit are negatively associated with ambulation (Capute, 1978; Sala & Grant, 1995). Inhibition of these reflexes by repositioning of the child so that tone is reduced and voluntary rather than obligate movements can be learned is the basis of the neurodevelopmental treatment of the Bobath (1980) approach. As these reflexes wane, antigravity protective and righting reflexes develop that can be built on to allow standing and ambulation.

The ability of a child to sit independently by 2 years correlates with a good prognosis for ambulation. Children who do not ambulate by 7–8 years are usually unable to do so. Ninety-eight percent of hemiplegics, 75% of diplegics, and 50% of quadriplegics will ambulate (Molnar & Gordon, 1976). Of those patients with quadriplegia, 25% will be independent, 50% will require assistance, and 25% will use wheelchairs. Most patients with ataxia ambulate. Hypotonic and rigid patients have the poorest prognosis for ambulation (Molnar, 1979). Children ambulate abnormally because of static and dynamic muscle dysfunction (Sutherland, 1984). Gaits are energy-inefficient, resulting in fatigability and limited endurance (Mossberg, Linton, & Friske, 1990).

Fine-motor, personal-social, and language skills also may be impaired to a variable degree. The Amiel-Tison scale, Milani-Comparetti scale, Denver Developmental Screening Test, and Bayley Scale of Infant Development may be employed for documentation of these dysfunctions.

Therapeutic Intervention

Direct treatment for cerebral palsy is unavailable. However, the use of prenatal glucocorticoid (dexamethasone) treatment administered to mothers of preterm infants may reduce the risk of intraventricular hemorrhage and periventricular leukomalacia. Secondarily, the risk of cerebral palsy in such a group may be reduced from 22% to 10% (Salokor et al., 1997). Research has suggested that use of free-radical scavengers and blockers of receptors of excitatory amino acids could limit the tissue damage sustained by neonates with perinatal asphyxia (Vannucci, 1990). Other, secondary treatments include therapy, tone-altering medications, provision of adaptive equipment to enhance patients' level of function, and orthopedic and neurosurgical procedures that correct deformities and normalize tone (Diamond, 1986; Lord, 1984).

Therapeutic systems share the goals of maintenance of joint range, prevention of contractures, normalization of tone, improvement in interaction with the environment, postural control, assumption of antigravity postures, development of muscular control and coordination, and education of the family (Deaver, 1956; Kottke, Halpern, Easton, Ozel, & Burrill, 1978). Many systems are axiomatic, being based on neuroplasticity in the child, avoidance of abnormal movement patterns, and the importance of sensorimotor learning in cognitive development (Matthews, 1988). Controlled studies are difficult to design, as parents are unwilling to assign their child to a nontreatment group (Guyatt et al., 1986; Martin & Epstein, 1976; Tirosh & Rabino, 1989). It has also been problematic to document the clinical effectiveness of early intervention programs, but there is a strong sense of the clinical validity of such treatment (Palmer et al., 1990; Resnick, Eyler, Nelson, Eitman, & Bucciarelli, 1987). The developmental stimulation, rather than physical therapy alone, may be responsible for enhancement of gross motor and cognitive skills (Palmer, Shapiro, & Wachtel, 1988). This is the rationale offered by proponents of the system of conductive education (Hill, 1990).

Systems have been proposed by Rood, Knott and Voss, and Brunstron, Temple Fay, and Dolman-Delacato (patterning) (Halpern, 1984), but the Bobath treatment generally prevails. By placing the child in a position in which the effects of abnormal tone and posture are deemphasized, voluntary muscular control may develop in a proximal-to-distal fashion, paving the way for more functional activities and the use of the upper extremities for something other than support (Finnie, 1974). Secondary reductions in tone may result in improvement in oromotor control, feeding, speech, and respiration (Nwaobi & Smith, 1986).

Other systems have been developed to deal with the visual-manual and spatial learning difficulties that may coexist (Bachrach & Greenspun, 1990). Additional options include training the patient in age-appropriate self-care skills and behavior modification. Traditionally, strengthening programs were felt to be contraindicated in spastic conditions such as cerebral palsy, as such efforts were felt to reinforce the patterns of spasticity that already existed. However, newer studies do not support this notion. Studies of ambulatory, teenage patients documented that a strengthening program for the quadriceps and hamstrings was effective in treating a crouch gait and improving the speed of ambulation without any negative effects (Damiano, Kelly, & Vaughan, 1995; Damiano, Vaughan, & Abel, 1995). These studies are also of note because they document the efficacy of physical therapy intervention in older patients in whom intervention was no longer felt to be of efficacy due to previous neurological maturation.

A variety of modalities, including shaking and cold, are believed to exert effects at the level of the vestibular receptors, muscle spindles, and the Golgi tendon apparatus. Nerve and motor point blocks and biofeedback also have been employed (Halpern, 1982; Kassover, Tauber, Au, & Pugh, 1986). Botulinum A toxin injected into the muscles of cerebral palsy patients transiently reduces spasticity for a period of about 4 months by blocking neuromuscular transmission to a variable degree. This temporary reduction in tone may permit reduction of dynamic deformities such as talipes equinus and a concomitant functional improvement, including enhancement of gait as a result of strengthening of agonist muscle groups. Both upper and lower extremities may be treated. Tendon-lengthening procedures may be deferred on this basis until the patient is older, but it is uncertain if this will obviate the need for a given procedure entirely (Korman, Mooney, Smith, Goodman, & Mulvaney, 1993). The long-term effects of repetitive treatment are unknown, although development of antibodies have been demonstrated (Goschel, Wohlfarth, Frevert, Dengler, & Bigalke, 1997) and distant atrophy of muscle groups reported (Ansved, Odergren & Borg, 1997). The use of tone-reducing orthotics (Bronkhorst & Lamb, 1987; Hinderer & Harris, 1988) may have a direct effect on muscle ultrastructure (Tardieu, de la Tour, Bret, & Tardieu, 1982).

The effect of anoxia on the spinal cord has recently been described (Clancy, Sladsky, & Rorke, 1989; Harrison, 1988). This lends credence to the use of antispastic medications such as Baclofen, an inhibitor of the neurotransmitter γ-aminobutyric acid at the spinal cord level (Young & Delwaide, 1981). It may be used orally but there are dosage limitations because lethargy may result. It also may be utilized intrathecally (Albright, Cervi, & Singletary, 1991) via an implantable pump, allowing for titration of dosage with decreased risk of side effects (Albright, 1996). Documented benefits in hamstring motion, upper-extremity function, and activities of daily living have been associated with this treatment (Albright, Barron, Fasick, Polinko, & Janosky, 1993). Selective dorsal rhizotomy, which reduces tone by surgical lesioning of sensory input at the spinal cord level (Fasano, Barolat-Romana, Zeme, & Squazzi, 1979) also may be utilized to this goal, as detailed below.

Appropriate prescription of seating devices for nonambulatory patients permits positioning in an upright manner, improved eye contact, enhanced interaction with the environment, decreased effect of hypertonicity (which pushes the patient out of the chair and adducts the hips), and enhanced feeding, respiration, and ability to use communication devices (Bergen & Colangelo, 1982). Helmets, bed rails, and cushions are used to prevent injury. Orthotics are provided to prevent progression of deformities, provide stability, and enhance function (Gold, 1991).

Traditional leather and metal braces have given way to custom-molded plastic orthoses, as they are light and can more easily control angular (varus/valgus) deformities. Full-control hip-knee-ankle-foot orthoses are generally used for positioning but are too heavy for functional ambulation. Variations of these devices that exclude the medial metal upright and thigh cuffs are lighter and may be helpful for children with toe walking and dynamic internal rotation at the hips. Ankle-foot orthoses are indicated to improve ankle dorsiflexion and control equinus deformities. Spring-assisted devices are contraindicated, as rapid stretch may exacerbate spasticity. Orthoses employed to maintain muscle length must be worn for at least 6 hours per day to achieve a physiological effect (Tardieu & Lespargot, 1988). This must be explained in order to achieve compliance with the wearing schedule. Ankle-foot orthoses can have hinges incorporated at the ankle to allow for active ankle dorsiflexion and to facilitate movements from sitting to standing (Wilson, Haideri, Song, & Telford, 1997). Orthoses that extend to just above the ankles (supramalleolar orthoses) can control foot alignment but do not control the ankle joints (Carlson, Vaughan, Damiano, & Abel, 1997).

For maximally involved children, the use of a walking frame with casters provides truncal alignment and support in conjunction with hip-knee-ankle foot orthoses. Although functional ambulation is not possible with such devices, their utilization permits tolerance of the upright posture, increased weight bearing, and a sense of movement for the child, which may be psychologically rewarding (Stallard, Major, & Farmer, 1996). Therapeutic electrical stimulation can be utilized as an adjunct to traditional therapeutic intervention. Low-intensity transcutaneous stimulation can be applied to a variety of weak muscles, nocturnally. Theoretically, the resultant increase in blood flow to these muscles at a time when growth hormone levels are the highest encourages their growth. This then permits the traditional strengthening efforts applied during the day to be more effective. Improvement in gait (enhanced tibialis anterior function, better balance, and improved gait pattern) has been demonstrated in a few studies (Hazlewood, Brown, Rowe, & Salter, 1994; Pape et al., 1993). However, the long-term effect of this treatment and any possible associated reduction in the subsequent need for surgical intervention have not yet been determined.

Surgical Options

Prevention of deformities resulting from inequalities in muscle tone and strength is the best option; however, orthopedic surgery should not be perceived as failure of previous treatment. Early tendon releases may initially interfere with acquisition of motor milestones and mobility and may increase the need for repeat surgery with growth. Conversely, a delay in surgery may necessitate more extensive procedures (i.e., osteotomies rather than muscle lengthenings). Psychological support services to both parent and child, to cope with fears and expectations, is most important. At least 6 months of extensive postoperative physical rehabilitation may be required to see signs of functional improvement because of transient deconditioning (Reimers, 1990). The separation of the parent from the child and the financial burdens encountered are other factors to be considered.

A full discussion of orthopedic deformities and their surgical treatment may be found in several excellent texts (Bleck, 1987; Samilson, 1981). Common lower-extremity deformities include hip flexion contractures, femoral anteversion with medial rotation of the legs, hip adduction with subluxation, pelvic asymmetry with secondary scoliosis, hamstring spasticity with kyphosis and knee flexion contractures, and equinovarus or equinovalgus deformities with hemiplegia and diplegia, respectively. Typical upper-extremity deformities include internal rotation contractures of the shoulders, flexion contractures at the elbows, wrist flexion contractures, ulnar deviation, finger flexion contractures, and thumb-in-palm deformities. For dependent patients, surgery may be performed to facilitate perineal care, reduce pain associated with dislocation, and correct pelvic asymmetry that may exacerbate a scoliosis and reduce supported sitting tolerance (Carr & Gage, 1987; Cooperman, Bartucci, Dietrick, & Millar, 1987). For children with better gross motor function, surgery is indicated to improve lower-extremity alignment and correct a progressively crouched gait.

Procedures include adductor tenotomies and varus derotation osteotomies of the femur (Bleck, 1990). Hamstring lengthenings are performed to correct knee flexion contractures, avoiding overlengthening which could result in hyperextension at the knees (Gage, 1990). Achilles tendon lengthenings are the most commonly performed procedure; with correction of the equinus deformity, toe walking is corrected, a stable base of support on a flat foot is established, and walking speed and stride length are increased (Shapiro & Susa, 1990). A posterior tibial tendon transfer may be indicated to correct equinovarus and to elevate the foot when walking; the indication may be supported by computerized gait analysis (Perry & Hoffer, 1976). For more resistant deformities at the foot, an extraarticular (Grice) procedure or other arthrodesis may be required (Fulford, 1990).

Surgery for the upper extremities is performed less frequently, as results may be limited by cognitive and sensory impairments. Procedures include release of the internal rotators of the shoulder, release of the biceps tendon and anterior capsulotomy to correct elbow flexion contractures, transfer of wrist flexors to function as wrist extensors, and release of the thumb-in-palm deformity (Mital & Sakellarides, 1981). Spinal fusion may be required to control scoliosis. Luque and other new spinal instrumentations permit some patients to forgo postoperative immobilization in a body jacket (Lonstein & Akbamia, 1983). Neurosurgical procedures, including stereotactic surgery to control intractable seizures and implantation of a cerebellar pacemaker, have been developed but are not employed in any large numbers (Penn, Mykleburst, Gottlieb, Agarwal, & Etzel, 1980).

The selective dorsal rhizotomy procedure to decrease lower-extremity tone has recently been implemented. Spinal nerve rootlets that have been determined as being electrically abnormal (Cahan & Kundi, 1987) are surgically lesioned in purely spastic patients. With modulation of abnormal sensory input, there is a resetting of muscle sensitivities with reduction in tone. Electromyographic monitoring is employed intraoperatively to assess which spastic rootlets should be lesioned, although responses may be less consistent than previously thought. In conjunction with a well-delineated postoperative program, improvements in tone, range, posture and sitting balance, and function may occur in 85%–90% of appropriately selected candidates (Abbott, Johann-Murphy, & Gold, 1991; Peacock & Staudt, 1991) to an extent greater than would be anticipated on the basis of the physical therapy intervention alone (Steinbok, Reiner, Beauchamp, Armstrong, & Cochrane, 1997). Improvement in gait is characterized by improved dynamic range of motion at the hips, improved velocity, and improved stride length (Thomas, Aiona, Pierce, & Piatt, 1996). Over time this may result in a decreased need for Achilles tendon lengthening, adductor releases, and hamstring releases but may not affect the subsequent rates of ankle-foot operations, femoral osteotomies, and iliopsoas releases in these patients (Chicoine, Park, & Kaufman, 1997). Although not a specific indication for performance of the procedure, secondary improvements in upper-extremity function and reduction in bladder spasticity also may result (Sweetser, Badell, Schneider, & Badlin, 1995). Complications may include dysesthesias, sensory deficits, and on long-term follow-up, spinal stenosis (Gooch & Walker, 1996).

Psychological, Vocational, and Medical Problems of Adults

Therapeutic services may enhance acquisition of gross motor skills, but cognitive improvement and emotional maturity are more elusive to treat. The severity of the physical disability does not correlate with the physical or psychological health of the parents (Wallander, Varni, et al., 1989). Sibling and spousal support are more pertinent predictors of achieving mental health and improvement in physical performance (Craft, Lakin, Oppliger, Clancy, & Vanderlinden, 1990). Lives of 50% of adolescents with cerebral palsy (and spina bifida) may be characterized by dependence on parents for personal care, lack of responsibility for home chores, lack of information about sexuality, and limited participation in social activities and sexual relationships (Blum, Resnick, Nelson, & St. Germaine, 1991; Hirst, 1989). This does not encourage independent living, marriage, or employment. Only 30%–50% of cerebral palsy patients are employed full-time at maturity; diplegic and hemiplegic patients are more successful (Bleck, 1987).

It has not been established what therapeutic services are necessary for adult cerebral palsy patients to maintain function. It is sobering to acknowledge that deterioration of gait in the presence of a static encephalopathy may begin prior to 14 years of age and is manifested by an increase in double-support time and a decrease in knee, ankle, and pelvic motion (Johnson, Dammiano, & Abel, 1997). Medical complications in an aging population (Bachrach & Greenspun, 1990) include cervical and lumbar radiculopathies (Ebara et al., 1990; Fuji et al., 1987; Reese, Msall, & Owens, 1991), carpal tunnel syndrome (Alvarez, Larkin, & Roxborough, 1981), and arthritis at major joints, each of which may require surgical intervention for restitution of function. Specifically, cervical disc disease is eight times more frequent in the adult athetoid patient than in the general population (Harade et al., 1996). There is an overall 63% incidence of degenerative arthritis in cerebral palsy patients under the age of 50 years. Seizure disorders persist into adulthood. Neurogenic bladder and unrecognized problems with toileting accessibility also may be problematic. Little in the way of organized and proactive treatment is available for this population (Murphy, Molnar, & Lankasky, 1995).

Ninety percent survival into adulthood is seen with cerebral palsy (Evans, Evans, & Alberman, 1990). Earlier demise occurs in patients who have severe mental deficiency, are totally dependent, have poorly controlled seizures, require gastrostomy feeding, have no means of communication, and whose illness is primarily respiratory in nature (Evans & Alberman, 1990). Demise is often coincident with the "aging-out" of parents and relocation from the home to an institutional facility (Eyman & Grossman, 1990). These findings should prompt the reexamination of public policies for provision of medical benefits to handicapped adults whose parents wish them to retain the family domicile and other financial assets that would permit continuation of home-based care.

SPINA BIFIDA

Spina bifida, or myelomeningocele, denotes a condition in which there are congenital abnormalities of the vertebral elements in association with extrusion of abnormally formed neural elements. Patients present with various lower-extremity motor and sensory deficits concomitant with variable bowel and bladder control, hydrocephalus, and other medical problems. The resultant condition impinges on normal motor development and may alter fine-motor, perceptual, linguistic, and cognitive function. A discussion of treatment strategies reflects not only technical advancements but the changes in advocacy for treatment of the handicapped child. This is not a static disorder but one in which progressive neurological and other organ system dysfunction may occur over time in up to 40% of the patients (Spindel, Bauer, & Dyro, 1987).

Anatomical Abnormalities

Failure of fusion of the posterior elements of the lumbosacral spine without associated neurological abnormalities is known as spina bifida occulta and occurs in 20%–25% of the population. Should such findings be noted in a patient with incontinence, cavus (high-arched) feet, and/or a hairy tuft of hemangioma over the lower spine, an associated malformation of the spinal cord may be present. In its most severe or manifest form, spina bifida is associated with exposure of the neural plaque, leakage of cerebrospinal fluid, and susceptibility of the meninges to infection (Brocklehurst, 1976). Abnormally formed neural elements with cystic structures within the spinal cord result in a picture of both upper and lower motor neuron deficits (Stark & Baker, 1967). Defects at the lumbosacral level are the most common; thoracic and cervical lesions occur less frequently. Because of the imbalance of muscle pull on major joints of the lower extremities, paresis/paralysis and severe orthopedic deformities occur.

The Lorber Criteria and Their Abandonment

In the past, severely deformed infants with myelomeningocele succumbed, without treatment, to meningitis, hydrocephalus, and/or renal failure in the interest of not prolonging the lives of children who would be cognitively subnormal, nonambulatory, and chronically ill. The mortality rate within the first month of life was 63% and was 89% by the sixth month. Lorber (1971) advised no treatment for those infants who would be totally plegic in the lower extremities, had severe hydrocephalus, had severe kyphoscoliosis that would not permit an erect posture, and/or had severe congenital malformations such as extrophy of the bladder or congenital heart disease. He felt that only 18% of the population would be ambulatory, cognitively normal, and able to earn an income. It was not recognized that survivors would be more compromised than necessary (McLaughlin & Shurtleff, 1979) nor that there was inability to predict which of cognitively normal patients would be sacrificed by lack of treatment. Adoption of these criteria implied that life in a wheelchair was one without quality. Other assumptions have recently proved invalid with more advanced treatments (Khoury, Erickson, & James, 1982; McClone, Dias, Kaplan, & Sommers, 1985).

Neurosurgery in the neonate to drain the collection of excessive cerebrospinal fluid associated with hydrocephalus can result in restoration of a relatively normal head circumference and reexpansion of the cerebral mantle. With appropriate treatment, a 5-year survival rate of 86% has been reported; however, patients with brain stem dysfunction had a greater mortality (Worley, Schuster, & Oakes, 1996). The severe gibbus deformity associated with kyphoscoliosis may be surgically corrected (Linter & Lindseth, 1994), as may other congenital abnormalities. Mental retardation is not intrinsic to spine bifida nor to the Arnold-Chiari malformation, which results in hydrocephalus. Up to 75% of patients may have normal intelligence (McClone, Czyzewski, Raimondi, & Sommers, 1982), but the incidence of learning disabilities will be high, with arithmetic and design copying skills frequently being compromised (Wills, Holmbeck, Dillon, & McClone, 1990). Functional bowel and bladder continence may ideally be achieved in 80% of school-age children. Eighty percent of school-age children will be community ambulators. Only 10%–15% of patients will require supportive care. The emotional and psychological costs for delaying treatment are high. Hence, early and aggressive treatment of these infants is now the rule.

Incidence, Embryology, and Etiology

The incidence of spina bifida manifesta in the United States is approximately 4.6 cases per 10,000 births (Lary & Edmonds, 1996). The lesion is most common in White females (Greene, Terry, DeMasi, & Herrington, 1991). A multifactorial genetic basis for explaining such variability is likely. The undefined insult to the embryo occurs at 21–26 days of gestation, when the neural tube that will become the central nervous system is invaginating. There may be a failure of fusion or a disruption of the tissue column caused by abnormalities in cerebrospinal fluid pressure (Streeter, 1942). The incidence of neural tube defects can be reduced by up to 86% by the intake of folic acid in the periconceptual period at a dosage of 0.4 mg/day. Control of obesity (maternal weight less than 31 kg/M^2) prior to the onset of pregnancy also may reduce the risk of neural tube defects (Waller et al., 1995). There is an increased familial tendency toward the disorder, with a 5% chance of recurrence in subsequent pregnancies and in patients with spina bifida who sire offspring. Other, nonfamilial etiologies proposed include exposure to potato blight, vitamin B and mineral deficiencies (Homes, 1988), maternal fever/infection, hormonal exposures, zinc deficiencies, subfertility, twinning, high sound intensity exposure, ethanol, and use of phenytoin and valproic acid (Khoury et al., 1982; Leck, 1974).

Prenatal diagnosis can be made by ultrasound (Robinson, Hood, Adam, Gibson, & Ferguson-Smith, 1980). Prenatal anatomic level as determined on high-resolution ultrasound can reliably be utilized to discuss functional motor outcome with the parents (Coniglio, Anderson, & Ferguson, 1996). Analysis of amniotic fluid and/or maternal serum for elevated alpha-fetoprotein, a substance that is liberated by fetal blood vessels of the uncovered neural elements, is also indicative of the disorder. Analyses are performed in the second trimester so that termination of pregnancy, if desired, is possible. False-positive results may occur in association with the gastrointestinal malformations (Milunsky & Alpert, 1976a, 1976b). Anencephaly and skin-covered lesions cannot be identified by chemical analysis, so ultrasound is very important. Theses tests are not consistently performed during pregnancy; therefore, the majority of cases are not diagnosed in utero. At present, 39.9% of all neural tube defects so identified result in termination of pregnancy (Bower, Raymond, Lumley, & Bury, 1993). For those pregnancies that go to completion, a cesarean section is indicated to lessen the risk of trauma to the exposed neural elements and hydrocephalic head.

ANTENATAL AND NEONATAL TREATMENT

In utero repair of myelomeningocele is still a very experimental option for attempting to reduce subsequent neurological dysfunction. Interposition of latissimus dorsi muscle flaps over the neurological lesion may prevent further in utero damage to the spinal cord and nerve roots or the damage that occurs at the time of delivery (Meuli et al., 1997; Meuli-Simmen, Meuli, Adzick, & Harrison, 1997).

The deformities of spina bifida manifesta are obvious at birth. The spinal defect is closed at 24 to 48 hours, and a ventriculoperitoneal shunt is placed in the 80% in whom it is required at that time or at a variable time thereafter. In the interim, the infant should be transferred to a tertiary care facility where a multidisciplinary team is available, kept abdomen-down in a warmer, and placed on intravenous antibiotics. The patient should be assessed for other congenital anomalies and also should have urological and orthopedic assessments (Alexander & Steg, 1989). The hiatus from birth to surgical treatment permits parents to be supplied with information about their child's condition, which will facilitate their ability to select suitable treatment options (Charney, 1990). Pediatricians who are unfamiliar with the diagnosis may offer an unnecessarily dire prognosis (Siperstein, Wolraich, Reed, & O'Keefe, 1988). Parents should handle the infant's range joint contracture, learn how to deal with the infant's insensate skin, and be instructed in intermittent urinary catheterization (Boytim, Davidson, Charney, & Melchionne, 1991).

The Arnold-Chiari Malformation and Hydrocephalus

The Arnold-Chiari II malformation, seen in up to 90% of patients (Badell-Ribera, Swinyard, Greenspan, & Deaver, 1964), is characterized by a downward displacement of a portion of the cerebellum through the foramen magnum into the spinal canal, with secondary compression of the fourth ventricle and development of hydrocephalus (Lemire, 1988). Untreated, this condition results in progressive expansion of the ventricles, with compression of cerebral tissue, spasticity, retardation, blindness, stridor, dysphagia, apnea, and death (Charney, Rorke, Sutton, & Schut, 1991). A shunt is placed from the ventricles into the peritoneal space to decompress the hydrocephalus. Shunted patients and those in whom shunting is not required have normal IQs (95 and 102, respectively). However, for each episode of bacterial ventriculitis that occurs, there is a 10–15-point decrement in the IQ, with an average score of 72 (Hunt & Holmes, 1976). Shunt surgery also may be complicated by breakage, infection, distal blockage, nephritis, and hydrocele. A newly developed alternative for the management of hydrocephalus is endoscopic third ventriculostomy. At present, its application may be best suited for patients over the age of 6 months. Long-term shunt dependence with late complications may thereby be avoided (Teo & Jones, 1996). Seizures may occur in up to 21% of patients with spina bifida. All of these patients have shunted hydrocephalus. However, most also have evidence of other central nervous system pathology, such as encephalomalacia, and other malformations or calcifications (Talwar, Baldwin, & Horbatt, 1995).

Neurological Level: Functional Implications

The performance of a neurological exam on the neonate is challenging because of lack of cooperation and existence of spinal shock (Chiaramonte, Horowitz,

Kaplan, & Brook, 1986). Stimulation of the arms and the upper trunk rather than the lower extremities may more reliably evoke volitional rather than reflexogenic movements (Stark & Baker, 1967). Somatosensory evoked potentials also may be performed to document the level of innervation. This determination is crucial, as it will indicate, with good reliability, ambulatory status and risk for the development of orthopedic deformities, those with the lowest neurological levels having the best prognosis (DeSouza & Carroll, 1976; Hoffer, Feiwell, Perry, Perry, & Bonnett, 1973). Further delineation is on strength of the muscles at a given level (McDonald, Jaffe, Mosca, Shurtleff, & Menelaus, 1991), especially the strength of the hip flexors and knee extensors, and the presence of orthopedic deformities, especially scoliosis, which may occur in up to 50% of the population (Drennan, 1976). Factors of lesser importance include age, sitting balance, height, sex, motivation, presence of spasticity, adequacy of bracing, appropriateness of orthopedic surgery, and motor planning abilities (Asher & Olsen, 1983). Infants with a thoracic-level lesion will have no voluntary movements in their lower extremities. With training and surgical correction of lower-extremity contractures, 50% of this group become therapeutic or community ambulators in childhood with extensive bracing (Charney, Melchionni, & Smith, 1991). With age, increasing weight, upward displacement of the center of gravity, and underlying trunk and respiratory muscle dysfunction, energy expenditure increases (Findley & Agre, 1988). By adulthood, this group is usually reliant on wheelchairs for mobility but capable of independent transfers, dressing, bowel and bladder management, and employment (Carroll, 1977). Despite the transient nature of their ambulation, walking should be attempted to provide patients with a vertical orientation, to permit performance of tabletop activities in standing, to improve the respiratory excursion and urinary drainage, and to lessen the possibilities of skin breakdown, contractures, and osteoporosis-related fractures.

Patients with innervation at the lumbar 1, 2, and 3 levels have motor power in hip flexors and adductors (which bring the legs into midline) and to a variable degree in the knee extensors. There is no ability to extend or abduct the hips or to move the feet. At this level, there is the highest risk of hip dislocation, given the imbalance in muscle pull. Hip dislocation may be an impediment to continued ambulation (Crandall, Birkeback, & Wintor, 1989; Curtis, 1973). Surgical procedures, such as iliopsoas transfer (Sharrard, 1964) or osteotomy of the femoral head, can be anticipated but are not obligatory for ambulation to continue (Sherk, Uppal, Lane, & Melchionni, 1991). Release of hip flexion contractures of greater than 30 degrees also can be considered in this group (Frawley, Broughton, & Menelaus, 1996). Such infants can be provided with footdrop splints to prevent progressive equinus deformities and may require hip adduction devices to maintain stability at those joints.

In nonambulatory children with high-level myelomeningocele lesions, unilateral hip dislocation may cause little functional disability, and surgical intervention is less frequently indicated than in years past. In ambulatory patients with lower level lesions, leg length discrepancy and its effect on functional problems mandates surgical correction (Fraser, Bourke, Broughton, & Menelaus, 1995). Patients with higher level lesions are generally braced with full-control devices necessitated not only by their lower-extremity weakness but by their hydrocephalus-related hypotonia. They can be supplied with a standing device known as a parapodium at about 18 months (Letts, Fulford, Eng, & Robson, 1976). A spina bifida cart also can be provided for independent mobility (Charney, Rorke, et al., 1991). By 2–3 years, hip-knee-ankle-foot orthoses can be provided and gait training with a rollator commenced (Lough & Nielsen, 1986). Alternatively, an Orlau parawalker can be considered (Major, Stollard, & Farmer, 1997). Depending on praxis and eye-hand coordination, crutches may be supplied at 4–5 years, with household and some community ambulation anticipated. Reciprocating gait (cable) orthoses may help to facilitate ambulation and reduce energy consumption by up to 50% in the group when compared with the use of traditional knee-ankle-foot orthoses used with a four-point gait pattern (Cuddeford et al., 1997).

With full innervation at the lumbar 4 level, knee extensors are stronger, and patients may be advanced to knee-ankle-foot orthoses. Some patients may have imbalance between knee flexors and extensors, requiring surgical release of the hamstrings to improve gait (Marshall, Broughton, Menelaus, & Graham, 1996). With innervation at the lumbar 5 level, muscle power about the hip is more balanced. The ankle dorsiflexors, but not the plantar flexors, are functioning, usually resulting in a calcaneal deformity, with ambulation on an insensate heel. Transfer of the tibialis anterior muscle, which dorsiflexes the foot, may be required to achieve a stable standing position; this is generally performed at about 5 years. A variety of other foot deformities, including planovalgus, may occur at this and other levels. Triple arthrodeses (ankle fusions) may be required at about 12 years (Menelaus, 1980; Shafer & Dias, 1983). However, this procedure has become less popular because of the resultant stiffness of the foot and the propensity for skin breakdown. Other surgical procedures considered for correction of valgus deformities include subtalar arthrodesis (or Grice procedure), talectomy, calcaneal-lengthening osteotomy, fibula–Achilles tendon tenodesis, distal medial tibial epiphysiodesis, and supramalleolar osteotomy (Abraham, Lubicky, Sanger, & Millar, 1996).

Patients with such lower lumbar lesions can be anticipated to pull to standing by 1 year and ambulate in the community with or without orthoses despite gait deviations. For patients with sacral level lesions, only minor foot deformities would be anticipated. These patients may require shoe modifications or ankle-foot orthoses but would be able to ambulate without them. They would be expected to have bowel and bladder incontinence. It is very important to follow patients with such low lesions as almost one third may show a decline in ambulatory ability over time, declines related to skin breakdown, osteomyelitis and the need for amputations in association with underrecognized tethering, and syringomyelia as discussed below (Brinker et al., 1994).

Scoliosis and Tethering of the Spinal Cord

Management of a paralytic spinal curvature is difficult. As posterior vertebral elements are lacking, surgical fixation with metal rods usually has to be performed anteriorly and posteriorly (Banta & Park, 1983). Surgical procedures require a period of immobilization, with the risk of further neurological compromise and development of pseudoarthroses. Unchecked, scoliosis causes restrictive pulmonary disease with decreased endurance. The uneven posture that results disturbs sitting balance, the upper extremities being used as tripods. The listing to one side, especially in tandem with hip dislocation, may result in formation of intractable decubiti.

Scoliosis may occur in response to unequal innervation of the paraspinal muscles and may be compounded by vertebral anomalies, but rapid progression may herald the development of neurological complications. Prior to the development of MRI, many of these conditions went undetected, and many childhood ambulators were using wheelchairs by adolescence. Other factors that may negatively affect ambulatory performance include obesity, joint stiffness with arthritic changes, and lack of motivation.

The two primary conditions responsible for the deterioration are tethering of the spinal cord and syringomyelia. With tethering, the spinal cord is subject to repeated microtrauma with flexion/extension, to which it is predisposed by scar tissue that keeps the cord firmly adherent at lower lumbar levels (Yamada, Zinke, & Sanders, 1981). Patients exhibit decreased lower-extremity strength, spasticity frequently associated with a crouched gait, dysesthesias or progressive sensory deficits, and/or decompensation of a previously well-managed neurogenic bowel and bladder (Peacock, Arens, & Berman, 1987). MRI studies and somatosensory evoked potentials may be helpful in objectifying the changes noted on physical examination (Li, Albright, Sclabassi, & Pang, 1996). Surgical release of the tether can result in restoration of function or can stop further neurological progression in most cases (Clancy et al., 1989; Reigel, 1983). Surgical techniques should permit the neural elements to remain free in the cerebrospinal fluid, preventing the risk of retethering (Zide, Constantini, & Epstein, 1995). An expanding fluid-filled cyst may distend the cord at any level and be associated with increasing weakness and sensory deficits, frequently involving the upper extremities. This is known as syringomyelia; it can be treated by surgical drainage of the cyst and placement of a shunt.

Therapeutic Assessment and Intervention

Assessment should include evaluation and description of joint contractures and deformities, neurological level and muscle power, pressure sores, mobility, and self-care skills. Treatment includes gentle, active, assistive range-of-motion exercises for the lower extremities, strengthening of innervated musculature, transfer training, gait training, and instruction in self-care skills (U.K. Collaborative Study, 1977). Physical activity programs aimed at improving cardiovascular fitness, and strength may improve the self-image of the disabled child (Andrade, Kramer, Garber, & Longmuir, 1991).

In general, infants with myelomeningocele are less active (Morrow, 1995). This coupled with low tone, weakness, and upper-extremity dysfunction, is a compelling reason for referral to an early intervention program. Initial studies of patients so referred suggest subsequent enhancement of functional ambulatory abilities and cognitive abilities so that educational mainstreaming is more apt to occur.

Hypo- or hypertonia may exist in the trunk and upper extremities in association with hydrocephalus. Even children with sacral lesions may have delays in performance of erect activities, integration of primitive reflexes, and acquisition of automatic reactions (Wolf & McLaughlin, 1992). The infant should be encouraged to assume antigravity positions, such as quadruped with weight bearing on extended forearms. These attempts may have to be augmented by placing the child over a bolster in prone position and/or by provision of a scooter board. As the child progresses, he can be set on a bolster to work on trunk and abdominal strengthening and sitting balance. Later, a standing table can be utilized. Depending on the neurological level, the child can then progress to rising from sitting to half-kneeling and from half-kneeling to standing, utilizing adaptive equipment as needed.

Appropriate orthoses are either of metal or of the newer, custom-molded plastic variety (Krebs, Edelstein, & Fishman, 1988). Ambulation, especially with hip-knee-ankle-foot orthoses, is energy-inefficient; caloric expenditures are about six times normal. The use of reciprocating cable orthoses should therefore be considered to reduce energy consumption and improve endurance (McCall & Schmidt, 1986). Upper-extremity dysfunction and perceptual motor problems correlate with the severity of the hydrocephalus and the level of the lesion. Hand function should be assessed in terms of preference; tactile discrimination; ability to perform activities such as page turning, grasp, and manipulation of small objects; handling of feeding utensils, stacking of blocks and checkers, praxis, graphesthesia, and two-point discrimination (Brunt, 1980; Grimm, 1976; Wallace, 1973). Older children must be assessed in terms of figure copying, graphomotor skills, and academic difficulties. Letter reversals and difficulty in sequencing tasks are not uncommon. Visual problems of astigmatism, nystagmus, and hyperopia seen in association with hydrocephalus may be contributory factors (Mankinen-Heikkinen & Mustonene, 1987). Remediation of perceptual motor difficulties may require occupational therapy and special education services (Gluckman & Barling, 1980). Upper-extremity dysfunction may adversely affect the ability to use crutches (Radke & Gosky, 1981; Wallace, 1973), accounting for the discrepancies in ambulation that occur among patients of the same neurological level.

Activities of daily living skills in spina bifida patients are likely to be below age level (Sousa, Gordon, & Shurtleff, 1976). This may be related to praxis and motor planning difficulties and to parental overprotection and time constraints. Preparation for adulthood and independent living may be restricted by these factors rather than lack of intelligence. The development of standardized pediatric assessments of self-care, such as the Functional Independence Measure for Children (WeeFIM; Granger, Hamilton, & Kayton, 1987) and the Pediatric Evaluation of Disability Inventory (PEDI; Feldman, Haley, & Coryell, 1990), will help to clarify the specific areas of training required.

Up to 61% of spina bifida patients may have strabismus. There is a high incidence of amblyopia as well, likely related to the presence of hydrocephalus. Such deficits require treatment, and their amelioration may permit better upper extremity and perceptual-motor function (Biglan, 1995). Respiratory problems may occur as a result of brain stem dysfunction, either on the basis of a congenital malformation or as a result of repeated traction on that area. Loss of central ventilatory function may present with stridor, intermittent loss of consciousness, and apnea. Sleep studies with analysis of respiratory gases document the lack of chemoregulatory ability, which can result in hypercarbia and anoxia (Swaminathan et al., 1989). Respirator support may be required, in association with a tracheostomy necessitated by vocal cord paralysis; some children gradually improve over time. Some centers advocate a posterior decompression of the cervical spine, although ultimate survival may not be improved (Worley, Schuster, & Oakes, 1991). Similarly, brain stem dysfunction may lead to oromotor incoordination, feeding difficulties, and aspiration. Seizures may occur in up to 20% of the population.

Praxis and sequencing problems of children with spina bifida also may be reflected in their delay in speech and language skills. Vocabulary deficits and distractibility may further compromise communication skills (Horn, Lorch, Lorch, & Culatta, 1985). Verbal output may not be reduced, resulting in superficial "cocktail party" patter. Therapeutic efforts addressing development of pragmatic, step-by-step verbal skills are indicated in such children: This is a prerequisite for instruction in dressing, self-catheterization, and other ADL skills.

Bowel and bladder incontinence results from lack of innervation at the sacral 2, 3, and 4 levels—paralysis and incoordination of the bladder and urinary sphincter on the basis of upper and lower motor neuron involvement. Urinary incontinence, stasis, and reflux of urine back into the kidneys may result in chronic infections with a potential for urosepsis, chronic renal acidosis, hypertension, renal failure, and death (Mundy, Shah, Borzyskowski, & Saxton, 1985). Until 20 years ago, upper-tract deterioration was inevitable, resulting in surgical correction of an ileal conduit. Currently, intermittent urinary catheterization is the mainstay of treatment, decreasing the risk of infection and stasis and permitting functional urinary continence (Peterson, 1987) and maintenance of good renal function (Peeker, Damber, Hjalmas, Sjodin, & Von Zweigbergle, 1997). Catheterization may be required in infancy to prevent hydronephrosis, which can be present in up to 81% of patients by 5 years of age (Charney, Snyder, & Melchionni, 1991). Earlier initiation of catheterization also may prevent irreversible bladder dysfunction and reduce the number of children indicated for bladder augmentation from 27% to 11% (Iwu, Baskin, & Kogan, 1997). Depending on sitting balance, hand function, and cognitive skills, self-catheterization can begin as early as 5 years (Smith, 1991). Perceptual problems may make the technique difficult; anatomically correct dolls may be employed to facilitate training.

Continence can be further enhanced by use of uropharmacological agents that relax bladder tone to prevent voiding or improve contraction of the urinary sphincter to prevent leakage. Low-dose antibiotic therapy may be required to prevent recurrent infections. In males, external collecting devices can be used as a backup measure, but females must rely on diapers or pads. Attention should be paid to the development of latex allergies in up to 35% such patients, possibly because of prolonged and repeated exposures to the material from multiple surgeries and intermittent catheterization regimens (Slater, 1989). Yearly renal ultrasound studies and blood tests to monitor renal function are mandatory. Surgical techniques developed to permit continence include bladder augmentation to increase bladder capacity between catheterization and the placement of an artificial urinary sphincter (Kaplan, 1985). In patients with some residual sensation, biofeedback techniques also may be successful (Kaplan & Richards, 1988). Low-intensity transcutaneous therapeutic electrical stimulation may be a method for increasing bladder capacity, improving a subjective sense of fullness, and achieving urinary and fecal continence (Balcom, Wiatrak, Biefeld, Rauen, & Langenstroer, 1997). Bowel continence is generally managed by the use of stool softeners, diet, and suppositories or enemas given at a consistent time. The olfactory stigma of an incontinent child may result in ostracism; this is a compelling reason for the early implementation of an effective bowel and bladder program.

Until recently, endocrinological dysfunction has been overlooked in this population. Up to 15% of patients may have reduction in growth hormone as manifested by a decrease in longitudinal height and in arm span. This is likely hydrocephalus-related, with secondary pressure effects being exerted on the hypothalamus and/or pituitary gland (Hochhaus, Butenadl, Schwarz, & Ring-Mrozik,

1997). Higher level spina bifida lesions may result in a greater degree of growth impairment (Rotenstein & Reigel, 1996). Not only are such reductions in height stigmatizing, but the associated changes in bony maturation may alter the standard surgical timetable. Supplementation of growth hormone is a treatment option; its long-term functional effect in terms of accentuating linear growth, elevation of the center of gravity, and increasing the incidence of symptomatic tethering of the spinal cord, has not yet been determined (Gold, 1996).

Provision of general medical care to patients with spina bifida is usually not problematic in the pediatric age range. However, because of patients' increased risk of recurrent infections and concern with administration of pertussis vaccine to neurologically compromised children, up to 24% of such children may be delayed in their immunizations at school entry. Accordingly, an immunization history is an important part of each clinic visit (Raddish, Goldman, Kaplan, & Perrin, 1998).

Given the increased longevity of the spina bifida patient, and the possibility of late complications, it is essential that team management is continued throughout the adult years. Without such services well over half of the patients might not receive any specialized services and some might receive no medical care at all (Kaufman et al., 1994). With ongoing care, potentially preventable complications, including pyelonephritis, renal calculi, decubitus formation with an underlying infection of the bone, and occult, late shunt malfunctions, can be avoided (Kinsman & Doehring, 1996). In this setting, patients also can be monitored for a possible increased risk of colorectal cancer (Tomlinson & Sugarman, 1995). Instead of treating complications, proactive procedures such as release of a tethered spinal cord, tendon releases, and bladder augmentation can be considered (Begeer & Staal-Schreinemachers, 1996).

Psychological and Vocational Implications

In the setting of multiple physical and medical problems, it is admirable that patients with spina bifida can function as well as has been described. Acknowledgment of psychological differences in myelomeningocele patients may be seen as early as in the preschool period. Figure drawings by such children reveal fewer portrayals of lower extremities than in the general population. Children tend to rate themselves as significantly different in terms of physical and cognitive competence but not on maternal or peer acceptance (Mobley, Harless, & Miller, 1996).

The secondary disability of social isolation results from the time allocated to medical care and hospitalization. Thus, by midchildhood, children so afflicted have up to a fourfold risk of developing a psychiatric disorder, primarily neurotic in nature. Hence, early intervention, socialization, and family counseling are warranted (Connell & McConnel, 1981). Dorner (1976, 1977) detailed the social dysfunction of the group. Teenagers were found to be lonely and unhappy and to have limited exposure to the nonhandicapped population, sexual experiences, and community resources. These factors, rather than the extent of the physical disability, determine subsequent dysfunctional behavior (Wallander, Feldman, & Varni, 1989). New studies reflect similar findings, although academic achievement may be somewhat improved on the basis of mainstreaming (Borjeson & Logergren, 1990; Lord, Varzos, Behrman, Wicks, & Wicks, 1990). Adult males with spina bifida have decreased understanding of sexual function, decreased fertility, and difficulty in maintaining erections.

Conversely, females often achieve fertility early because of the premature onset of puberty associated with their hydrocephalus. Pregnant females may be predisposed to premature labor due to a contracted pelvis and urinary tract anomalies. Ventriculoperitoneal shunts may dysfunction during this period. If a C-section is indicated for delivery, then prophylactic antibiotics and peritoneal irrigation should be performed (Rietberg & Lindhout, 1993). Sexual education in either circumstance is exceedingly important.

Despite good cognitive skills and educational opportunities, it is not uncommon for patients to remain in the homes of their parents past maturity. This may not only be a sign of prolonged emotional dependence but may be an economic necessity, as only 20% of adults are likely to be employed (Castree & Walker, 1981). The survival rate for the majority of patients with spina bifida now exceeds 90%. This provides the medical community with a mandate to expand the range of services available to such adults.

REFERENCES

Abbott, R., Johann-Murphy, M., & Gold, J. T. (1991). Selective functional rhizotomy for the treatment of spasticity in children. In M. Sindou (Ed.), *Neurosurgery for spasticity* (pp. 149–157). New York: Springer-Verlag.

Abraham, E., Lubicky, J. P., Sanger, M. N., & Millar, E. A. (1996). Supramalleolar osteotomy for ankle valgus in myelomeningocele. *Journal of Pediatric Orthopaedics, 16,* 774–781.

Albright, A. L. (1996). Baclofen in the treatment of cerebral palsy. *Journal of Child Neurology, 11,* 77–83.

Albright, A. L., Barron, W. B., Fasick, D., Polinko, P., & Janosky, J. (1993). Continuous intrathecal Baclofen infusion for spasticity of cerebral origin. *Journal of the American Medical Association, 270,* 2475–2477.

Albright, A. L., Cervi, A., & Singletary, J. (1991). Intrathecal Baclofen for spasticity in cerebral palsy. *Journal of the American Medical Association, 265,* 1418–1422.

Alexander, M. A., & Steg, N. L. (1989). Myelomeningocele: Comprehensive treatment. *Archives of Physical Medicine and Rehabilitation, 70,* 637–641.

Alvarez, N., Larkin, C., & Roxborough, J. (1981). Carpal tunnel syndrome in athetoid-dystonic cerebral palsy. *Archives of Neurology, 39,* 311–326.

Andrade, C. K., Kramer, J., Garber, M., & Longmuir, P. (1991). Changes in self-concept, cardiovascular endurance and muscular strength of children with spina bifida aged 8 to 13 years in response to a 10-week physical activity programme: A pilot study. *Child: Care, Health and Development, 17,* 183–196.

Ansved, T., Odergren, T., & Borg, K. (1997). Muscle fiber atrophy in leg muscles after botulinum toxin type A treatment of cervical dystonia. *Neurology, 48,* 1440–1442.

Asher, M., & Olson, J. (1983). Factors affecting the ambulatory status of patients with spina bifida cystica. *Journal of Bone and Joint Surgery, 65A,* 350–356.

Ashton, B., Piper, M. C., Warren, S., Stewin, L., & Byrne, P. (1991). Influence of medical history on assessment of at-risk infants. *Developmental Medicine and Child Neurology, 33,* 412–418.

Bachrach, S., & Greenspun, B. (1990). Care of the adult with myelomeningocele. *Delaware Medical Journal, 62,* 1287–1295.

Badell-Ribera, A., Swinyard, G. A., Greenspan, L., & Deaver, G. G. (1964). Spina bifida with myelomeningocele: Evaluation of rehabilitation potential. *Archives of Physical Medicine and Rehabilitation, 45,* 443–453.

Balcom, A. H., Wiatrak, M., Biefeld, T., Rauen, K., & Langenstroer, P. (1997). Initial experience with home therapeutic electrical stimulation for continence in the myelomeningocele population. *Journal of Urology, 158,* 1272–1276.

Banker, B., & Larroche, J. C. (1962). Periventricular leukomalacia of infancy: A form of neonatal anoxic encephalopathy. *Archives of Neurology, 7,* 386–410.

Banta, J. V., & Park, S. M. (1983). Improvement in pulmonary function in patients having combined anterior and posterior spine fusion for myelomeningocele scoliosis. *Spine, 8,* 765–770.

Begeer, I. H., & Staal-Schreinemachers, A. L. (1996). The benefits of team treatment and control of adult patients with spinal dysraphism. *European Journal of Pediatric Surgery, 6,* 15–16.

Benedict, M. I., White, R. B., Wulff, L. M., & Hall, B. J. (1990). Reported maltreatment in children with multiple disabilities. *Child Abuse and Neglect, 14,* 207–217.

Bergen, A. F., & Colangelo, C. (1982). *Positioning of the client with central nervous system deficits: The wheelchair and other adaptive equipment.* Valhalla, NY: Valhalla Rehabilitation.

Biglan, A. W. (1995). Strabismus associated with meningomyelocele. *Journal of Pediatric Ophthalmology and Strabismus, 32,* 309–314.

Blair, E., & Stanley, F. (1990). Intrauterine growth retardation and spastic cerebral palsy: 1. Association with birth weight for gestational age. *American Journal of Obstetrics and Gynecology, 162,* 229–237.

Bleck, E. E. (1987). Orthopaedic management of cerebral palsy. In *Clinical developmental medicine* (Vol. 99/100). Oxford: MacKeith.

Bleck, E. E. (1990). Management of the lower extremities in children with cerebral palsy. *Journal of Bone and Joint Surgery, 72A,* 140–144.

Blum, R. W., Resnick, M. D., Nelson, R., & St. Germaine, A. (1991). Familial and peer issues among adolescents with spina bifida and cerebral palsy. *Pediatrics, 88,* 280–285.

Bobath, B., & Bobath, K. (1975). *Motor development in the different types of cerebral palsy*. London: Heineman.

Bobath, K. (1980). *A neurophysiologic basis to the treatment of cerebral palsy*. Laveham, U.K.: Spastics International.

Borjeson, M. C., & Logergren, J. (1990). Life conditions of adolescents with myelomeningocele. *Developmental Medicine and Child Neurology, 32,* 698–706.

Bower, C., Raymond, M., Lumley, J., & Bury, G. (1993). Trends in neural tube defects 1980–1989. *Medical Journal of Australia, 158,* 152–154.

Boytim, M. J., Davidson, R. S., Charney, E., & Melchionne, J. B. (1991). Neonatal fractures in myelomeningocele patients. *Journal of Pediatric Orthopedics, 11,* 28–30.

Brinker, M. R., Rosenfeld, S. R., Feiwell, E., Granger, S. P., Mitchell, D. C., & Rice, J. C. (1994). Myelomeningocele at the sacral level. *Journal of Bone and Joint Surgery, 76-A,* 1293–1300.

Brocklehurst, G. (Ed.). (1976). *Spina bifida for the clinician.* Philadelphia: J. B. Lippincott.

Bronkhorst, A. J., & Lamb, G. A. (1987). Orthosis to aid in the reduction of lower extremity spasticity. *Orthotics and Prosthetics, 41,* 23–28.

Brunt, A. (1980). Characteristics of upper limb movements in a sample of myelomeningocele children. *Perceptual and Motor Skills, 51,* 431–437.

Cahan, L. D., & Kundi, M. S. (1987). Electrophysiological studies in selective dorsal rhizotomy for spasticity in children with cerebral palsy. *Applied Neurophysiology, 50,* 459–460.

Capute, A. J. (1978). *Primitive reflex profile.* Baltimore: University Park Press.

Capute, A. J., Shapiro, B. K., & Palmer, F. B. (1981). Spectrum of developmental disabilities. *Orthopedic Clinics of North America, 12,* 3–22.

Carlson, W. E., Vaughan, C. L., Damiano, D. L., & Abel, M. F. (1997). Orthotic management of gait in spastic diplegia. *American Journal of Physical Medicine and Rehabilitation, 76,* 216–225.

Carr, C., & Gage, J. R. (1987). The fate of the non-operated hip in cerebral palsy. *Journal of Pediatric Orthopedics, 7,* 262–267.

Carroll, N. C. (1977). The orthotic management of spina bifida children: Present status, future goals. *Prosthetics and Orthotics International, 1,* 39–42.

Castree, B. J., & Walker, J. H. (1981). The young adult with spina bifida. *British Medical Journal, 283,* 1040–1042.

Charney, E. B. (1990). Parental attitudes toward management of newborns with myelomeningocele. *Developmental Medicine and Child Neurology, 32,* 14–19.

Charney, E. B., Melchionni, J. B., & Smith, D. R. (1991). Community ambulation by children with myelomeningocele and high-level paralysis. *Journal of Pediatric Orthopedics, 11,* 579–582.

Charney, E. B., Rorke, L. B., Sutton, L. N., & Schut, L. (1991). Management of Chiari II complications in infants with myelomeningocele. *Journal of Pediatrics, 111,* 364–371.

Charney, E. B., Snyder, H. M., & Melchionni, J. B. (1991). Upper urinary tract deterioration with myelomeningocele. *Developmental Medicine and Child Neurology, 33*(Suppl. 64), 18–37.

Chiaramonte, R. M., Horowitz, R. M., Kaplan, G. M., & Brook, W. A. (1986). Implications of hydronephrosis in newborns with myelodysplasia. *Journal of Urology, 136,* 427–429.

Chicoine, M. R., Park, T. S., & Kaufman, B. A. (1997). Selective dorsal rhizotomy and rates of orthopaedic surgery in children with spastic cerebral palsy. *Journal of Neurosurgery, 86,* 34–39.

Clancy, R. R., Sladsky, J. T., & Rorke, L. B. (1989). Hypoxic-ischemic spinal cord injury following perinatal asphyxia. *Annals of Neurology, 25,* 185–189.

Coniglio, S. J., Anderson, S. M., & Ferguson, J. E. (1996). Functional motor outcome in children with myelomeningocele. Correlation with anatomic prenatal ultrasound. *Developmental Medicine and Child Neurology, 38,* 675–680.

Connell, H. M., & McConnel, T. S. (1981). Psychiatric sequelae in children treated operatively for hydrocephalus in infancy. *Developmental Medicine and Child Neurology, 23,* 505–517.

Cooperman, D. R., Bartucci, E., Dietrick, E., & Millar, E. A. (1987). Hip dislocation in spastic cerebral palsy: Long-term consequences. *Journal of Pediatric Orthopedics, 7,* 268–276.

Coorsen, E. A., Msall, M. E., & Duffy, L. C. (1991). Multiple minor manifestations as a marker for prenatal etiology of cerebral palsy. *Developmental Medicine and Child Neurology, 33,* 730–736.

Craft, M. J., Lakin, J. A., Oppliger, R. A., Clancy, G. M., & Vanderlinden, D. W. (1990). Siblings as change agents for promoting the functional status of children with cerebral palsy. *Developmental Medicine and Child Neurology, 32,* 1049–1057.

Crandall, R. C., Birkeback, C. R., & Wintor, B. R. (1989). The role of hip location and dislocation in the functional status of the myelodysplastic patient. *Orthopedics, 12,* 675–683.

Cuddeford, T. J., Freeling, R. P., Thomas, S. S., Aniona, M. D., Rex, D., Sirolli, H., Elliott, J., & Magnusson, M. (1997). Energy consumption in children with myelomeningocele: A comparison between reciprocating gait orthosis and hip-knee-ankle-foot orthosis ambulators. *Developmental Medicine and Child Neurology, 39,* 239–242.

Curtis, B. H. (1973). The hip in the myelomeningocele child. *Clinical Orthopedics, 90,* 11–21.

Damiano, D. L., Kelly, L. E., & Vaughan, C. L. (1995). Effects of quadriceps femoris muscle strengthening on crouch gait in children with spastic diplegia. *Physical Therapy, 75,* 658–667.

Damiano, D. L., Vaughan, C. L., & Abel, M. F. (1995). Muscle response to heavy resistance exercise in children with spastic cerebral palsy. *Developmental Medicine and Child Neurology, 37,* 731–739.

Deaver, G. (1956). Cerebral palsy: Methods of beating the neuromuscular disability. *Archives of Physical Medicine and Rehabilitation, 37,* 363–378.

DeSouza, L. L., & Carroll, N. (1976). Ambulation of the braced myelomeningocele patient. *Journal of Bone and Joint Surgery, 58A,* 1112–1118.

Diamond, M. (1986). Rehabilitation strategies for the child with cerebral palsy. *Pediatric Annals, 15,* 230–236.

Dorner, S. (1976). Adolescents with spina bifida: How they view their situation. *Archives of Disease in Childhood, 51,* 439–444.

Dorner, S. (1977). Sexual interest and activity in adolescents with spina bifida. *Journal of Child Psychology, 18,* 229–237.

Drennan, J. C. (1976). Orthotic management of the myelomeningocele spine. *Developmental Medicine and Child Neurology, 18,* 97–103.

Drvaric, D. M., Roberts, J. M., Burke, S. W., King, A. G., & Falterman, K. (1987). Gastroesophageal evaluation in totally involved cerebral palsy patients. *Journal of Pediatric Orthopedics, 7,* 187–190.

Ebara, S., Yamazaki, Y., Harada, T., Hosono, N., Morimoto, Y., Tang, L., Seguchi, Y., & Ono, K. (1990). Motion analysis of the cervical spine in athetoid cerebral palsy. *Spine, 15,* 1097–1103.

Ellenberg, J. H., & Nelson, K. B. (1981). Early recognition of infants at risk for cerebral palsy: Examination at age 4 months. *Developmental Medicine and Child Neurology, 23,* 705–714.

Evans, D. M., & Alberman, E. (1990). Certified cause of death in children and young adults with cerebral palsy. *Archives of Disease in Childhood, 66,* 325–329.

Evans, D. M., Evans, J. W., & Alberman, E. (1990). Cerebral palsy: Why we must plan for survival. *Archives of Disease in Childhood, 65,* 1329–1333.

Eyman, R. K., & Grossman, H. J. (1990). The life expectancy of profoundly handicapped people with mental retardation. *New England Journal of Medicine, 323,* 584–589.

Farmer, S. F., Harrison, L. M., Ingram, D. A., & Stephens, J. A. (1991). Plasticity of central motor pathways in children with hemiplegic cerebral palsy. *Neurology, 41,* 1505–1510.

Fasano, V. A., Barolat-Romana, G., Zeme, S., & Squazzi, A. (1979). Electrophysiological assessment of spinal circuits in spasticity by direct dorsal root stimulation. *Neurosurgery, 4,* 146–151.

Feldman, A. B., Haley, S. M., & Coryell, J. (1990). Concurrent and construct validity of the Pediatric Evaluation of Disability Inventory. *Physical Therapy, 70,* 602–610.

Findley, T. W., & Agre, J. C. (1988). Ambulation in the adolescent with spina bifida: Oxygen cost of mobility. *Archives of Physical Medicine and Rehabilitation, 69,* 855–861.

Finnie, N. R. (1974). *Handling the young cerebral palsied child at home.* New York: E. P. Dutton.

Ford, G. W., Kitchen, W. H., Doyle, L. W., Richards, A. L., & Kelly, E. (1990). Changing diagnosis of cerebral palsy in very low birth weight children. *American Journal of Perinatology, 7,* 178–181.

Fraser, R. K., Bourke, H. M., Broughton, N. S., & Menelaus, M. B. (1995). Unilateral dislocation of the hip in spina bifida: A long-term follow-up. *Journal of Bone and Joint Surgery, 77-B,* 615–619.

Frawley, P. A., Broughton, N. S., & Menelaus, M. B. (1996). *Journal of Bone and Joint Surgery, 78-B,* 299–302.

Fuji, T., Yonebu, K., Fujiwara, K., Yamashita, K., Ebara, S., Ono, K., & Okada, K. (1987). Cervical radiculopathy or myelopathy secondary to athetoid cerebral palsy. *Journal of Bone and Joint Surgery, 69A,* 815–821.

Fulford, G. E. (1990). Surgical management of ankle and foot deformities in cerebral palsy. *Clinical Orthopaedics, 253,* 55–61.

Gage, J. R. (1990). Surgical treatment of knee dysfunction in cerebral palsy. *Clinical Orthopaedics, 253,* 45–54.

Gisel, E. G., & Patrick, J. (1988). Identification of children with cerebral palsy unable to maintain a normal nutritional state. *Lancet, 1,* 283–286.

Gluckman, S., & Barling, J. (1980). Effect of remedial program on visual-motor perception in spina bifida children. *Journal of General Psychology, 136,* 195–202.

Gold, J. T. (1991). Orthotic management and rehabilitation of the foot and ankle in the neurologically impaired child. In M. H. Jahss (Ed.), *Disorders of the foot and ankle.* Philadelphia: W. B. Saunders.

Gold, J. T. (1996). Growth hormone treatment of children with neural tube defects [letter; comment]. *Journal of Pediatrics, 129,* 771.

Gooch, J. L., & Walker, M. L. (1996). Spinal stenosis after total lumbar laminectomy for selective dorsal rhizotomy. *Pediatric Neurosurgery, 25,* 28–30.

Goschel, H., Wohlfarth, K., Frevert, J., Dengler, R., & Bigalke, T. T. (1997). Botulinum A toxin therapy: Neutralizing and nonneutralizing antibodies—therapeutic consequences. *Experimental Neurology, 147,* 96–102.

Graham, L., Levene, M. I., & Trounce, J. Q. (1987). Prediction of cerebral palsy in very low birth weight infants: Prospective ultrasound study. *Lancet, 2,* 593–596.

Granger, C. V., Hamilton, B. B., & Kayton, R. (1987). Guide for the use of the Functional Independence Measure for Children (WeeFIM) of the Uniform Data Set for medical rehabilitation. Buffalo, NY: Research Foundation, State University of New York.

Grant, A., O'Brien, N., Joy, M. T., Hennessy, E., & MacDonald, D. (1989). Cerebral palsy among children born during the Dublin randomized trial of intrapartum monitoring. *Lancet, 2,* 1233–1236.

Greene, W. B., Terry, R. C., DeMasi, R. A., & Herrington, R. T. (1991). Effect of race and gender on neurological level in myelomeningocele. *Developmental Medicine and Child Neurology, 33,* 110–117.

Grimm, R. A. (1976). Hand preference and tactile perception in a group of children with myelomeningocele. *American Journal of Occupational Therapy, 30,* 234–250.

Guyatt, G., Sackett, D., Taylor, D. W., Chong, J., Roberts, R., & Dugsley, S. (1986). Determining optimal therapy: Randomized trials in individual patients. *New England Journal of Medicine, 314,* 889–892.

Hagberg, B., & Hagberg, G. (1989). The changing panorama of cerebral palsy in Sweden: 5. The birth year period 1979–82. *Acta Paediatrica Scandinavica, 78,* 283–290.

Hagberg, B., & Hagberg, G. (1996). The changing panorama of cerebral palsy: Bilateral spastic forms in particular. *Acta Paedictrica, 416,* 48–52.

Halpern, D. (1982). Duration of relaxation after intramuscular neurolysis with phenol. *Journal of the American Medical Association, 247,* 1473–1476.

Halpern, D. (1984). Therapeutic exercises for cerebral palsy. In J. V. Basmajian (Ed.), *Therapeutic exercises* (pp. 118–143). Baltimore: Williams and Wilkins.

Harade, T., Ebara, S., Anwar, M. M., Okawa, A., Kajiura, I., Hiroshima, K., & Ono, K. (1996). The cervical spine in athetoid cerebral palsys: A radiological study of 180 patients. *Journal of Bone and Joint Surgery, 78-B,* 613–619.

Harris, S. R. (1989). Early diagnosis of spastic diplegia, spastic hemiplegia and quadriplegia. *American Journal of Diseases of Children, 143,* 1356–1360.

Harrison, A. (1988). Spastic cerebral palsy: Possible spinal interneuronal contributions. *Developmental Medicine and Child Neurology, 30,* 769–780.

Hazlewood, M. I., Brown, J. K., Rowe, P. J., & Salter, P. M. (1994). The use of therapeutic electrical stimulation in the treatment of hemiplegic cerebral palsy. *Developmental Medicine and Child Neurology, 36,* 661–673.

Hill, A. E. (1990). Conductive education for physically handicapped children. *Ulster Medical Journal, 59,* 41–45.

Hinderer, K. A., & Harris, S. R. (1988). Effects of tone reducing versus standard plaster casts on gait improvement in children with cerebral palsy. *Developmental Medicine and Child Neurology, 30,* 370–377.

Hirst, M. (1989). Patterns of impairment and disability related to social handicap in young people with cerebral palsy and spina bifida. *Journal of Biosocial Science, 21,* 1–12.

Hochhaus, F., Butenandl, O., Schwarz, H. P., & Ring-Mrozik, E. (1997). *European Journal of Pediatrics, 156,* 597–601.

Hoffer, M. M., Feiwell, E., Perry, R., Perry, J., & Bonnett, C. (1973). Functional ambulation in patients with myelomeningocele. *Journal of Bone and Joint Surgery, 55A,* 137–148.

Holm, V. A. (1982). The causes of cerebral palsy. *Journal of the American Medical Association, 247,* 1473–1475.

Homes, L. B. (1988). Does taking vitamins at the time of conception prevent neural tube defects? *Journal of the American Medical Association, 260,* 3181–3183.

Horn, D. G., Lorch, E. P., Lorch, R. F., & Culatta, B. (1985). Distractibility and vocabulary deficits in children with spina bifida and hydrocephalus. *Developmental Medicine and Child Neurology, 27,* 713–720.

Hunt, G. M., & Holmes, A. E. (1976). Factors relating to intelligence in treated cases of spina bifida cystica. *American Journal of Diseases of Children, 130,* 823–827.

Ingram, T. S. S. (1955). Early manifestations and course of diplegia in childhood. *Archives of Disease in Childhood, 30,* 244–250.

Iwu, H. Y., Baskin, L. S., & Kogan, B. A. (1997). Neurogenic bladder dysfunction due to myelomeningocele: Neonatal versus childhood treatment. *Journal of Urology, 157,* 2295–2297.

Johnson, D. C., Damiano, D. L., & Abel, M. F. (1997). The evolution of gait in childhood and adolescent cerebral palsy. *Journal of Pediatric Orthopaedics, 17,* 392–396.

Kaplan, W. E. (1985). Management of myelomeningocele. *Urology Clinics of North America, 12,* 93–101.

Kaplan, W. E., & Richards, I. (1988). Intravesical bladder stimulation in myelodysplasia. *Journal of Urology, 140,* 1282–1284.

Kassover, M., Tauber, C., Au, J., & Pugh, J. (1986). Auditory biofeedback in spastic diplegia. *Journal of Orthopaedic Research, 4,* 246–249.

Kaufman, B. A., Terbrock, A., Winters, N., Ito, J., Klosterman, A., & Park, T. S. (1994). Disbanding a multidisciplinary clinic: Effects on health care of myelomeningocele patients. *Pediatric Neurology, 21,* 36–44.

Keating, J. C., McCarron, K., James, J., Gruenberg, J., & Lonczak, R. S. (1985). Urobehavioral intervention in the rehabilitation of lower urinary tract dysfunction: A case report. *Journal of Manipulative and Physiological Therapeutics, 8,* 185–189.

Khoury, M. J., Erickson, J. D., & James, L. M. (1982). Etiologic heterogenicity of neural tube defects: Clues from epidemiology. *American Journal of Epidemiology, 115,* 538–548.

Kinsman, S. L., & Doehring, M. C. (1996). The cost of preventable conditions in adults with spina bifida. *European Journal of Pediatric Surgery, 6,* 17–20.

Korman, L. A., Mooney, J. F., Smith, B., Goodman, A., & Mulvaney, T. (1993). Management of cerebral palsy with botulinum-A toxin: Preliminary investigation. *Journal of Pediatric Orthopaedics, 13,* 489–495.

Kottke, F. J., Halpern, D., Easton, J. K. M., Ozel, A. T., & Burrill, C. A. (1978). The training of coordination. *Archives of Physical Medicine and Rehabilitation, 59,* 567–578.

Kraus, F. T. (1997). Cerebral palsy and thrombi in placental vessels of the fetus: Insights from litigation. *Human Pathology, 28,* 246–248.

Krebs, D. E., Edelstein, J. E., & Fishman, S. (1988). Comparison of plastic/metal and leather metal knee-ankle-foot orthoses. *American Journal of Physical Medicine, 67,* 175–185.

Lary, J. M., & Edmonds, L. D. (1996). Prevalence of spina bifida at birth—United States, 1983–1990: A comparison of two surveillance systems. *Morbidity and Mortality Weekly Report CDC Surveillance Summaries, 45*(2), 15–26.

Leck, I. (1974). Causation of neural tube defects: Clues from epidemiology. *British Medical Bulletin, 30,* 158–163.

Lemire, R. J. (1988). Neural tube defects. *Journal of the American Medical Association, 259,* 558–562.

Letts, R. M., Fulford, D., Eng, B., & Robson, D. A. (1976). Mobility aids for the paraplegic child. *Journal of Bone and Joint Surgery, 58A,* 38–41.

Levine, M. S. (1980). Cerebral palsy diagnosis in children over 1 year of age: Standard criteria. *Archives of Physical Medicine and Rehabilitation, 61,* 385–392.

Li, V., Albright, A. L., Sclabassi, R., & Pang, D. (1996). The role of somatosensory evoked potentials in the evaluation of spinal cord retethering. *Pediatric Neurosurgery, 24,* 126–133.

Lingam, S., & Joester, J. (1994). Lesion of the week: Spontaneous fractures in children and adolescents with cerebral palsy. *British Medical Journal, 309,* 265–268.

Lintner, S. A., & Lindseth, R. E. (1994). Kyphotic deformity in patients who have a myelomeningocele: Operative treatment and long-term follow-up. *Journal of Bone and Joint Surgery, 76-A,* 1301–1307.

Lonstein, J. E., & Akbamia, B. (1983). Operative treatment of spinal deformities in patients with cerebral palsy or mental retardation. *Journal of Bone and Joint Surgery, 63A,* 43–57.

Lorber, J. (1971). Results of treatment of myelomeningocele: An analysis of 524 selected cases with special references to possible selection for treatment. *Developmental Medicine and Child Neurology, 13,* 279–303.

Lord, J., Varzos, N., Behrman, B., Wicks, J., & Wicks, D. (1990). Implications of mainstream classrooms for adolescents with spina bifida. *Developmental Medicine and Child Neurology, 32,* 20–29.

Lord, J. P. (1984). Cerebral palsy: A clinical approach. *Archives of Physical Medicine and Rehabilitation, 65,* 542–556.

Lough, L. K., & Nielsen, D. H. (1986). Ambulation of children with myelomeningocele: Parapodium versus parapodium with Orlau swivel modification. *Developmental Medicine and Child Neurology, 28,* 489–497.

Major, R. E., Stollard, J., & Farmer, S. E. (1997). A review of 42 patients of 16 years and over using the Orlau Parawalker. *Prosthetics and Orthotics International, 21,* 147–152.

Mankinen-Heikkinen, A., & Mustonene, E. (1987). Ophthalmologic changes in hydrocephalus. *Acta Ophthalmologica, 65,* 81–86.

Mannino, F. L., & Traunor, D. (1983). Stroke in neonates. *Journal of Pediatrics, 102,* 605–609.

Marshall, P. D., Broughton, N. S., Menelaus, M. B., & Graham, H. K. (1996). Surgical release of knee flexion contractures in myelomeningocele. *Journal of Bone and Joint Surgery, 78-B,* 912–916.

Martin, J. E., & Epstein, L. H. (1976). Evaluating treatment effectiveness in cerebral palsy. *Physical Therapy, 56,* 285–293.

Matthews, D. (1988). Controversial therapies in the management of cerebral palsy. *Pediatric Annals, 17,* 762–765.

McCall, R. E., & Schmidt, W. T. (1986). Clinical experience with the reciprocating gait orthosis in myelodysplasia. *Journal of Pediatric Orthopedics, 16,* 157–161.

McClone, D. G., Czyzewski, D., Raimondi, A., & Sommers, R. (1982). Central nervous system infections as a limiting factor in the intelligence of children with myelodysplasia. *Pediatrics, 70,* 338–342.

McClone, D. G., Dias, L., Kaplan, W., & Sommers, M. (1985). Concepts in the management of spina bifida. *Concepts in Pediatric Neurosurgery, 5,* 97–106.

McDonald, C. M., Jaffe, K. M., Mosca, V. S., & Shurtleff, D. B. (1991). Ambulatory outcome of children with myelomeningocele: Effect of lower extremity strength. *Developmental Medicine and Child Neurology, 33,* 482–490.

McDonald, C. M., Jaffe, K. M., Mosca, V. S., Shurtleff, D. B., & Menelaus, M. B. (1991). Modifications to the traditional description of neurosegmental innervation in myelomeningocele. *Developmental Medicine and Child Neurology, 33,* 473–481.

McLaughlin, J. F., & Shurtleff, D. B. (1979). Management of the newborn with myelodysplasia. *Clinical Pediatrics, 18,* 463–476.

McNeal, D., Hawtrey, C. E., Wolraich, M. L., & Mapel, J. R. (1983). Symptomatic neurogenic bladder in a cerebral palsy population. *Developmental Medicine and Child Neurology, 25,* 612–621.

Menelaus, M. B. (1980). *Orthopaedic management of spina bifida cystica* (2nd ed.). Edinburgh: Churchill-Livingstone.

Milunsky, A., & Alpert, E. (1976a). Prenatal diagnosis of neural tube defects: 1. Problems and pitfalls: Analysis of 2495 cases using the alpha-fetoprotein assay. *Journal of Obstetrics and Gynecology, 48,* 1–5.

Milunsky, A., & Alpert, E. (1976b). Prenatal diagnosis of neural tube defects: 2. Analysis of false positive and false negative alpha-fetoprotein results. *Journal of Obstetrics and Gynecology, 48,* 6–12.

Meuli, M., Meuli-Simmen, C., Hutchins, G. M., Seiler, M. J., Harrison, M. R., & Adzick, N. S. (1997). The spinal cord lesion in human fetuses with myelomeningocele. Implications for fetal surgery. *Journal of Pediatric Surgery, 32,* 448–452.

Meuli-Simmen, C., Meuli, M., Adzick, N. S., & Harrison, M. R. (1997). Latissimus dorsi flap procedures to cover myelomeningocele in utero: A feasibility study in human fetuses. *Journal of Pediatric Surgery, 32,* 1154–1156.

Missuna, C., & Pollack, N. (1991). Play deprivation in children with physical disabilities: The role of the occupational therapist in preventing secondary disability. *American Journal of Occupational Therapy, 45,* 882–888.

Mital, M. A., & Sakellarides, H. (1981). Surgery of the upper extremity in the retarded individual with spastic cerebral palsy. *Orthopedic Clinics of North America, 12,* 127–136.

Mobley, C. E., Harless, L. S., & Miller, K. L. (1996). Self-perception of preschool children with spina bifida. *Journal of Pediatric Nursing, 11,* 217–224.

Molnar, G. E. (1979). Cerebral palsy prognosis and how to judge it. *Pediatric Annals, 8,* 10–24.

Molnar, G. E., & Gordon, S. U. (1976). Cerebral palsy: Predictive value of selective clinical signs for early prognostication of motor function. *Archives of Physical Medicine and Rehabilitation, 57,* 153–159.

Molnar, G. E., & Taft, L. T. (1977). Pediatric rehabilitation: Part 1. Cerebral palsy and spinal cord injuries. *Current Problems in Pediatrics, 7,* 6–11.

Morrow, J. D. (1995). Temperament of the infant with myelomeningocele. *Journal of Pediatric Nursing, 10,* 99–104.

Mossberg, K. A., Linton, K. A., & Friske, K. (1990). Ankle-foot orthoses: Effect on energy expenditure of gait in spastic diplegic children. *Archives of Physical Medicine and Rehabilitation, 71,* 490–494.

Mundy, A. R., Shah, P. J. R., Borzyskowski, M., & Saxton, H. M. (1985). Sphincter behavior in myelomeningocele. *British Journal of Urology, 57,* 647–651.

Murphy, K. P., Molnmar, G. E., & Lankasky, K. (1995). Medical and functional status of adults with cerebral palsy. *Developmental Medicine and Child Neurology, 37,* 1075–1084.

Naeye, R. L., & Peters, E. C. (1989). Origins of cerebral palsy. *American Journal of Diseases of Children, 143,* 1154–1160.

Nelson, K. B. (1989). Relationship of intrapartum and delivery events to long-term neurologic outcome. *Clinical Perinatology, 16,* 995–1007.

Nelson, K. B., & Ellenberg, J. H. (1979). Neonatal signs as predictors of cerebral palsy. *Pediatrics, 64,* 2–14.

Nelson, K. B., & Ellenberg, J. H. (1981). Apgar scores as predictors of chronic neurologic disability. *Pediatrics, 68,* 36–46.

Nelson, K. B., & Ellenberg, J. H. (1986). Antecedents of cerebral palsy. *New England Journal of Medicine, 315,* 81–86.

Noetzel, M. J., & Blake, J. N. (1991). Prognosis for seizure control and remission in children with myelomeningocele. *Developmental Medicine and Child Neurology, 33,* 803–810.

Nwaobi, O. M., & Smith, P. D. (1986). Effects of adaptive seating on pulmonary function in children with cerebral palsy. *Developmental Medicine and Child Neurology, 28,* 351–354.

Palmer, F. B., Shapiro, B. K., Allen, M. C., Mosher, B. S., Bilker, S. A., Harryman, S. E., Meinert, C. L., & Capute, A. J. (1990). Infant stimulation curriculum for infants with cerebral palsy: Effects on infant temperament, parent infant interaction and home environment. *Pediatrics, 85,* 411–415.

Palmer, F. B., Shapiro, B. K., & Wachtel, R. C. (1988). Effects of physical therapy on cerebral palsy. *New England Journal of Medicine, 318,* 803–808.

Pape, K. E., Kirsch, S. E., Galil, A., Boulton, J. E., White, M. A., & Chipman, M. (1993). Neuromuscular approach to the motor deficits of cerebral palsy: A pilot study. *Journal of Pediatric Orthopaedics, 13,* 628–633.

Park, T. S., Cail, W. S., & Maggio, W. M. (1985). Progressive spasticity and scoliosis in children with myelomeningocele. *Journal of Neurosurgery, 62,* 367–375.

Peacock, W. J., Arens, L. J., & Berman, B. (1987). Cerebral palsy spasticity: Selective posterior rhizotomy. *Pediatric Neuroscience, 13,* 61–66.

Peacock, W. J., & Staudt, L. A. (1991). Functional outcomes following selective posterior rhizotomy in children with cerebral palsy. *Journal of Neurosurgery, 74,* 380–385.

Peeker, R., Damber, J. E., Hjalmas, K., Sjodin, J. G., & Von Zweigbergk, M. (1997). The urological fate of young adults with myelomeningocele: A three decade follow-up study. *European Urology, 32,* 213–217.

Penn, R. D., Mykleburst, B. M., Gottleib, G. L., Agarwal, G. C., & Etzel, M. E. (1980). Chronic cerebellar stimulation for cerebral palsy. *Journal of Neurosurgery, 53,* 160–169.

Perlstein, M. A. (1952). Infantile cerebral palsy: Classification and clinical correlations. *Journal of the American Medical Association, 149,* 30–37.

Perry, J., & Hoffer, M. M. (1976). Pre-operative and post-operative dynamic electromyography as an aid in planning tendon transfer in children with cerebral palsy. *Journal of Bone and Joint Surgery, 58A,* 531–543.

Petersen, T. (1987). Management of urinary incontinence in children with myelomeningocele. *Acta Neurologica Scandinavica, 75,* 52–55.

Raddish, M., Goldman, D. A., Kaplan, D. C., & Perrin, J. M. (1998). The immunization status of children with spina bifida. *American Journal of Diseases of Children, 147,* 849–853.

Radke, J., & Gosky, G. A. (1981). Hearing and speech screening in a hydrocephalus myelodysplasia population. *Spina Bifida Therapy, 3,* 25–26.

Reese, M. E., Msall, M. E., & Owens, S. (1991). Acquired cervical spine impairment in young adults with cerebral palsy. *Developmental Medicine and Child Neurology, 33,* 153–166.

Reigel, D. H. (1983). Tethered spinal cord. *Concepts in Pediatric Neurosurgery, 4,* 142–164.

Reimers, J. (1990). Functional changes in the antagonists after lengthening of the agonists in cerebral palsy. *Clinical Orthopaedics, 253,* 30–37.

Resnick, M. B., Eyler, F. D., Nelson, R. M., Eitman, D. V., & Bucciarelli, R. L. (1987). Developmental intervention for low birth weight infants: Improved early developmental outcome. *Pediatrics, 80,* 68–74.

Rietberg, C. C., & Lindhout, D. (1993). Adult patients with spina bifida cystica. *European Journal of Obstetrics, Gynecology and Reproductive Biology, 52,* 63–70.

Robinson, H. P., Hood, V. D., Adam, A. H., Gibson, A. A. M., & Ferguson-Smith, M. A. (1980). Diagnostic ultrasound: Early detection of fetal neural tube defects. *Obstetrics and Gynecology, 56,* 705–710.

Robinson, R. O. (1973). The frequency of other handicaps in children with cerebral palsy. *Developmental Medicine and Child Neurology, 15,* 305–316.

Rosenstein, S. N. (1982). *Dentistry in cerebral palsy and related handicapping conditions.* Springfield, IL: Charles C Thomas.

Rotenstien, D., & Reigel, D. H. (1996). Growth hormone treatment of children with neural tube defects: Results from 6 months to 6 years. *Journal of Pediatrics, 128,* 184–189.

Rothman, J. G. (1978). Effects of respiratory exercises on the vital capacity and forced volume in children with cerebral palsy. *Physical Therapy, 58,* 421–425.

Sala, D. A., & Grant, A. D. (1995). Prognosis for ambulation in cerebral palsy. *Developmental Medicine and Child Neurology, 37,* 1020–1026.

Salakor, P. T., Sajaniemi, N., Hallback, H., Kari, A., Rila, H., & von Wendt, L. (1997). Randomization study of the effects of antenatal dexamethasone on growth and development of premature children at the corrected age of two years. *Acta Paediatrica, 86,* 294–298.

Samilson, R. L. (1981). Current concepts of surgical management in the lower extremities in cerebral palsy. *Clinical Orthopaedics, 158,* 99–113.

Shafer, M. F., & Dias, L. S. (1983). *Myelomeningocele: Orthopaedic treatment.* Baltimore: Williams and Wilkins.

Shapiro, A., & Susa, K. Z. (1990). Pre-operative and post-operative gait evaluation in cerebral palsy. *Archives of Physical Medicine and Rehabilitation, 71,* 236–240.

Sharrard, W. J. W. (1964). Posterior iliopsas transplantation in the treatment of paralytic dislocation of the hip. *Journal of Bone and Joint Surgery, 46B,* 426–444.

Sherk, H. H., Uppal, G. S., Lane, G., & Melchionni, J. (1991). Treatment versus non-treatment of hip dislocations in ambulatory patients with myelomeningocele. *Developmental Medicine and Child Neurology, 33,* 491–494.

Siperstein, G. N., Wolraich, M. L., Reed, D., & O'Keefe, P. (1988). Medical decisions and prognostications of pediatricians for infants with myelomeningocele. *Journal of Pediatrics, 113,* 835–840.

Slater, J. E. (1989). Rubber anaphylaxis. *New England Journal of Medicine, 320,* 1126–1129.

Smith, K. A. (1991). Bowel and bladder management of the child with myelomeningocele in the school setting. *Journal of Pediatric Health Care, 4,* 175–180.

Sousa, J. C., Gordon, L. H., & Shurtleff, D. B. (1976). Assessing the development of daily living skills in patients with spina bifida. *Developmental Medicine and Child Neurology, 37*(Suppl. 18), 134–143.

Spindel, M. R., Bauer, S. B., & Dyro, I. M. (1987). The changing lesion in myelodysplasia. *Journal of the American Medical Association, 258,* 1630–1633.

Staheli, L. T. L., Duncan, W. R., & Schaefer, E. (1960). Growth alterations in the hemiplegic child. *Clinical Orthopaedics, 60,* 205–212.

Stallard, J., Major, R. E., & Farmer, S. E. (1996). The potential for ambulation by severely handicapped cerebral palsy patients. *Prosthetics and Orthotics International, 20,* 122–128.

Stanley, F., & Blair, E. (1991). Why have we failed to reduce the frequency of cerebral palsy? *Medical Journal of Australia, 154,* 623–626.

Stark, G. D., & Baker, G. C. W. (1967). The neurologic involvement of the lower limb in myelomeningocele. *Developmental Medicine and Child Neurology, 9,* 732–743.

Steinbok, P., Reiner, A. M., Beauchamp, R., Armstrong, R. W., & Cochrane, D. D. (1997). A randomized clinical trial to compare selective posterior rhizotomy plus physiotherapy with physiotherapy alone in children with spastic diplegic cerebral palsy. *Developmental Medicine and Child Neurology, 39,* 178–184.

Streeter, G. L. (1942). Developmental horizons in human embryos: Description of age group XI, 13 to 20 somites, and age group XII, 21–29 somites. *Contributions in Embryology, 30,* 211–245.

Sutherland, D. H. (1984). *Gait disorders of childhood and adolescence.* Baltimore: Williams and Wilkins.

Swaminathan, S., Paton, J. Y., Ward, S. D. L., Jacobs, R. A., Sargent, C. W., & Keens, T. G. (1989). Abnormal control of ventilation in adolescents with myelodysplasia. *Journal of Pediatrics, 115,* 898–903.

Sweetser, P. M., Badell, A., Schneider, S., & Badlin, G. H. (1995). Effects of sacral dorsal rhizotomy on bladder function in patients with spastic cerebral palsy. *Neuroradiology and Urodynamics, 14,* 57–64.

Talwar, D., Baldwin, N. A., & Horbatt, C. I. (1995). Epilepsy in children with meningomyelocele. *Pediatric Neurology, 13,* 29–32.

Tardieu, C., de la Tour, H., Bret, M. D., & Tardieu, G. (1982). Muscle hypoextensibility in children with cerebral palsy. *Archives of Physical Medicine and Rehabilitation, 63,* 97–110.

Tardieu, C., & Lespargot, A. (1988). For how long must the soleus muscle be stretched each day to prevent contracture? *Developmental Medicine and Child Neurology, 30,* 3–10.

Tardorf, K. (1986). Spontaneous remission in cerebral palsy. *Neuropediatrics, 17,* 19–22.

Teo, C., & Jones, R. (1996). Management of hydrocephalus by endoscopic third ventriculostomy in patients with myelomeningocele. *Pediatric Neurosurgery, 25,* 57–63.

Thomas, S. S., Aiona, M. D., Pierce, R., & Piatt, J. H. (1996). Gait changes in children with spastic diplegia after selective dorsal rhizotomy. *Journal of Pediatric Orthopaedics, 16,* 747–752.

Tirosh, E., & Rabino, S. (1989). Physiotherapy for children with cerebral palsy. *American Journal of Diseases of Children, 143,* 551–553.

U.K. collaborative study on alpha-fetoprotein measurement in antenatal screening for anencephaly and spina bifida in early pregnancy. (1977). *Lancet, 1,* 1323–1332.

Tomlinson, P., & Sugarman, I. D. (1995). Complications in shunts in adults with spina bifida. *American Journal of Diseases of Children, 143,* 551–553.

Vannucci, R. C. (1990). Experimental biology of cerebral hypoxic ischemia: Relationship of perinatal brain damage. *Pediatric Research, 27,* 317–326.

Vaughn, C. W., Neilson, P. D., & O'Dwyer, N. J. (1988). Motor control deficits of orofacial muscles in cerebral palsy. *Journal of Neurology, Neurosurgery, and Psychiatry, 51,* 534–539.

Vohr, B. R., & Msall, M. E. (1997). Neuropsychological and functional outcomes of very low birth weight infants. *Seminars in Perinatology, 21,* 202–220.

Wallace, S. J. (1973). The effect of upper-limb function on mobility of children with myelomeningocele. *Developmental Medicine and Child Neurology, 15,* 84–91.

Wallander, J. L., Babani, L., Varni, J. W., Banis, H. T., & Wilcox, K. T. (1989). Family resources as resistance factors for psychological maladjustment in chronically ill and handicapped children. *Journal of Pediatric Psychology, 14,* 157–173.

Wallander, J. L., Feldman, W., & Varni, J. W. (1989). Physical status and psychological adjustment in children with spina bifida. *Journal of Pediatric Psychology, 14,* 89–102.

Wallander, J. L., Varni, J. W., Babani, L., Deltaan, C. B., Wilcox, K. T., & Banis, H. T. (1989). The social environment and the adaptation of mothers of physically handicapped children. *Journal of Pediatric Psychology, 14,* 371–387.

Waller, D. K., Mills, J. L., Simpson, J. L., Cunningham, G. C., Conley, M. R., Lassman, M. R., & Rhoads, G. G. (1995). Are obese women at greater risk for producing malformed offspring? *American Journal of Obstetrics and Gynecology, 172,* 245–247.

Williams, M. D., Lewandowski, L. J., Coplan, J., & D'Eugenio, D. B. (1987). Neurodevelopmental outcome of preschool children born preterm with and without intracranial hemorrhage. *Developmental Medicine and Child Neurology, 29,* 243–249.

Wills, K. E., Holmbeck, G. N., Dillon, K., & McClone, D. G. (1990). Intelligence and achievement in children with myelomeningocele. *Journal of Pediatric Psychology, 15,* 161–176.

Wilson, H., Haideri, M. E., Song, K., & Telford, D. (1997). Ankle foot orthoses for preambulatory children with spastic diplegia. *Journal of Pediatric Orthopaedics, 17,* 310–376.

Wolf, L. S., & McLaughlin, J. F. (1992). Early motor development in infants with meningomyelocele. *Pediatric Physical Therapy, 3,* 12–17.

Worley, G., Rosenfeld, L. R., & Lipscomb, J. (1991). Financial counselling for families of children with chronic disabilities. *Developmental Medicine and Child Neurology, 33,* 679–689.

Worley, G., Schuster, J. M., & Oakes, W. J. (1991). The influence on survival of cervical laminectomy for children with meningomyelocele who have potentially lethal brainstem dysfunction due to the Chiari II malformation. *Developmental Medicine and Child Neurology, 33*(Suppl. 64), 19–26.

Worley, G., Schuster, J. M., & Oakes, W. J. (1996). Survival at 5 years of a cohort of newborn infants with myelomeningocele. *Developmental Medicine and Child Neurology, 38,* 816–822.

Yamada, S., Zinke, D. E., & Sanders, D. (1981). Pathophysiology of tethered cord syndrome. *Journal of Neurosurgery, 54,* 494–503.

Yokochi, K. (1997). Thalamic lesions revealed by M.R.I. associated with periventricular leukomalacia and clinical profiles of suspect. *Acta Paediatrica, 86,* 493–496.

Young, R. R., & Delwaide, P. J. (1981). Drug therapy: Spasticity. *New England Journal of Medicine, 304,* 28–43.

Zide, B., Constantini, S., & Epstein, F. J. (1995). Prevention of recurrent tethered spinal cord. *Pediatric Neurosurgery, 22,* 111–114.

Chapter 19

Peripheral Vascular Disorders

Glenn R. Jacobowitz and Thomas S. Riles

Peripheral vascular disease (PVD) encompasses not only diseases of arteries and veins but also multiple underlying medical conditions such as coronary artery disease, diabetes, and renal insufficiency, which are associated with and are often the cause of the vascular pathology. Such a broad range of diseases involves the entire body, literally from head to toe. The brain, abdominal viscera, lungs, and upper and lower extremities are all end organs affected by vascular disease. It is not uncommon for one patient to manifest different aspects of vascular disease. There are various functional presentations that must be recognized. After treatment of PVD, patients are often left with disabilities that require extensive rehabilitation, both physical and psychological. Ambulation and activities of daily living must often be relearned following either revascularization or amputation of an extremity. Cerebrovascular disease may lead to central cognitive and/or motor deficits. A wide range of services may be required for these patients, including physical therapy, occupational therapy, and psychosocial support services. In addition, rehabilitation physicians and staff must be aware of the chronic nature of PVD. In the rehabilitation phase of recovery, patients may have recurrence of their disease (e.g., leg ischemia, transient ischemic attack), which must be recognized and expeditiously treated. Therefore, it is critical for the rehabilitation physician to have an understanding of the functional presentation and treatment of PVD.

The broad scope of PVD may be separated into several areas. A practical organization should include (a) lower extremity peripheral arterial occlusive disease, (b) cerebrovascular disease, (c) venous disease, and (d) peripheral and abdominal arterial aneurysmal disease. All of these entities are associated with specific medical presentations, indications for operation, treatment modalities, recovery regimens, and disabilities that warrant separate attention and will therefore be reviewed individually.

FUNCTIONAL PRESENTATION

Lower Extremity Peripheral Arterial Occlusive Disease

There are several disease processes, associated disorders, and degrees of disability related to lower extremity PVD. The most common is atherosclerotic occlusive disease. Patients with chronic lower extremity ischemia have been divided into two groups. The first includes patients with intermittent claudication, who are considered to have a good prognosis, benign course, and low rate of amputation or need for surgical intervention. The second group, in contrast, includes patients with limb-threatening ischemia. These patients have been thought to have a poor prognosis with almost certain amputation if no intervention could be performed. The definition of limb-threatening ischemia is rest pain or the presence of gangrene in the extremity.

In the past, the presence of limb-threatening ischemia was the primary indication for surgical intervention and the appropriate angiographic studies. However, as the diagnostic and interventional armamentarium has expanded in recent years, previous indications for intervention and imaging have been reevaluated. The advent of balloon angioplasty, intraarterial stenting, thrombolytic agents, and endovascular prostheses have revolutionized the treatment of PVD. Imaging techniques, including both conventional angiography and magnetic resonance angiography (MRA) have greatly improved. There is now a multitude of treatment options for vascular disease, and physicians caring for patients with vascular disease should be aware of these options and the indications for their use.

The term *claudication* is derived from the Latin verb *claudicare*, meaning "to limp." Intermittent claudication is defined as the inability to mount an appropriate augmentation of blood supply in response to exercise. It consists of three essential features: the pain is in a functional muscle unit, it is reproducibly precipitated by a consistent amount of exercise, and it is promptly relieved by a cessation of exercise. At least 10% of the population above the age of 70 have intermittent claudication, as well as 1%–2% of younger patients (Peabody, Kannel, & McNamara, 1974). However, the vast majority of patients can be treated nonoperatively. A thorough understanding of the natural history of lower extremity ischemia and the available treatment options form the basis of sound clinical decision making.

The most important studies on the natural history of intermittent claudication have focused not only on patient history but also on objective evidence of arterial obstruction by arteriography or noninvasive means such as ankle-brachial blood pressure indices. Some of these studies document that up to 80% of such patients remain stable or improve over 2.5–6 years (Imparato, Kim, Davidson, & Crowley, 1975; Jonason & Ringquiest, 1985). Other studies have shown only 40%–60% of claudication improvement over time (Cronenwett et al., 1984; Rosenbloom et al., 1988). Risk factors of worsening ischemia include cigarette smoking and diabetes. The single worst prognostic factor is the severity of arterial occlusive disease at the time of initial presentation (Cronenwett et al., 1984; Imparato et al., 1975; Jonason & Ringquiest, 1985; Rosenbloom et al., 1988).

Limb-threatening ischemia occurs when resting blood flow is unable to meet baseline metabolic demands because of arterial occlusion. Clinically, this presents as rest pain (typically in the most distal portion of the extremity, such as the forefoot or toes), ulceration, or gangrene. The pain is typically exacerbated by elevation of the extremity and alleviated by placing the leg in a dependent position from which arterial pressure is increased by gravity. Ischemic ulceration may occur when minor traumatic lesions fail to heal because of inadequate blood flow. Gangrene occurs when arterial blood flow is so poor that areas with the least perfusion undergo spontaneous necrosis (Figure 19.1).

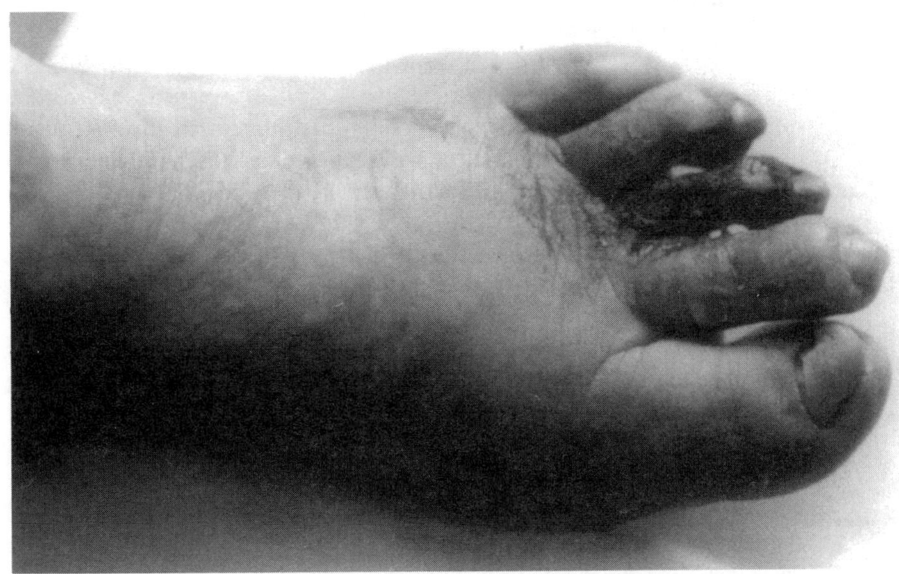

FIGURE 19.1 Gangrene of the left third toe resulting from ischemia.

The assumption that rest pain or tissue loss results in uniform limb loss is not entirely valid, as shown by several studies using nonoperative therapy (Rivers, Veith, Ascer, & Gupta, 1986; Schuler et al., 1984). Chronic ischemia represents a spectrum of levels of disease from fairly benign, mild intermittent claudication to the gangrenous extremity. The likelihood of limb loss remains related to the severity of the ischemia at initial presentation, as measured both angiographically and via arterial Doppler signals. Absent Doppler signals carry a poor prognosis for the limb in question if no intervention is performed (Felix, Siegel, & Gunther, 1987).

The success of exercise and cessation of smoking makes nonoperative therapy the first treatment option in patients with intermittent claudication. An additional reason is the observation (although controversial) that a failed bypass graft may acutely induce limb-threatening ischemia or ultimately obligate a higher level of amputation than a nonoperated limb (Dardik, Kahn, Dardik, Sussman, & Ibrahim, 1982; Schlenker & Wolkoff, 1975). Operative management is thus reserved for threatened limb loss as determined by clinical and angiographic parameters.

Extracranial Cerebrovascular Disease

Cerebrovascular disease may include disease of the aortic arch, carotid arteries, or the vertebrobasilar system. Functional presentation of extracranial cerebrovascular disease may be asymptomatic, a transient ischemic attack (e.g., amaurosis fugax or other neurological deficit resolving within 24 hours), or following a completed stroke. Depending on the degree of disability, patients may require various types of rehabilitation and support services. It is extremely important to evaluate the extracranial circulation in patients presenting for rehabilitation after strokes so that further strokes may be prevented when possible by surgical or medical intervention.

The diagnosis and treatment of extracranial cerebrovascular disease begins at the aortic valve. The decrease in annual stroke rate in the United States has paralleled the increase in the frequency of carotid endarterectomy (Lamparello & Riles, 1975). Currently, more than 100,000 carotid endarterectomies are performed annually in this country. Over the past 40 years, the safety of carotid surgery has progressed, with most large centers reporting perioperative morbidity and mortality rates of less than 2%. Indications for extracranial cerebral revascularization have been well defined for both symptomatic and asymptomatic patients in large prospective, randomized trials. The North American Symptomatic Carotid Endarterectomy Trial (NASCET) established that symptomatic patients with greater than 70% diameter reduction of the internal carotid artery have a significant reduction in the incidence of stroke with surgery, compared to medical management alone (NASCET Collaborators, 1991). Similarly, the Asymptomatic

Carotid Atherosclerosis Study (ACAS) demonstrated better stroke prevention in patients with greater than 60% stenosis treated with endarterectomy versus those treated medically (Executive Committee for ACAS, 1995). As noted above, such patients may present after completed strokes, with a history of a transient ischemic attack, or they may be asymptomatic, with carotid stenoses detected on duplex examinations performed as part of a workup for a bruit heard on physical exam or for nonspecific neurological symptoms.

Upper extremity ischemia, too, is often related to aortic arch disease. Emboli to the hands or fingers may originate in the chambers of the heart, aortic arch, or axillary and subclavian arteries. Transesophageal echocardiography (TEE) and aortic arch and upper extremity angiography are the tests of choice for identifying a potential source of emboli. Magnetic resonance angiography also may be useful. Functional presentation is similar to that in the lower extremity, with sudden onset of pain and cyanosis of the distal hand or fingers. Pulses may be absent. Collateral circulation of the upper extremity is usually excellent, often allowing the hand to remain viable during workup.

Venous Disease

Patients with venous disorders frequently exhibit a chronic course and are not often dramatically improved by surgical procedures. Chronic venous insufficiency is the most common form of venous disease, and nonoperative therapy remains the mainstay of treatment. The other form of venous disease seen commonly, especially in the nonambulatory patient, is acute deep venous thrombosis. This is more sudden in onset and requires systemic anticoagulation or occasionally placement of a vena cava filter. These two forms of venous disease will be discussed separately.

Chronic Venous Insufficiency

The functional presentation of chronic venous insufficiency (CVI) includes swelling, pain and ulceration of the lower extremity. This is caused by valvular incompetence of the venous system, resulting in increased hydrostatic pressure. Typically, CVI presents as swelling of the distal lower extremity with thickening of the subcutaneous tissue in the perimalleolar "gaiter" distribution. Mild CVI is associated with mild to moderate ankle edema. Often the patients complain of a feeling of heaviness or pain in the legs. This mild form of insufficiency is usually limited to the superficial veins. Moderate CVI has hyperpigmentation of the skin, moderate brawny edema, and subcutaneous fibrosis without ulceration. Severe CVI is associated with ulceration, eczemoid skin changes (stasis dermatitis), and severe edema. Extensive involvement of the deep venous system and diffuse loss of valvular function is present.

The venous anatomy consists of a superficial and a deep system. In the lower extremity, the longest superficial vein, the greater saphenous vein, is located anterior to the medial malleolus and courses along the medial aspect of the leg until it reaches the saphenofemoral junction in the medial aspect of the proximal thigh. Connecting the superficial system to the deep system are the perforating veins.

The perforating veins are variable in location. However, the most important set is in the medial aspect of the lower leg, called Cockett's perforators. Insufficiency of the valves in these perforators lead to the characteristic physical findings of CVI in the posteromedial malleolar area. Blood flow in the leg is from the superficial to the deep system via the perforating veins. Blood is propelled to the heart via the deep veins. Failure of any of the venous valves, perforators, or calf muscle pump (which acts to force blood against gravity) will create a situation in which the lower leg is exposed to the pressure created by a column of blood. The sustained venous hypertension is felt to be the cause of CVI. The venous hypertension is transmitted to the skin, causing dermal proliferation. Eventually, lymphatic destruction occurs, with the subsequent accumulation of colloid materials in the subcutaneous tissue. The resulting edema and fibrin deposition causes cellular damage and eventual ulceration.

Bed rest and limb elevation have universally been accepted as effective therapy for CVI. However, they are impractical for most patients, particularly those in a rehabilitation program promoting ambulation. Effective therapy must control the symptoms of CVI, promote healing, and prevent recurrence of venous stasis ulcers while allowing for normal ambulation.

Several studies have shown the benefits of compression stockings in the treatment of CVI and venous ulceration (Dinn & Henry, 1992; Mayberry, Moneta, & Taylor, 1991). Cellulitis may be associated with CVI and often requires oral or intravenous antibiotic therapy. Hydrocortisone cream may help surround stasis dermatitis. Typical compression stockings have 30 to 40 torr of elastic compression at the level of the ankle, which gradually decreases more proximally. This type of stocking may be used with normal arterial circulation. If arterial circulation is compromised, a stocking with less compression must be used. In addition, Ace bandages may be used. There are multiple brands of compression stockings on the market, with different designs to make application possible for the patient with disability.

Acute Deep Venous Thrombosis

Acute deep venous thrombosis may occur in the upper or (more commonly) the lower extremity. In the upper extremity, thrombus may occur in the axillosubclavian vein, and the most common causes are thoracic outlet syndrome and catheter-related thrombosis. Under most circumstances, one or more of the features of Virchow's triad for venous thrombosis is present. The triad includes endothelial injury (as by a catheter), stasis (as by thoracic outlet obstruction), and a hypercoagulable state (as with some malignancies).

Functional presentation of upper extremity deep venous thrombosis includes swelling of the extremity, usually to the level of the axilla, and prominence of the subcutaneous veins over the shoulder girdle and the anterior chest wall, which become engorged with collateral venous flow resulting from obstruction of the deep vein (Figure 19.2). Pain of an aching or stabbing type may include the shoulder and axilla but can also be felt in the arm. These classic symptoms are particularly common in patients who thrombose acutely due to thoracic outlet compression. This can occur after weight lifting or similar exertional activity by the upper extremity. Axillosubclavian vein thrombosis may also present after sleeping, probably due to sleeping with the arm overhead (with the thoracic outlet partially obstructed).

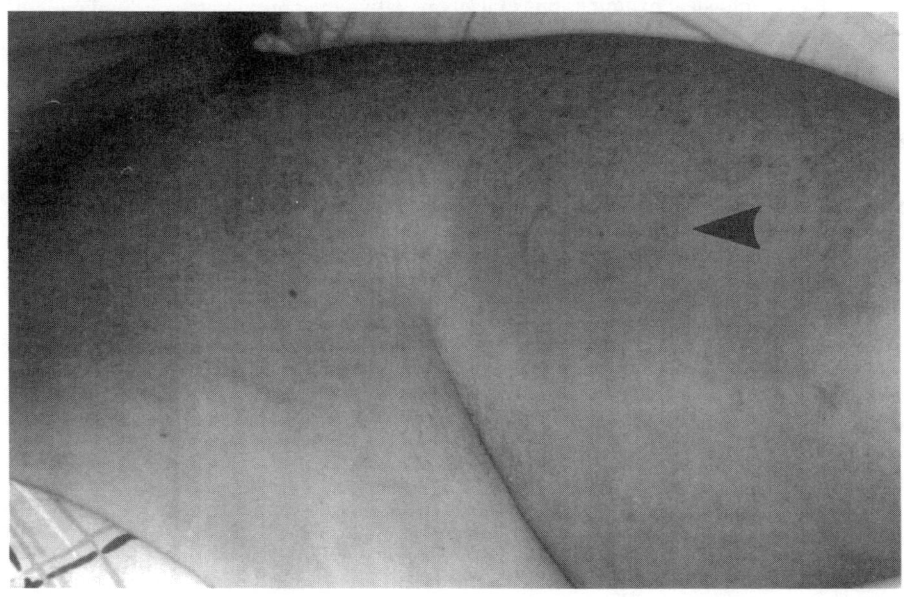

FIGURE 19.2 Swollen proximal left upper arm in patient with axillosubclavian thrombosis. Arrow shows engorged subcutaneous veins over anterior shoulder.

Initial diagnosis of axillosubclavian vein thrombosis is by venous duplex examination. If this is negative but there is a high clinical index of suspicion, then a venogram should be performed. Similarly, if the duplex is positive and thrombolytic therapy is being considered, venography is indicated. The reported incidence of pulmonary embolism with untreated upper extremity deep venous thrombosis is about 9%–12% (Becker, Philbrick, & Walker, 1991). Patients should be treated with heparin anticoagulation followed by a 3–6-month course of Coumadin. Persistent symptoms are least likely in patients with catheter-related thrombosis. Chronic symptoms (arm swelling with exercise) occur in about 38% of patients treated with anticoagulation and 15% receiving thrombolytic therapy (intraarterial urokinase infusion), compared with 64% receiving no therapy (Becker et al., 1991). When axillosubclavian vein thrombosis is recognized, a vascular surgeon should be consulted to further direct therapy. Unless contraindicated, anticoagulation should be started promptly to prevent further propagation of thrombus.

The signs and symptoms of lower extremity deep venous thrombosis are similar to that of the upper extremity. They include swelling of the limb, prominence of superficial veins, and pain, which is usually dull in character. Unfortunately, physical examination is falsely negative in approximately 50% of patients with acute deep venous thrombosis, as well as falsely positive in patients with symptoms related to conditions other than deep venous thrombosis.

The acute complication of deep venous thrombosis is pulmonary embolism and the late complication is the postthrombotic syndrome. This syndrome is that of chronic swelling and venous insufficiency resulting from valvular damage caused by the thrombus. Anticoagulation will reduce the risk of pulmonary embolus from approximately 25% if left untreated to less than 5% (Hyers, Hull, & Weg, 1992). In patients with a contraindication to anticoagulation, a vena cava filter may be placed (usually percutaneously). These devices will lower the incidence of pulmonary embolus to 2%–4%.

Abdominal Aortic and Peripheral Arterial Aneurysmal Disease

Abdominal aortic aneurysm (AAA) is defined as a focal dilation of the aorta at least 50% greater than the expected normal diameter (Johnston, Rutherford, & Tilson, 1991; see Figure 19.3). The main complication of AAA is rupture, for which the mortality may exceed 90%. The 5-year risk of rupture for AAA of 5 cm or greater in diameter ranges from 25%–40%. This may be as high as 20% per year for aneurysms greater than 7 cm in diameter. Aneurysms measuring between 4 cm and 5 cm in diameter have lower 5-year rupture rates, about 3%–12% (Brown, Pattenden, & Gutelius, 1992). Aneurysms less than 4 cm in

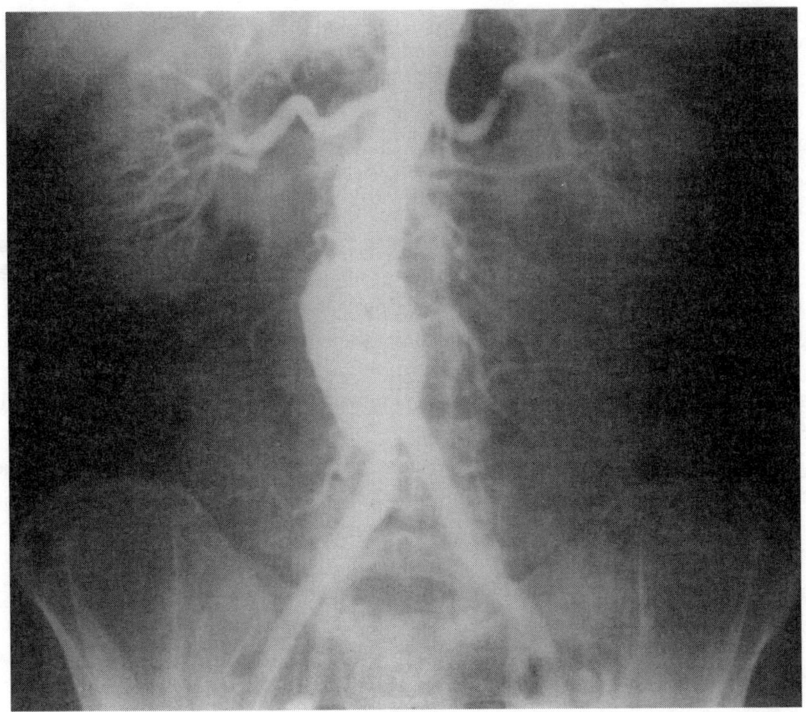

FIGURE 19.3 Angiogram of an infrarenal abdominal aortic aneurysm.

diameter have about a 2% rate of rupture. Overall elective surgical mortality is about 2%–4% (Ernst, 1993). Therefore, repair of AAA is reserved for asymptomatic aneurysms greater than 5 cm in diameter, symptomatic aneurysms (abdominal or back pain), or a ruptured AAA. Rarely, a laminated thrombus from the inner lining of an aneurysm sac may embolize to the lower extremities. This is also an indication for repair regardless of aneurysm diameter. Standard surgical repair is by replacement of the aneurysmal segment with a synthetic graft, usually Dacron. Recent technological advances have included the successful use of transfemorally placed vascular endografts that exclude the aneurysmal segment from arterial pressure.

AAA usually presents as a finding on routine physical examination (pulsatile abdominal mass) or as an incidental finding on a radiological study (abdominal ultrasound, CT scan, or magnetic resonance image) obtained for other reasons. Any aneurysm greater than 3 cm in diameter should be brought to the attention of an internist or vascular surgeon, who can follow the patient with yearly ultrasound examination to monitor the aneurysm size. Average annual growth of AAA is about 0.4 cm in diameter per year.

Popliteal artery aneurysms (PAA) are the most common peripheral artery aneurysm. There is a strong association of PAA with AAA. A patient with a unilateral PAA has a 50% chance of having a contralateral PAA and a 30% chance of having a AAA. More than 90% of PAAs occur in men (Szilagyi, Schwartz, & Reddy, 1981).

A popliteal artery is considered aneurysmal if its diameter exceeds 2 cm or 1.5 times the diameter of the proximal, nonaneurysmal segment. The clinical presentation is variable. Almost 30% of PAAs are symptomatic. They are usually found on physical examination (pulsatile mass or wide pulse at popliteal fossa) or incidentally on ultrasound, CT scan, or magnetic resonance imaging of the popliteal fossa. Results of surgical management in this group of patients is excellent.

Symptomatic PAAs usually present with distal embolization to the tibial arteries. Rupture is rare. This embolization is often severe, with lower limb ischemia occurring in up to 70% of patients and amputation rates as high as 20% (Reilly, Abbott, & Darling, 1983). Elective repair of all PAAs is recommended because of the high rate of limb loss once these aneurysms become symptomatic.

PSYCHOLOGICAL AND VOCATIONAL IMPLICATIONS

Peripheral vascular disease can leave patients with severe vocational impairment and psychological stress. Partial or complete amputation of a limb and the ramifications of strokes can be tremendously disabling, both physically and psychologically.

Two thirds of all lower-extremity amputations are currently performed as a result of complications of PVD or diabetes. As a result, a majority of lower-extremity amputations are being performed by vascular surgeons. The purpose of amputation is to remove gangrenous tissue, relieve pain, obtain primary healing of the most distal amputation possible, and obtain maximum rehabilitation after amputation.

It has been shown that the greatest chance of successful ambulation is with expeditious rehabilitation, either by immediate postoperative prosthesis or accelerated conventional programs utilizing a temporary prosthesis until a permanent prosthesis can be made (Folsom, King, & Rubin, 1992). Advantages of early ambulation include decreased hospital time, increased rates of rehabilitation, a reduction in the complications of amputation, and an improvement in the psychological outcome of the patient after amputation (Bradway, Racy, & Malone, 1984). Early ambulation alleviates a sense of loss and inadequacy experienced by many amputees. It is clear that a full rehabilitation team provides the best outcome. This should include the rehabilitation physician, prosthetist, patient family, physical and occupational therapists, social services, and community services.

Peripheral vascular disease is present in many patients who have had strokes, and it is commonly the underlying cause of those strokes. Fortunately, the perioperative stroke rate for carotid endarterectomy in most major centers is less than 3%. However, many patients present with a completed stroke prior to carotid endarterectomy, and the operation serves only to prevent further infarction. As a result, many patients with PVD, and in particular those with extracranial cerebrovascular disease, may require rehabilitation from stroke.

Major factors affecting rehabilitation of stroke victims include motivation and family support (Evans & Northwood, 1983). In addition, depression may be a significant complication of stroke, and it can inhibit patient motivation (Parikh, Lipsey, & Robinson, 1987). Anxiety and fear are also common among stroke victims. This distress can be eased by an empathic rehabilitation team. The recovery of physical function and motor skills is often enhanced by the emotional stability of the patient. In turn, the return of function enhances psychosocial functioning. Thus, psychosocial, recreational, and vocational interventions must all be provided. Peer support also may be helpful. All of these services should be provided in the setting of a directed stroke rehabilitation program, which has been shown to enhance functional ability beyond that of natural recovery (Kalra, 1994).

Age alone probably does not play a major role in determining the recovery of a patient with stroke. However, it may be associated with significant medical comorbidities (such as PVD) that may make recovery more difficult. Consequently, older patients may have longer recovery times and require increased psychosocial support.

CONCLUSIONS

Patients with PVD usually have multiple medical problems, and the nature of their disease may be chronic and involve multiple organ systems. Because of the high incidence of limb surgery, limb loss, and stroke, patients with PVD are in particular need of rehabilitation medicine and services. The chronic nature of PVD requires the rehabilitation team to be keenly aware of its functional presentation, as recurrences or progression of disease are not uncommon. It is only with a full range of physical and psychological rehabilitation services that patients with PVD may be completely treated.

REFERENCES

Becker, D. M., Philbrick, J. T., & Walker, F. B. (1991). Axillary and subclavian venous thrombosis: Prognosis and treatment. *Archives of Internal Medicine, 151,* 1934–1943.

Bradway, J. P., Racy, J., & Malone, J. M. (1984). Psychological adaptation to amputation. *Orthotics and Prosthetics, 38,* 46–50.

Brown, P. M., Pattenden, R., & Gutelius, J. R. (1992). The selective management of small abdominal aortic aneurysms: The Kingston study. *Journal of Vascular Surgery, 15,* 21–27.

Cronenwett, J. L., Warner, K. G., Zelenock, G. B., Whitehouse, W. M., Graham, L. M., Lindenhauser, S. M., & Stanley, J. C. (1984). Intermittent claudication: Current results of non-operative management. *Archives of Surgery, 119,* 430–436.

Dardik, H., Kahn, M., Dardik, I., Sussman, B., & Ibrahim, I. (1982). Influence of failed bypass procedures on conversion of below-knee to above-knee amputation levels. *Surgery, 91,* 64–69.

Dinn, E., & Henry, M. (1992). Treatment of venous ulceration by injection sclerotherapy and compression hosiery. *Phlebology, 7,* 23–26.

Ernst, C. B. (1993). Abdominal aortic aneurysm. *New England Journal of Medicine, 328,* 1167–1173.

Evans, R. L., & Northwood, L. (1983). Social support needs in adjustment to stroke. *Archives of Physical Medicine and Rehabilitation, 64,* 61–64.

Executive Committee for the Asymptomatic Carotid Atherosclerosis Study. (1995). Endarterectomy for asymptomatic carotid artery stenosis. *Journal of the American Medical Association, 273,* 1421–1428.

Felix, W. R., Jr., Siegel, B., & Gunther, N. L. (1987). The significance for morbidity and mortality of Doppler absent pedal pulses. *Journal of Vascular Surgery, 5,* 849–855.

Folsom, D., King, T., & Rubin, J. (1992). Lower extremity amputation with immediate postoperative prosthetic placement. *American Journal of Surgery, 164,* 320–322.

Hyers, T. M., Hull, R. D., & Weg, J. G. (1992). Antithrombotic therapy for venous thromboembolic disease. *Chest, 102*(Suppl.), 408–425.

Imparato, A. M., Kim, G. E., Davidson, T., & Crowley, J. G. (1975). Intermittent claudication: Its natural course. *Surgery, 78,* 795–799.

Johnston, K. W., Rutherford, R. B., & Tilson, M. D. (1991). Suggested standards for reporting on arterial aneurysms. *Journal of Vascular Surgery, 13,* 452–458.

Jonason, T., & Ringquiest, I. (1985). Factors of prognostic importance for subsequent rest pain in patients with intermittent claudication. *Acta Medica Scandinavica, 218,* 27–33.

Kalra, L. (1994). The influence of stroke unit rehabilitation on functional recovery from stroke. *Stroke, 25,* 821–825.

Lamparello, P. J., & Riles, T. S. (1975). MR angiography in carotid stenosis: A clinical perspective. *MRI Clinics of North America, 3,* 455–465.

Mayberry, J. C., Moneta, G. L., & Taylor, L. M. (1991). Fifteen-year results of ambulation compression therapy for chronic venous ulcers. *Surgery, 109,* 573–581.

North American Symptomatic Carotid Endarterectomy Trial Collaborators. (1991). Beneficial effect of carotid endarterectomy in symptomatic patients with high-grade stenosis. *New England Journal of Medicine, 325,* 445–453.

Parikh, R. M., Lipsey, J. R., & Robinson, R. G. (1987). Two-year longitudinal study of poststroke mood disorders: Dynamic changes in correlates of depression at one and two years. *Stroke, 18,* 579–584.

Peabody, C. N., Kannel, W. B., & McNamara, P. M. (1974). Intermittent claudication: Surgical experience. *Archives of Surgery, 109,* 693–697.

Reilly, M. K., Abbott, W. M., & Darling, R. C. (1983). Aggressive surgical management of popliteal artery aneurysms. *American Journal of Surgery, 145,* 498–502.

Rivers, S. P., Veith, F. J., Ascer, E., & Gupta, S. K. (1986). Successful conservative therapy of severe limb threatening ischemia: The value of nonsympathectomy. *Surgery, 99,* 759–762.

Rosenbloom, M. S., Flanigan, D. P., Schuler, J. J., Meyer, J. P., Durham, J. P., Edrup-Jorgensen, J., & Schwarcz, T. H. (1988). Risk factors affecting the natural history of claudication. *Archives of Surgery, 123,* 867–870.

Schlenker, J. D., & Wolkoff, J. S. (1975). Major amputation after femoropopliteal bypass procedures. *American Journal of Surgery, 129,* 495–499.

Schuler, J. J., Flanigan, D. P., Holcroft, J. W., Ursprung, J. J., Mohrland, J. S. A., & Pyke, J. (1984). Efficacy of prostaglandin E1 in the treatment of lower extremity ischemic ulcers secondary to peripheral vascular occlusive disease: Results of a prospective randomized double-blind multicenter clinical trial. *Journal of Vascular Surgery, 1,* 160–170.

Szilagyi, D. E., Schwartz, R. I., & Reddy, D. L. (1981). Popliteal arterial aneurysms. *Archives of Surgery, 116,* 724–728.

Chapter 20

Psychiatric Disabilities

Gary R. Bond

The term *psychiatric disability* has been used by the vocational rehabilitation (VR) system to describe a range of psychiatric disorders interfering with the capacity to work and function successfully in the community. The VR disability coding system distinguishes three types of psychiatric disability: psychotic disorders, psychoneurotic disorders, and other character disorders. Derived from the psychiatric diagnostic system in practice four decades ago, these categories are now archaic. Currently, the diagnostic standards in the mental health field are codified in the *Diagnostic and Statistical Manual of Mental Disorders*, fourth edition (*DSM-IV*). This compendium of mental disorders is the culmination of work by the American Psychiatric Association (APA) begun in 1952 and updated periodically (APA, 1994).

Unlike earlier diagnostic systems, *DSM-IV* has adopted a descriptive, atheoretical stance toward defining disorders. It attempts to define symptoms of mental disorders through the use of observable criteria. To increase specificity, DSM-IV uses a *multiaxial system* of diagnosis, with assessment on five distinct dimensions. Axis I, which describes clinical syndromes, is most pertinent to psychiatric disability, although the personality disorders on Axis II are also relevant. Substance use disorders (on Axis I) and developmental disorders (on Axis II) are grouped separately from the psychiatric disabilities, not only by VR but also by most state mental health systems. The remaining axes concern physical disorders (III), severity of psychosocial stressors (IV), and level of functioning (V).

Proper assessment requires a trained diagnostician who administers a structured interview and has access to records of the patient's psychiatric history. In practice, many rehabilitation clients receive diagnoses based on far less rigorous assessment procedures. Not only is the VR disability coding system archaic, it does not reflect the limited role of psychiatric diagnoses in rehabilitation practice. Although important for treatment planning, particularly medication decisions, diagnosis is less relevant to rehabilitation planning than a functional assessment of the individual's strengths and weaknesses in specific environments (Anthony, Cohen, & Cohen, 1984).

Information on psychiatric diagnosis is widely available in many sources, ranging from technical manuals (APA, 1994) to less technical but detailed sources, such as abnormal psychology textbooks and guides for the general public (Andreasen, 1984; Bernheim, Lewine, & Beale, 1982; Mueser & Gingerich, 1994; Torrey, 1995). Space does not permit more than a general description of only a few of the major diagnoses, falling under the groupings of psychotic disorders, anxiety disorders, and personality disorders.

PSYCHOTIC DISORDERS

A psychotic episode is a period of time in which an individual is grossly out of touch with reality, as indicated by disorientation and confusion, odd sensory experiences, false beliefs, and/or severe disturbances of mood accompanied by behaviors that sometimes are life-threatening (e.g., not eating). Psychotic disorders have many different patterns of episodes. Some psychotic episodes are brief and nonrecurrent (as in brief reactive psychosis); in other individuals there are acute episodes interspersed with normal or near-normal adjustment, and in still other instances the disturbance is relatively continuous, punctuated by periods of temporary improvement and deterioration.

Disorders that represent major variants in behavior and can include psychotic symptoms historically have been placed into two categories: *organic* and *functional*. Organic mental disorders are so labeled because they are known or presumed to have a specific brain dysfunction (e.g., those caused by brain tumors, senility, and alcohol abuse). Those disorders are not discussed in this chapter. The etiology of the functional psychotic disorders is not clearly established, although it is now widely accepted that this latter group of disorders also can be traced to specific brain abnormalities. There are two main types: disorders of *thought* (schizophrenia) and of *mood* (mood disorders). Among the remaining psychotic diagnoses, a common one is *schizoaffective* disorder, which applies to individuals who have symptoms of both these major types.

Schizophrenia

The lifetime prevalence rate for schizophrenia in the general population is approximately 1%. A major epidemiological study found a 1-month prevalence rate of

0.6% among community residents in 5 American cities (Robins & Regier, 1991). The first episode of schizophrenia usually occurs between the ages of 15 and 30. Males are as likely as females to develop schizophrenia, but males are more likely to have their first psychiatric hospitalization before the age of 25, whereas after 25 the opposite is true.

The presentation of schizophrenia includes *positive symptoms*—behaviors that are notably odd and socially deviant, such as hallucinations (sensory experiences in the absence of any environmental stimuli) and delusions (false beliefs, often bizarre, typically firmly held even in the face of disconfirming evidence). Schizophrenic hallucinations are most often auditory, frequently in the form of hearing voices. In a major study of schizophrenia, 74% of the sample reported auditory hallucinations (Sartorius, Shapiro, & Jablonsky, 1974). Delusions range from innocuous confusions to extensive paranoid delusions involving perceived threats from conspiracies of seemingly unrelated people and events. Delusions often involve *ideas of reference*, in which a person attaches personal significance to unrelated activities of others (e.g., concluding that an overheard conversation between strangers refers to oneself). *Paranoid* delusions may be combined with delusions of grandeur, an exaggerated belief in one's own powers and sometimes the assumption of the identity of a famous person. *Thought broadcasting* (belief in the ability to transmit thoughts directly from one's mind to another person) and *thought insertion* (belief in the reception of thoughts in this fashion) are also positive symptoms of schizophrenia.

Other common symptoms relate to peculiar patterns of speech, such as loose associations (odd juxtaposition of topics and ideas), incoherence, neologisms (invented words with private meanings), and poverty of speech (conversation conveying little information). Persons with schizophrenia have difficulty with words that have more than one meaning; a word they interpret with the wrong meaning may lead them off on a tangent. Also, they are often baffled by simple analogies, as suggested by their poor performance in diagnostic tests requiring that they interpret common proverbs. Green (1996) concluded that deficits in verbal memory and vigilance are common in people with schizophrenia and that these neurocognitive deficits affect their everyday functioning. In addition to cognitive problems, peculiar motor behaviors—odd posture, gait, gestures, and facial expressions—also are common in schizophrenia.

In contrast, the *negative symptoms* of schizophrenia consist of patterns of nonresponsivity: passivity, a lack of spontaneity, *flat affect* (a lack of emotional responsivity), social withdrawal, a lack of motivation, and *anhedonia* (an inability to experience pleasure). Flat affect is especially common, found in 66% of the participants in one study of schizophrenia (Sartorius et al., 1974). The negative symptom of *ambivalence* (difficulty making decisions) may perpetuate a pattern of inaction. Family members often find negative symptoms the most distressing aspect of schizophrenia and more burdensome than positive symptoms (Mueser & Glynn, 1995).

Mood Disorders

The two major types of mood disorders (also known as affective disorders) are *depressive disorders* and *bipolar disorders*. Mood disorders are very common: lifetime prevalence rates for an episode of *major depression* (the most common diagnosis of mood disorder) are 9% to 26% in females and 5% to 12% in males. Bipolar disorders affect 0.4% to 1.2% of the population, in equal proportion of men and women (APA, 1994). Approximately 5% of the population is suffering from a mood disorder at any given time (Robins & Regier, 1991). The age of onset for depression is highly variable. The average age of onset of bipolar disorder is in the late 20s (APA, 1994).

Depression is probably the widest ranging psychiatric disorder in terms of severity and duration. There are vexing diagnostic problems, for example, in deciding if depressed feelings accompanying a physical disability qualify as a separate psychiatric diagnosis. Moreover, one type of depression, *dysthymia*, is never accompanied by psychotic symptoms, nor are psychotic symptoms required for major depression. Thus, the boundaries between different types of depressive disorders are often hard to draw.

The cognitive symptoms of depression include negative, pessimistic beliefs; distorted, negative self-image (including feelings of guilt and worthlessness); suicidal thoughts; and trouble in concentrating. Whereas disordered thought in schizophrenia is often bizarre and puzzling, the distortions accompanying major depression are usually coherent, albeit often magnifying difficulties and jumping to distorted conclusions from incomplete information or selective attention to details. Beck (1967) has termed these distortions *faulty logic*. Depression also includes physical symptoms, such as lethargy, difficulty in sleeping, loss of appetite, lack of energy, and lack of sexual interest. Paradoxically, depression also can be accompanied by excesses in sleeping and eating. Severe depression can be termed psychotic when it includes hallucinations or delusions (e.g., "I am dead").

Bipolar disorder, also known as manic-depressive disorder, differs symptomatically from major depression primarily by the presence of episodes of *mania* in addition to depressive episodes. Each episode lasts from several days to several months. In its most severe form (*rapid cycling*), bipolar disorder involves frequent alternation between manic and depressive episodes, but there are many different patterns, including those in which either mania or depression rarely occurs. Persons experiencing a manic episode are expansive, unrealistically happy (although they can also be irritable when thwarted), impulsive, and easily distracted.

They often have an exaggerated belief in their own abilities and make reckless decisions (e.g., extravagant purchases). Another common symptom is nonstop talking (pressured speech), even when others try to break in or when no one is listening. Their conversation may show *flight of ideas*, in which they jump from one unfinished topic to another.

ANXIETY DISORDERS

In contrast to psychotic disorders, persons with anxiety disorders usually recognize their symptoms and are not out of touch with reality. These conditions, however, can be severely debilitating. Anxiety disorders include *generalized anxiety disorder* (a condition of constant worry and fretting across many situations), *phobic disorder* (an intense fear of an object or situation representing no real danger), *panic disorder* (sudden and unanticipated attacks of intense fear or discomfort, accompanied by symptoms such as increased heart rate, difficulty in breathing, dizziness, and terror), *obsessive-compulsive disorder* (characterized by intrusive and recurring thoughts and impulses, known as *obsessions*, and ritualistic repetitions of illogical behaviors in response to these obsessions, known as *compulsions*), and *posttraumatic stress disorder* (PTSD). Phobic disorders run the gamut from childhood fears (e.g., of the dark), which often disappear spontaneously, to more pervasive and enduring conditions, such as a social phobia, involving exaggerated shyness.

One of the most debilitating anxiety disorders is *agoraphobia*, which may take the form of a fear of leaving home, even to do simple errands or for outside employment. Despite its name, agoraphobia is grouped with panic disorders in DSM-IV because it has been found to be closely associated with them. PTSD is an extreme emotional reaction to a life trauma, such as combat, rape, or an accident, in which the individual reexperiences the feared event in nightmares and flashbacks. Symptoms include a reduced interest in previous activities, estrangement from others, poor concentration, and an inability to recall aspects of the trauma. Although often overlooked, PTSD is a common co-occurring disorder in people with other severe psychiatric disorders (Mueser et al., 1998).

PERSONALITY DISORDERS

Personality disorders are defined by the presence of long-standing, extreme, inflexible personality traits that are maladaptive although not accompanied by a loss of contact with reality. The one best described is the *antisocial personality*. Persons with this disorder, although often superficially charming, violate norms of human behavior and decency, showing no remorse for their hurtful actions.

The remaining personality disorders fall into three clusters: an *odd-eccentric* cluster (e.g., *schizoid personality*), which includes disorders sharing some of the symptoms of schizophrenia but is not as extreme; a *dramatic-impulsive* cluster (e.g., *borderline personality*), and an anxious-fearful cluster (e.g., *passive-aggressive personality*). Except for the antisocial personality, the diagnostic reliability for personality disorders is poor, and the utility of these diagnoses is questionable (Beck, Ward, Mendelson, Mock, & Erbaugh, 1962).

FUNCTIONAL PRESENTATION OF PSYCHIATRIC DISABILITY

Psychiatric disabilities include a heterogeneous group of disorders. Even within a single diagnosis there are wide variations in the severity and chronicity of the illness and the success in coping with the symptoms. The pattern of symptoms within any one individual tends to be quite consistent, however. One further distinction is crucial to the rehabilitation field: the difference between *disabling* psychiatric disorders and those in which individuals are still relatively capable of functioning in major life roles. Of most interest to the rehabilitation field, then, is *severe (and persistent) mental illness* (abbreviated as SMI; previously referred to as chronic mental illness), as defined by three criteria: diagnosis, disability, and duration (Goldman, 1984). These criteria have been widely accepted within the mental health field, although the specific operational definitions have varied.

The majority of persons with SMI have a diagnosis of schizophrenia, and a sizable minority have mood disorders. Severe cases of personality disorder or anxiety disorder also may fulfill this criterion. Disability is defined by role impairment, typically in several of the following areas of functioning: self-care, self-direction, interpersonal relationships, learning and recreation, independent living, and economic self-sufficiency. The criterion for sufficient duration is usually met by at least one admission to a psychiatric hospital or other restrictive setting (e.g., group home) within a 5-year period. A 1980 study estimated that 800,000 to 1,500,000 adult Americans with SMI were living outside institutions (Goldman, 1984). A more recent study estimated that 4.8 million Americans (2.6% of the population) were severely and persistently mentally ill ("Estimation Methodology," 1997). The comments in the remainder of this chapter apply to people with SMI.

Severe mental illness is accompanied by many challenging psychological and social difficulties. These often include the threat of suicide, difficulties coping with interpersonal situations, problems in following instructions, adherence to treatment, substance use, poverty, and involvement with the criminal justice system, as described below.

Feelings of worthlessness and self-hatred are very common in persons with SMI and are associated with suicidal ideation and suicide attempts. The lifetime suicide rate for mood disorders is approximately 15%, over 30 times the rate in the general population. The suicide rate for persons with schizophrenia has been estimated to be between 10% and 13% (Caldwell & Gottesman, 1990).

Persons with SMI tend to function poorly in emotionally charged, critical social situations. In particular, persons with schizophrenia are much more likely to have an exacerbation of psychotic symptoms if they live in families with high expressed emotion, that is, those that are hostile and critical (Brown, Birley, & Wing, 1972). Similar findings have been reported for depression and bipolar disorder (Mueser & Glynn, 1995). More generally, persons with SMI typically have limited tolerance for stress of any kind (e.g., noise, weather, and everyday hassles).

Many persons with SMI are withdrawn and avoid contact with others; 75% have been found to be moderately to very isolated (Minkoff, 1978). They may lack assertiveness in even routine social transactions (e.g., receiving correct change at a store). They often are not inclined to initiate or continue conversations. Lack of spontaneity and other negative symptoms interfere with the formation and maintenance of intimate relationships. In most studies of SMI, the rate of those currently married is 20% or less (Rogers, Anthony, & Jansen, 1988), with particularly low rates reported for men with schizophrenia.

Not surprisingly, persons with SMI have impoverished social networks. If asked to name whom they depend on, they may mention someone they just met. Often a parent or therapist provides the only continuous social contact. Such relationships tend to be nonreciprocal. A person with SMI may show little gratitude or awareness of the effort put forth by the caregiver, despite a pattern of excessive dependency. An estimated 40% of all persons with SMI live with their parents or other family members, often imposing a considerable burden on their families (Torrey, Erdman, Wolfe, & Flynn, 1990).

Another aspect to forming extremely dependent relationships is vulnerability to exploitation as a result of using poor judgment in selecting friends. Increased risk of human immunodeficiency virus (HIV) infection and other sexually transmitted diseases is a logical correlate of this behavior, although statistical data are currently not available.

Persons with SMI are often concrete and literal ("Do you think you could take out the trash?" "I don't think about the trash at all."). Transfer of training from one context to another (e.g., applying skills learned in a hospital setting to a community setting) is often poor (Stein & Test, 1980).

Treatment is difficult when clients act uncooperatively, for example, by refusing to share personal information or take medications as prescribed. Treatment noncompliance should be understood in context: secretive or suspicious attitudes are characteristic of approximately two thirds of all persons with schizophrenia (Sartorius et al., 1974). Moreover, this same survey found that 97% of the sample lacked insight about their illness.

Persons with schizophrenia range widely in their intelligence, following a distribution similar to the nonschizophrenic population. Their capacity to apply their intellectual abilities, however, is impaired by the disorder. After the onset of schizophrenia they often do not attain or regain the level of accomplishment predicted by their premorbid educational achievement. When the onset occurs in adolescence, not only is the individual's peer group affiliation disrupted but also the educational process.

Substance use is a complicating factor in SMI because of its interaction with the mental illness and with psychotropic medications. Prevalence rates vary widely across studies, but at least 20% of persons with SMI also have a co-occurring substance use disorder, with higher rates in young adults (Drake, Osher, & Wallach, 1989).

Poverty is another common consequence of SMI. Among clients with SMI attending mental health programs, it is common for 80% or more to have government entitlements as their main source of support (Rogers et al., 1988). Another substantial segment of the SMI population is homeless. Estimates of mental illness within the homeless population range from 28% to 37% (Dennis, Buckner, Lipton, & Levine, 1991).

The rate of major mental illness is twice as high in jail populations as in the general population (Teplin, 1990). An estimated 67,000 prison inmates in the United States suffer from SMI (Torrey, 1988). Of the 1.1 million individuals held in state and federal prisons in 1995, the 1-year prevalence rates were 5% for schizophrenia, 6% for bipolar disorder, and 9% for unipolar depression (SAMSHA, 1997).

Although many of the characteristics described above are directly related to psychiatric symptoms, they are also influenced by external factors (e.g., institutionalization, societal attitudes, and medications). For example, the stultifying effects of hospital and nursing homes undoubtedly reinforce the passivity and withdrawal so prominent in SMI (Goffman, 1961). At the societal level, the labeling process in mental illness is demoralizing and discriminatory (Estroff, 1989). Because of diagnostic preconceptions, the label of schizophrenia is "sticky"; once obtained, even normal behavior cannot easily eradicate it (Rosenhan, 1973). Moreover, employers attach more stigma to psychiatric disabilities than to physical disabilities (Berven & Driscoll, 1981). In the housing domain, the NIMBY (not in my back yard) prejudice against persons with SMI is intense; group homes are especially likely to meet with community resistance if located in conservative, middle-class neighborhoods (Segal & Aviram, 1978). Stigma continues to be a significant barrier to community integration (Wahl, 1997).

The belief that mental illness leads to increased risk of violent behavior is a popular and damaging stereotype, reinforced by dramatic examples (e.g., the assassination attempt on President Reagan by John Hinkley, who has a diagnosis of schizophrenia). The research findings are complex and ambiguous. One study found more self-reported violent behavior by persons with schizophrenia and other major mental illnesses than by those with no psychiatric diagnosis (Swanson, Holzer, Ganju, & Jono, 1990). However, another study found that the rate of violence by recently discharged patients from psychiatric hospitals who had no symptoms of substance abuse was no different than the rate by community residents living in the same neighborhoods who also were without symptoms of substance abuse (Steadman et al., 1998). Moreover, most persons with SMI are more at risk of being victimized by violence and crime than of being perpetrators.

PROGNOSIS AND TREATMENT

Prognosis

The prognosis for schizophrenia is clearly worse than for other major mental illnesses. For many it is a lifelong disabling condition. However, contrary to what was formerly thought, schizophrenia does not follow a relentless downward course; rather, decline in psychosocial functioning typically plateaus approximately 5 to 10 years after onset (McGlashan, 1988). Traditionally, the prognostic rule of thumb was that one third of patients were expected to show a sharp decline in functioning; one third, to achieve a marginal adjustment; and one third, to recover to essentially former levels of functioning. With appropriate community support and rehabilitation, a substantially larger percentage may approach former levels of functioning (Harding, Brooks, Ashikaga, Strauss, & Breier, 1987). Among persons with schizophrenia, approximately half (and two thirds of their families) recognize the prodromal symptoms (i.e., the warning signs of an impending psychotic episode specific to each individual) as much as a week in advance (Herz, 1984). Psychoeducational groups are designed to assist clients to recognize these symptoms and to employ coping responses (e.g., reducing stress, seeking additional support).

Persons with major depression sometimes recover spontaneously; an estimated 40% of depressed patients recover with no treatment. Approximately half of all patients recover with no recurrence in a 10-year period; most of the remainder will be symptom-free for several years. Between episodes, individuals with mood disorders may be highly competent and nondisabled, as illustrated by the historical examples of Winston Churchill and Abraham Lincoln. With proper treatment, the prognosis is good for the majority of those with depressive disorders. By contrast, bipolar disorder is generally far more debilitating than major depression; untreated, it has a poor prognosis.

History of Treatment Approaches

Prior to the 1950s there were numerous somatic treatments for SMI (Isaac & Armat, 1990). None was effective, except for electroconvulsive therapy (ECT), and although also used with schizophrenia, ECT's demonstrated effectiveness has been limited to accelerating improvement in some severe depressions (Crow & Johnstone, 1986). Psychiatric hospitalization providing little more than custodial care (and often neglect) was standard practice.

Beginning in the 1950s, a combination of economic, legal, and humanitarian factors, in addition to the widespread use of psychotropic medications, led to *deinstitutionalization*, that is, the process of releasing mental patients from state hospitals (Talbott, 1978). The number of residents in state mental hospitals has declined from more than 550,000 to fewer than 90,000 over the past four decades (Torrey, 1995). In 1963 the Community Mental Health Centers Act authorized the creation of a network of community mental health centers (CMHCs), with a broad mission to address the mental health needs of the nation, including the care and treatment of discharged patients with mental disorders (Mental Retardation Facilities, 1963). Altogether, 789 CMHCs were eventually funded, providing the bulk of public mental health services for people with SMI (Torrey, 1995).

Initially, most CMHCs were unprepared to serve people with SMI for several reasons: First, many professionals incorrectly assumed that antipsychotic medications, by themselves, would be sufficient to enable people with SMI to return to the community. Second, CMHCs typically were limited to office-based services, on the assumption that discharged patients would seek CMHC services as necessary. This assumption also proved wrong. A 1986 national survey found that 937,000 (78%) of 1.2 million persons with schizophrenia living outside institutions were not receiving any CMHC outpatient treatment (Torrey, 1988). Other studies showed that clients with SMI receiving outpatient treatment had a high dropout rate (Axelrod & Wetzler, 1989). Finally, CMHCs failed to address a wide range of needs relating to housing, employment, socialization, and other areas of functioning discussed above. The phenomenon of *revolving-door clients*—persons who return frequently to psychiatric hospitals—was one consequence of this limited treatment focus. Over half of all psychiatric patients released from state hospitals returned within 2 years (Anthony, Cohen, & Vitalo, 1978). Four decades later, the problem of revolving-door clients still had not been fully solved; Weiden and Olfson (1993) reported a national annual rate of 250,000 short-term hospitalizations. These trends suggested the need for new, comprehensive approaches to augment traditional CMHC services (Talbott, 1978).

Drug Treatments

Medications for Schizophrenia

Until recently, the main psychopharmacological treatment for schizophrenia was a group of "traditional" antipsychotic medications (also called neuroleptics), including chlorpromazine (Thorazine), thioridazine (Mellaril), and haloperidol (Haldol). The efficacy of these traditional neuroleptics in reducing the relapse rate and the positive symptoms of schizophrenia is well established (Davis, 1980). About two thirds of people with schizophrenia benefit from neuroleptics.

Unfortunately, traditional neuroleptics have troubling side effects, summarized by the mnemonic, THE SEA: *t*ardive dyskinesia, *h*ypotension, *e*xtrapyramidal symptoms, *s*edation, *e*ndocrine effects, and *a*nticholinergic symptoms (Wittlin, 1988). *Tardive dyskinesia,* the most serious of the side effects, involves stereotyped, involuntary movements of the mouth and face. Occurring more commonly after long use of antipsychotic drugs, it is usually irreversible. Hypotension refers to abnormally low blood pressure, which may be experienced as dizziness. *Extrapyramidal symptoms,* prominent during the first week of drug treatment, include tremors of the arms, rigidity of extremities, *akinesia* (listlessness), and *akathisia* (internal restlessness). Sedation is experienced as drowsiness. Endocrine disturbances include sexual dysfunction and weight gain. Among anticholinergic symptoms are dry mouth and blurred vision. Treatment of side effects includes reducing dosage levels, changing medications, and in the case of extrapyramidal effects, the use of antiparkinsonian drugs, such as benztropine (Cogentin). Another limitation to traditional antipsychotics is their lack of impact on negative symptoms of schizophrenia.

Recently, a number of new "atypical" neuroleptics have been developed. Their main advantage over traditional neuroleptics is that they produce fewer motor side effects. Moreover, they also may reduce negative symptoms (Tamminga, 1997). Three of these new drugs and their year of approval by the Food and Drug Administration for use in the United States are clozapine (Clozaril), 1990; risperidone (Risperdal), 1994; and olanzapine (Zyprexa), 1996. Several others are in the final stages of approval: sertindole (Serdolect), quetiapine (Seroquel), and ziprasidone (Zeldox). Clozapine has been used for people with schizophrenia who have not responded to other medications. Approximately 30% of patients not helped by other medications improve with clozapine (Safferman, Lieberman, Kane, Szymanski, & Kinon, 1991). Clozapine requires that patients have frequent blood tests because of the life-threatening risk of *agranulocytosis* (high white blood count). Neither risperidone nor olanzapine has the risk of agranulocytosis, and both appear to have advantages over traditional antipsychotics. In some states, olanzapine and risperidone are being used as first-line medications for schizophrenia; that is, they are prescribed when schizophrenia is first diagnosed (Simon & Toprac, 1997). The atypical neuroleptics are rapidly replacing traditional neuroleptics as the most prescribed medications for schizophrenia. One major drawback of these medications is that they are priced many times higher than traditional neuroleptics. Also, experience with these new medications in routine practice is needed before drawing definitive conclusions about their value (Binder, McNiel, & Sandberg, 1998).

Medications for Mood Disorders

A range of drugs has been used in the treatment of mood disorders. Lithium is used to treat bipolar disorder, particularly during the manic phases, although it is also used by patients who have never had manic episodes. It is effective in 63% to 90% of all cases of mania (Noll, Davis, & DeLeon-Jones, 1985). Lithium is lethal in high doses; thus, patients require careful blood monitoring. Various antidepressant drugs have been used for depression. Before the 1990s, the most common were the tricyclics, including amitriptyline (Elavil) and imipramine (Tofranil). The side effects of the tricyclics include anticholinergic effects, sedation, and irregularities in the cardiovascular system. A group of new antidepressants known as *selective serotonin reuptake inhibitors* (SSRIs), including fluoxetine (Prozac), are relatively free of side effects (Glod, 1996; Möller & Volz, 1996). SSRIs have become enormously popular in a short period of time. They are widely prescribed for depression and a wide array of other psychiatric disorders (Kramer, 1993), although they are not without their detractors (Kirsch & Sapirstein, 1998).

Medications for Anxiety Disorders

Persons with anxiety are often prescribed antianxiety drugs, including diazepam (Valium), which at one time was the most prescribed medication in the United States (Lickey & Gordon, 1991). Research on the psychopharmacology of antianxiety drugs has been rapidly expanding in recent years with the attempt to find specific agents to reduce the symptoms of specific disorders. For example, alprazolam (Xanax) has been used in the treatment of panic disorders. Major drawbacks of some antianxiety drugs are that they are addictive and that they are dangerous if taken in combination with alcohol. Buspirone (BuSpar) is an antianxiety medication that appears to avoid both of these problems.

Medication Nonadherence

Medication nonadherence is a major barrier to effective drug treatment of psychotic disorders, with as many as 50% of patients not taking drugs as prescribed

(Streicker, Amdur, & Dincin, 1986). One review concluded that patients on antipsychotics took an average of 58% of the recommended amount of medications, with higher adherence rates for patients on antidepressants (Cramer & Rosenheck, 1998). Medication education is one strategy used to increase adherence (Wallace, Liberman, MacKain, Blackwell, & Eckman, 1992). Strategies specific to schizophrenia have focused on modifying medications. One common way to ensure adherence is to substitute long-acting injectable forms of medications, such as fluphenazine decanoate (Prolixin), for the usual oral administration (Kane, Woerner, & Sarantakos, 1986). Another strategy is to reduce dosage levels. Some research has suggested that, with careful monitoring, the use of much lower dosage levels than usually prescribed can reduce side effects while retaining the positive effects of neuroleptics (Hogarty et al., 1988). Finally, because the atypical neuroleptics have fewer side effects, it appears that adherence is better for these medications than for traditional neuroleptics.

Recently, *practice guidelines* have been developed in many fields of medicine to systematize knowledge about "best practices" in the treatment of medical disorders, including schizophrenia (Herz et al., 1997) and other psychiatric disorders. Practice guidelines covering medications for psychiatric disorders are evolving.

Psychosocial Interventions

It is now widely accepted that drug treatment of SMI works best in conjunction with practical psychosocial interventions (Hogarty, Goldberg, & Collaborative Study Group, 1973). However, there is no single "best" therapeutic approach for clients with psychiatric disabilities, partly because of the heterogeneity of the population. The foundation for all successful interventions is a therapeutic relationship. This principle applies to people with SMI (McGrew, Wilson, & Bond, 1996), as well as to individuals with less severe psychiatric disorders. Psychotherapeutic approaches emphasizing insight and self-examination are most helpful for individuals who are least disabled. The literature demonstrating the efficacy of psychotherapy for relieving distress in persons with mild anxiety and depression is substantial (Lipsey & Wilson, 1993). No specific psychotherapeutic approach (e.g., client-centered, rational-emotive) appears to be differentially more effective in relieving distress, but behavioral approaches seem more effective in modifying specific behaviors, such as phobic reactions. Both cognitive-behavioral therapy and interpersonal therapy have been used successfully in the treatment of depression (Elkin et al., 1989). Insight-oriented psychotherapy is of limited use in treating schizophrenia and is sometimes harmful (Drake & Sederer, 1986).

Among the ingredients that are crucial for effective interventions for people with SMI are direct, unambiguous communication; supportive, noncritical attitudes; and a focus on problem-solving and skill training (Mueser & Gingerich, 1994). Brief sessions appear to be more effective than the traditional 50-minute hour. The helper should be energetic, supplying "dynamic hopefulness," especially when the client appears unresponsive (Dincin, 1975).

However, a supportive relationship by itself is not a sufficient response to the psychosocial problems of SMI. A comprehensive approach is needed. In the 1970s a national conference of mental health experts culminated in the conceptualization of a "community support program" (CSP) (Turner & TenHoor, 1978). The CSP approach assumes that nontraditional roles for mental health providers are necessary for successful intervention with this population, including outreach to clients not receiving services, assistance in housing and other basic needs, development of permanent supportive networks, vocational rehabilitation, and advocacy. A number of approaches compatible with CSP principles have been developed, including the clubhouse model, assertive community treatment, skills training, family approaches, and self-help.

Clubhouse Model. The psychosocial approach known as the clubhouse originated with the Fountain House program in New York City (Beard, Propst, & Malamud, 1982). In the 1940s the precursor to Fountain House was a self-help group for patients discharged from the state psychiatric hospital. Subsequently, the group sought a professional to serve as center director. Under his direction, the group evolved into an innovative program for helping clients with SMI adjust to community living. Operating outside the mental health system, the program became known as a *clubhouse* because its identity revolved around a central meeting place for members to socialize. Fountain House pioneered many innovations, including two key vocational concepts: the *work-ordered day* and *transitional employment.* With the work-ordered day, members are in prevocational work crews, doing chores around the clubhouse. The clubhouse model emphasizes informal and experiential learning, as opposed to more structured approaches found in skills training. Transitional employment consists of temporary, part-time community jobs located by the clubhouse staff.

Assertive Community Treatment. In the 1970s, Stein and Test (1980) developed an intensive approach known as assertive community treatment (ACT). ACT programs are staffed by a group of professionals working as a team. They serve clients on an individual basis, having contact mostly in clients' homes and neighborhoods rather than in agency offices. The ACT team keeps in frequent contact with clients, typically averaging two visits per week. The nature of the contact depends on the needs of a client on a given day. ACT teams help in such things as budgeting money, shopping, finding housing, and taking medications. ACT teams attempt to anticipate crises, for example, by paying attention to the warning signs of a relapse. ACT programs exemplify assertive outreach in that the staff initiates contacts with clients, rather than depending on clients to keep appointments. Another feature of ACT is its emphasis on continuity and consistency. Clients are not discharged from ACT teams, but continue to receive services on a time-unlimited basis (Test, 1992).

Skills Training. The rationale for skills training is based on the finding that people with SMI often experience difficulties in interpersonal situations, ranging from intimate relationships to everyday contacts in public settings. The goal of social skills training is to systematically teach the component skills necessary for effective social interactions. Typically, the steps in skills training are as follows: (1) give a rationale for learning the skill, (2) role-play the skill, (3) provide an exercise in which the client role-plays the skill, (4) give specific positive and corrective feedback on the client's role play, (5) have the client practice the skill, and (6) give a homework assignment in a real-life situation (Mueser, Drake, & Bond, 1997). Although skills training typically focuses on social skills, it also has been used for a range of other skills needed for independent living. There is little doubt that well-defined skills, including social skills, can be taught to persons with SMI (Wallace et al., 1992). However, most of the extensive research on skill training suffers from a failure to show whether the skills taught in classroom settings generalize to everyday settings (Dilk & Bond, 1996).

Family Approaches. Behavioral family management (BFM) involves intervening with families that have a child or other family member with SMI either living with them or in frequent contact (Falloon et al., 1982). BFM programs include psychoeducation, providing families with factual information about SMI and a frame of reference for understanding the burden of mental illness. BFM therapists train families in behavioral techniques for dealing with their relatives with SMI. The programs draw on the expressed emotion literature and on basic behavioral techniques. Family members are taught, for example, about creating a noncritical atmosphere, setting limits, being concrete and direct, having realistic expectations, and developing problem-solving strategies. Most of the contact with the family is in the home, where in vivo assessments provide more reliable information. McFarlane, Dushay, Stastny, Deakins, and Link (1996) have developed a variation of BFM involving therapy with several families together. It offers advantages similar to those of BFM but in a more cost-effective manner.

Self-help. In the past decade the consumer movement has prompted major changes in the conception of mental health services. Over 500 self-help groups have formed nationwide (Chamberlin, Rogers, & Sneed, 1989). These groups have been active in developing drop-in centers, which provide friendship, social and recreational activities, and concrete assistance (Mowbray, Chamberlain, Jennings, & Reed, 1988). Since its inception in 1979, the National Alliance for the Mentally Ill (NAMI), an organization for families, has grown to a membership of 140,000 (NAMI, n.d.).

Effectiveness of Psychosocial Approaches. Among the various psychosocial treatment approaches, ACT and family approaches have the most empirical support (Mueser et al., 1997). Controlled research on these interventions suggests specific benefits in the areas of relapse and rehospitalization, housing stability, social functioning, and psychotic symptoms. Mueser et al. (1997) identify five characteristics of successful psychosocial interventions: (1) they are usually direct and behavioral; (2) they have specific effects on outcomes they are intended for, with limited generalization to other domains; (3) they are more effective when delivered close to clients' natural environments; (4) short-term interventions are less effective than long-term interventions; (5) effective programs often combine skills training and environmental support.

Access. Access to quality programs is clearly limited (Torrey, 1995). The capacity of exemplary programs is dwarfed by the size of the population in need. For example, Meisler (1997) identified 397 ACT programs in 14 states serving an estimated 24,000 clients. A 1996 directory identified 229 clubhouses in the United States; a survey of 173 programs found that clubhouses averaged an active membership of 118 clients, with average daily attendance of 48 clients (Macias, Jackson, Schroeder, & Wang, in press). Underfunding of mental health services is one major factor in this disparity between need and program capacity.

VOCATIONAL IMPLICATIONS

Unemployment is a major issue for persons with SMI, with less than 15% competitively employed at any time (Rogers et al., 1988). Most clients do not have access to any vocational programs (Noble, Honberg, Hall, & Flynn, 1997), partly because vocational rehabilitation counselors and mental health professionals often regard persons with SMI as poor prospects for employment. The barriers to access to the VR system are substantial (Drake, Becker, Xie, & Anthony, 1995). Moreover, people with SMI have far more difficulty than persons with physical disabilities in obtaining any VR services (Marshak, Bostick, & Turton, 1990). Reviews of the vocational literature have pessimistically concluded that none of the traditional psychiatric rehabilitation approaches (including vocational counseling approaches, skills training, sheltered workshops, job clubs, and transitional employment) are effective in helping people with SMI achieve permanent jobs in the community (Bond, 1992).

Recently, a new vocational approach has been introduced that has more encouraging outcomes. *Supported employment* is intended for people with the most severe handicaps; it is defined as paid work that takes place in normal work settings, with provision for ongoing support services (Wehman & Moon, 1988). It was developed originally for people with developmental disabilities as a more effective, humane, and cost-effective alternative to sheltered workshops (Wehman & Moon, 1988), but subsequently was exported to the psychiatric rehabilitation field. Although first described in the psychiatric rehabilitation literature only recently (Mellen & Danley, 1987), supported employment has been disseminated to many mental health and rehabilitation programs serving psychiatric populations. By 1995 a national survey had identified 36,000 people with mental illness employed in supported employment positions (Wehman, Revell, & Kregel, 1997).

Bond, Drake, Mueser, and Becker (1997) have summarized the research on supported employment for people with SMI. Overall, they found a mean competitive employment rate of 58% for supported employment clients, compared to 21% for clients in control groups receiving traditional vocational assistance. Other indicators of vocational success (such as earnings from employment and job tenure) also favored supported employment. Several studies have shown that day treatment programs can be closed down and replaced with supported employment, leading to better employment outcomes and greater community integration, with no observed negative outcomes (Drake et al., 1994; Drake, Becker, Biesanz, Wyzik, & Torrey, 1996). Among the various supported employment approaches, the *Individual Placement and Support* (IPS) model (Drake, McHugo, Becker, Anthony, & Clark, 1996) has been the most extensively studied. It is based on the following principles:

1. *Competitive employment as goal*: The goal is competitive employment in work settings integrated in a community's economy.
2. *Rapid job search*: Consumers are expected to obtain jobs directly, rather than following lengthy preemployment training.
3. *Integration of rehabilitation and mental health*: Rehabilitation is an integral component of mental health treatment, rather than a separate service.
4. *Attention to consumer preferences*: Services are based on consumers' preferences and choices, rather than on providers' judgments.
5. *Continuous and comprehensive assessment*: Assessment is continuous and based on real work experiences, starting from initial contact with consumers and continuing after a consumer is employed.
6. *Time-unlimited support*: Follow-along supports are continued indefinitely.

Research has been conducted supporting each of these principles (Bond, 1998). For example, rapid job search approaches are more effective than stepwise approaches (Drake, McHugo, et al., 1996). Integration of rehabilitation and mental health services avoids the lack of communication found in brokered approaches (Drake et al., 1995). Long-term support leads to better employment outcomes than do time-limited approaches (Test, 1992). Clients who obtain jobs matching their initial preferences have longer job tenure and greater job satisfaction (Becker, Drake, Farabaugh, & Bond, 1996).

Unfortunately, one key limitation of supported employment is that, in practice, it is limited mostly to entry-level jobs (Bond et al., 1997). Educational programs are one option for higher functioning clients, who may not be challenged sufficiently by traditional psychiatric rehabilitation programs (Hatfield, 1989).

Supported education helps clients obtain education and training in order to have the skills and credentials necessary for obtaining jobs with career potential (Moxley, Mowbray, & Brown, 1993). Unger, Danley, Kohn, and Hutchinson (1987) were among the first to pilot the concept of supported education. Starting in the late 1980s, this concept was applied to training clients to work as mental health paraprofessionals (Sherman & Porter, 1991). This idea has been widely emulated (Mowbray, Moxley, Jasper, & Howell, 1997).

Community integration entails helping people to move out of patient roles, treatment centers, segregated housing arrangements, and work enclaves for people with disabilities, and enabling them to move toward illness self-management, normal adult roles, and normal adult settings in their communities. Like others with long-term illnesses, people with SMI want to manage their own illnesses, to work with and relate to a range of other people, and to live in normal housing situations. Progress has been made toward realizing these goals, although many changes are needed in the mental health system before exemplary services are available to everyone desiring them.

REFERENCES

American Psychiatric Association. (1994). *Diagnostic and statistical manual of mental disorders* (4th ed.). Washington, DC: American Psychiatric Press.

Andreasen, N. C. (1984). *The broken brain.* New York: Harper & Row.

Anthony, W. A., Cohen, M. R., & Cohen, B. F. (1984). Psychiatric rehabilitation. In J. A. Talbott (Ed.), *The chronic mental patient: Five years later* (pp. 137–157). Orlando, FL: Grune & Stratton.

Anthony, W. A., Cohen, M. R., & Vitalo, R. (1978). The measurement of rehabilitation outcome. *Schizophrenia Bulletin, 4,* 365–383.

Axelrod, S., & Wetzler, S. (1989). Factors associated with better compliance with psychiatric aftercare. *Hospital and Community Psychiatry, 40,* 397–401.

Beard, J. H., Propst, R. N., & Malamud, T. J. (1982). The Fountain House model of rehabilitation. *Psychosocial Rehabilitation Journal, 5*(1), 47–53.

Beck, A. T. (1967). *Depression: Clinical, experimental, and theoretical aspects.* New York: Harper & Row.

Beck, A. T., Ward, C. H., Mendelson, M., Mock, J. E., & Erbaugh, J. K. (1962). Reliability of psychiatric diagnosis: 2. A study of consistency of clinical judgments and ratings. *American Journal of Psychiatry, 119,* 351–357.

Becker, D. R., Drake, R. E., Farabaugh, A., & Bond, G. R. (1996). Job preferences of clients with severe psychiatric disorders participating in supported employment programs. *Psychiatric Services, 47,* 1223–1226.

Bernheim, K. F., Lewine, R. R., & Beale, C. T. (1982). *The caring family: Living with chronic mental illness.* Chicago: Contemporary Books.

Berven, N. L., & Driscoll, J. H. (1981). The effects of past psychiatric disability on employer evaluation of a job applicant. *Journal of Applied Rehabilitation Counseling, 12,* 50–55.

Binder, R. L., McNiel, D. E., & Sandberg, D. A. (1998). A naturalistic study of clinical use of risperidone. *Psychiatric Services, 49,* 524–526.

Bond, G. R. (1992). Vocational rehabilitation. In R. P. Liberman (Ed.), *Handbook of psychiatric rehabilitation* (pp. 244–275). New York: Macmillan.

Bond, G. R. (1998). Principles of the Individual Placement and Support model: Empirical support. *Psychiatric Rehabilitation Journal, 22*(1), 11–23.

Bond, G. R., Drake, R. E., Mueser, K. T., & Becker, D. R. (1997). An update on supported employment for people with severe mental illness. *Psychiatric Services, 48,* 335–346.

Brown, G. W., Birley, J. L., & Wing, J. K. (1972). Influence of family life on the course of schizophrenic disorders: A replication. *British Journal of Psychiatry, 121,* 241–258.

Caldwell, C. B., & Gottesman, I. I. (1990). Schizophrenics kill themselves too: A review of risk factors for suicide. *Schizophrenia Bulletin, 16,* 571–589.

Chamberlin, J., Rogers, J. A., & Sneed, C. S. (1989). Consumers, families, and community support systems. *Psychosocial Rehabilitation Journal, 12*(3), 93–106.

Cramer, J. A., & Rosenheck, R. (1998). Compliance with medication regimens for mental and physical disorders. *Psychiatric Services, 49,* 196–201.

Crow, T. J., & Johnstone, E. C. (1986). Controlled trials of electroconvulsive therapy. In S. Malitz & H. A. Sackeim (Eds.), *Electroconvulsive therapy: Clinical and basic research issues* (pp. 12–29). New York: New York Academy of Sciences.

Davis, J. M. (1980). Antipsychotic drugs. In H. I. Kaplan, A. M. Freedman, & B. J. Sadock (Eds.), *Comprehensive textbook of psychiatry* (Vol. 3, pp. 2257–2289). Baltimore: Williams & Wilkins.

Dennis, D. L., Buckner, J. C., Lipton, F. R., & Levine, I. S. (1991). A decade of research and services for homeless mentally ill persons. *American Psychologist, 46,* 1129–1138.

Dilk, M. N., & Bond, G. R. (1996). Meta-analytic evaluation of skills training research for individuals with severe mental illness. *Journal of Consulting and Clinical Psychology, 64,* 1337–1346.

Dincin, J. (1975). Psychiatric rehabilitation. *Schizophrenia Bulletin, 1,* 131–147.

Drake, R. E., Becker, D. R., Biesanz, J. C., Torrey, W. C., McHugo, G. J., & Wyzik, P. F. (1994). Rehabilitation day treatment vs. supported employment: 1. Vocational outcomes. *Community Mental Health Journal, 30,* 519–532.

Drake, R. E., Becker, D. R., Biesanz, J. C., Wyzik, P. F., & Torrey, W. C. (1996). Day treatment versus supported employment for persons with severe mental illness: A replication study. *Psychiatric Services, 47,* 1125–1127.

Drake, R. E., Becker, D. R., Xie, H., & Anthony, W. A. (1995). Barriers in the brokered model of supported employment for persons with psychiatric disabilities. *Journal of Vocational Rehabilitation, 5,* 141–149.

Drake, R. E., McHugo, G. J., Becker, D. R., Anthony, W. A., & Clark, R. E. (1996). The New Hampshire study of supported employment for people with severe mental illness: Vocational outcomes. *Journal of Consulting and Clinical Psychology, 64*, 391–399.

Drake, R. E., Osher, F. C., & Wallach, M. A. (1989). Alcohol use and abuse in schizophrenia. *Journal of Nervous and Mental Disease, 177,* 408–414.

Drake, R. E., & Sederer, L. I. (1986). The adverse effects of intensive treatment of chronic schizophrenia. *Comprehensive Psychiatry, 27,* 313–326.

Elkin, I., Shea, T., Watkins, J. T., Imber, S. D., Sotsky, S. M., Collins, J. F., Glass, D. R., Pilkonis, P. A., Leber, W. R., Docherty, J. P., Fiester, S. J., & Parloff, M. B.

(1989). National Institute of Mental Health Treatment of Depression Collaborative Research Program: General effectiveness of treatment. *Archives of General Psychiatry, 46,* 971–982.

Estimation methodology for adults with serious mental illness. (1997). *Federal Register, 62,* 14928–14923.

Estroff, S. E. (1989). Self, identity, and subjective experiences: In search of the subject. *Schizophrenia Bulletin, 15,* 189–196.

Falloon, I. R. H., Boyd, J. L., McGill, C. W., Razani, J., Moss, H. B., & Gilderman, A. M. (1982). Family management in the prevention of exacerbations of schizophrenia. *New England Journal of Medicine, 306,* 1437–1440.

Glod, C. A. (1996). Recent advances in the pharmacotherapy of major depression. *Archives of Psychiatric Nursing, 10,* 355–364.

Goffman, E. (1961). *Asylums: Essays on the social situation of mental patients and other inmates.* Chicago: Aldine.

Goldman, H. H. (1984). Epidemiology. In J. A. Talbott (Ed.), *The chronic mental patient: Five years later* (pp. 15–31). Orlando, FL: Grune & Stratton.

Green, M. F. (1996). What are the functional consequences of neurocognitive deficits in schizophrenia? *American Journal of Psychiatry, 153,* 321–330.

Harding, C. M., Brooks, G. W., Ashikaga, T., Strauss, J. S., & Breier, A. (1987). The Vermont longitudinal study of persons with severe mental illness: 2. Long-term outcome of subjects who retrospectively met DSM-III criteria for schizophrenia. *American Journal of Psychiatry, 144,* 727–735.

Hatfield, A. B. (1989). Serving the unserved in community rehabilitation programs. *Psychosocial Rehabilitation Journal, 13*(2), 71–82.

Herz, M. I. (1984). Recognizing and preventing relapse in patients with schizophrenia. *Hospital and Community Psychiatry, 35,* 344–349.

Herz, M. I., Liberman, R. P., Lieberman, J. A., Marder, S. R., McGlashan, T. H., & Wang, P. (1997). Practice guideline for the treatment of patients with schizophrenia. *American Journal of Psychiatry, 154*(Suppl.), 1–63.

Hogarty, G., Goldberg, S., & Collaborative Study Group (1973). Drug and sociotherapy in the aftercare of schizophrenia patients: One-year relapse rates. *Archives of General Psychiatry, 28,* 54–64.

Hogarty, G. E., McEvoy, J. P., Munetz, M., DiBarry, A. L., Bartone, P., Cather, R., Cooley, S. J., Ulrich, R. F., Carter, M., & Madonia, M. J. (1988). Dose of fluphenazine, familial expressed emotion, and outcome in schizophrenia. *Archives of General Psychiatry, 45,* 797–805.

Isaac, R. J., & Armat, V. C. (1990). *Madness in the streets: How psychiatry and the law abandoned the mentally ill.* New York: Free Press.

Kane, J. M., Woerner, M., & Sarantakos, S. (1986). Depot neuroleptics: A comparative review of standard, intermediate, and low-dose regimens. *Journal of Clinical Psychiatry, 47*(Suppl.), 30–33.

Kirsch, I., & Sapirstein, G. (1998). Listening to Prozac but hearing placebo: A meta-analysis of antidepressant medication. *Prevention & Treatment, 1*(0002a), http://journals.apa.org/prevention.

Kramer, P. D. (1993). *Listening to Prozac.* New York: Viking Penguin.

Lickey, M. E., & Gordon, B. (1991). *Medicine and mental illness.* New York: W. H. Freeman.

Lipsey, M. W., & Wilson, D. B. (1993). The efficacy of psychological, educational, and behavioral treatment: Confirmation from meta-analysis. *American Psychologist, 48,* 1181–1209.

Macias, C., Jackson, R., Schroeder, C., & Wang, Q. (in press). What is a clubhouse? Report on the ICCD 1996 survey of USA clubhouses. *Community Mental Health Journal.*

Marshak, L. E., Bostick, D., & Turton, L. J. (1990). Closure outcomes for clients with psychiatric disabilities served by the vocational rehabilitation system. *Rehabilitation Counseling Bulletin, 33,* 247–250.

McFarlane, W. R., Dushay, R. A., Stastny, P., Deakins, S. M., & Link, B. (1996). A comparison of two levels of family-aided assertive community treatment. *Psychiatric Services, 47,* 744–750.

McGlashan, T. H. (1988). A selective review of recent North American long-term followup studies of schizophrenia. *Schizophrenia Bulletin, 14,* 515–542.

McGrew, J. H., Wilson, R., & Bond, G. R. (1996). Client perspectives on helpful ingredients of assertive community treatment. *Psychiatric Rehabilitation Journal, 19*(3), 13–21.

Meisler, N. (1997). Assertive community treatment initiatives: Results from a survey of selected state mental health authorities. *Community Support Network News, 11*(4), 3–5.

Mellen, V., & Danley, K. (1987). Special issue: Supported employment for persons with severe mental illness. *Psychosocial Rehabilitation Journal, 9*(2) [whole issue].

Mental Retardation Facilities and Community Mental Health Centers Construction Act of 1963. Pub. L. 88-164 (1963).

Minkoff, K. (1978). A map of chronic mental patients. In J. A. Talbott (Ed.), *The chronic mental patient* (pp. 11–37). Washington, DC: American Psychiatric Association.

Möller, H., & Volz, H. (1996). Drug treatment of depression in the 1990s: An overview of achievements and future possibilities. *Drugs, 52,* 625–638.

Mowbray, C. T., Chamberlain, P., Jennings, M., & Reed, C. (1988). Consumer-run mental health services: Results from five demonstration projects. *Community Mental Health Journal, 2,* 151–156.

Mowbray, C. T., Moxley, D. P., Jasper, C. A., & Howell, L. L. (Eds.). (1997). *Consumers as providers in psychiatric rehabilitation.* Columbia, MD: International Association of Psychosocial Rehabilitation Services.

Moxley, D. P., Mowbray, C. T., & Brown, K. S. (1993). Supported education. In R. W. Flexer & P. L. Solomon (Eds.), *Psychiatric rehabilitation in practice* (pp. 137–153). Boston: Andover Medical Publishers.

Mueser, K. T., Drake, R. E., & Bond, G. R. (1997). Recent advances in psychiatric rehabilitation for patients with severe mental illness. *Harvard Review of Psychiatry, 5,* 123–137.

Mueser, K. T., & Gingerich, S. (1994). *Coping with schizophrenia: A guide for families.* Oakland, CA: New Harbinger Publications.

Mueser, K. T., & Glynn, S. M. (1995). Families as members of the treatment team. In *Behavioral family therapy for psychiatric disorder* (pp. 1–29). Needham Heights, MA: Allyn & Bacon.

Mueser, K. T., Goodman, L. B., Trumbetta, S. L., Rosenberg, S. D., Osher, F. C., Vidaver, R., Auciello, P., & Foy, D. W. (1998). Trauma and posttraumatic stress disorder in severe mental illness. *Journal of Consulting and Clinical Psychology, 66,* 493–499.

National Alliance for the Mentally Ill. (n.d.). *Understanding schizophrenia: What you need to know about this medical illness.* Arlington, VA: Author.

Noble, J. H., Honberg, R. S., Hall, L. L., & Flynn, L. M. (1997). *A legacy of failure: The inability of the federal-state vocational rehabilitation system to serve people with severe mental illness.* Arlington, VA: National Alliance for the Mentally Ill.

Noll, K. M., Davis, J. M., & DeLeon-Jones, F. (1985). Medication and somatic therapies in the treatment of depression. In E. E. Beckham & W. R. Lebe (Eds.), *Handbook of depression: Treatment, assessment and research* (pp. 220–315). Homewood, IL: Dorsey Press.

Robins, L. N., & Regier, D. A. (1991). *Psychiatric disorders in America: The Epidemiologic Catchment Area study.* New York: Free Press.

Rogers, E. S., Anthony, W. A., & Jansen, M. A. (1988). Psychiatric rehabilitation as the preferred response to the needs of individuals with severe psychiatric disability. *Rehabilitation Psychology, 33,* 5–14.

Rosenhan, D. L. (1973). On being sane in insane places. *Science, 179,* 250–258.

Safferman, A., Lieberman, J. A., Kane, J. M., Szymanski, S., & Kinon, B. (1991). Update on the clinical efficacy and side effects of clozapine. *Schizophrenia Bulletin, 17,* 247–261.

SAMHSA. (1997). *Just the facts: The prevalence of co-occurring mental and substance disorders in the criminal justice system.* Rockville, MD: National GAINS Center, Substance Abuse and Mental Health Services Administration.

Sartorius, N., Shapiro, R., & Jablonsky, A. (1974). The international pilot study of schizophrenia. *Schizophrenia Bulletin, 2,* 21–35.

Segal, S. P., & Aviram, U. (1978). *The mentally ill in community-based sheltered care: A study of community care and social integration.* New York: Wiley-International.

Sherman, P. S., & Porter, R. (1991). Mental health consumers as case management aides. *Hospital and Community Psychiatry, 42,* 494–498.

Simon, S., & Toprac, M. (1997, December). *Texas Medication Algorithm Project.* Paper presented at the Fourth Annual Florida Conference on Behavioral Healthcare Evaluation, Orlando.

Steadman, H. J., Mulvey, E. P., Monahan, J., Robbins, P. C., Appelbaum, P. S., Grisso, T., Roth, L. H., & Silver, E. (1998). Violence by people discharged from acute psychiatric inpatient facilities and by others in the same neighborhoods. *Archives of General Psychiatry, 55,* 393–404.

Stein, L. I., & Test, M. A. (1980). Alternative to mental hospital treatment: 1. Conceptual model, treatment program, and clinical evaluation. *Archives of General Psychiatry, 37,* 392–397.

Streicker, S. K., Amdur, M., & Dincin, J. (1986). Educating patients about psychiatric medications: Failure to enhance compliance. *Psychosocial Rehabilitation Journal, 9*(4), 15–28.

Swanson, J. W., Holzer, C. E., Ganju, V. K., & Jono, R. T. (1990). Violence and psychiatric disorder in the community: Evidence from the Epidemiologic Catchment Area surveys. *Hospital and Community Psychiatry, 41,* 761–770.

Talbott, J. A. (Ed.). (1978). *The chronic mental patient.* Washington, DC: American Psychiatric Association.

Tamminga, C. A. (1997). The promise of new drugs for schizophrenia treatment. *Canadian Journal of Psychiatry, 42,* 265–273.

Teplin, L. A. (1990). The prevalence of severe mental disorder among male urban detainees: Comparison with the Epidemiologic Catchment Area program. *American Journal of Public Health, 80,* 663–669.

Test, M. A. (1992). Training in community living. In R. P. Liberman (Ed.), *Handbook of psychiatric rehabilitation* (pp. 153–170). New York: Macmillan.

Torrey, E. F. (1988). *Nowhere to go.* New York: Harper and Row.

Torrey, E. F. (1995). *Surviving schizophrenia: A manual for families, consumers, and providers* (3rd ed.). New York: HarperCollins.

Torrey, E. F., Erdman, K., Wolfe, S. M., & Flynn, L. M. (1990). *Care of the seriously mentally ill: A rating of state programs* (3rd. ed.). Arlington, VA: National Alliance for the Mentally Ill.

Turner, J. C., & TenHoor, W. I. (1978). The NIMH community support program: Pilot approach to a needed social reform. *Schizophrenia Bulletin, 4,* 319–348.

Unger, K. V., Danley, K. S., Kohn, L., & Hutchinson, D. (1987). Rehabilitation through education: A university-based continuing education program for young adults with psychiatric disabilities on a university campus. *Psychosocial Rehabilitation Journal, 10*(3), 35–49.

Wahl, O. (1997). *Consumer experience with stigma: Results of a national survey.* Alexandria, VA: NAMI.

Wallace, C. J., Liberman, R. P., MacKain, S. J., Blackwell, G., & Eckman, T. A. (1992). Effectiveness and replicability of modules for teaching social and instrumental skills to the severely mentally ill. *American Journal of Psychiatry, 149,* 654–658.

Wehman, P., & Moon, M. S. (Eds.). (1988). *Vocational rehabilitation and supported employment.* Baltimore: Paul Brookes.

Wehman, P., Revell, G., & Kregel, J. (1997). Supported employment: A decade of rapid growth and impact. In P. Wehman, J. Kregel, & M. West (Eds.), *Supported employment research: Expanding competitive employment opportunities for persons with significant disabilities* (pp. 1–18). Richmond, VA: VCU Rehabilitation Research and Training Center.

Weiden, P. J., & Olfson, M. (1993). The cost of relapse in schizophrenia. *Schizophrenia Bulletin, 21,* 419–428.

Wittlin, B. J. (1988). Practical psychopharmacology. In R. P. Liberman (Ed.), *Psychiatric rehabilitation of chronic mental patients* (pp. 117–145). Washington, DC: American Psychiatric Association.

Chapter 21

Pulmonary Disorders

Frederick A. Bevelaqua and
Francis V. Adams

Chronic obstructive pulmonary disease (COPD) affects as many as 30 million Americans. It encompasses a spectrum of disorders from asthmatic bronchitis and chronic obstructive bronchitis, which are largely diseases of the airways, to emphysema, which affects both the alveoli and the airways. COPD is the fifth leading cause of death in the United States and a major source of morbidity. It is estimated that more than 5.5 million Americans 55 years and older have COPD (Hodgkin, 1990). The financial impact of obstructive airway disease in the United States is enormous and increasing. The economic effect of these disorders can be estimated in terms of the costs of treatment, reduced productivity because of morbidity, and reduced productivity because of mortality. With proper treatment and rehabilitation many individuals may achieve a degree of comfort and physical capability that will allow them to return to work. Although bronchial asthma is a separate disorder from COPD, it is also a disease of the airways and has many features similar to COPD.

Likewise, other chronic pulmonary disorders, such as the occupational lung diseases, interstitial lung diseases, and cystic fibrosis, have some characteristics in common with COPD. Therefore, an understanding of the clinical characteristics, pathology, and physiology of COPD is crucial to an understanding of the other disorders. In this chapter we will discuss these points in detail and review the management, prognosis, and vocational and psychological implications involved.

CHRONIC OBSTRUCTIVE PULMONARY DISEASE

Disease Description and Definitions

Chronic obstructive pulmonary disease is characterized by decreased expiratory airflow. Reduction in expiratory airflow has two causes: decreased expiratory air flow pressure (decrease in driving pressure) and increased resistance to expiratory air flow. In the lung the driving pressure for expiratory airflow is caused by the elastic recoil pressure of the lung. Increased resistance to airflow results from narrowing of the airways. COPD patients seldom have only one type of lesion, but often one may predominate. In chronic bronchitis, obstruction to airflow is predominantly due to disease of the airways, which results in increased resistance to airflow. In emphysema, airflow obstruction or limitation to airflow primarily results from loss of elastic recoil pressure, which decreases airflow driving pressure. The anatomical changes in the lung associated with the loss of alveoli in emphysema also result in premature compression or closure of the bronchioles on exhalation, which contributes to airflow obstruction. In chronic bronchitis, obstruction to airflow is caused by chronic inflammation of the bronchial passageways, with increased mucus production, smooth muscle hyperplasia, increased bronchomotor tone, and bronchial wall thickening.

The term "asthmatic bronchitis" is often used to refer to a variation of chronic bronchitis in which there is a variable degree of airflow obstruction superimposed on a chronic or fixed degree of obstruction. The variable portion of the airway obstruction is reminiscent of asthma in that there is some reversibility with the use of bronchodilator drugs. However, although in this respect there is some similarity to asthma, which will be discussed in detail later, there is unlikely to be the major reversibility with bronchodilator therapy that is seen in most forms of asthma. The pathophysiology of asthmatic bronchitis is quite similar to that of chronic bronchitis and is characterized by varying degrees of airflow obstruction due to inflammation and increased bronchomotor tone. Indeed, asthmatic bronchitis is thought to be a form of chronic bronchitis, and the distinction between the two may not be relevant. In emphysema the primary pathological process is loss of alveolar walls, with consequent loss of alveolar surface area. This results in hyperinflation, but airflow obstruction or airflow limitation during expiration also occurs because anatomical changes in the lung associated with the loss of alveoli also predisposes to collapse of the smaller airways during expiration.

Emphysema and chronic bronchitis are often considered together under the term COPD because most patients have a combination of chronic bronchitis (or asthmatic bronchitis) and emphysema. In other words, they have both airway disease and alveolar disease. The classic textbook criterion for chronic bronchitis, a chronic productive cough for at least 3 months of the year for 2 consecutive years, is not adequate. The underlying pathophysiology also must be considered. By the time the patient has advanced and irreversible airflow obstruction, particularly at an older age, there is little point in seeking a more specific diagnosis than COPD. However, there is a great deal of importance in identifying those patients who have a major potential for reversibility in response to therapy because they often have a much better prognosis with bronchodilator therapy than do those with more fixed and progressive airflow obstruction.

Other disease states also are characterized by chronic airflow obstruction, for example, cystic fibrosis, bronchiectasis, bronchiolitis obliterans, and interstitial lung diseases. However, they should not be designated as COPD because they have different prognoses, etiologies, and therapies. Because they are not as common as COPD, they will be discussed separately and in less detail later in this chapter.

Etiology, Pathophysiology, and Clinical Features

Several factors are involved in the pathogenesis of COPD, but smoking is the most important. Inflammation of the respiratory tract produced by smoking promotes bronchoconstriction and interferes with the protective antibacterial function of the alveolar macrophages. It also inhibits the normal clearance mechanisms of the tracheobronchial tree. Occupational exposure to dust and fumes also promotes inflammation, bronchospasm, and edema of the airways. Epidemiological data suggest a close relationship between air pollution and COPD, but these factors are usually less common than smoking as a cause of COPD. Inflammation, hypersecretion, and bronchoconstriction increase susceptibility to subsequent infection, which in turn leads to further bronchial obstruction, alveolar destruction, and emphysema. Bronchial obstruction creates a mismatch of ventilation to perfusion that may lead to hypoxia and hypercapnia. If the hypoxia is severe and chronic, it may lead in turn to pulmonary hypertension because hypoxia causes pulmonary vasoconstriction and induces secondary polycythemia. This may eventually progress to right heart failure. Hypercapnia causes respiratory acidosis to develop, which further worsens pulmonary vasoconstriction and bronchoconstriction. A cycle is set up that may eventually lead to respiratory failure.

In addition to all of the above, the development and progression of COPD is largely related to genetic predisposition. In one particular form of COPD, familial emphysema is associated with an inherited deficiency of a proteolytic enzyme inhibitor, α_1-antitrypsin deficiency. Severe α_1-antitrypsin deficiency is associated with emphysema beginning at a relatively early age, usually under 40. The mechanism accounting for this type of familial emphysema is thought to be lysis of elastic lung tissue by enzymes released from blood leukocytes, alveolar macrophages, and bacteria. In the presence of normal levels of this inhibitor the enzymes are prevented from causing lung damage, but when the levels are insufficient, the lung tissue is unprotected from the destructive effects of these enzymes.

Many factors combine to produce airway obstruction in COPD. Spasm of the smooth muscles of the respiratory tract, edema of the airways, excess mucus production, and compression or collapse of bronchial walls are all involved in producing obstruction to airflow. With the loss of alveoli in emphysema, there is a decrease in the supporting framework in which the terminal bronchioles are suspended. Therefore, during expiration, pressure in the alveoli exceeds the pressure in the bronchioles, so the bronchioles are exposed to a compressive force that overwhelms the radial traction forces of the remaining alveoli that tend to keep the bronchioles open. This leads to airway collapse during expiration, known as dynamic compression of the airways. In chronic bronchitis, inflammation of the bronchial mucosa is the primary pathological process. The inflammation may be caused by a variety of infections or irritants, resulting in damage to the mucosa lining the respiratory tract. As a result of this damage, excess amounts of mucus are secreted. The mucosa and smooth muscle lining of the respiratory tract become hypertrophic or enlarged. The mucociliary system that moves mucus upward is impaired, and the normal protective function of the mucus, which is to trap bacteria and irritants, is therefore compromised.

In addition to damaging the mucosa and causing excess mucus production, this inflammation stimulates the parasympathetic nervous system, which enhances spasm of the smooth muscle lining the respiratory tract. Thus, there are two basic types of airway obstruction in chronic bronchitis. One involves direct blockage of the airway due to inflammation and swelling of the mucosa, with subsequent accumulation of mucus in the bronchial tubes and smooth muscle hypertrophy. The other involves narrowing of the bronchial lumen by smooth muscle spasm resulting from inflammation and irritation. Both types of bronchial obstruction also occur in patients with asthma, which will be discussed later, and contribute to the airflow obstruction in emphysema as well.

Although the clinical and pathophysiological features of chronic bronchitis and emphysema often overlap, as discussed above, some patients with COPD have characteristics that more clearly place them in one category or the other. The Type A, or "pink puffer," is considered to have predominantly emphysema, whereas the Type B, or "blue bloater," is considered to have predominantly chronic bronchitis. The reason some patients develop a predominantly Type A clinical profile and others a Type B profile is unclear. As mentioned previously, overlap is so common that it is difficult to consider emphysema (alveolar disease) and chronic bronchitis (airway disease) as separate entities. However, for the sake of simplicity, patients are often labeled as having either chronic bronchitis or emphysema. The patients who have predominantly chronic bronchitis are characterized by a more prominent cough and sputum production. They are more likely to be hypoxic and hypercapnic and to develop cor pulmonale (enlargement of the right ventricle of the heart) secondary to pulmonary hypertension from chronic vasoconstriction of the pulmonary arterioles. Pathological changes in the large airways are more extensive in chronic bronchitis, including mucus gland hyperplasia, smooth muscle hypertrophy, and increased mucus. Disease in the smaller airways is even more important in limiting airflow. These smaller airways may undergo obliteration, resulting in a decrease in the total cross-sectional area of the airways.

Clinically, the patients who predominantly have emphysema have less cough and sputum production. The loss of alveoli is more pronounced. They also tend to be less hypoxic and hypercapnic until the disease is very far advanced. In emphysema the loss of alveoli results in a decreased elastic recoil of the lung, which in turn results in hyperinflation of the lung. This tends to flatten the diaphragm, placing it at a mechanical disadvantage, so that it does not contract properly. Loss of elastic recoil also results in limitation of airflow because it facilitates compression of the airways during expiration (dynamic compression). In severe cases, flow is limited even during quiet breathing because of the easy compression or collapsibility of the airways during exhalation. Such a severely compromised patient would have marked dyspnea even at rest.

Airflow limitation in emphysema is also affected by pathological changes in the small airways themselves. Small airways are normally responsible for 10%–20% of the airway resistance in the respiratory tract. In obstructive lung disease, the resistance to air flow in the small airways resulting from these pathological changes can increase tremendously. In patients with emphysematous lung disease, such small airway disease can also greatly increase the airflow limitation caused by the dynamic compression of the airways. Thus, in patients with emphysema, airflow limitation has two causes. First, the loss of elastic recoil (due to loss of alveoli) causes dynamic compression of the airways during expiration. Second, the pathological changes in the small airways themselves produce increases in airway resistance.

In patients with COPD the loss of alveoli is associated with loss of alveolar capillaries, so emphysematous lungs contain many areas with higher than normal ratios of ventilation to blood perfusion (increased physiological "dead space"). As this happens, the minute ventilation (liters per minute of air moved in and out of the lung) required to produce adequate levels of alveolar ventilation (liters per minute of air actually involved with gas exchange in functioning alveoli) increases, and therefore the total work of breathing increases as well. As the disease progresses, the patient becomes less able to compensate even with increased work of breathing. An even more severe impairment in gas exchange may occur in areas where there is underventilation in relation to perfusion. This is the major cause of hypoxia in COPD.

Patients with emphysema also have areas of low ventilation-to-perfusion matchup and resultant hypoxia because of obstructive inflammatory changes in the airways. This is most striking in patients who present clinically with features of both chronic bronchitis and emphysema. Patients who predominantly have emphysema usually maintain an arterial oxygen level remarkably close to normal, despite a marked degree of airflow limitation, until the disease is very far advanced. Such preservation of arterial oxygen is unusual in patients with severe chronic bronchitis, bronchiectasis, or cystic fibrosis. For an equivalent degree of airflow limitation, the patient who predominantly has emphysema is less likely to develop a low blood oxygen level and high blood carbon dioxide (CO_2) level than is the patient who predominantly has chronic bronchitis. This also reflects a relatively intact ventilatory response to CO_2 in the emphysema patient. This preservation of CO_2 responsiveness in emphysema and the apparently impaired responsiveness in chronic bronchitis are not well understood. Although the patient with emphysema tends to have less severe hypoxemia than does the patient with chronic bronchitis, hypercapnia often becomes a feature, late in the course of even relatively pure emphysema, and again the distinctions between emphysema and chronic bronchitis become blurred.

When emphysema exists in relatively pure form (i.e., no major pathological changes in the airways), there is dyspnea on minimal exertion, but the patient is generally free from productive cough or bronchospasm. Cyanosis and clubbing are usually absent. Use of accessory muscles of respiration and pursed-lip breathing occur. By restricting the airway opening, pursed-lip breathing serves to maintain pressure within the airway itself and helps to minimize the external dynamic compression of the airways during expiration that is characteristic of emphysema. In classic chronic bronchitis there is also dyspnea with minimal exertion, but the patient usually has a more productive cough, often associated with bronchospasm, and cyanosis is more common. Use of the accessory muscles and pursed-lip breathing may also occur, but it is less pronounced than in the more emphysematous type patient. On physical examination the emphysematous lung is hyperresonant. Diaphragmatic excursion and breath sounds are diminished. Wheezes and rhonchi are the result of turbulence associated with obstructive airway pathology and not of the emphysema (loss of alveoli) per se.

When chronic bronchitis predominates, the wheezes and rhonchi are often much more noticeable. Inspection of the thorax and chest x-rays of patients with emphysema usually give the impression of an increased front-to-back diameter of the chest. Clinicians often diagnose pulmonary emphysema from chest x-rays based on the findings of low, flat diaphragms, increased retrosternal air space, elongated mediastinum, enlarged hilar vessels, and bullous changes. These are relatively insensitive findings, and in general the clinician should place much more emphasis on physical examination and pulmonary function studies when evaluating patients with suspected airflow obstruction of any type.

Other Types of COPD

Asthma, bronchiectasis, and cystic fibrosis are other forms of COPD in which the major pathology involves the airways. Asthma and cystic fibrosis will be discussed in more detail later in this chapter because they are important disorders, with characteristic features deserving special attention.

Bronchiectasis is characterized pathologically by chronic and irreversible dilation and distortion of the bronchi. These changes usually follow some sort of inflammatory insult to the respiratory tract (e.g., severe pneumonia or respiratory tract infection) and may be more likely seen if the infection or inflammation occurs in early childhood or infancy, before the development of the respiratory tract has been completed. Anatomical bronchial abnormalities that are congenital in nature may also lead to the development of bronchiectasis. The clinical manifestations depend on the severity of the pathology and the degree of vascularity associated with the anatomical distortion of the bronchi. Patients usually have a chronic cough that is productive of mucopurulent sputum and often have hemoptysis, which at times may be severe and life-threatening. Chronic sinusitis and clubbing of the fingers are also common clinical characteristics.

Functional Disabilities

The earliest manifestations of COPD may be relatively mild, but as time goes on, dyspnea becomes the most important limiting factor. Years may pass before the degree of dyspnea is severe enough to limit routine daily activities such as walking. As time progresses, activities such as dressing, bathing, speech, and even eating cannot be accomplished without severe shortness of breath. Until disease is extremely far advanced, relatively sedentary activities may be accomplished without too much difficulty. Driving may be possible, but walking even limited distances may not be, particularly if an incline or stairs are involved.

Nonetheless, there are some patients even with severe lung disease who maintain a good level of activity despite reduced oxygen levels and elevated CO_2 levels. Such individuals may be able to remain at work in a sedentary capacity, although physical activity such as walking more than a few feet on a level plane or stair climbing may be totally beyond their capabilities. Therefore, assessment of a given patient's functional capability may be difficult to determine based on pulmonary function studies and blood gases alone. Depression, fear, and anxiety are potent factors that may further exacerbate the patient's physical limitations. Many such patients are unaware that medical treatment and rehabilitation may greatly improve their functional capacities. Recurrent respiratory tract infections and continuation of smoking greatly enhance the progress of disease. Preparation for a sedentary occupation would be wise even at the time of relatively mild disease because the rate of progression is variable.

Medical Evaluation

In general, patients with symptomatic respiratory disease should be examined and evaluated by a specialist in internal medicine or pulmonary diseases. Appropriate therapy can sometimes make a tremendous difference in a patient's functional capacity. A chest x-ray should be obtained to rule out cancer and infections such as tuberculosis. Although a chest x-ray may often show the changes characteristic of emphysema, often there is not a very close correlation between x-ray findings and the patient's functional capacity or rehabilitation potential.

Pulmonary function studies are particularly important. The forced vital capacity (FVC), which is the maximum amount of air that can be inspired and expired, and the forced expired volume in one second (FEV_1) are important parameters to follow in COPD. The volume exhaled with a forced expiratory maneuver during the first, second, and third seconds (FEV_1, FEV_2, FEV_3) is often measured. The FVC, FEV_1, FEV_2, and FEV_3 are all reduced in obstructive lung disease, but restrictive lung diseases (see "Interstitial Lung Disease," below) can also reduce them. However, in obstructive lung disease the ratios of FEV_1, FEV_2, and FEV_3 to FVC are reduced, whereas in the restrictive lung diseases these ratios tend to be normal or above normal. The maximum voluntary ventilation (MVV) is another parameter that is often used in evaluating physical capacity. This maneuver records the maximal volume of air the patient can breathe in 12 seconds while breathing in and out as rapidly and forcefully as possible.

Pulmonary function studies are useful in evaluating patient performance only when patient cooperation is complete and a competent technician is performing the study. The tests should be carried out as least three times, using equipment approved by the Disability Determination Unit of the Social Security Administration. The best result obtained from the patient is the one reported. Arterial blood gas determinations and lung volume measurements are often helpful in the evaluation. On occasion the blood gases are significantly worse than one would expect based on the pulmonary function abnormalities alone. The reverse is also sometimes true. Knowing the arterial oxygen and carbon dioxide levels, particularly with exercise, may be quite helpful in evaluating the patient's functional capacity. Motivation and conditioning are also extremely important in assessing the patient. Highly motivated and well-conditioned patients may be much more capable of physical activity than poorly motivated, deconditioned patients even though their pulmonary function studies are comparable.

Treatment

Many patients with chronic pulmonary disorders may have a potential for some reversibility, which can be achieved with proper medical management. Periodic exacerbations caused by a variety of factors, including infection, may also occur. Such exacerbations may cause an acute deterioration in function that will improve as the acute process is treated. A variety of antibiotics are available to treat these respiratory tract infections. There are also a number of medications that can help relieve the bronchospasm found in many patients with COPD. Theophylline-type drugs have been commonly used in the past to relieve bronchospasm, as have β-adrenergic drugs such as albuterol, terbutaline, metaproterenol, and salbutamol. Aerosols can be used to deliver β-adrenergic drugs directly to the lung via metered-dose inhalers (small pressurized hand-held canisters) or nebulizers (small air compressors). Ipratropium bromide is an atropine derivative in aerosol form that has marked bronchodilating potential.

Glucocorticoid-type steroids have marked antiinflammatory effects that can be extremely useful in the management of severe bronchospasm. However, these drugs when given orally or parenterally are difficult to use on a long-term basis because of associated side effects, including osteoporosis, weight gain, muscle weakness, enhancement of diabetes mellitus, cataract formation, peptic ulcer disease, and others. Inhaled glucocorticoid steroids such as beclomethasone, triamcinalone, budesonide, and others may be particularly useful for long-term management of steroid-responsive bronchospasm because of their minimal side effects, but they are not very effective for acute, severe bronchospasm. Newer medications such as the antileukotrienes, although primarily developed to reduce the inflammation in asthma, may be helpful in reducing the inflammatory response in patients who have chronic obstructive lung disease with a bronchospastic component.

Adequate fluid intake and the use of expectorants helps to facilitate the clearance of respiratory tract secretions. Chest physical therapy and pulmonary rehabilitation programs are very useful in a variety of ways. The physical therapist can assist the patient, through postural drainage and percussion techniques, to expel mucus from the respiratory tract. Breathing exercises and relaxation techniques may help the patient in activities of daily living. Exercise reconditioning can help increase endurance and improve work capacity even though conventional lung function tests may change little if at all.

Patients in graded exercise programs should be monitored closely because oxygen desaturation can occur during exercise, along with arrhythmias or myocardial ischemia. Supplemental oxygen may be necessary during such programs. Nocturnal oxygen supplementation may also be useful in patients who have arterial oxygen desaturation at night. The improved oxygen saturation may have beneficial effects on the pulmonary circulation and cardiac function. It may also enhance the patient's sense of well-being. Continuous oxygen therapy may be needed in patients who are chronically hypoxic. Judicious use of oxygen therapy may help such patients remain active. However, oxygen use requires careful monitoring and supervision. Arterial blood gases should be obtained periodically to assess the efficacy of the oxygen administration and to make sure patients are not developing excessive levels of CO_2 retention in response to the elevated oxygen levels.

Vocational Implications

It is extremely important that patients and their families develop an understanding of the illness in order to deal with it effectively. In many instances patients may be inadequately treated or may not be taking their medications properly. Frequently, with the proper use of medications, patients can derive significant relief of their symptoms and may be able to resume some if not all of their routine activities. Smoking cessation may be crucial in helping to delay the progression of disease. Proper nutrition, exercise reconditioning, and chest physical therapy sometimes prove invaluable in helping the patient to resume a more active life. Psychological counseling often helps the patient deal with the anxiety and stress associated with diseases that can cause frightening shortness of breath and marked limitation of activity. Learning to deal effectively with these problems and to make satisfactory adaptations in lifestyle may mean the difference between a productive life and a desperate one.

Patients may have to change their employment goals. Cough and expectoration can preclude some occupations requiring close personal interaction. For patients who are severely compromised (e.g., FEV_1 of 1 L or less), slow walking on the level is often possible, whereas stair climbing or rapid movement is impossible. Likewise, resting hypoxemia (PaO_2 of 60 torr or lower) can be adequate for a sedentary job, but even minimally strenuous activity can cause a significant decrease in oxygen level that would preclude employment. Access to supplemental oxygen often allows the chronically hypoxemic patient or the patient who desaturates with minimal exertion to remain employed at a sedentary activity. However, even sedentary activities may periodically require greater levels of activity than are feasible. Traveling to and from work sometimes poses a level of exertion beyond the patient's capability.

Most methods employed in assessing disability or impairment from respiratory disease consider several factors, including a clinical examination and diagnostic tests. The nature of the underlying disease is extremely important. For example, patients with asthma may be terribly incapacitated during acute attacks but quite functional between attacks. On the other hand, patients with severe chronic bronchitis or emphysema are much less likely to have dramatic remissions of their symptoms. The progressive deterioration of lung function in COPD produces a progressive disability. Some disorders, on the other hand, are acute but nonprogressive. For example, the patient who has lung cancer and undergoes a lung resection may develop impairment of lung function, but the resultant disability remains relatively stable providing the remaining lung stays healthy. Some objective means of classifying pulmonary impairment is necessary. In 1982 and in an update in 1986, the American Thoracic Society (ATS) formulated guidelines for the evaluation and classification of impairment and disability due to pulmonary disease. These guidelines, which are based on spirometry, diffusion capacity, and cardiopulmonary exercise testing, have been endorsed by the American Medical Association (1993). Criteria for impairment as defined by the Social Security Administration also have been revised to incorporate some of the ATS recommendations.

In evaluating pulmonary impairment, the FVC, the FEV_1, and the FEV_1/FVC ratio are particularly important parameters. The equipment, techniques, and standards used must meet the criteria approved by the ATS (1993). The diffusion capacity for carbon monoxide (DLCO) is sometimes useful when the patient's symptoms are more severe than one would expect on the basis of spirometry alone. This test might detect abnormalities in gas exchange that would not otherwise be apparent. Arterial blood gases are also quite useful in this regard but are relatively invasive. The MVV may be of some help in estimating exercise capacity, but the result is very effort-dependent and as such requires a very cooperative patient. It is no longer recommended and should probably be omitted from most evaluations. For more accurate assessment of exercise capacity, actual measurement of the patient's oxygen consumption (VO_2) with exercise may be undertaken. Tables listing the oxygen demands for various activities or occupations allow the evaluator to get an idea as to which activities the patients can tolerate.

The ATS (1986) divides the degree of impairment by pulmonary function testing into mild, moderate, and severe. Mild impairment is usually not correlated with diminished ability to perform most jobs. Moderate impairment is correlated with a decreased ability to meet the demands of many jobs. Severe impairment prevents the patient from meeting the demands of most jobs. The American Medical Association (1993) considers not only pulmonary function abnormalities but also the degree of dyspnea and the VO_2 in its classification of respiratory impairment. The Social Security Administration utilizes the FEV_1, blood gas analysis, and DLCO in its determinations (USDHHS, 1986). Whereas most of these methods serve a purpose in evaluating the disability or impairment of a patient, they may not adequately evaluate the patient's actual capacity to do physical work. Measurement of VO_2 during exercise is sometimes the best indicator of whether or not a specific patient can perform a specific activity. Therefore, exercise testing with measurement of aerobic parameters can offer a more accurate means of estimating a patient's physical capacity to do work, and this information may be as important in the total evaluation of the patient as the determination of the degree of disability.

ASTHMA

Disease Description, Etiology, Pathophysiology, and Clinical Features

Asthma is now regarded as an inflammatory disease of the airways that is characterized by reversible airway obstruction and bronchial hyperreactivity. Both the number of cases and the mortality rate have increased without clear explanation. Asthma is often divided into either an allergic, or extrinsic, type, which commonly has its onset in childhood, and an adult-onset, or intrinsic, type. In extrinsic asthma, exposure to an allergen (pollen, dust, animal dander, mold, foods, medication) may clearly precipitate an attack. Intrinsic asthma attacks are more often precipitated by infection. There is considerable overlap between the two groups, with the majority of patients demonstrating clinical features of both. Because bronchial hyperreactivity or hyperresponsiveness is present in all asthma attacks, they may be precipitated by environmental stimuli of many types (air temperature, humidity, ozone levels, particulate levels, cigarette smoke, cooking odors, insecticides, etc.). Exercise has been demonstrated to produce bronchoconstriction in many asthma patients, as can a simple cough or laugh. Aspirin and food additives such as sulfites are also well-known potential triggers of asthmatic attacks.

In the asthma attack there is constriction of bronchial smooth muscle, mucus hypersecretion, and "plugging" of small airways, as well as inflammation and shedding of the bronchial lining or epithelium. The end result is airway obstruction. The frequency, duration, and severity of the asthmatic attack varies markedly from patient to patient. There is increasing emphasis on dividing the asthmatic attack into an early, or immediate, phase and a late phase that may develop hours after the initial onset. This late, or delayed, phase may explain why asthma attacks may last for days or weeks.

Although there are differences from patient to patient, the asthma attack is typically characterized by shortness of breath and wheezing. Cough and mucus production also may be present. In a small number of patients cough may be the only symptom of bronchial asthma. The patient demonstrates a rapid rate of respiration, often requiring the use of accessory muscles of the neck or chest.

Severe attacks may end in exhaustion, with an ominous slowing of the respiratory rate and arrest of breathing.

Functional Disability

During an asthma attack the patient is totally disabled. Even speech may be impossible because of severe breathlessness. The patient may be totally consumed by the effort to breathe and unable to eat or dress. The patient is restless and unable to lie flat. Severe cough may produce musculoskeletal pain that aggravates the condition. Depending on the severity of the patient's disease, the attack may be totally or partially reversible, allowing the patient to assume normal activities between episodes. Patients with severe asthma remain symptomatic at all times and resemble chronic bronchitis and emphysema patients, described above, with similar levels of disability.

Medical Evaluation

The standard evaluation will resemble that of the COPD patient. In addition, an allergy evaluation is also required regardless of age of onset or clear precipitating factors of the patient's attacks. As in the COPD patient, pulmonary function testing is used in diagnosis and in follow-up of patients. Laboratory evaluation also should include consideration of immunodeficiency and cystic fibrosis, especially in children and young adults. Psychological evaluation may be important because emotional factors can precipitate attacks. In children and young adults, social service evaluation may be helpful in identifying developmental and environmental factors as well as parental influences.

Treatment

Current medical therapy is focused on both the treatment and prevention of an asthma attack. The emphasis on prevention stems from the view of asthma as an inflammatory process and has been aided by the development of antiinflammatory agents.

Asthma medications are now divided into "controllers" (antiinflammatory agents or long-acting bronchodilator spray), which are taken on a regular basis, and "relievers" (short-acting bronchodilator), which are used as needed. Patients with mild, intermittent asthma may be treated with a rapid-acting bronchodilator alone, taken infrequently. Patients with more frequent symptoms that define mild, moderate, and severe asthma are treated with an antiinflammatory agent such as a topical steroid spray in combination with a bronchodilator. Patients with severe asthma may require oral bronchodilator medications or oral corticosteroid given intermittently or, in the most severe disease, continuously.

Self-monitoring with a home peak flow meter has aided in determining the degree of airway obstruction, allowing the patient and physician to recognize the severity of an attack and adjust medication. In this way, emergency room treatment or hospitalization may be avoided. Severe asthma attacks (status asthmaticus), however, often require hospitalization despite appropriate outpatient treatment. Selected patients with allergic asthma may be helped by desensitization with specific allergens. Careful avoidance of environmental allergens should be practiced at home and at work.

Vocational Implications

The degree of disability secondary to asthma will, of course, vary from patient to patient, depending on the severity of disease and the frequency of attacks. The vocational counselor should confer with the client's physician to determine the severity of disease. This information should be used as a guide to determine the suitability of various occupations. In general, the asthma patient should avoid adverse environmental conditions such as outdoor work, temperature changes, heavy particulates, fumes, cigarette smoke, and the like. Physical labor is not contraindicated but should be limited to patients with mild disease who are well controlled on medication and under medical supervision. The counselor also should interact with employers to attempt to ensure the avoidance of environmental irritants and to achieve recognition of the client's illness and potential for absenteeism.

Asthma may develop as a result of exposure to certain occupational materials. This occupational asthma has been documented in meat packers, woodworkers, and agriculture workers and can occur in virtually any industry that creates exposure to organic dusts, fibers, or fungal spores. Industrial asthma also can occur where workers are exposed to chemical fumes or powders. A change of vocation or workplace may clearly be necessary for the asthmatic patient. The counselor must consider the client's potential for retraining and additional education. The asthmatic population is usually a younger age group, compared to COPD patients, and therefore has more potential for career changes.

INTERSTITIAL LUNG DISEASE

A large number of lung diseases involve the supporting structure (interstitium) of the gas-exchanging units (alveoli) of the lung and are termed interstitial lung disease (ILD). Although ILD represents a heterogeneous group of diseases in which there may be inflammation and fibrosis of alveolar walls (alveolitis), vascular components, and small airways, there are many common features. One striking common feature is loss of lung volume, which is often described as "restrictive" lung disease in contrast to the "obstructive" pattern of COPD and asthma.

Disease Description

Inhalation of organic dusts may result in hypersensitivity pneumonitis. These dusts originate from animal proteins, agricultural products, or bacteria or fungi that contaminate food, wood, or detergents. The illnesses are often named after the occupation in which they occur. Farmer's lung results from exposure to fungi in moldy hay; bird breeder's lung results from inhalation of avian proteins.

Inhalation of inorganic dusts results in another form of occupational lung disease, termed pneumoconiosis ("dusty lungs"). Silica (silicosis) and silicates (asbestosis) are two examples of dusts that may produce pulmonary fibrosis. Other potential offenders are aluminum, beryllium, and cobalt. In pneumoconiosis the duration and intensity of exposure to the offending material, as well as smoking history, are important factors in determining etiology. It should be noted that pulmonary fibrosis in pneumoconiosis often occurs 10 to 20 years after exposure began, and symptoms frequently occur after the patient has left the occupation in which he or she was exposed.

Idiopathic pulmonary fibrosis is a well-described ILD in which the cause of fibrosis is unknown. At times an identical form of pulmonary fibrosis will coexist with a systemic disease such as rheumatoid arthritis ("rheumatoid lung"). Sarcoidosis is another idiopathic inflammatory disease that may result in pulmonary fibrosis. Although often a benign disease of young adults that may present with eye or skin lesions, the pulmonary involvement may result in severe fibrosis and disability.

Functional Disability

The common clinical feature of patients with interstitial lung disease is dyspnea or shortness of breath. Depending on the severity of fibrosis or inflammation, the patient may be symptomatic at rest or only on exertion. Difficulty in walking will often be noted, first in increased distress on stair climbing. Simple daily activities of eating, dressing, and bathing may become difficult. Patients with severe disease demonstrate striking "air hunger," with rapid respiratory rates and obvious respiratory distress. Cough also may be a predominant feature. Patients with hypersensitivity pneumonitis may present with constitutional symptoms such as fever or with wheezing. The patient with rheumatoid arthritis and pulmonary fibrosis will typically have severe joint disease. The patient with severe pulmonary fibrosis secondary to sarcoidosis will typically have extrapulmonary disease involving the skin, eyes, and bones.

As in the COPD patient, significant psychosocial disabilities may result from severe breathlessness. Anxiety and depression are common, not only as a result of the air hunger but also from the drastic change in lifestyle and activities. Household family members often are affected by concern over the patient's health and by financial and social problems that stem from the patient's inability to function. Spouses often have specific concerns regarding sexual activity.

Medical Evaluation

The medical evaluation will resemble that of the COPD patient, as detailed above. A thorough and detailed occupational history will be necessary and is essential to the diagnosis of hypersensitivity pneumonitis and of pneumoconiosis. Diagnosis also will depend on patterns of chest x-ray abnormality in many of these disease entities. In pneumoconiosis the chest x-ray may be used to grade severity and intensity of exposure, whereas in silicosis and asbestosis it can form the basis of the diagnosis. The roentgenographic manifestations of pulmonary fibrosis may be nonspecific in terms of etiology but yet reflect the severity of disease.

As with the COPD patient and the asthma patient, pulmonary function testing is essential in determining disability. As noted above, the characteristic pattern in patients with ILD is restrictive, with a loss of vital capacity (VC) and lung volumes (functional residual capacity [FRC], residual capacity [RV], total lung capacity [TLC]). In early stages of inflammation and fibrosis and occasionally in patients with more advanced disease, little change in lung volumes may be noted but more significant reduction will be seen in diffusion capacity and blood gases. Resting arterial oxygen tensions, however, may be within normal limits in patients with significant functional limitations. In these patients and in patients with interstitial disease in general, an exercise evaluation can be extremely helpful in demonstrating a marked reduction in oxygen tension on minimal exertion and may clearly demonstrate the functional disability.

In view of the large number of diseases that may produce ILD, a lung biopsy is often necessary to establish a definite diagnosis. As in the COPD patient, a psychological evaluation may be useful to assess anxiety and depression. Social service evaluation of the patient's family is also helpful in determining the extent of support mechanisms in the home. Family members may require psychosocial evaluation and treatment.

Treatment

Knowledge of the natural history of each disease entity is essential in its management. In this heterogeneous group of diseases the ability to reverse the disease process will vary considerably according to the nature of the injury (e.g., inhalation of organic dust) and the stage at which the disease is detected. In hypersensitivity pneumonitis, withdrawal of the offending material is necessary and may have dramatic results. In pneumoconiosis, reduction of intensity and duration of exposure will reduce the severity of disease.

For the diseases that may be reversible, introduction of drug therapy during the earliest inflammatory stage is essential. In general, the decision to treat is often based on the presence of symptomatology (e.g., dyspnea). Because immunologically mediated inflammation is characteristic of many of the interstitial diseases, corticosteroids are considered the drug of choice. Other immunosuppressive agents also have been used, either in conjunction with corticosteroids or alone.

Vocational Implications

In the occupational lung diseases, the counselor should work with the physician and employer in determining the offending substances that must be avoided. Retraining and extension of education will be necessary for those with occupationally induced disease.

As in the COPD patient, dyspnea will reduce functional ability. Pulmonary function testing should provide guidance in the determination of disability. Patients with lung volumes and/or diffusion capacities reduced to 50% or less of predicted values are usually totally disabled. Patients with significant reductions in oxygen tension at rest or on exercise are equally limited. Those with less severe disease may perform sedentary activities but may require shortened workdays or work weeks. Again, the counselor may have to work with employers to obtain these adjustments in the workplace. Supplemental oxygen and rehabilitation programs can increase functional abilities, although the results of these measures are not as helpful as they are in the COPD group.

CYSTIC FIBROSIS

Disease Description

Cystic fibrosis (CF) is a commonly lethal, genetic deficiency disease that is characterized by recurrent respiratory tract infection and progressive respiratory insufficiency. It is estimated that 1 of every 20 people is a carrier of the defect. It occurs more often in White children (1 in 2,500 births) than in other racial groups. The disease is usually diagnosed by age 6 and limits life expectancy to 29 years. Survival into adulthood is increasingly common with medical and scientific advances and has created the need for increased social and psychological support mechanisms for these patients.

The specific gene responsible for CF was discovered in 1989. Scientists have now discovered hundreds of mutations in this gene. Because of these varied abnormalities, the severity of CF may vary from person to person. The genetic defect in CF affects the mechanism by which chemicals such as sodium and chloride (salt) pass out of cells. In CF, the epithelial cells that line the surface passages of many organs, such as the lung and pancreas, retain increased amounts of sodium and chloride. The high concentration of these chemicals draws water from the airways of the lung (or pancreatic ducts), producing a thick, dehydrated mucus. The highly viscous mucus obstructs and plugs the passageways, producing secondary infection and destruction of tissue. Although pulmonary involvement is the most striking feature of CF, multiple organs may be affected, including the pancreas, liver, intestine, and genitalia.

Functional Disability

Recurrent respiratory tract infection (including sinuses) is characteristic of the disease. In children, poor nutrition, slow growth, and delayed puberty are common. The patient has a chronic cough, with wheezing and recurrent bronchitis, pneumonitis, and sinusitis. Hemoptysis and bronchiectasis are evident, and as a result dyspnea is present and progressive. The pancreatic and intestinal involvement create malabsorption and abdominal discomfort. Hepatic involvement creates jaundice and cirrhosis. Sodium loss in sweat may lead to circulatory collapse. There is considerable variation in time of presentation of these symptoms. Although 75% of patients with CF are diagnosed before age 6, they may not exhibit symptoms until adolescence or later.

Medical Evaluation

The diagnosis of CF is usually made clinically by the presence of pancreatic insufficiency and recurrent respiratory tract infection. The laboratory finding of elevated sodium in sweat has been the diagnostic standard for CF for many years. Genetic testing (DNA analysis) is likely to replace the sweat test in the near future. A reliable genetic screening test for newborns is currently available as well as prenatal screening.

The chest x-ray typically reflects the disease with evidence of cystic bronchiectasis, fibrosis, mucus plugging, and hyperinflation. Pulmonary function testing is useful in documenting the progress of the disease. As in the patient with COPD or asthma there is evidence of airway obstruction and ultimately "air trapping" and hyperinflation. Blood gases reveal a decrease in oxygen tension early in the disease, with elevation of CO_2 tension noted later. Progressive pulmonary insufficiency will ultimately lead to cardiac failure.

Treatment

Advances in antibiotic therapy, nutritional support, and chest physiotherapy have markedly increased survival in CF patients. Heart-lung transplantation has been applied to patients with cystic fibrosis. Five-year survival for patients undergoing transplantation has reached more than 50% in some centers. Genetic engineering may offer another approach that will further increase survival.

Patients with CF require daily chest physiotherapy to loosen secretions and prevent stagnation and secondary infections. Antibiotics are essential in treating infection and usually must be given intravenously for prolonged periods. Techniques for intravenous therapy now permit treatment outside the hospital and frequently permit the patient to remain functional. Nutritional support may also be administered via this route in malnourished patients.

Vocational and Psychological Implications

Patients with CF have excellent educational success and are typically productive individuals. Achievements in virtually all vocations have been noted and confirm the need to provide health-sustaining support for these patients. The counselor will have to work with employers to provide the support mechanisms that will allow the patient to remain in the workplace. This may include the provision of time for chest physiotherapy or antibiotic therapy during the workday. Also, the work environment must be reviewed to ensure the absence of irritants that might exacerbate the disease. Supplemental oxygen may be necessary to allow the patient to continue to be productive and ambulatory.

Psychological outcome in CF patients appears to depend on factors such as altered physical appearance, loneliness, and family strife that the patients attribute to their illness. Faced with these factors and concerns over their sexual function, individuals may develop anxiety or depression. Psychological evaluation and treatment will be necessary. Despite the fact that CF is an accepted disability, these patients appear to be disadvantaged in employment and in social relationships. The counselor must work with patients' families to improve support at home that will allow the patient to increase social and vocational activities.

REFERENCES

American Medical Association. (1993). The respiratory system. In *Guides to the evaluation of permanent impairment* (4th ed., rev.) (pp. 53–67). Chicago: Author.

American Thoracic Society. (1982). Evaluation of impairment/disability secondary to respiratory disease. *American Review of Respiratory Disease, 126,* 945–951.

American Thoracic Society. (1986). Evaluation of impairment/disability secondary to respiratory disorders. *American Review of Respiratory Disease, 133,* 1205–1209.

American Thoracic Society. (1993). Guidelines for the evaluation of impairment/disability in patients with asthma. *American Review of Respiratory Disease, 147,* 1056–1061.

Hodgkin, J. E. (1990). Pulmonary rehabilitation. In J. E. Hodgkin (Ed.), Chronic obstructive pulmonary disease. *Clinics in Chest Medicine, 11,* 447–461.

U.S. Department of Health and Human Services. (1986). Disability evaluation under Social Security (SSA Publication No. 05-10089). Washington, DC: U.S. Government Printing Office.

Chapter 22

Chronic Renal Failure

Kotresha Neelakantappa and
Jerome Lowenstein

Chronic renal failure poses a singular challenge for health professionals who deal with illness-related disability and rehabilitation. The course of progressive renal disease leading to renal failure often spans many years; during the period before dialysis or renal transplantation is undertaken, the patient may experience disabilities related to cardiovascular disease, anemia, malnutrition, metabolic bone disease, neuropathy, muscle wasting, and acid-base and electrolyte disturbances. Dialysis treatment and transplantation significantly prolong the lives of patients with renal failure but often allow some of the most disabling features of renal disease to persist or progress. Better understanding of the pathophysiological basis for many of the disabling aspects of chronic renal failure has led to therapies that may reduce the frequency and/or severity of these manifestations. Prevention of disability and rehabilitation have become increasingly important as dialysis therapy and renal transplantation have extended the life expectancy of patients with chronic renal failure.

DISEASE DESCRIPTION

Chronic Renal Failure and Its Progression

Most renal parenchymal diseases, regardless of the etiology of the underlying disease, exhibit progressive scarring and loss of function over a period of many years. In some instances, progression occurs because of persistent disease or repeated recurrences of the primary disease, but more frequently progression occurs without evidence of activity of the original disease. Surgical ablation of a critical mass of renal tissue in rats and in dogs results in progressive loss of nephrons in the remaining, previously healthy tissue. This form of progression is characterized by glomerular sclerosis and obsolescence of some nephrons and hypertrophy of the remaining nephrons. Studies of the mechanisms underlying this "nonimmunologic" progression have provided therapeutic strategies for delaying the onset of renal failure.

Micropuncture studies in the remnant kidney model have shown that single-nephron plasma flow and glomerular capillary hydrostatic pressure are increased in the remaining nephrons. The factors responsible for glomerular hypertrophy and glomerular hemodynamic alterations are not well understood. Increased levels of growth hormone, certain dietary amino acids, vasodilator renal prostaglandins, increased local concentrations of angiotensin II, and autoregulation of glomerular blood flow leading to glomerular hypertension have all been implicated. The increase in glomerular hydrostatic pressure may occur in the absence of systemic hypertension. Increased surface area of the glomerular filtering bed and glomerular hypertension, while maintaining glomerular filtration rate (GFR) close to normal, appear to lead to accelerated glomerular injury and fibrosis. Treatment with antihypertensive agents is beneficial in slowing the rate of progression in a variety of renal diseases in both experimental animals and humans. Low-protein diet prevents the compensatory increase in flow, glomerular hypertension, and hypertrophy and leads to marked attenuation of sclerosis in rats with the remnant kidney model of progressive renal disease. Most studies of protein restriction in humans with both diabetic and nondiabetic chronic renal disease also demonstrated a similar benefit. However, the largest study to date (Klahr et al., 1994), which examined the effect of protein restriction on progression of nondiabetic renal disease in 585 patients, did not show a statistically significant benefit. This finding was surprising, and it has been suggested that the beneficial effects of good control of hypertension and the use of angiotensin converting enzyme inhibitor (ACEi) may have masked the effects of dietary protein restriction on disease progression.

Functional Adaptation to Nephron Loss

Adaptive changes in residual nephrons permit the kidney to perform most of its function despite marked reduction in nephron number. Systemic and intrarenal hemodynamic changes, hormonal stimuli, and possibly structural changes along the nephron lead to increase in single-nephron GFR and to changes in tubular reabsorption and tubular secretion of various metabolites in the surviving nephrons. With further nephron loss, compensatory changes in the residual nephrons fail to maintain normal total renal function, and abnormalities in blood composition become evident.

Minute changes in body composition resulting from retention of some substances trigger mechanisms that result in compensatory increase in their excretion with little change in the internal milieu. These mechanisms themselves are associated with varying degrees of untoward but less harmful effects than those of retention of the substance in question. This is referred to as the trade-off hypothesis. It is well illustrated by the compensatory responses that maintain external balance of sodium, potassium, hydrogen ion, calcium, and phosphorus.

Sodium

Under normal circumstances, approximately 25,000 mEq of Na^+ are filtered daily. All except about 150 mEq (average daily intake) are reabsorbed. As the GFR and the filtered load of sodium decline with progressive renal disease, there is a reciprocal increase in the fraction of filtered sodium that escapes reabsorption. Despite marked reduction in filtered sodium in advanced renal failure, edema is not usually observed. The mechanism responsible for rejection of an increased fraction of the filtered sodium may directly or indirectly be related to increased systemic blood pressure. Hypertension may be the trade-off for maintaining sodium balance in the face of declining GFR. The same mechanisms that maintain sodium excretion when GFR is reduced may be responsible for impaired sodium conservation when dietary sodium intake is reduced or extrarenal losses of sodium occur.

Potassium

Filtered potassium is completely reabsorbed before the glomerular filtrate reaches the distal convoluted tubule. Potassium balance is maintained mainly by secretion by the principal cells in the late distal convoluted tubule and cortical collecting duct. Tubular secretion of potassium is dependent on the negative electrical charge in the lumen created by sodium reabsorption and sodium conductance across the epithelium of the collecting duct, which in turn is dependent on aldosterone. Although plasma aldosterone concentration is not usually elevated in chronic renal disease, patients with moderately advanced renal failure are prone to develop hyperkalemia if drugs that antagonize aldosterone (spironolactone), reduce angiotensin II production, leading to decreased aldosterone secretion (ACE inhibitors and nonsteroidal antiinflammatory drugs), or block angiotensin effect on the adrenal (angiotensin II receptor antagonists) are given. Hyperkalemia is usually not seen until GFR drops to less than 10%–15% of normal.

Hydrogen Ion

Daily metabolism leads to generation of fixed acids (predominantly sulfuric acid), which dissociate into their respective anions (e.g., sulfate) and the cation, H^+ (protons). Daily metabolic production averages about 1 mEq/kg/day. The protons titrate the body buffers, predominantly bicarbonate. The kidney excretes the anions of the acids and regenerates the bicarbonate (and other body buffers). The regeneration of bicarbonate stores and the "back titration" of other body buffers (predominantly proteins) is accomplished by the renal tubular secretion of H^+ and by renal ammoniagenesis. The renal secretion of H^+, formed from the breakdown of H_2CO_3 ($H_2CO_3 \rightleftarrows H^+ + HCO_3^-$) generates an equimolar quantity of bicarbonate, which is absorbed across the basolateral membrane of the renal tubule. Renal ammoniagenesis results in the formation of NH_4^+ and glutamate or α-ketoglutarate. The NH_4^+ is excreted, and the organic anions are metabolized to yield bicarbonate.

Renal acid excretion is only modestly reduced despite marked reduction in nephron number as renal disease progresses. This is the result of increased proton secretion and increased renal ammonia production per residual nephron. Although total ammonia generation is reduced, increased ammonia generation in remaining nephrons leads to an increase in local NH_4^+ concentration. In experimental animals this has been shown to cause activation of complement components and tubulointerstitial damage. Prevention of increased local ammonia concentration by bicarbonate administration ameliorates tubulointerstitial damage. One can view tubulointerstitial damage as another example of trade-off, in which adaptation (i.e., increased ammonia generation per residual nephron) results in increased ammonia concentration, leading to complement activation and tissue injury.

Calcium and Phosphorus

Calcium and phosphorus metabolism are markedly altered in progressive renal disease. The concentration of 1,25$(OH)_2$ vitamin D_3, the active form of vitamin D, is governed by the enzymatic hydroxylation of 25(OH) vitamin D_3 by the kidneys. The concentration of 1,25$(OH)_2$ vitamin D_3 is reduced in advanced renal failure, and calcium absorption by the intestine decreases, resulting in hypocalcemia. The filtration of phosphorus decreases as the GFR falls. Normally 80%–95% of the filtered phosphorus is reabsorbed. In renal failure, the reabsorption of phosphate may be reduced to 15%, but beyond this point, phosphate balance can be maintained only by increased plasma phosphate concentration. Phosphate retention contributes to hypocalcemia by deposition of calcium phosphate in tissues. Despite these perturbations in calcium and phosphorus balance, serum calcium and phosphorus concentrations are maintained in the normal range until GFR is markedly reduced. In large part this is attributable to increased parathyroid hormone (PTH) secretion. PTH not only reduces tubular reabsorption of phosphate, but also mobilizes calcium from the skeletal system. The pathogenesis of this "secondary hyperparathyroidism" involves several mechanisms. Hypocalcemia stimulates PTH release from parathyroid cells. Reduced vitamin D concentration leads to parathyroid hyperplasia by removing the normal suppressive effect it exerts on the parathyroid, with a concomitant down-regulation of vitamin D receptors on parathyroid cells. The trade-off for maintenance of calcium and phosphorus concentrations is the development of parathyroid bone disease characterized by osteomalacia and osteitis fibrosa cystica.

TREATMENT OF CHRONIC RENAL FAILURE

Management of chronic renal disease involves both delaying progression of the renal disease and correcting the metabolic abnormalities.

Hypertension

Although hypertension is almost always a result rather than a cause of renal disease, it leads to accelerated progression of the underlying disease, creating a vicious circle. The control of hypertension in renal disease is directed at both a reduction in cardiovascular morbidity and slowing the progression of the underlying renal disease. Antihypertensive drugs have selective actions on afferent or efferent arterioles and differ in their ability to reduce glomerular hypertension. ACE inhibitors, which lower glomerular capillary pressure (P_{GC}), have been shown to reduce proteinuria and delay progression in both diabetic nephropathy and IgA nephropathy, the two most common forms of progressive parenchymal renal diseases. Calcium channel blockers differ in their effect on the kidney. Dihydropyridines, which are potent vasodilators, lead to an increase in proteinuria, perhaps because afferent arteriolar dilatation leaves P_{GC} unchanged or increased. Nondihyropyridines have been shown to result in a reduction in proteinuria that is additive to that brought about by ACE inhibitors.

Metabolic Acidosis

Metabolic acidosis in chronic renal disease is generally well tolerated and is usually not treated unless it is severe. The arguments against treatment have included the risk of sodium overload associated with sodium bicarbonate therapy; reduction in ionized calcium concentration, resulting in tetany and seizures; and perhaps diminished oxygen (O_2) delivery to tissues due to reversal of an adaptive change in the O_2 dissociation curve. More recent evidence suggests that the benefits of treatment outweigh these objections. Treatment of metabolic acidosis with bicarbonate or a metabolizable anion that can act as a substitute for bicarbonate (e.g., citrate) has been shown to prevent growth retardation in children with renal tubular acidosis. It has been noted that correction of metabolic acidosis by increasing dialysate bicarbonate concentration in patients with end stage renal disease (ESRD) improves bone mineralization, diminishes bone resorption, and reduces the severity of secondary hyperparathyroidism.

Chronic metabolic acidosis is associated with muscle weakness and decreased lean body mass. Forearm muscle studies in patients with chronic renal disease, utilizing phenylalanine appearance rate as a measure of protein degradation and disposal rate as a measure of protein synthesis, have demonstrated that protein catabolic rate is directly related to the degree of acidosis. Further, albumin synthesis is diminished and negative nitrogen balance increased in patients with chronic renal disease made acidotic by the administration of ammonium chloride. The down-regulation of protein catabolic rate, normally seen in patients with chronic renal failure placed on a protein-restricted diet, is impaired in those who also have metabolic acidosis; this can be corrected by treatment of acidosis with bicarbonate.

Anemia

Although there are many causes of anemia in chronic renal disease, reduced erythropoietin (EPO) production seems to be the most important factor. Both Type I renal interstitial cells and proximal tubular epithelial cells are known to produce EPO. A heme protein acts as the oxygen sensor in the kidney. When stimulated by diminished oxygen delivery, this sensor leads to synthesis of a protein that binds to the enhancer region of the EPO gene, leading to an increase in the production of EPO. EPO levels are markedly reduced in patients with anemia of chronic renal failure. Administration of recombinant human erythropoietin (rHuEPO) corrects the anemia of renal disease in a dose-dependent manner. Ninety percent of patients on dialysis in the United States and many patients with chronic renal disease who are not yet on dialysis receive rHuEPO therapy. The target hematocrit of 32%–38% is reached in a majority of patients at a dose of 50–100 U/kg given 3 times a week. Seventy percent of patients respond to a dose of 50 U/kg three times a week (TIW) and 90% respond to 100 U/kg TIW. The most common cause of resistance to rHuEPO is iron deficiency. Other causes of resistance to EPO include bone marrow fibrosis, inflammatory conditions, poor nutrition, and underdialysis.

Anemia has been found to be an independent predictor of the de novo occurrence of congestive heart failure and increased mortality in ESRD. Left ventricular hypertrophy also has been found to be associated with increased mortality in ESRD. Successful treatment of anemia with rHuEPO has been shown to reverse cardiovascular and hemodynamic abnormalities such as left ventricular hypertrophy, increased cardiac output, and decreased peripheral vascular resistance. Clinically, amelioration of angina, congestive heart failure, and fatigue have been observed. Patients report improved vitality and exercise tolerance. Other beneficial effects of EPO therapy include improvement in platelet dysfunction of uremia, uremic pruritus, impaired carbohydrate and cortisol metabolism, and sexual function in male patients.

Renal Osteodystrophy

Although symptomatic renal osteodystrophy (e.g., bone pain and fractures) seldom occurs prior to the onset of ESRD, altered mineral metabolism is present early in the course of renal failure. The two classic forms of renal osteodystrophy are osteitis fibrosa, characterized by an increased rate of bone turnover secondary to hyperparathyroidism, and osteomalacia, in which bone turnover is diminished and there is an increased volume of unmineralized bone (osteoid). Although osteomalacia was initially thought to result from vitamin D deficiency in patients with ESRD, it is now believed that the major cause is aluminum toxicity. More recently, a third entity, adynamic bone disease or aplastic bone disease, has been described. It is characterized by diminished skeletal turnover and reduced rate of osteoid formation. This condition may be caused by excessive suppression of PTH by 1,25$(OH)_2$ vitamin D_3.

The administration of synthetic 1,25$(OH)_2$ vitamin D_3 plays a major role in the prevention of hyperparathyroidism and renal osteodystrophy. Together with the control of hyperphosphatemia with non-aluminum-containing antacids and the use of deionized water for dialysate, calcitriol replacement has resulted in a marked reduction in the incidence of both osteitis fibrosa and osteomalacia in the past 20 years. In certain instances, the parathyroid hyperplasia is nodular and so severe that it is not possible to suppress it medically, a condition referred to as tertiary hyperparathyroidism; this may necessitate surgical parathyroidectomy.

Uremic Neuropathy

Uremic neuropathy can present as either a polyneuropathy or a mononeuropathy involving both sensory and motor fibers. It generally occurs in advanced renal failure and is an indication to start dialysis for ESRD. When it occurs in patients who are already on dialysis, one needs to consider inadequate dialysis as a cause. Pathologically, uremic polyneuropathy is associated with demyelination and axonal degeneration, and the involvement is directly proportional to axonal length, affecting longer axons first. It is usually symmetrical in nature. The metabolic and chemical defects leading to these changes are not well understood. Clinically, it first presents as paresthesias, burning sensation and pain in distal areas such as feet. Sensory symptoms usually precede motor symptoms. The onset of motor symptoms reflects advanced disease, which, unlike the sensory neuropathy, may not reverse with the institution of dialysis. Electrophysiological studies are very useful in detecting subclinical neuropathy. Uremic mononeuropathy usually involves median and ulnar nerves. Other nerves involved include seventh and eighth cranial nerves and peroneal nerves. Carpal tunnel syndrome is common in ESRD. It results from compression of the median nerve at the wrist between carpal bones and transverse carpal ligament. Deposition of β_2-microglobulin-related amyloid fibrils in the carpal tunnel plays an important role in the pathogenesis of the syndrome. Early initiation of dialysis, the use of better dialysis membranes with higher clearance for β_2-microglobulin, and close attention to adequacy of dialysis have reduced the incidence of uremic neuropathy. The extent of recovery is directly related to the degree of dysfunction prior to initiation of dialysis. Restoration of renal function with renal transplantation results in remarkable recovery from even the most severe sensory and motor neuropathy.

Sexual Dysfunction

Erectile dysfunction and a decrease in libido and frequency of intercourse are present in over half the men with uremia. This is organic in nature, as evidenced by a decline in nocturnal penile tumescence. Such decline is more marked than in normal controls and patients with other chronic illness, suggesting that it is the effect of uremia; yet it does not improve with hemodialysis. Factors other than uremia that can contribute to erectile dysfunction include peripheral neuropathy, autonomic dysfunction, and peripheral vascular disease. Psychological and physical stress also may play a role.

Lack of ovulation and scant menstruation are common in women with chronic renal failure. Some women may have hypermenorrhagia, leading to worsening of anemia. Pregnancy occurs rarely in chronic renal failure, and fetal loss is the rule. Elevated prolactin levels also are seen in women with chronic renal disease. Although suppression of very high prolactin levels with bromocriptine improves the clinical syndrome of amenorrhea and galactorrhea in women with normal renal function, it fails to restore normal menstruation or correct galactorrhea in uremic women. Successful renal transplantation leads to restoration of fertility and sexual function in most patients.

TREATMENT OF END STAGE RENAL FAILURE

When Willem Kolff introduced hemodialysis a little over 50 years ago, its use was restricted to treatment of patients with acute reversible renal failure. Today, hemodialysis and peritoneal dialysis can support and rehabilitate patients with end stage, irreversible renal failure. In 1995, the last year for which such data are available, 257,000 patients were being treated for ESRD (United States Renal Data System [S40–S53], 1997). Approximately 60% of these were treated with hemodialysis, 10% had peritoneal dialysis, and 27% had a successful renal transplantation. Thirty-four percent of patients were over the age of 65, and 31% were diabetics. The cost of treatment of ESRD for the year 1995 was $13 billion, which exceeded the projected cost for the year 2000 by $3 billion. In the United States, most medical expenses for dialysis treatment are reimbursed by Medicare.

Hemodialysis

Hemodialysis is typically performed three times a week. The procedure involves diffusion of solutes between the plasma and the dialysis bath (dialysate) across the semipermeable dialyzer membrane and down a concentration gradient. Fluid (usually equal to the volume retained from one dialysis to the next) is removed by ultrafiltration, by regulating the dialyzer transmembrane hydrostatic pressure. Blood flow rates through the dialyzers in excess of 200 ml/min are necessary to obtain sufficient clearance of solutes over a reasonably short period of time (2–4 hours). Because the normal blood flow rates in peripheral veins are insufficient for this purpose, it is necessary to have some form of access to the circulation where the blood flow rate is of this magnitude. A simple catheter placed in a central vein or an arteriovenous fistula/shunt, with or without the interposition of a synthetic tubular graft, is the most common form of hemodialysis access.

Peritoneal Dialysis

In this technique the patient's peritoneum substitutes for the dialyzer membrane. When the peritoneal cavity is filled with dialysate solution, diffusion of solutes occurs between the plasma flowing in the capillaries supplying the peritoneum and the dialysate until concentration equilibrium is reached. In 1976, Popovich, Moncrief, Decherd, and Pyle (1976) described the basic concept of continuous ambulatory peritoneal dialysis (CAPD). They made use of the fact that some solute transfer continued to occur for as long as 4–5 hours, and one could achieve sufficient solute clearance with four to five 2-L exchanges of dialysis fluid a day. Negative fluid balance is achieved by increasing the osmotic concentration of the dialysis fluid. This forms the basis for the use of peritoneal dialysis as a treatment option for patients with ESRD. The incidence of peritonitis as a complication of this procedure has been markedly reduced by improvements in techniques and in the design of catheters and connections.

Survival of ESRD Patients

Although maintenance dialysis prevents death from uremia, patient survival is still limited. USRDS data (USRDS, 1997) show a mean expected remaining life span of 7.98 years for patients beginning dialysis between the ages of 40 and 44 and 4.38 years for those beginning between the ages of 60 and 64 years. These are 22.3%, and 22.5%, respectively, of the expected life span for the general U.S. population of comparable age groups. Understandably, survival depends on comorbid conditions. For the year 1994, diabetics had a death rate of 27 per 100 patient years, compared to 18.1 per 100 patient years for patients with glomerulonephritis as the etiology of ESRD. Although most of these data are from patients on hemodialysis (60% of the ESRD population), similar observations hold true for the peritoneal dialysis population.

Cardiovascular events (strokes and heart attack) account for about 50% of deaths in ESRD. The other important causes of death in ESRD are infections, most often stemming from hemodialysis access sites or peritonitis in those on peritoneal dialysis. About 5%–10% of deaths are caused by withdrawal from dialysis.

Adequacy of Dialysis

The National Cooperative Dialysis Study (NCDS), a prospectively randomized and controlled study, demonstrated that the "dose of dialysis," as measured by urea clearance, correlated with morbidity (Lowrie, Parker, & Sargent, 1981). The dose-of-dialysis therapy can be expressed as the virtual volume of plasma completely cleared of urea during dialysis, relative to the volume of distribution. This is expressed by the formula Kt/V, where K is urea clearance, t is duration of dialysis, and V is volume of distribution. The urea reduction ratio (URR) is also a correlate of Kt/V. The Work Group of National Kidney Foundation—Dialysis Outcomes Quality Initiative (NKF-DOQI, 1997) recommended a prescribed minimum of 1.3 for Kt/V and 70% for URR. Several studies (Hakim, Breyer, Ismail, & Schulman, 1994; Held et al., 1996; Parker, Husni, Huang, Lew, & Lawrie, 1994) have shown that increasing the dose of dialysis reduces the mortality, which in one study (Held et al., 1996) was 7% for each 0.1 unit increment in Kt/V.

However, it is unclear if increasing Kt/V to greater than 1.4 is associated with further reduction in mortality. Similar observations have been made regarding adequacy of dialysis and mortality and morbidity for patients on maintenance peritoneal dialysis. The Canada–USA (CANUSA) Peritoneal Dialysis Study Group (1996), in a prospective cohort study, found that a decrease of 0.1 unit Kt/V was associated with a 5% increase in the relative risk of death. A weekly Kt/V of 2.1 and a weekly creatinine clearance of 70 L/1.73 m^2 were both associated with a 2-year survival of 78%.

Nutrition

Malnutrition is common in chronic renal disease. It not only results from protein restriction in an attempt to slow the progression of renal disease but also as a function of advancing renal disease. Analysis of the data from Modification of Diet in Renal Disease (MDRD) study showed that body mass index, anthropometric measurements, and urinary creatinine excretion (an index of muscle mass) were lower than expected in patients with moderately advanced renal disease entering the study (Klahr et al., 1994). Several indices of nutrition, such as dietary protein intake, serum cholesterol, transferrin, insulin-like growth factor 1 (IGF-1), percent body weight, and urinary creatinine excretion, decline as the renal function deteriorates (Ikizler, Greene, Wingard, Parker, & Hakim, 1995). Mild to moderate protein-calorie malnutrition is present in a third of the patients on maintenance dialysis. Factors contributing to malnutrition in the dialysis population include poor nutrient intake, intercurrent illness, and dialysis itself. Concentrations of plasma proteins such as albumin, prealbumin, transferrin, and IGF-1, as well as markers of tissue protein stores, such as predialysis creatinine concentration, lean body mass, and anthropometrics (measurement of skin fold thickness at the triceps or subscapular area as an index of body fat and mid-arm circumference as an index of muscle mass), are reduced. Although several markers of malnutrition, such as low blood urea, serum cholesterol, creatinine, potassium, and phosphorus, have been associated with increased risk of mortality, low serum albumin concentration seems to be the strongest predictor of mortality. The odds ratio for the risk of death is inversely related, exponentially, to serum albumin concentration in patients maintained on either hemo- or peritoneal dialysis. Significant hypoalbuminemia (< 3.7 g/dl) is present in approximately 25% of patients on maintenance hemodialysis. Even though peritoneal losses contribute to hypoalbuminemia in CAPD patients, Lowrie et al. (Lowrie, Huang, & Lew, 1995) found that the relative risk of death was the same for hemodialysis patients and CAPD patients with hypoalbuminemia, suggesting that regardless of the mechanism, hypoalbuminemia carried the same risk.

Various interventions, ranging from simple nutritional supplements to administration of intradialytic parenteral nutrition, may be of value in correcting malnutrition in patients with ESRD. Experimentally, recombinant human growth hormone (rhGH) and recombinant human insulin-like growth factor 1 (rhIGF-1) have been shown to lead to positive nitrogen balance.

PHYSICAL REHABILITATION

As in any other chronic illness, rehabilitation is extremely important if patients with ESRD are to live as normal a life as possible. Even though hemodialysis and peritoneal dialysis provide means to sustain life in the absence of kidney function, patients are generally weak and disabled to a variable extent. The trend in favor of institution of dialysis before severe debility is incurred has made rehabilitation more effective.

The availability of synthetic $1{,}25(OH)_2$ vitamin D_3 and better understanding of the pathophysiology of renal osteodystrophy, including the importance of aluminum toxicity, have reduced the incidence of severe skeletal disease to a great extent. The incidence of dialysis-related amyloidosis, causing carpal tunnel syndrome and arthropathy, has markedly decreased since the introduction of synthetic dialysis membranes with better β_2-microglobulin clearance. In addition to these advances in medical care, flexibility and range of movement exercises will help improve patients' ability to perform activities of daily living, such as stooping, bending, and reaching. Although strengthening (isometric) exercises such as weight lifting have been shown to increase blood pressure, well-selected exercises in moderation help maintain muscle strength, which is important for activities of daily living such as lifting and carrying objects.

Maximal aerobic capacity as measured by peak oxygen uptake (VO_2 peak) is reduced in patients with ESRD to roughly half of that seen in normal sedentary individuals. The determinants of VO_2 peak are (1) oxygen delivery to the muscles, which is dependent on arterial oxygen content and blood supply to the muscle, and (2) oxygen extraction by the muscle. Hemodialysis patients demonstrate a limitation in both cardiac output (mainly as a blunted response of heart rate to exercise) and diminished ability to extract oxygen at the muscle level. These abnormalities continue to worsen because of disease progression, development of comorbid conditions, and deconditioning. Correction of anemia with rHuEPO results in an increase in the arterial oxygen content and improves VO_2 peak by an average of 28%, but the change in VO_2 peak is much smaller than that expected for the change in hemoglobin and arterial oxygen content. The resultant VO_2 peak is only 65% of that of age-matched sedentary controls. Painter and Moore (1994) have analyzed the available data and compared the improvement in VO_2 peak relative to the rise in hemoglobin in dialysis patients and normal subjects whose hemoglobin was varied by phlebotomy and reinfusion of packed cells. They concluded that the increase in VO_2 for a given rise in hemoglobin concentration in patients with chronic renal failure was only one half that seen in normal subjects. They suggested that there may be an underlying limitation in maximal oxygen extraction by skeletal muscles in dialysis patients. Skeletal muscle abnormalities described in dialysis patients have included reduced oxidative enzyme activity, decreased Type I to Type II muscle fiber ratio, atrophy of fibers, low capillary density, mitochondrial dysfunction, low carnitine content, and accumulation of acylated metabolites of carnitine. Utilizing phosphorus 31 magnetic resonance spectroscopy (^{31}PMRS), measurements of pH and the ratio of phosphocreatine to phosphocreatine plus inorganic phosphorus have revealed that the intrinsic metabolic capacity of muscles during static hand grip, when blood flow through capillaries and O_2 delivery cease, is similar in hemodialysis patients, successful transplant recipients, and normal controls. However, rhythmic hand grip which is dependent on both intrinsic muscle function and oxygen delivery, led to increased intracellular acidosis and phosphocreatine depletion in hemodialysis patients. These studies suggest a reduction in oxidative generation of adenosine triphosphate (ATP), a need for more ATP for the same amount of muscle function or the utilization of more ATP for nonmuscular activity such as ion pumping. Exercise training alone has been shown to improve VO_2 peak by 25%.

Remarkable effects of exercise training combined with EPO treatment are exemplified by two athletes who participated in the 1991 California Transplant Games (Painter & Moore, 1994). One had diabetes and was on peritoneal dialysis for 4 years, and the other, with glomerulonephritis, had been on hemodialysis for 8 years. They finished in the top two places in the 1-mile run and had VO_2 max. of 40.2 and 36.1 ml/kg/min, respectively. These values were better than those of age- and sex-matched normal sedentary individuals. Although these are exceptional examples, they serve as reminders of what can be achieved by training. The mechanisms by which aerobic exercise training leads to improved oxygen utilization in normal individuals (Saltin & Rowell, 1980) include increased oxidative enzyme number and activities, increased Type I fibers, increased capillary to fiber ratio, and increased total muscle blood flow. Moore et al. (1993) reported that 5 of 11 hemodialysis patients increased VO_2 peak by 26% after exercise training. This change resulted from an increase in aVO_2 difference (oxygen extraction); there was no change in cardiac output, stroke volume, heart rate, or hemoglobin concentration. Even patients who did not show an increase in VO_2 peak showed an increase in peak work load achieved, suggesting that exercise training improves efficiency of work at a given VO_2.

As is well appreciated in the general population, exercise training offers other health benefits in dialysis patients. Endurance exercise training in hemodialysis patients offers cardiovascular risk benefits: lowering of both systolic and diastolic blood pressure sufficient to withdraw antihypertensive therapy in a number of patients and a decline in plasma triglycerides and very low density lipoprotein (VLDL) levels while increasing high-density lipoprotein (HDL) level (Hagberg et al., 1983; Harter & Goldberg, 1985). Plasma insulin declines, and glucose tolerance improves. Exercise training has also been shown to improve hemoglobin concentration. Psychosocial functioning, including Beck Depression Score, the frequency of pleasant activities, and participation in enjoyable events are reported to improve after exercise training (Harter & Goldberg, 1985). Although psychosocial function is better with exercise, improvement in vocational rehabilitation, which is dependent on many other issues, such as economic incentives, needs to be demonstrated.

Although the best time for exercise in relation to hemodialysis is not clear, exercise training during dialysis sessions has the advantages of supervision and encouragement by the staff as well as a productive use of dialysis time. One can expect improved compliance with the exercise program. Flexibility, strengthening, and aerobic exercises, utilizing a stationary bicycle, can all be performed effectively during dialysis. Because of the likelihood of hypotension and muscle cramps during the latter part of dialysis, exercise is best performed in the first hour of dialysis. It has been suggested that exercise during dialysis might improve dialysis efficiency (Mustata et al., 1997). Although there are some risks of musculoskeletal injury associated with participation in an exercise program for a patient with ESRD, proper patient selection makes this risk negligible.

Carnitine

Carnitine is an important intermediary in fat metabolism. It combines with toxic acyl-CoA to form acylcarnitine and transports long-chain fatty acids such as acylcarnitine into mitochondria for β-oxidation, providing energy. Carnitine is synthesized by the liver, kidney, and brain and is also derived from dietary red meat and dairy products. About 95% of carnitine is stored in the muscle. Free carnitine is filtered freely at the glomerulus but is reabsorbed almost totally by the renal tubule. On the other hand, acylcarnitine is also filtered but is not reabsorbed. Renal clearance of acylcarnitine is four to eight times greater than that of free carnitine. Although the levels of both free and acylcarnitine are elevated in chronic renal failure, the ratio of free to acyl form is markedly reduced. Hemodialysis removes free carnitine preferentially and leads to very high levels of acylcarnitine relative to free carnitine. Low plasma levels of free carnitine are also reported in patients on CAPD. Because many of the manifestations of carnitine deficiency mimic those of uremia and do not correlate with plasma carnitine profiles, response to carnitine supplementation has been used to define its effective deficiency. A multicenter double-blind, placebo-controlled study of L-carnitine administration in 82 hemodialysis patients (Ahmad et al., 1990) found that intradialytic hypotension and muscle cramps were significantly reduced in the carnitine group. This group also showed a decline in the predialysis urea, creatinine, and phosphorus levels, suggesting a decreased muscle catabolism. Measurement of mid-arm circumference and triceps skin fold thickness showed an increase in the calculated mid-arm muscle area in the carnitine group. VO_2 peak also increased in the carnitine group. Other uncontrolled studies have shown that L-carnitine supplementation improves plasma lipid profile, muscle strength, exercise capacity, cardiac function, anemia, response to rHuEPO, and a sense of well-being. Although, routine administration of L-carnitine to all dialysis patients was not recommended at a recent Consensus Conference, its use in patients with intradialytic hypotension and cramps, skeletal muscle weakness and myopathy, lack of energy, cardiomyopathy, and anemia unresponsive to large doses of rHuEPO was suggested (Consensus Group Statement, 1994).

PSYCHOLOGICAL AND VOCATIONAL REHABILITATION

In addition to the appropriate management of the gamut of abnormalities resulting from chronic renal failure outlined above, one must also address the issue of the patient returning to living a full life. For some this may not mean returning to work but feeling well enough to enjoy the family and the surroundings. The goal should be to help the patient to resume all the duties, responsibilities, and benefits he or she enjoyed prior to the illness. Psychological problems stemming from chronic illness, dependence on dialysis, sexual dysfunction, and the change in status from an earning and supporting member of the family to a dependent person should be identified and addressed. Gainful employment is extremely important for an adult in the earning period of his or her life, to regain self-esteem and to interact with society confidently. However, the fear of losing financial benefits such as Social Security Disability Insurance (SSDI) and Supplemental Security Income (SSI) may deter some patients from seeking employment, even if they are able to return to work. In several states, there are work incentive programs whereby the state agencies waive the termination of financial benefits to persons with disability if they seek employment ("Work Incentives," 1997). Assistance by a knowledgeable social worker in the field is extremely helpful in this regard. Valuable information may be obtained on a case-by-case basis from the Life Options Rehabilitation Resource Center (RRC) at (800) 468-7777. The USRDS Dialysis Morbidity and Mortality Study: Wave 2 (USRDS, 1997) found that almost 50% of patients with ESRD reported that they were disabled. Only 17.9% were employed full-time, 5.1% were employed part-time, 9.5% were keeping house, and 3.5% were looking for work. Rasgon et al. (1993, 1996) have shown that multidisciplinary predialysis intervention leads to maintenance of employment in a larger number of patients starting dialysis, both in the in-center setting and in the home hemodialysis and CAPD population. The quality of life is significantly better after a successful transplantation. A recent long-term study (Matas et al., 1996) showed that more than 40% of transplant recipients were employed part-time or full-time 8 years after transplantation.

Life Options Rehabilitation Advisory Council (LORAC), which was formed in 1993 by a group of patients, health care providers, researchers, government representatives, and private business persons, has played a major role in bringing the rehabilitation and quality-of-life issues into focus. *Renal Rehabilitation Report*, its newsletter for patients and professionals, has been an important publication, devoted to all the issues concerning rehabilitation for the ESRD patient.

REFERENCES

Ahmad, S., Robertson, H. T., Golper, T. A., Wolfson, M., Kurtin, P., Katz, L. A., Hirschberg, R., Nicora, R., Ashbrook, D. W., & Kopple, J. D. (1990). Multicenter trial of L-carnitine in maintenance hemodialysis patients: 2. Clinical and biochemical effects. *Kidney International, 38*, 912–918.

Canada–USA (CANUSA) Peritoneal Dialysis Study Group. (1996). Adequacy of dialysis and nutrition in continuous peritoneal dialysis: Association with clinical outcomes. *Journal of the American Society of Nephrology, 7*, 198–207.

Consensus Group Statement. (1994). Role of L-carnitine in treating renal dialysis patients. *Dialysis and Transplantation, 23*, 177.

Hagberg, J. M., Goldberg, A. P., Ehsani, A. A., Heath, G. W., Delmez, J. A., & Harter, H. R. (1983). Exercise training improves hypertension in hemodialysis patients. *American Journal of Nephrology, 3*, 209–212.

Hakim, R. M., Breyer, J., Ismail, N., & Schulman, G. (1994). Effect of dose of dialysis on mortality and morbidity. *American Journal of Kidney Diseases, 2*, 661–669.

Harter, H. R., & Goldberg, A. P. (1985). Endurance exercise training: An effective therapeutic modality for hemodialysis patients. *Medical Clinics of North America, 69*, 159–175.

Held, P. J., Port, F. K., Wolfe, R. A., Stannard, D. C., Carroll, C. E., Daugirdas, J. T., Bloembergen, W. E., Greer, J. W., & Hakim, R. M. (1996). The dose of hemodialysis and patient mortality. *Kidney International, 50*, 550–556.

Ikizler, T. A., Greene, J., Wingard, R. L., Parker, R. A., & Hakim, R. M. (1995). Spontaneous dietary protein intake during progression of chronic renal failure. *Journal of the American Society of Nephrology, 6,* 1386–1391.

Klahr, S., Levy, A. S., Beck, G. J., Caggiula, A. W., Hunsicker, L., Kusek, J. W., & Striker, G. (Modification of Diet in Renal Disease Study Group). (1994). The effects of dietary protein restriction and blood pressure control on the progression of chronic renal disease. *New England Journal of Medicine, 330,* 877–884.

Lowrie, E. G., Huang, W. H., & Lew, N. L. (1995). Death risk predictors among peritoneal dialysis and hemodialysis patients: A preliminary comparison. *American Journal of Kidney Diseases, 26*, 220–228.

Lowrie, E. G., Laird, N. M., Parker, T. F., & Sargent, J. A. (1981). Effect of the hemodialysis prescription on patient morbidity. *New England Journal of Medicine, 305*, 1176–1180.

Matas, A. J., Lawson, W., McHugh, L., Gilligham, K., Payne, W. D., Dunn, D. L., Gruessner, R. W. G., Sutherland, D. E. R., & Najarian, J. S. (1996). Employment patterns after successful kidney transplantation. *Transplantation, 61*, 729–733.

Moore, G. E., Parsons, D. B., Stray-Gundersen, J., Painter, P. L., Brinker, K. R., & Mitchell, J. H. (1993). Uremic myopathy limits aerobic capacity in hemodialysis patients. *American Journal of Kidney Diseases, 22,* 277–287.

Mustata, S., Goh, S. T., Goh, S. L., Sanchez, M., Amodeo, M., Conolly, A., Walker, M., Silverstein, A., Mailis, A., & Richardson, R. M. A. (1997). The effect of an exercise program on fitness, quality of life and Kt/V in hemodialysis patients. *Journal of the American Society of Nephrology, 8*, 204A–205A.

National Kidney Foundation—Dialysis Outcomes Quality Initiative (NKF-DOQI). (1997). Clinical practice guidelines for hemodialysis adequacy. *American Journal of Kidney Diseases, 30*(Suppl. 2), S32–S37.

Painter, P. L., & Moore, G. E. (1994). The impact of recombinant human erythropoietin on exercise capacity in hemodialysis patients. *Advances in Renal Replacement Therapy, 1*, 55–65.

Parker, T. F., III., Husni, L., Huang, W., Lew, N., & Lowrie, E. G. (1994). Survival of hemodialysis patients in the United States is improved with a greater quantity of dialysis. *American Journal of Kidney Diseases, 23*, 670–680.

Popovich, R. P., Moncrief, J. W., Decherd, J. F., & Pyler, R. (1976). The definition of a novel portable/wearable equilibrium peritoneal dialysis technique. *Transactions of the American Society of Artificial Internal Organs (Abstracts), 5,* 64.

Rasgon, S. A., Chemleski, B. L., Ho, S., Widrow, L., Yeoh, H. H., Schwankovsky, L., Idroos, M., Reddy, C. R., Agudelo-Dee, L., James-Rogers, A., & Butts, E. (1996). Benefits of a multidisciplinary predialysis program in maintaining employment among patients on home dialysis. *Advances in Peritoneal Dialysis, 12,* 132–135.

Ragson, S., Schwankovsky, L., James-Rogers, A., Widrow, L., Glick, J., & Butts, E. (1993). An intervention for employment maintenance among blue-collar workers with end-stage renal disease. *American Journal of Kidney Disease, 22,* 403–412.

Saltin, B., & Rowell, L. B. (1980). Functional adaptations to physical activity and inactivity. *Federation Proceedings, 39*, 1506–1513.

United States Renal Data System. (1997). Annual data report [Special issue]. *American Journal of Kidney Diseases, 30*(2).

Work incentives: Thoughts from an expert. (1997). *Renal Rehabilitation Report, 5*(5), 3.

Chapter 23

Rheumatic Diseases

Sicy H. Lee and Steven B. Abramson

Rheumatic diseases encompass all disorders in which some portion of the musculoskeletal system, including synovial joints, periarticular structures, or muscles, is involved. Arthritis is the general term used when the joint disease predominates in the patient's illness. Examples of some inflammatory arthritides include rheumatoid arthritis, Reiter's syndrome, and psoriatic arthritis. In other conditions, the periarticular soft tissue or muscle disease is the primary concern, and the joint complaints are only a minor component. Some examples of these diseases include fibromyalgia, polymyositis, polymyalgia rheumatica, and scleroderma.

The classification of rheumatic diseases established by the American College of Rheumatology (ACR), the professional medical organization of the subspecialty of rheumatology, lists 116 rheumatic diseases under 10 major general classes of disorders. The current classification is based on known pathological changes induced in affected tissues, clinical patterns, and/or causative agents of each disease. The classification of the rheumatic diseases is a dynamic process that undergoes periodic review as important new information and concepts concerning pathophysiological mechanisms of these diseases are discovered.

According to the latest estimates derived from numerous surveys and published by the Arthritis Foundation in 1990, there are over 37 million persons suffering from some form of arthritis or related diseases in the United States. Among these individuals at least 26% are partially disabled, and about 10% are totally disabled. Arthritis and related diseases resulted in at least 45 million lost workdays yearly. These figures underscore the magnitude and the problems in diagnosis and management of these diseases. Furthermore, because most rheumatic diseases are chronic disabling conditions, these diseases as a group have significant social and economic ramifications. The rheumatic diseases detailed in this chapter—rheumatoid arthritis, spondyloarthropathies, and degenerative joint disease—are important because they are chronic disabling diseases that occur with relative frequency among individuals within the working population.

RHEUMATOID ARTHRITIS

The prevalence of rheumatoid arthritis in most White populations approaches 1% among adults age 18 and older and increases with age, approaching 2% and 5% in men and women, respectively, by age 65. The incidence also increases with age, peaking between the fourth and sixth decades. The annual incidence for all adults has been estimated at 67/100,000. Both prevalence and incidence are two and three times greater in women than in men (Hochberg, 1981). Racial factors appear to be important in rheumatoid arthritis. American Blacks, native Japanese, and Chinese may have a lower prevalence of rheumatoid arthritis than do Whites, whereas several North American Indian tribes (the Yakima of central Washington State and the Mille-Lac Band of Chippewa in Minnesota) have a high prevalence of rheumatoid arthritis (Cunningham & Kelsey, 1984). Reasons for these differences are unknown but may relate to both genetic and environmental factors.

Genetic factors have an important role in the susceptibility to rheumatoid arthritis. The concordance among monozygotic twins is 25%–50%, whereas the concordance among dizygotic twins is only 10%. Studies have demonstrated a strong association between the major histocompatibility complex (MHC) Class II antigen HLA-DR4 and rheumatoid arthritis across several racial groups. Furthermore, a 5-amino-acid sequence on the beta-1 chain of the DR antigen appears to be shared among DR4 and non-DR4 individuals with rheumatoid arthritis, suggesting that the susceptibility to rheumatoid arthritis appears to be more specifically conferred by this 5-amino-acid sequence than by the entire DR4 molecule (Gregersen, Lee, Silver, & Winchester, 1987). The role of environmental factors, particularly infectious agents, as a causal factor in rheumatoid arthritis remains under active investigation.

Etiology and Pathogenesis

Rheumatoid arthritis is an autoimmune disease in which the normal immune response is directed against an individual's own tissue, including the joints, tendons, and bones, resulting in inflammation and destruction of these tissues.

The cause of rheumatoid arthritis is not known, but current evidence suggests that the initiating event is an immune reaction to a foreign antigen, such as a virus. In an individual with the genetic susceptibility for rheumatoid arthritis, this normal immune response is unchecked, perpetuating the inflammatory response. This theory is supported by the existence of an antibody called the rheumatoid factor, which is initially formed in the synovial fluid and can be found in the serum of about 80% of patients who have had rheumatoid arthritis for several months. This antibody is unique in that it interacts with normal immunoglobulin G, which is itself an antibody. An experimental arthritis in animals similar to rheumatoid arthritis can be induced following inoculation of protein substances similar to these antibodies, supporting this hypothesis in part (Holmdahl, Nordling, Rubin, Tarkowski, & Klareskog, 1986).

During this process of inflammation, cells of the immune system, including monocytes, T lymphocytes, B lymphocytes, and neutrophils, are activated to secrete a variety of chemical substances. These chemicals further stimulate proliferation of the synovial cells that normally line the joints, causing fluid accumulation in the joints (effusion), destruction of cartilage, and erosion of bone. The erosions in the bone can be observed radiographically and are characteristic of rheumatoid arthritis. Pathologically, the typical feature is the invasion of the cartilage and bone by the pannus, a vascular granulation tissue composed of various numbers of inflammatory cells, synovial cells, and new blood vessels. The tendons and ligaments can be similarly affected.

Description of Disease

Rheumatoid arthritis is a systemic disease manifested primarily as polyarthritis. Although the diagnosis is made on clinical grounds, the most recent criteria, established by the ACR in 1987, afford a sensitivity of 91.2% and a specificity of 89.3% for diagnosing rheumatoid arthritis (Arnett et al., 1988). These include (1) morning stiffness lasting at least 1 hour before maximal improvement; (2) arthritis of three or more joints or joint areas simultaneously for more than 6 weeks; (3) involvement of at least one of the following: the wrist, metacarpophalangeal joints (MCPs), or proximal interphalangeal joints (PIPs); (4) symmetrical pattern of joint involvement; (4) subcutaneous nodules over bony prominence or extensor surfaces; (5) positive rheumatoid factor tested by any method that has been positive in less than 5% of normal control subjects; (6) radiographic changes that are typical of rheumatoid arthritis on posteroanterior (PA) views of the hand and wrists, including periarticular osteopenia and/or erosions.

Rheumatoid arthritis usually has a slow, insidious onset over weeks to months. About 15%–20% of individuals have a more rapid onset that develops over days to weeks. About 8%–15% actually have acute onset of symptoms that develop over days. The initial symptoms may be systemic or articular. In some patients, fatigue, malaise, low-grade fever, or diffuse musculoskeletal pain may be the first nonspecific complaints. Morning stiffness is frequently the first presenting symptom prior to onset of joint pain. Although a symmetric pattern is common, asymmetric presentation is not unusual. The usual involvement is oligoarthritis progressing to polyarthritis in an additive but not migratory pattern. The most common joints involved in rheumatoid arthritis are MCPs (87%), PIPs (82%), and wrists (63%). Among larger joints, knees are most commonly involved (56%), followed by the shoulders (47%) and the hips. Medium-size joints are the least commonly involved, with the ankles (53%) affected more frequently than the elbows (21%) (Harris, 1997). The natural history of rheumatoid arthritis is varied. In a minority of patients the intermittent course is marked by partial to complete remission without need for continuous therapy. This pattern of disease is usually mild. Initially, only a few joints are involved. Insidious return of the disease is often marked by progressive joint involvement. The majority of patients develop persistent disease requiring chronic therapy. At least 50% will develop erosive disease of cartilage in bone, which in a significant minority of patients is progressive and debilitating. Recent studies by Pincus and Callahan (1992) and others underscore the increased mortality and morbidity among patients with RA.

Functional Presentation and Disability

In the initial stages of each joint involvement, there is warmth, pain, and redness, with corresponding decrease of range of motion of the affected joint. In the hand, soft tissue swelling occurs as an early finding in rheumatoid arthritis and usually appears as fusiform enlargement of the PIPs. Patients describe difficulty in activity requiring motion of these joints, particularly in the morning. Progression of the disease results in reducible and later fixed deformities, including ulnar deviation, swan neck, or boutonniere deformities (Figures 23.1–23.3). The distal interphalangeal joints (DIPs) are seldom involved in rheumatoid arthritis. Many patients are able to continue performing activities of daily living as well as various nondextrous vocational tasks. The most severe form is arthritis mutilans, in which there is complete bone and joint destruction and all movement is severely limited. At the wrist, there is decreased ability to extend or flex, with progression toward eventual fusion. An exaggerated flexion with near dislocation (subluxation) can occur in severe disease.

Deformities also occur at other joints. At the neck, there can be limitation in extension/flexion as well as rotation. The more serious deformities are those that result in neurological problems such as weakness and paralysis. The transverse ligaments that stabilize C-1 and C-2 vertebrae can become eroded. This results

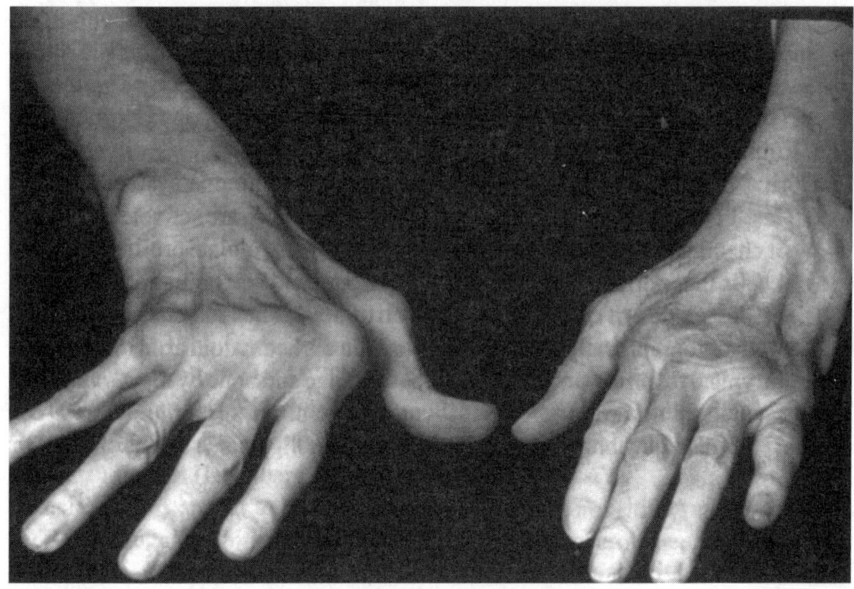

FIGURE 23.1 Rheumatoid arthritis with synovitis of the MCPs and ulnar deviation. (Reproduced with permission from the American College of Rheumatology clinical slide collection.)

in C1–2 (atlantoaxial) subluxation and can cause instability with possible compression of the spinal cord or upward migration of the cervical spine and impingement of the medulla (brain). Such neurological involvement requires surgical intervention. The knees can decrease in flexion and can also develop flexion contracture. The hip may become limited in rotation or flexion extension. The ankle can be affected, with decreased ability to invert/overt or flex/extend. With inflammation or rupture of certain tendons, the foot can become flat. The toes mirror what occurs in the hands with involvement of the MTPs and PIPs. The most common deformities are hammer or cockup toes with metatarsal phalangeal joint (MTP) subluxation and callus formation of the planter surface.

Muscle weakness and atrophy develop early in the course of the disease in many patients. The exact cause of these problems is not clear. One observation is that perhaps the patients are unable to move because of pain, and this lack of movement can cause further muscle atrophy and weakness. The combination of pain and muscle atrophy further diminishes the patient's ability to perform activities requiring both strength and dexterity. Therefore, the vocational and functional

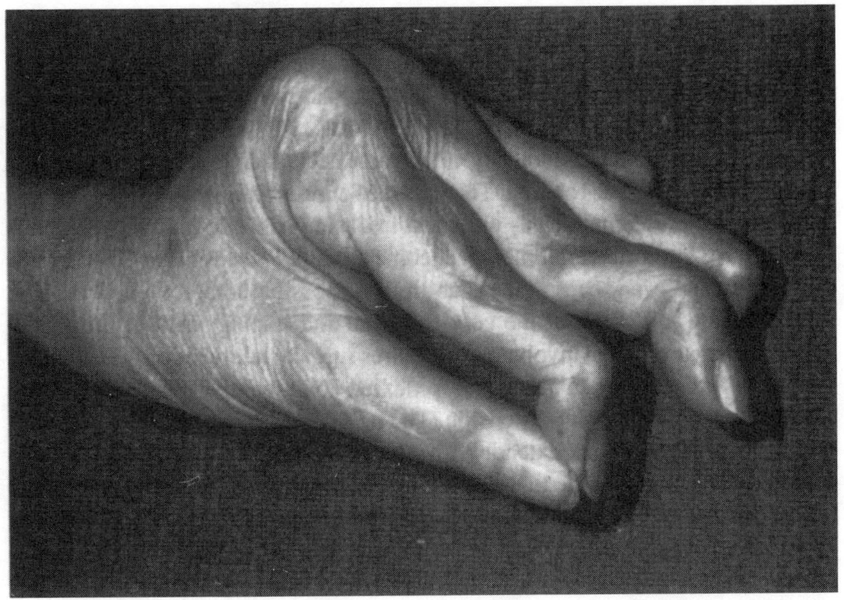

FIGURE 23.2 Rheumatoid arthritis with swan-neck deformity.

skills of the patient may be impaired early by pain, inflammation, and weakness. If the inflammation clears after several weeks and no damage has been done to the bone or cartilage, there usually will be no residual impairment. If the inflammation persists, permanent deformities can develop, such that the mechanics of the joint are altered and the joint cannot function well, even though pain and inflammation may subside eventually.

Complications

There are a number of complications in rheumatoid arthritis. These include carpal tunnel syndrome, Baker's cyst, vasculitis, subcutaneous nodules, Sjögren's syndrome, peripheral neuropathy, cardiac and pulmonary involvement, Felty's syndrome, and anemia (Hurd, 1984). With the exception of carpal tunnel syndrome and Baker's cyst, these complications usually occur in the presence of seropositive, progressive, and destructive disease.

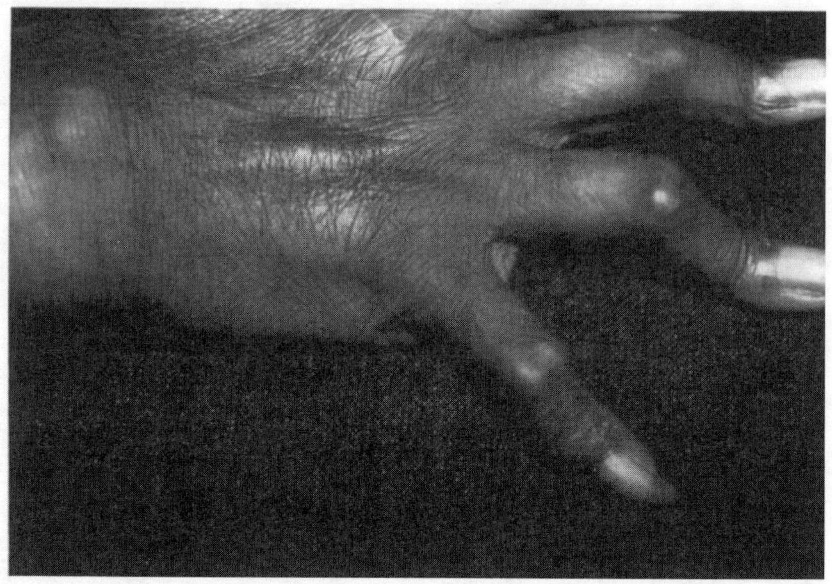

FIGURE 23.3 Rheumatoid arthritis with boutonnier deformity.

Carpal tunnel syndrome occurs when the proliferating synovial tissue compresses on the median nerve as it travels through the narrow space in the flexor surface of the wrist. It is characterized by numbness and tingling and eventual loss of feeling in the thumb and the second and third fingers. The small muscles of the thumb may weaken and atrophy when the compression is not relieved. Baker's cyst occurs when the synovial fluid escapes from the knee and collects in the space behind the knee, with extension into the calf. Rupture of the Baker's cyst can occur abruptly and cause sudden pain and swelling in the calf. These symptoms must be distinguished from venous thrombophlebitis by ultrasound studies.

Vasculitis is the inflammation of blood vessel, affecting capillaries and small and medium-size blood vessels. It can lead to skin lesions such as ulcers and subcutaneous nodules and to more severe problems, such as mononeuritis multiplex. Subcutaneous nodules may develop in approximately 20%–25% of patients. They typically occur in areas subject to pressure, such as the elbows, occiput, or sacrum. They may occasionally break down or become infected but generally are asymptomatic.

In Sjögren's syndrome, lymphocytes invade the glandular tissue of the mouth, nose, eyes, throat, and lungs, resulting in dry eyes (keratoconjunctivitis sicca) and dry mouth (xerostomia). The loss of glandular function may cause ulcers of the eye tissue, dental caries, and an inability to chew food normally. When dry eyes and dry mouth occur alone, the sicca syndrome is said to be present. When sicca syndrome is accompanied by rheumatoid arthritis, the condition is termed Sjögren's syndrome. Lymphocytes can also invade the kidney, liver, lungs, and other internal organs, resulting in their dysfunction.

Many patients with rheumatoid arthritis can develop peripheral neuropathy and complain of mild numbness and tingling in their fingers and toes. Rarely, they can develop mononeuritis and lose complete function of a major nerve. This loss of nerve function is due to inflammation of the blood vessels that supply the nerve. When more than one nerve is involved, it is termed mononeuritis multiplex.

The most common cardiac involvement in rheumatoid arthritis is pericardial effusion, which is reported in about 40% of patients at autopsy but is usually clinically asymptomatic. When symptomatic pericarditis occurs, it will rarely proceed to pericardial tamponade. Sometimes a focal myocarditis may be recognized. Lesions similar to rheumatoid nodules may be found involving the myocardium and the valves. Valvular insufficiency, conduction abnormalities, and myocardial infarction secondary to these inflammatory lesions may occasionally be seen as clinical manifestations of rheumatoid heart disease.

Several forms of pulmonary disease can occur in patients with rheumatoid arthritis. Rheumatoid pleural disease, though frequently found at autopsy, is most commonly asymptomatic. Pleural effusions can develop, but rarely will they accumulate to significant size and cause respiratory distress. Multiple pulmonary nodules may occur bilaterally. Another, more serious pulmonary manifestation of rheumatoid arthritis is interstitial fibrosis with pneumonitis. This may progress to a honeycomb appearance on x-rays, with bronchiectasis, chronic cough, and progressive dyspnea. Lung biopsy can show chronic inflammatory cell infiltration accompanied by neutrophils and eosinophils. Laryngeal obstruction can be caused by arthritis of the cricoarytenoid joint.

Felty's syndrome is characterized by splenomegaly, lymphadenopathy, anemia, thrombocytopenia, and neutropenia in association with chronic active rheumatoid arthritis. Systemic manifestations such as fever, fatigue, anorexia, and weight loss are common. Hyperpigmentation and leg ulcers may accompany Felty's syndrome.

The anemia of rheumatoid arthritis can result either from chronic inflammation that primarily affects the production of red blood cells in the bone marrow or from iron deficiency secondary to occult blood loss among individuals treated with medications that can cause gastritis or peptic ulcer disease. Frequently, a combination of both factors can be present.

Treatment and Prognosis

A variety of medications are available in the treatment of rheumatoid arthritis (Harris, 1997). They can be divided into several broad categories: nonsteroidal antiinflammatory drugs (NSAIDs); steroids; slow-acting, disease-modifying drugs (DMARDs); and immunosuppressive agents. The specific drugs in each group are summarized in Table 23.1 (Solomon, 1991). The choice of therapeutic agents is individualized and dictated by a careful analysis of the severity of the patient's disease and rate of progression of the disease. Clinical assessment is supplemented by laboratory and radiographic assessment. Because articular cartilage or bone in humans cannot be replaced, the goal of the therapy must be to arrest the synovitis prior to any irreversible damage. Early disease can be directly and effectively managed on NSAIDs alone, but these drugs do not arrest the disease process or prevent damage to the cartilage or bone. In individuals who have apparent complete response to NSAIDs alone, follow-up radiographs are imperative to ascertain that there is no occult progression of the disease. Radiographic evidence of progression indicates that DMARDs should be initiated. In individuals with evidence of erosive disease at the initial assessment, DMARDs should be given immediately. Because all DMARDs are slow-acting agents, requiring 2–6 months to be effective, NSAIDs should be given simultaneously. In patients with extensive synovitis who do not obtain relief from NSAIDs, low-dose steroids can be given for temporary relief until DMARDs become effective. Once the disease is controlled or improved on DMARDs, steroid therapy should be tapered and discontinued. Steroids alone should be never be the mainstay of medical therapy because they do not prevent cartilage damage and because they have major side effects. Long-term steroid use can result in early cataract formation, osteoporosis, peptic ulcer disease, augmentation or initiation of hypertension and diabetes, increased skin and vascular fragility, delayed wound healing, muscle weakness, unsightly weight gain and fat accumulation on the face and the trunk, and poor resistance to bacterial and other opportunistic (e.g., fungal) infections.

There is now an increasing tendency to begin DMARDs earlier and more aggressively in the course of the patient's illness. This tendency resulted from the emerging view that there is a brief window of opportunity early in the patient's illness to reverse the inflammatory process. Once articular damage occurs, the destructive process appears to self-perpetuate and cannot be reversed with medications. Methotrexate, sulfasalazine, hydroxychloroquine, parenteral gold and D-penicillamine are the most frequently used medications. Gold and D-penicillamine have potential major side effects, including nephrosis (protein in the urine), anemia, leukopenia, thrombocytopenia, stomatitis, skin rash, and interstitial pulmonary fibrosis. Therefore, close laboratory and clinical monitoring is required while patients are on these medications. In order for the patients to accept these

TABLE 23.1 Agents Used to Treat Rheumatoid Arthritis

Agent	Dose[a]
Antiinflammatory agents	
Salicylates	1000–5000 mg/day (adjusted based on serum salicylate levels)
Aspirin	
Sodium salicylate	
Salicylic acid (Trilisate)	
Diflunisal (Dolobid)	
NSAIDs	
Ibuprofen (Motrin)	400–800 mg t.i.d.–q.i.d.
Sulindac (Clinoril)	150–200 mg b.i.d
Piroxicam (Feldene)	10–20 mg q.d.
Indomethacin (Indocin)	25–50 mg b.i.d.–q.i.d., 75 mg SR
Meclofenamate (Meclomen)	50–100 mg b.i.d.–q.i.d.
Naproxen (Naprosyn/Naprelene)	25–500 mg b.i.d.
Ketoprofen (Orudis/Oruvail)	50–75 mg b.i.d.–q.i.d., 200 mg q.d.
Oxaprozin (Daypro)	1200–1800 mg q.d.
Tolmetin (Tolectin)	200–400 mg b.i.d.–q.i.d
Diclofenac (Voltaren/Cataflam)	25–75 mg b.i.d.
Flurbiprofen (Ansaid)	50–100 mg b.i.d.
Corticosteroids	5.0–15 mg q.d. for arthritis
Oral prednisone	Higher doses for extraarticular disease
Intraarticular	Varies with joint size
Disease-modifying agents (slow-acting agents)	
Gold	
Oral (Ridaura)	3 mg q.i.d.–b.i.d.
Parenteral (Solganol)	
D-penicillamine (Depen, Cupramine)	125–1000 mg q.d.
Hydroxychloroquine (Plaquenil)	200–600 mg q.d.
Sulfasalazine (Azulfidine)	1000–1500 mg b.i.d.
Immunosuppressive agents	
Methotrexate (PO, IM, IV)	5.0–30 mg/week
Azathioprine (Imuran)	25–150 mg q.d.
Cyclophosphamide (Cytoxan)	25–150 mg q.d.

(continued)

TABLE 23.1 *(continued)*

Agent	Dose[a]
Biological agents	
TNF receptor antagonist (Embrel)	
IL-10	
IL-2 fusion toxin	
IL-1 receptor antagonist	
Monoclonal antibodies	
Anti-CD4	
Anti-CD5	
Miscellaneous	
Leflunomide (Arava)	
Levamisole	
Mecophenolic acid	
Cyclosporin A (Neoral)	
Dapsone	
Thalidomide	

[a]q.d. = once daily; b.i.d. = twice a day; t.i.d. = three times a day; q.i.d. = four times a day; SR = slow release.

Adapted from "Inflammatory Arthritis" by G. Solomon (1991), in M. Jahss (Ed.), *Disorders of the Foot and Ankle* (2nd ed.), Vol. 2, New York: W. B. Saunders. Adapted with permission.

potentially toxic medications, the physician must adequately explain the necessity for their use. Oral gold and antimalarials have less toxic side effects but are also less likely to be effective. Because of the potential damage to the retina, regular ophthalmological examination is necessary while the patient is on antimalarials. Methotrexate is gaining widespread use and is relatively easy to administer, as it is given once a week. The drug is effective, but there are concerns about long-term toxicity, particularly pulmonary and hepatic fibrosis (Tugwell, Bennett, & Gent, 1987). Sulfasalazine has gained popularity in Europe as an effective DMARD (Pinals, Kaplan, Lawson, & Hepburn, 1986). The adverse effects associated with the use of this drug include blood dyscrasias, drug fever, hepatitis, allergic pneumonitis, drug-induced lupus, vasculitis, and significant cutaneous reaction, including exfoliative dermatitis. Very few serious reactions have been reported in rheumatoid arthritis patients, and the adverse events appear to occur more commonly among slow acetylators. Leflunomide (Arava) is an isoxazole drip recently approved by the FDA for treatment for RA, and appears similar to methotrexate and sulfasalazine in efficacy; the major potential side effect is hepatotoxicity, and monitoring is required monthly.

Other cytotoxic drugs (azathioprine, cyclophosphamide) appear effective but also have many potential side effects and require careful monitoring (Hunter, Urowitz, & Gordon, 1975). Other antirheumatic agents whose long-term benefits have not been fully established include dapsone, cyclosporin A, levamisole, amiprilose hydrochloride (Therafectin) (Caldwell, Saville, & Bedsole, 1987; Fowler, Shadforth, Crook, & Lawton, 1984; Miller, Demerieux, & Srinivasan, 1980; Yocum, Klippel, & Wilder, 1988).

The newest class of drugs under active investigation in the treatment of rheumatoid arthritis comprises the biological agents, including tumor necrosis factor (TNF)-receptor antagonists, interleukin (IL)-10, anti-CD5 and anti-CD4 monoclonal antibodies (Ackerman & Strand, 1990; Dayer, 1990; Merkel, Letourneau, & Polisson, 1995; Saunders, 1991; Waldman, 1991). These agents are unique in that they target a specific arm or subpopulation of cells within the immune system so that the inflammatory response in rheumatoid arthritis is abrogated. The soluble TNF antagonist (Embrel) has been preliminarily approved by the FDA for treatment in RA. Other therapies include nonpharmacological interventions such as lymphoid irradiation, lymphopheresis, and radiation synovectomy. Dietary modifications of endogenous prostaglandin synthesis with fish oil supplements is currently under investigation at many centers and appears to be of some clinical benefit. Another emerging trend in the medical management of rheumatoid arthritis is the use of combination drug therapy. Smaller doses of multiple drugs with synergistic effects are used, in effect lowering the level of toxicity of individual drugs and enhancing the efficacy of treatment. Few controlled studies for various regimens of combination therapy are available, and the selection of the best combination remains to be established. The ultimate challenge for the future is to devise safe and effective therapies that can be administered in early stages of the disease.

Surgical treatment in rheumatoid arthritis should be used in combination with medical therapy. For patients with severe synovitis, in whom the slow-acting agents have not yet taken effect, early synovectomy (removal of the synovial tissue to as great a degree as possible) can be considered for the elbows and knees. When permanent deformities have developed despite medical therapy, surgery can be performed to correct these deformities to decrease pain and improve the patient's functional status. These procedures include joint fusions (e.g., wrist fusion to provide a stable and painless wrist), resections (e.g., resection of the distal ends of the metatarsal heads to reduce foot pain and improve comfort and walking), and joint prosthesis. The most successful total joint replacements are the hips and knees; joint replacement for the shoulder, elbow, and ankle are available but less successful.

Rehabilitation therapy is an integral part of treatment in rheumatoid arthritis. In early disease, the goal is to reduce pain and inflammation and to prevent deformities and muscle atrophy. As the disease progresses, it is an important modality to correct deformities and increase strength. The major goal at each stage is to improve functional skills in the patient. Modalities that are used to reduce pain and inflammation include moist heat, paraffin baths, and cold packs that allow more activities to be performed with less discomfort. The choice of treatment depends largely on patient preference because there are few data on which one can base the choice. The pain relief is temporary, lasting perhaps 2 hours. It is important, therefore, that the patient be taught how to perform these treatments at home. Placing a joint in plastic, fiberglass, or plaster splints will protect the joint and diminish the inflammation. There must be balance between exercise and rest, however, to prevent deterioration of motion and muscle atrophy. Splints are most conveniently placed on the wrists or hands. For some, night use alone may be sufficient.

Exercise is important to prevent as well as preserve and increase muscle strength. Non-weight-bearing and isometric exercises will allow improvement in strength without joint inflammation. Passive range-of-motion exercises will help preserve motion without stress on the joints. Physical and occupational therapists should also evaluate the patient's functional limitation in activities of daily living and ambulation. Patients should be taught ambulation and transfer techniques. Devices such as reachers, hooks, and built-up utensil handles can be provided. The occupational therapist may also make energy- or labor-saving recommendations for the home, such as the raising or lowering of table tops or changing to more easily activated faucet handles. All of these measures aim to allow the patient to be more functional and independent.

The majority of patients with rheumatoid arthritis respond partially to some form of therapy, but few go into true remission, defined as absence of radiographic progression and of clinical symptoms. The general course of rheumatoid arthritis, then, is generally gradual diminution of inflammation but progression of deformities (Pincus & Callahan, 1992). The speed with which the deformities occur varies from patient to patient. Factors associated with poor prognosis include persistent inflammation despite aggressive medical therapy of more than 1 year's duration; onset of disease below age 30; presence of extraarticular manifestation of rheumatoid arthritis, including subcutaneous nodules, vasculitis, Sjögren's syndrome, and neuropathy; and high-titer rheumatoid factor.

Psychological and Vocational Implications

Patients with rheumatoid arthritis undergo several stages of psychological adjustments. In the early stages of disease, it is common for patients with rheumatoid arthritis to be frightened because of the uncertainty of the prognosis of the disease and the degree of disability. Many patients also tend to blame themselves or a particular incident for the onset of the disease. Along with this feeling of guilt, there is also denial. Many patients do not give up hope that one day the disease and pain will miraculously vanish. This type of denial may lead to unrealistic expectations and resistance to medical treatment. As the disease progresses, the patient may express various degrees of anger, frustration, resentment, and depression. Some patients adapt to their disease and disability and function well with limited abilities, whereas other patients seem incapacitated by fairly minimal involvement. Adaptation to rheumatoid arthritis requires the patient to have self-confidence and the willingness to adjust certain aspects of lifestyle without sacrificing independence. This adaptation is difficult and may be thwarted by pain denial, anger, and depression. Another reaction to the disease is hopelessness and increased dependency. Faced with the prospect of progressive deformities and apparent deterioration, the patient may give up trying to remain active by increasingly depending on others for care.

Not all individuals with rheumatoid arthritis progress unremittingly to disability. In the minority of patients with mild disease, fewer adjustments are required and vocational goals can be easily met. However, in individuals in whom the disease is an evolving and dynamic process, the vocational counselor should make frequent assessment of the patient's functional ability as the disease progresses and provide realistic goals and support through the more difficult periods so that employment can be sustained.

In general, motor coordination, finger and hand dexterity, and eye-hand-foot coordination are adversely affected by rheumatoid arthritis. Vocational goals dependent on fine, dexterous, or coordinated movement of the hand are therefore not ideal for patients with rheumatoid arthritis. Loss of motion and pain on motion slow the patient's movements and diminish coordination. Therefore, the operation of machines requiring repetitive, dexterous, and rapid movements is also not a desirable choice. However, if the force required is quite low, dexterous tasks such as the use of an electric typewriter or computer are quite possible.

Most jobs requiring medium to heavy physical activity are also not desirable. Although most patients may be able to perform medium manual labor (i.e., lift 25–30 lb), that level of activity will not be sustainable as the disease progresses. In addition, such a workload may be harmful to the joints. Activities such as climbing, balancing, stooping, kneeling, standing, or walking are all hampered by pain on weight bearing or with motion. Although these activities can be accomplished by most individuals with milder forms of rheumatoid arthritis, jobs requiring such activities repetitively and without periods of rest cannot be sustained and indeed may damage joints.

It is usual for patients with rheumatoid arthritis to detect changes in humidity, temperature, or barometric pressure. Therefore, extremes of weather or abrupt changes in temperature should be avoided, and an indoor climate in which the environment is relatively controlled is recommended. Excessive noise, vibration, fumes, gases, dust, and poor ventilation have no specific effects on patients with rheumatoid arthritis except for those individuals with appreciable pulmonary involvement.

Advanced or additional educational goals, such as vocational training and/or college courses of 2 to 4 years, should be strongly considered for individuals with recent-onset rheumatoid arthritis and those with long-standing disease despite increased mortality and morbidity among the latter. Educational goals should be guided by the patient's interest and aptitude. It is important to realize that the individual with rheumatoid arthritis does not have a permanent invariant disability but rather a changing disability with chronic pain (which can vary from day to day) that generally results in a progressive and unfavorable outcome. Such individuals require ongoing coordinated counseling that provides a combination of empathy, encouragement, and adequate evaluation and treatment.

SERONEGATIVE SPONDYLARTHROPATHIES

The seronegative spondyloarthropathies consist of a group of related disorders that include Reiter's syndrome, ankylosing spondylitis, psoriatic arthritis, and arthritis in association with inflammatory bowel disease. This group of diseases occurs more commonly among young men, with a mean age at diagnosis in the third decade and a peak incidence between ages 25 and 34. The prevalence appears to be approximately 1%. The male-to-female ratio approaches 4 to 1 among adult Caucasians (Hochberg, 1992).

Genetic factors play an important role in the susceptibility to each disease. Among Caucasians, over 90% of patients with ankylosing spondylitis are HLA-B27-positive, and approximately 20% of individuals with the HLA-B27 antigen will develop some form of spondyloarthritis. In addition, disease concordance for ankylosing spondylitis among monozygotic twins exceeds 50%. Linkage to other MHC Class I antigens that are cross-reactive with B27 (B7, B22, B40, B42) also has been observed, particularly among Blacks, in whom the association between ankylosing spondylitis and HLA-B27 (40%–50%) is not as striking as that in Caucasians (Arnett, 1984).

Etiology and Pathogenesis

The cause of spondyloarthritis is unclear, but there is strong evidence that the initial event involves interaction between genetic factors determined by Class I MHC genes and environment factors, particularly bacterial infections. The onset of musculoskeletal symptoms following exposure to infections suggest an immunologically mediated process, as does the finding of lymphocytes at the sites of inflammation.

Reiter's syndrome may follow a wide range of gastrointestinal infections, including species of *Salmonella*, *Shigella*, *Yersinia*, *Campylobacter*, and *Escherichia coli* (Arnett, 1984). Recent work by Schumacher has identified chlamydia organisms in the synovial tissue. *Giardia*, *Brucella*, and *Streptococcus* organisms also have been implicated, as well as amebae, and episodes of diarrhea in which no specific pathogen can be identified have been reported (Callin & Fries, 1976; Voltonen, Leirisalo, & Pentikainen, 1985). Arthritis also occurs in association with inflammatory bowel disease in patients who have undergone intestinal bypass operations for obesity and in Whipple's disease. Bowel inflammation has been implicated in the pathogenesis of endemic Reiter's syndrome, psoriatic arthritis, and ankylosing spondylitis. A putative link between these diverse conditions is the ability of enteric organisms to gain access to the systemic circulation and initiate an immune response in a genetically susceptible individual. The observation that some bacterial antigens share certain amino acid sequences with the HLA-B27 molecule suggests molecular mimicry as a plausible mechanism to explain the link between infection and arthritis in the presence of HLA-B27 (Inman, Chiu, Johnston, & Falk, 1992). This association, however, does not explain why only 20% of HLA-B27 individuals develop arthritis in the face of appropriate enteric infection. Whether there are fewer evident genetic differences between healthy and diseased HLA-B27-positive individuals remains under investigation.

Description of Disease

The spondyloarthropathies share certain common features, including the absence of serum rheumatoid factor, an oligoarthritis commonly involving large joints in the lower extremities, frequent involvement of the axial skeleton, familial clustering, and linkage to HLA-B27. Unlike rheumatoid arthritis, in which the predominant site of inflammation is the synovium, these disorders are characterized by inflammation at sites of attachment of ligament, tendon, fascia, or joint capsule to bone (enthesopathy).

Because the musculoskeletal presentation in each of the seronegative disorders is indistinguishable, current classification schemes are based on the presence of extraarticular features such as psoriasis, colitis, urethritis, aphthous stomatitis, inflammatory eye disease, nail changes, and keratoderma blenorrhagicum. Unfortunately, none of these features is unique to any particular disease. Psoriasis may occur in the setting of inflammatory bowel disease, aphthous stomatitis may occur in any of the seronegative disorders, keratoderma may be indistinguishable from pustular psoriasis, and axial changes in psoriatic or colitic arthritis can be indistinguishable from primary ankylosing spondylitis. Overlap syndromes are common. Finally, there are patients with oligoarthritis and enthesopathy who

TABLE 23.2 Clinical Criteria for Ankylosing Spondylitis (New York, 1966)

Diagnosis

1. Limitation of the lumbar spine in all three planes—anterior flexion, lateral flexion, and extension
2. History or the presence of pain in the dorsolumbar junction or in the lumbar spine
3. Limitation of chest expansion to 1 inch (2.5 cm) or less, measured at the level of the fourth intercostal space

Grading (requires radiographs of sacroiliac joints)

Definite AS

Grade 3–4 bilateral sacroiliitis with at least one clinical criterion

Grade 3–4 unilateral or grade 2 bilateral sacroiliitis with clinical criterion 1 or with clinical criteria 2 and 3

Probable AS

Grade 3–4 bilateral sacroiliitis with no clinical criteria

From P. H. Bennett and T. A. Burch (1967), "New Diagnostic Criteria," *Bulletin on the Rheumatic Diseases, 17*, p. 453. Reprinted by permission.

lack sufficient extraarticular features to allow a specific diagnosis by existing criteria. HLA typing may provide a means of establishing that these patients have a disorder that falls within the spectrum of spondyloarthropathy. Given these pitfalls, the most accurate way of classifying a given patient may be to delineate fully the clinical features of the disease as well as the immunogenetic background in which it occurs. Ankylosing spondylitis is the prototype disease among this group of disorders. The diagnosis is confirmed by clinical and radiographic findings. Existing criteria include the Rome and the New York criteria (Table 23.2) (P. H. Bennett & Burch, 1967). Ankylosing spondylitis is considered primary if no other rheumatological disorder is present and secondary if the patient has evidence of Reiter's syndrome, psoriasis, or colitis.

Reiter's syndrome was first described by Reiter in 1916 and consists of the triad of arthritis, urethritis, and conjunctivitis. Paronen (1948) subsequently pointed out the association of antecedent infectious urethritis or dysentery with the clinical triad. Arnett introduced the concept of incomplete Reiter's syndrome to describe those individuals who had only two of the features of the triad and underscored the association of the incomplete syndrome with HLA-B27 (Arnett, McClusky, & Schacter, 1976). The most current ACR criteria are much broader; they define Reiter's syndrome as a seronegative arthritis that follows urethritis, cervicitis, or dysentery. Possible associated features include balanitis, inflammatory eye disease, oral ulcers, and keratoderma. Callin has proposed a broader definition (Table 23.3) that gives added weight to these extraarticular features (Fox, Callin, Gerber, & Gibson, 1979).

Psoriatic arthritis is not a single disease entity but consists of many different patterns of musculoskeletal disorders occurring in individuals with psoriasis. Patients may present with disease that is clinically indistinguishable from rheumatoid arthritis, ankylosing spondylitis, or Reiter's syndrome. The most widely used criteria are those of Moil and Wright (Table 23.4; R. M. Bennett, 1979). Complicating this classification scheme is the observation that in up to 20% of patients the musculoskeletal disease antedates the onset of psoriasis. Therefore, an individual with dactylitis and radiographic evidence of pencil-in-cup deformities may be considered to have psoriatic arthritis even if the patient lacks skin disease. A family history of psoriasis or the presence of psoriasis-associated HLA alleles would further support this diagnosis (Mielants, Veys, & Cuvelier, 1985).

There are no distinct criteria for the enteropathic arthritis accompanying ulcerative colitis or Crohn's disease. A clinical spectrum of diseases similar to those seen in association with psoriasis may be observed. In an individual patient, axial disease, peripheral arthritis, or enthesopathy may predominate. Peripheral arthritis tends to parallel activity of bowel disease, whereas axial disease may progress independent of bowel activity. Complicating the concept of enteropathic arthritis as a distinct disease is the observation that low-grade bowel inflammation may be found on colonic or ileal biopsy in all of the seronegative disorders.

Patients with spondyloarthropathy may also develop inflammation of the aorta (aortitis) and the aortic valve, resulting in aortic insufficiency. Pulmonary fibrosis also may occur, resulting in diminished diffusion capacity and restrictive lung disease.

TABLE 23.3 Clinical Criteria for Reiter's Syndrome

Seronegative asymmetric arthropathy (predominately lower extremity)
Plus one or more of the following:
- Urethritis
- Cervicitis
- Inflammatory eye disease
- Mucocutaneous disease: balanitis, oral ulceration, or keratoderma

Exclusions
- Primary ankylosing spondylitis
- Psoriatic arthropathy
- Other rheumatic disease

From R. Fox, A. Callin, R. C. Gerber, & D. Gibson (1979), "The Chronicity of Symptoms and Disability in Reiter's Syndrome. An Analysis of 131 Consecutive Patients," *Annals of Internal Medicine, 91*, p. 190. Reprinted by permission.

TABLE 23.4 Diagnosis of Psoriatic Arthritis

Criterion I	Psoriatic skin or nail involvement
Criterion II	Peripheral arthritis
Clinical	Pain and soft-tissue swelling with or without limitation of motion of the distal interphalangeal joints for over 4 weeks
	Pain and soft-tissue swelling with or without limitation of motion of the peripheral joints involved in an asymmetric peripheral pattern for over 4 weeks; this category includes diffuse swelling of an entire digit, known as the "sausage" digit
	Symmetric peripheral arthritis for over 4 weeks, in the absence of rheumatoid factor or subcutaneous nodules
Radiologic	"Pencil-in-cup" deformity, "whittling" of terminal phalanges, "fluffy periostitis," and "bony ankylosis"
Criterion III	Axial involvement
Clinical	Spinal pain and stiffness with restriction of motion present for over 4 weeks
Radiologic	Grade II symmetrical sacroiliitis according to the New York criteria or Grade II or IV unilateral sacroiliitis

Definite diagnosis of psoriatic arthritis requires Criterion I and any of the subheadings under Criteria II and III.

From "Psoriatic Arthritis" by R. M. Bennett (1979), in D. J. McCarthy (Ed.), *Arthritis and Allied Conditions: A textbook on rheumatology* (9th ed.), Philadelphia: Lea & Febiger. Reprinted by permission.

Functional Presentation and Disability

When the axial skeleton is involved, the initial symptom is morning stiffness and lower back pain. As the disease worsens, there is progressive diminution of motion of the spine. Eventually, the sacroiliac joints, lumbar, thoracic, and cervical spine become fused, although the process may skip over parts. At this stage the spine is no longer painful, but the patient has lost all ability to flex or rotate the spine and generally develops a hunched-over posture with fused flexion of the cervical spine and flexion contracture of the hips to compensate for the loss of the lordosis curvature in the lumbar spine. The joints where the ribs attach to the vertebrae are also affected, and chest expansion and lung volume are decreased. Frequently, peripheral joints are involved, and the pattern is usually asymmetric oligoarthritis involving primarily the large or medium joints, including the hips, knees, and ankles. Rarely are smaller joints or the joints in the upper extremities involved. Enthesopathy can occur at multiple sites but more commonly presents as plantar fasciitis, Achilles tendinitis, and medial or lateral epicondylitis.

Loss of motion of the spine or pain in the spine with motion generally affects a patient's mobility, making certain chores difficult. Walking, however, remains unimpaired unless the hips and knees are affected. Frequent stooping and bending become impossible. Toilet activities and dressing may be difficult, but rarely does the patient become dependent. In fact, a patient with ankylosing spondylitis typically is able to continue vocational activity despite progressive stiffness, unless it requires significant back mobility or physical labor.

Treatment and Prognosis

NSAIDs are the initial primary agents in the treatment of seronegative spondyloarthritis. Indomethacin is commonly regarded as being the most effective. Phenylbutazone is probably equally effective, but its use is restricted by the risk of aplastic anemia. Other NSAIDs, including naproxen, piroxicam, meclofenamate, and flurbiprofen, are also efficacious. Salicylates generally are not effective treatment. Corticosteroids, when given at a significantly higher dose than that used in rheumatoid arthritis, also can be quite effective. If the inflammation does not completely resolve with NSAIDs alone or erosive disease is present at the initial evaluation, DMARDs should be given to prevent joint destruction and fusion. The more common DMARDs used in the treatment of spondyloarthritis include sulfasalazine and methotrexate (Nissila, Lehtinen, & Leirisalo-Repo, 1988). Parenteral gold has been found to be effective therapy in patients with the form of psoriatic arthritis that mimics rheumatoid arthritis. Surgical intervention includes either early synovectomy or total joint replacement in the later stages of disease. Physical therapy is also an integral part of treatment. Exercises should be done daily and should include those that enable the patient to maintain maximum chest expansion and erect posture as well as maximal axial flexibility.

Spondyloarthritis follows at least three different courses. The majority of patients experience recurrent episodes of arthritis. A minority have only one self-limiting episode of the disease. A smaller minority of patients suffer a continuous and unremitting aggressive course. Although most patients can continue to work, most are affected and become disabled as the disease progresses (Fox et al., 1979).

Vocational Implications

The patient with spondylitis should be considered for vocational or professional education as resources and interest dictate. Although motor coordination, eye-hand coordination, and eye-hand-foot coordination will not be impaired among individuals with minimum peripheral arthritis, a stiff back will limit the patient's rotation and flexion so that overall dexterity may be affected. Tasks that require reaching or bending will be difficult. Work requiring lifting of over 10 to 15 lb may cause increased back pain. Climbing and balancing skills, stooping, and kneeling may be tolerated initially but become difficult as the disease worsens. Even with sedentary tasks, the patient must be allowed the opportunity to stretch the spine frequently. Although many individuals describe joint pain in relation to weather changes, patients with spondylitis should not necessarily require an indoor environment. Some noise, vibration, fumes, gas, dust, and poor ventilation should not be more intolerable than they are to an individual without spondyloarthritis unless significant pulmonary involvement is present. In general, patients with advanced education or clerical skills will frequently be able to continue meaningful employment, whereas those with only manual skills will become disabled.

DEGENERATIVE JOINT DISEASE

Degenerative joint disease (osteoarthritis) is the most common rheumatic disease and is characterized by progressive loss of cartilage and reactive changes at the margins of the joint and in the subchondral bone. The disease usually begins in the fourth decade; prevalence increases with age, and the disease becomes almost universal in individuals aged 65 and older (Scott & Hochberg, 1984). It primarily affects weight-bearing joints such as the knees, hips, and lumbosacral spine. Frequently, the DIPs and PIPs are involved. Rarely, the shoulder also can be affected.

Etiology and Pathogenesis

The cause of degenerative arthritis is unclear. It is considered to be a "wear and tear" arthritis and is thought to occur as a consequence of some earlier damage or overuse of the joint. Obesity is frequently associated with degenerative joint disease in the weight-bearing joints (Hartz, Fischer, & Bril, 1986). Genetic factors play a role in the development of osteoarthritis of the PIPs and DIPs and appear to involve a single autosomal gene that is sex-influenced and dominant in females, resulting in an incidence 10 times greater than in men.

Degenerative changes begin as focal erosion of cartilage at various points of stress. There follows an increase in water content of the cartilage and quantitative and qualitative changes in the cartilage proteoglycans. Enzymes capable of degrading proteoglycans and collagen are increased in the osteoarthritis cartilage. As disease progresses, cartilage erosions become confluent and lead to large areas of denuded surface. The final outcome is full-thickness loss of cartilage down to bone. In contrast with this structural ulcerative breakdown, there is a proliferative cartilage and bone response leading to thickening of the subchondral bone and increased bony formation (osteophyte). Low-grade synovitis is common, particularly in advanced disease and is due to release of inflammatory mediators or humoral and cell-mediated immune responses to damaged joint components (Pelletier, Martel-Pelletier, & Howell, 1985).

Description of Disease

In early disease, pain occurs only after joint use and is relieved by rest. As disease progresses, pain occurs with minimal motion or even at rest. Nocturnal pain is commonly associated with severe disease. Acute inflammatory flares may be precipitated by trauma or, in some patients, by crystal-induced synovitis in response to crystals of calcium pyrophosphate, or apatite. Stiffness usually occurs only in affected joints. Local tenderness, pain on passive motion, and bony crepitus are prominent findings. Joint enlargement results from synovitis, synovial effusion, or proliferative changes in cartilage and bone (osteophyte formation). Clinical symptoms usually show positive correlation with radiological abnormalities. In a given patient, however, the lack of correlation between joint symptoms and radiographic findings may be striking.

Osteophytes formed at the DIPs are termed Heberden's nodes, and similar changes at the PIPs are called Bouchard's nodes. Flexor and lateral deviation of the DIPs are common. In most patients, Heberden's nodes develop slowly over months or years. These deformities are generally asymptomatic and primarily concern the patient for cosmetic reasons. In other patients, onset is rapid and associated with moderately severe inflammatory changes. This pattern of osteoarthritis is termed erosive osteoarthritis and frequently occurs during the fourth decade in women with a strong familial history. The first metacarpal (MP) joints are frequently involved, leading to tenderness at the base of the first MP bone and a squared appearance of the hand.

Osteoarthritis of the knee is characterized by localized tenderness over various components of the joint and by pain on passive or active motion. Crepitus is usually present, and muscle atrophy is seen secondary to disuse. Disproportionate losses of cartilage localized to the medial or lateral compartments of the knee lead to secondary genu varum or valgum deformity. Chondromalacia patellae is commonly detected and is associated with softening and erosion of the patellar articular cartilage. Pain, localized around the patella, is aggravated by activity such as climbing stairs.

Osteoarthritic changes in the hip present with an insidious onset of pain. Pain is usually localized to the groin or along the inner aspect of the thigh, although patients often complain of pain in the buttocks, sciatic region, or the knee due to pain referral along contiguous nerves. Physical examination shows loss of hip motion, initially most marked on internal rotation or extension. Osteoarthritis of the MTPs can lead to MTP subluxation with corresponding hammer toe deformities. In the first MTP, the most common change is hallux valgus deformities. The severity of these deformities is usually aggravated by inappropriate footwear such as high heels and narrow, pointed, tight shoes.

Osteoarthritis of the spine results from involvement of the intervertebral disks, vertebral bodies, or posterior apophyseal articulations. Associated symptoms include local pain and stiffness and radicular pain due to compression of contiguous nerve roots. Lumbar stenosis is the term used when compression of the spinal cord occurs at multiple levels. The presenting symptoms can be pain on walking and must be differentiated from claudication secondary to vascular incompetence. The presence of nocturnal pain can be a differentiating symptom for lumbar disease. In severe cases, myelopathy can develop, leading to muscle atrophy and disability. Surgical intervention is recommended when there are signs of neuropathy or myelopathy.

Functional Disabilities

Osteoarthritis affects the patient's performance by impeding use of the involved joint. Because the hips, knees, and lower back are common sites of degenerative joint disease, walking and transfer activities may be impaired. At first the patient will be able to function well in a limited area, but as the disease progresses, the patient's functional capability decreases. Generally, however, activities of daily living, including dressing and eating, will not be significantly impaired.

Treatment and Prognosis

The primary goal in the treatment of osteoarthritis is pain control and improvement of function in the affected joint. NSAIDs should be used in patients who show signs of inflammatory response in the affected joint. Analgesic agents such as acetaminophen may be used on a continuous basis, in combination with NSAIDs, to enhance pain control. Oral or parenteral therapy with corticosteroids is contraindicated in the treatment of osteoarthritis. Intraarticular injections of corticosteroids, however, may be beneficial when used judiciously in the management of acute flares, when inflammatory response appears to be a major component. Injections should be infrequent because joint deterioration may be accelerated by masking of pain and subsequent joint overuse or by a direct deleterious effect of these drugs on cartilage.

Newer therapies on the horizon are aimed at preserving the joint function and preventing further damage. These potential treatments can be divided into disease- or structure-modifying drugs and those that improve functional status only. The disease-modifying agents include tetracyclines, glycosaminoglycan polyuric acid, glycosaminoglycan-peptide complex, pentosan polysulfate, gene therapy, and the use of growth factors and cytokines (Howell & Altman, 1993). The mode of action is either through inhibition of collagenase activity, increase in the level of tissue inhibitor of metalloproteinases (TIMP), or manipulation of these factors via cytokines or gene therapy. Potential agents that are used only for symptomatic treatment of osteoarthritis include glucosamine sulfate, chondroitin sulfate, and intraarticular administration of hyaluronic acid derivatives. Glucosamine sulfate and chondroitin sulfate are available in the United States as nutritional supplements. Some evidence exists from Europe that these drugs may modify symptoms in selected patients, but no adequate controlled trial has been conducted to establish their effect in structural modification. Although hyaluronic acid derivatives are often mentioned as potential structure-modifying drugs, these products are currently considered to be long-acting, symptom-modifying drugs only (Peyron, 1993).

The goal in early physical therapy is to improve the functional status and prevent further deterioration of the affected joint. Patients should be instructed in daily non-weight-bearing exercise to strengthen muscles and thus protect joints from overuse. In addition, they should be taught weight-bearing techniques. Appliances such as canes are also beneficial. Surgical procedures in the treatment of osteoarthritis include arthroplasty, osteotomy, and total prosthetic replacement. Hip and knee replacement procedures produce striking symptomatic relief and improved range of motion. Advances in arthroscopic techniques have led to increased surgical management, such as debridement to remove loose bodies and abrasion chondroplasty, earlier in the disease.

Osteoarthritis is a slowly progressive disease. Although medical and rehabilitative treatment can lead to improvement of function and diminution of pain in most patients, the effect is generally temporary. There is currently no established disease-modifying drug in the treatment of osteoarthritis. The eventual outcome is complete destruction of the joint, and ultimately surgical intervention is required.

Vocational Implications

Because osteoarthritis is not a systemic disease, successful treatment of a single involved joint may result in continued employment in the patient's current job unless it requires dexterous or heavy use of the involved joint. Even if surgical or medical treatment results in an increased range of motion, diminished pain, and increased functional ability of the affected joint, the use of that joint should be limited. Heavy lifting, which repeatedly places stress on the hips, knees, or lumbosacral spine, should be avoided by those who have osteoarthritis in these areas. Light to medium work should be possible. Climbing, balancing skills, stooping, and kneeling will be impaired in many patients with osteoarthritis. The environment has no significant effect on patients with osteoarthritis even though changes in relative humidity and barometric pressures may cause transient joint discomfort.

Returning to work after undergoing successful surgery requires intensive postoperative rehabilitation and continued exercise to maintain muscle strength. As the patient's endurance and tolerance for activity normalize, work can be resumed. However, heavy manual work should be avoided, as the durability of the prosthetic implants is still limited. Stooping and kneeling may be accomplished without pain following surgery but should be limited. Certain motions involved with stooping and kneeling may cause dislocation of a prosthetic hip. Climbing and balancing can be accomplished, but such repetitive motions are hazardous and should also be limited. Most individuals with osteoarthritis are able to sustain gainful employment and a normal level of activity following successful medical and surgical therapy.

REFERENCES

Ackerman, S., & Strand, V. (1990). Use of an anti-CD-5 immunoconjugate in the treatment of rheumatoid arthritis. In V. Strand (Ed.), *Proceedings: Early decisions in DMARD development: 2. Biologic agents in autoimmune disease* (pp. 86–93). Atlanta, GA: Arthritis Foundation.

Arnett, F., McClusky, O. E., & Schacter, B. Z. (1976). Incomplete Reiter's syndrome: Discriminating features and HLA w27 in diagnosis. *Annals of Internal Medicine, 84,* 8–13.

Arnett, F. C. (1984). HLA and the spondylarthropathies. In A. Callin (Ed.), *Spondylarthropathies* (pp. 297–321). Orlando, FL: Grune & Stratton.

Arnett, F. C., Edworthy, S. M., Bloch, D. A., McShane, D. J., Fries, J. F., Cooper, N. S., Healey, L. A., Kaplan, S. R., Liang, M. H., Luthra, H. J. S., Medsger, T. A., Jr., Mitchel, D. M., Neustadt, D. H., Pinals, R. S., Schaller, J. G., Sharp, J. T., Wilder, R. L., & Hunder, G. G. (1988). The American Rheumatism Association 1987 revised criteria for the classification of rheumatoid arthritis. *Arthritis and Rheumatism, 31,* 315–324.

Bennett, P. H., & Burch, T. A. (1967). New York symposium on population studies in the rheumatic diseases: New diagnostic criteria. *Bulletin on the Rheumatic Diseases, 17,* 453–469.

Bennett, R. M. (1979). Psoriatic arthritis. In D. J. McCarthy (Ed.), *Arthritis and allied conditions* (9th ed., pp. 453–466). Philadelphia: Lea & Febiger.

Caldwell, J. R., Saville, P. P., & Bedsole, G. D. (1987). Therafectin (amiprilose HCl) in rheumatoid arthritis: A six month double blind placebo controlled study followed by a six month open extension. *Arthritis and Rheumatism, 30,* 538–543.

Callin, A., & Fries, J. F. (1976). An "experimental" epidemic of Reiter's syndrome, revisited: Follow-up evidence on genetic and environmental factors. *Annals of Internal Medicine, 84,* 564–574.

Cunningham, L. S., & Kelsey, J. L. (1984). Epidemiology of musculoskeletal impairments and associated disability. *American Journal of Public Health, 74,* 574–579.

Dayer, J. M. (1990). Use of an IL-1 inhibitor in inflammation. In V. Strand (Ed.), *Proceedings: Early decisions in DMARD development: 2. Biologic agents in autoimmune disease* (pp. 44–46). Atlanta: Arthritis Foundation.

Fowler, P. D., Shadfonh, M. F., Crook, P. R., & Lawton, A. (1984). Report on choloroquine and dapsone in the treatment of rheumatoid arthritis: A 6 month comparative study. *Annals of Rheumatic Diseases, 43,* 200–207.

Fox, R., Callin, A., Gerber, R. C., & Gibson, D. (1979). The chronicity of symptoms and disability in Reiter's syndrome: An analysis of 131 consecutive patients. *Annals of Internal Medicine, 91,* 190–207.

Gregersen, P. K., Lee, S., Silver, J., & Winchester, R. (1987). The shared epitope hypothesis: An approach to understanding the molecular genetics of rheumatoid arthritis susceptibility. *Arthritis and Rheumatism, 30,* 1205–1213.

Harris, H. D., Jr. (1997). The clinical features of rheumatoid arthritis and treatment of rheumatoid arthritis. In W. N. Kelly, E. D. Harris, S. Ruddy, & C. Sledge (Eds.), *Textbook of rheumatology* (pp. 898–950). Philadelphia: W. B. Saunders.

Hartz, A. J., Fischer, M. E., & Bril, G. (1986). The association of obesity with joint pain and osteoarthritis. *Journal of Chronic Diseases, 39,* 311–319.

Hochberg, M. C. (1981). Adult and juvenile rheumatoid arthritis: Current epidemiologic concepts. *Epidemiology Review, 3,* 27–41.

Hochberg, M. C. (1992). Epidemiology. In A. Callin (Ed.), *Spondylarthropathies.* Orlando, FL: Grune & Walton.

Holmdahl, R., Nordling, C., Rubin, K., Tarkowski, A., & Klareskog, L. (1986). Generation of monoclonal rheumatoid factors after immunization with collagen Il–anti-collagen 11 immune complexes: An anti-idiotype antibody to anti-collagen II is also a rheumatoid factor. *Scandinavian Journal of Immunology, 24,* 197–212.

Howell D. S., & Altman, R. D. (1993). Cartilage repair and conservation in osteoarthritis. *Rheumatic Diseases Clinics of North America, 19,* 713–724.

Hunter, T., Urowitz, M. B., & Gordon, D. A. (1975). Azathioprine in rheumatoid arthritis: A long-term follow-up study. *Arthritis and Rheumatism, 18,* 15–21.

Hurd, E. R. (1984). Extra-articular manifestations of rheumatoid arthritis. *Seminars in Rheumatic Diseases, 8,* 151–163.

Inman, R. D., Chiu, B., Johnston, M. E. A., & Falk, J. (1992). Molecular mimicry in Reiter's syndrome: Cytotoxicity and ELISA studies of HLA-microbial relationships. *Immunology, 58,* 501–512.

Merkel, P. A., Letourneau, E. N., & Polisson, R. P. (1995). Investigational agents for rheumatoid arthritis. *Rheumatic Diseases Clinics of North America, 21,* 779–796.

Mielants, H., Veys, E. M., & Cuvelier, C. (1985). HLA B27 related arthritis and bowel inflammation: Part 2. Colonoscopy and bowel histology in patients with HLA B27 related arthritis. *Journal of Rheumatology, 12,* 294–299.

Miller, B., Demerieux, P., & Srinivasan, R. (1980). Double-blind placebo-controlled crossover evaluation of levamisole in rheumatoid arthritis. *Arthritis and Rheumatism, 23,* 172–183.

Nissila, M., Lehtinen, K., & Leirisalo-Repo, M. (1988). Sulfasalazine in the treatment of ankylosing spondylitis: A 26-week placebo-controlled clinical trial. *Arthritis and Rheumatism, 31,* 1111–1117.

Paronen, A. (1948). Reiter's disease: A study of 344 cases observed in Finland. *Acta Medica Scandinavica, 131,* 1–143.

Pelletier, J. P., Martel-Pelletier, J., & Howell, D. S. (1985). Collagenase and nolytic activity in human osteoarthritic cartilage. *Arthritis and Rheumatism, 28,* 554–561.

Peyron, J. G. (1993). Intraarticular hyaluronan injection in the treatment of osteoarthritis: State-of the-art review. *Journal of Rheumatology, 20*(39), 10–15

Pinals, R. S., Kaplan, S. B., Lawson, J. G., & Hepurn, B. (1986). Sulfasalazine in rheumatoid arthritis. *Arthritis and Rheumatism, 29,* 1427–1434.

Pincus, T., & Callahan, L. F. (1992). Taking mortality in rheumatoid arthritis serious: Predictive markers, socio-economic status and co-morbidity. *Journal of Rheumatology, 13,* 841–845.

Saunders, M. (1991). The use of chimeric CD-4 monoclonal antibody for the treatment of rheumatoid arthritis. In International Business Communications (Organizers), *Advances in understanding and treatment of rheumatoid arthritis*. Philadelphia: IBC USA Conferences Inc. MASS.

Scott, J. C., & Hochberg, M. C. (1984). Osteoarthritis. *Maryland Medical Journal, 33,* 712–716.

Solomon, G. (1991). Inflammatory arthritis. In M. Jahss (Ed.), *Disorders of the foot and ankle* (2nd ed., pp. 1681–1702). New York: W. B. Saunders.

Tugwell, P., Bennett, K., & Gent, M. (1987). Methotrexate in rheumatoid arthritis: Indications, contraindications, efficacy, and safety. *Annals of Internal Medicine, 107,* 358–366.

Voltonen, V. V., Leirisalo, M., & Pentikainen, P. J. (1985). Triggering infections in reactive arthritis. *Annals of Rheumatic Diseases, 44,* 399–412.

Waldman, T. A. (1991). Interleukin-2 receptor directed therapy in autoimmune disease. In V. Strand (Ed.), *Proceedings: Early decisions in DMARD development: 2. Biological agents in autoimmune disease* (pp. 34–38). Atlanta: Arthritis Foundation.

Yocum, D. E., Klippel, J. H., & Wilder, R. L. (1988). Cyclosporin A treatment of refractory rheumatoid arthritis. *Annals of Internal Medicine, 1,* 863–873.

Chapter 24

Spinal Cord Injury

Allen W. Heinemann

This chapter summarizes recent advances in our understanding of the functional, psychological, and vocational aspects of spinal cord injury (SCI). It begins by reviewing the epidemiology of SCI, continues by describing the functional consequences, and concludes by exploring the psychological and vocational implications. A goal in writing the chapter was not to duplicate information reported about orthopedic and neuroanatomical issues (Donovan, 1981), medical rehabilitation processes (Matthews & Carlson, 1987; Nixon, 1985), or earlier summaries of psychological, social, and vocational aspects of SCI (Trieschmann, 1988; Wright, 1983). The purpose of the chapter is to provide rehabilitation professionals with an overview of spinal injury information that prepares them to delve deeper into the topic.

Traumatic SCI is a relatively uncommon impairment in the United States, with an incidence of about 30 to 40 cases per million sustaining permanent disability and a total prevalence of 183,000 to 230,000 (Go, DeVivo, & Richards, 1995). Motor vehicle crashes account for the largest proportion of injuries (44.5%), followed by falls (18.1%), acts of violence (16.6%), sports (12.7%), and other causes (8.1%). Reflecting larger societal changes, SCI resulting from acts of violence has increased since the inception of the Model SCI Systems in 1973, particularly for African Americans. Motor vehicle crashes are the leading cause of injury through age 45; falls account for the largest proportion of injuries after age 45. SCI has a strong seasonal variation; most injuries occur in summer months and the fewest in winter months. The rate of injury is greater on weekends than on weekdays. Behavioral factors are reflected in these data, given the higher rate of drinking and driving on weekends, resulting in motor vehicle crashes, and diving injuries in warm months.

Risk of SCI varies across age, gender, and socioeconomic groups. SCI occurs more often to persons 16 to 30 years of age than to all other age groups combined; the median age at injury is 26 years (Go et al., 1995). Men are disproportionately at risk of SCI; 82% of persons sustaining injuries reported to the National SCI Database were men. The proportion of African Americans and Native Americans in the national database is greater than their representation in the national population (19.6% vs. 12.1% for African Americans; 1.3% vs. 0.8% for Native Americans); conversely, Caucasians and Asian Americans are underrepresented. Location of Model SCI System facilities in urban centers where persons from minority backgrounds are concentrated may account in part for this observation. Education levels at injury tend to be somewhat lower than that of the general U.S. population, considering age. Specifically, 86% of the U.S. population between 18 and 21 years of age are high school graduates, compared to 66% in the National SCI Database. The unemployment rate at time of injury (14.3%) tends to be greater than for the general U.S. population. Given the relatively young age of persons who sustain SCI, it is not surprising that the majority (53.5%) are never married at the time of injury.

Functional Presentation

Spinal injury resulting in permanent paralysis and loss of sensation might seem to be one of the most devastating experiences imaginable. Yet the experience of persons who live with SCI is usually quite different. Advances in acute care and rehabilitation practices have reduced morbidity and mortality dramatically over the past few decades (Stover, DeLisa, & Whiteneck, 1995). People who sustain SCI are able to achieve independent and satisfying lives; the increasing use of assistive technology is responsible, in part, for improved quality of life (Scherer, 1988).

The World Health Organization's (WHO) model of disablement provides a fundamental advance in our understanding of how to distinguish various aspects of injury and chronic health consequences and the relationships among disablement concepts (WHO, 1993). This model defines three concepts: *impairment*, affecting performance at the organ level; *disability*, affecting performance at the person level; and *handicap*, affecting performance at the societal level. Impairment reflects any loss or abnormality of psychological, physiological, or anatomical structure or function (WHO, 1993). Level, or completeness, of SCI resulting in paralysis is an example of impairment. Impairment may result in disability, defined as any restriction or lack (resulting from an impairment) of ability to perform an activity in the manner or within the range considered normal for a human being (WHO, 1980). The Functional Independence Measure (FIM™; SUNY at Buffalo, 1993) and the Patient Evaluation Conference System (PECS; Harvey & Jellinek, 1981) were developed to describe the extent of independence in performing activities of daily living. These instruments assess activities such as eating, bathing, dressing, sphincter management, walking, and stair climbing. In turn, impairment or disability may result in handicap, defined as a disadvantage for a given individual that limits or prevents the fulfillment of a role that is normal (depending on age, sex, and social and cultural factors) for that individual (WHO, 1993). Social roles such as worker, homemaker, student, and community member are examples of roles that may be limited. The Craig Handicap Assessment and Reporting Technique (CHART; Whiteneck, Charlifue, Gerhart, Overholser, & Richardson, 1992) is a tool developed to assess extent of role limitation or, conversely, societal participation. Although other conceptual frameworks have been developed (Pope & Tarlov, 1991), the WHO model provides a clearly distinguished set of constructs by which we can understand distinct aspects of disablement.

Extent of impairment is characterized several ways in the National SCI Database. Complete neurological injuries, characterized by the absence of sensory or motor function below the level of injury, are incurred by about half of their sample (51.7%); however, the rate of complete injuries has declined over the years, reflecting improved emergency medical services and high-dose, methylprednisolone therapy (Bracken et al., 1990). Incomplete tetraplegia is the most common discharge neurological category (31.2%); complete paraplegia (26.0%), complete tetraplegia (21.9%), incomplete paraplegia (20.0%), and complete recovery (0.9%) comprise the other neurological groups (Ditunno, Cohen, Formal, & Whiteneck, 1995).

Clarity in disablement constructs has allowed the construction of measures with linear properties and adequate validity. Linear measurement is crucial to the advancement of rehabilitation practice. The raw scores obtained by summing item responses, such as lesion level or motor index scores (American Spinal Injury Association [ASIA], 1992), are ordinal in nature. Such unequal-interval numbers preclude their use in parametric statistical comparisons because these raw data only allow rank ordering of scores. A measurement procedure that can be used to develop reliable, valid, and interval-scaled measures from ordinal scores is rating-scale, or Rasch, analysis, named after the Danish mathematician whose work in the 1950s and 1960s has been widely applied in educational testing and more recently in rehabilitation outcome measurement (Rasch, 1960). Interval-level measures possess the advantage of having equal intervals between units of the scale. When distributed in a reasonably normal fashion, measures from an interval scale can be confidently subjected to parametric statistical analyses that relate independent and dependent variables. Transforming ordinal raw scores to interval measures allows one to quantify individuals' level of impairment, disability, or handicap along an equal-interval continuum; make quantitative comparisons within an individual across time; or compare individuals or groups.

Whereas most of the literature describes the neurological consequences of SCI categorically as complete and incomplete paraplegia or tetraplegia, rating-scale analysis allows us to describe severity of impairment resulting from SCI in equal-interval terms. Heinemann, Hamilton, and Johnston (1998) used this measurement methodology to evaluate the extent to which commonly used descriptors of SCI impairment cohere to define a unidimensional construct. Attending physicians characterized extent of neurological injury in a sample of 169 patients from four rehabilitation facilities at admission and discharge on commonly used descriptors of SCI consequences: motor and sensory level, completeness of SCI lesion using ASIA's (1992) International Impairment Scale, and bladder management. Nearly four strata of patients could be defined by the items (extremely impaired, severely impaired, moderately impaired, and mildly impaired); the corresponding reliability coefficient was .87. The item set could distinguish a potentially much broader range of impairment, as indicated by an item reliability of .99. The items cohered reasonably well to define a measure of SCI impairment; the "noisiest" items were bladder management and the ASIA impairment scale, with 180% and 160% of the expected amount of information, respectively. In contrast, the four items pertaining to neurological level tended to over-fit with only 50% to 60% of the expected amount of information. Figure 24.1 shows that the easiest items on which to be rated favorably were the two sensory-level items, followed by the two motor-level items. Considerably more difficult were the ASIA Impairment Scale item and bladder management. A measure ranging from 0 to 100 was defined, in which the lowest ratings on all items in this sample would correspond to a measure of 0, and the highest rating would correspond to 100. The distribution of patients on this measure shows that the six items are able to array a wide range of impairment. This distribution is apt to be representative of Model System facility contributors, given that two of the four facilities were Model System participants and three of the four had experience caring for patients who were dependent on ventilators.

The consequences of impairment define severity of disability. The FIM (Hamilton, Granger, Sherwin, Zielezny, & Tashman, 1987) is the most widely used measure of disability in the United States, as over 500 rehabilitation facilities subscribe to the Uniform Data System for Medical Rehabilitation (UDSmr). Heinemann and colleagues (Heinemann, Linacre, Wright, Hamilton, & Granger, 1993; Linacre, Heinemann, Wright, Granger, & Hamilton, 1994) used rating-scale analysis to evaluate the difficulty of FIM items, to examine the extent to which items relate to a single construct of disability, and to determine the similarity of scaled measures across impairment groups. We found that the FIM contains two fundamental subsets of items: one set of 13 items measures motor disability (feeding, grooming, bathing, dressing, toileting, transfers, locomotion, bladder and bowel management, and stair climbing), and the second measures cognitive function (comprehension, expression, social interaction, problem solving, and memory). The validity of the FIM was supported by the similar patterns of item difficulties across impairment groups. We also evaluated the motor and cognitive function gains from admission to discharge attained by inpatients undergoing medical rehabilitation. Using interval-level motor and cognitive measures derived from the FIM, we found that not only were patients in various impairment groups admitted with differing levels of function, but the gains they made were not equivalent. Specifically, patients with SCI had a high admission level of cognitive function and consequently made relatively small cognitive gains (Heinemann et al., 1994). In contrast, the gains in motor function were substantial.

Valid measures of disability allow us to predict the outcomes of rehabilitation and the resources required to achieve these outcomes. One study used linear measures of motor and cognitive function derived from the FIM with samples of patients with SCI and traumatic brain injury (TBI) undergoing initial rehabilitation to predict functional status at discharge and length of stay (Heinemann et al., 1994). Admission functional status was consistently related to discharge function and length of stay, though the strength of these associations varied with type of impairment. Motor function was a stronger predictor of length of stay than was cognitive function for both the SCI and the TBI group. However, the unique contribution of cognitive function was apparent for specific impairment groups. The predicted variance in discharge motor function averaged 55%; in discharge cognitive function, 70%; and in length of stay, 20%.

Burden of disability, measured in terms of the time nurses spend providing patient care, and length of stay are strongly correlated with admission motor function (Heinemann et al., 1997). Total minutes of care were assessed for a 24-hour period within the first week of admission for 47 patients with SCI. Decrease in nursing time was greatest for small improvements in motor function at the low end of the range of motor function (scaled to range from 0, corresponding to complete dependence, to 100, corresponding to complete independence). For example, an improvement from an FIM motor score of 10 to 20 was associated with an 18-minute decline in teaching time (from 70 to 52 minutes), while an equivalent 10-point improvement from 70 to 80 was associated with only a 3-minute decline (from 12 to 9 minutes). We also predicted length of stay. We found a curvilinear relationship between disability and length of stay showing that much longer stays were predicted for patients with low levels of motor function at admission.

It is important to monitor change in impairment concurrently with change in disability in order to modulate and guide rehabilitation interventions. If improvement in disability is dependent on improvement in impairment, then therapy

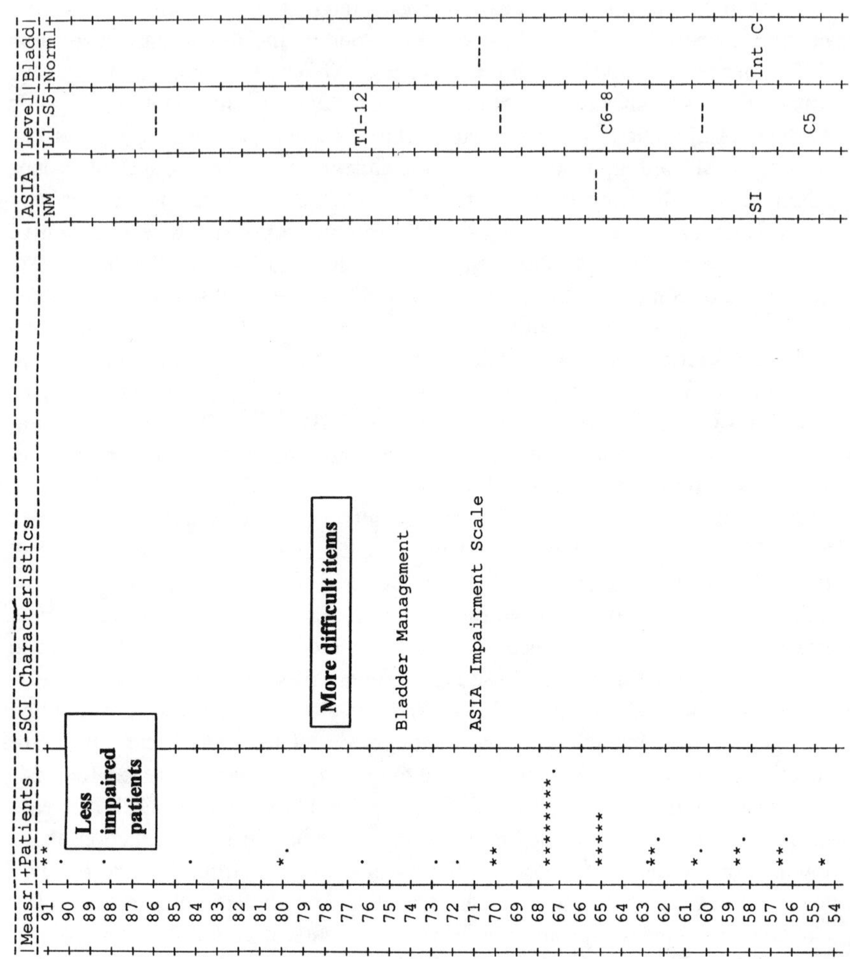

Measr
+Patients
-SCI Characteristics
ASIA
Level
Bladd
Less impaired patients
More difficult items
Bladder Management
ASIA Impairment Scale
NM
SI
L1-S5
T1-12
C6-8
C5
Norml
Int C

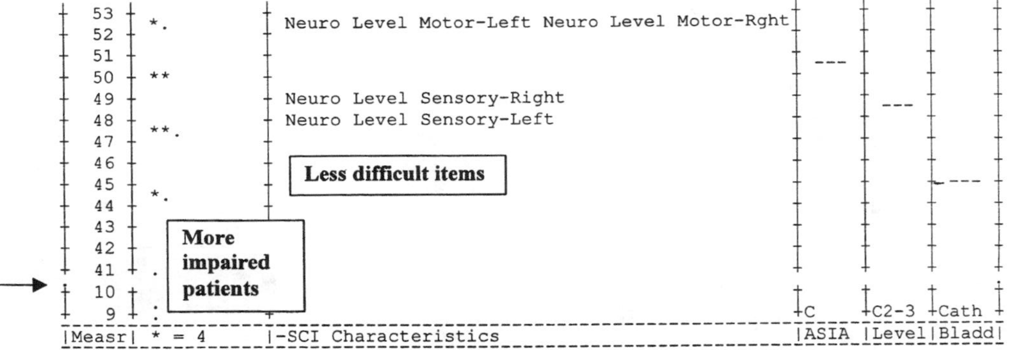

FIGURE 24.1 Map of spinal-cord-injury characteristics. The distribution of *patient measures* is shown on the left under the "Measr" heading; each asterisk represents four patients and each dot represents one patient. Patients with less severe impairment are shown at the top of the distribution. The distribution is truncated at the arrow (→) to allow the figure to fit on one page. The distribution of *item difficulties* is shown in the middle; the position of each item corresponds to its calibration (or difficulty). On the right are the average measures for each category of the three *rating scales*. The rating scale for the ASIA Impairment Scale (ASIA) was motor and sensory complete (C), sensory incomplete (SI), and nonfunctional motor (NM); no patient was rated as having functional motor skills. For neurological level (Level) the rating scale categories were C_1 (no patient rated at this level), C_{2-3}, C_4, C_5, C_{6-8}, T_{1-12}, and L_1–S_5. The rating scale categories for bladder management (Bladd) were indwelling catheter, suprapubic catheter, or spontaneous voiding (Cath), intermittent catheterization (Int C), and normal voiding (Norm l). A patient with the modal level of impairment, corresponding to a measure of 67, would have somewhat better than a sensory incomplete injury at the C_{6-8} level and use intermittent catheterization to manage bladder function. The authors thank Rita Bode, PhD, and Patrick Fisher for their assistance with this analysis.

could be better timed to coincide with such an opportunity. Alternatively, if there is little relationship between improvement in impairment and disability, then timing of therapy that targets disability may be less important. For example, patients with SCI may have little improvement in impairment but very large improvement in disability as they learn to use adapted equipment and tenodesis. An improved understanding of the rate of neurological recovery will allow us to time and sequence rehabilitation interventions more effectively.

The relationship between impairment and disability is striking. Ditunno, Cohen, Formal, and Whiteneck (1995) reported motor and cognitive FIM measures by level and completeness of spinal injury. Figure 24.2 summarizes the average measures for more than 2,000 cases reported to the National SCI Database. For FIM-measured motor function at rehabilitation discharge, consistent increases in functional status are observed across groups of persons classified with Frankel A (complete), B (incomplete, preserved sensation only), and C (incomplete, preserved motor nonfunctional) injury grades. In contrast, functional status is relatively equivalent across injury levels for persons classified with Frankel D (incomplete, preserved motor functional) injuries. The same minimal variation across injury level and completeness is observed for cognitive function. Figure 24.2 shows only slight variation in cognitive status at discharge regardless of injury level or completeness, in contrast to other impairment groups.

One important outcome of impairment, disability, and handicap is the person's self-perceived quality of life. Relationships between quality of life and

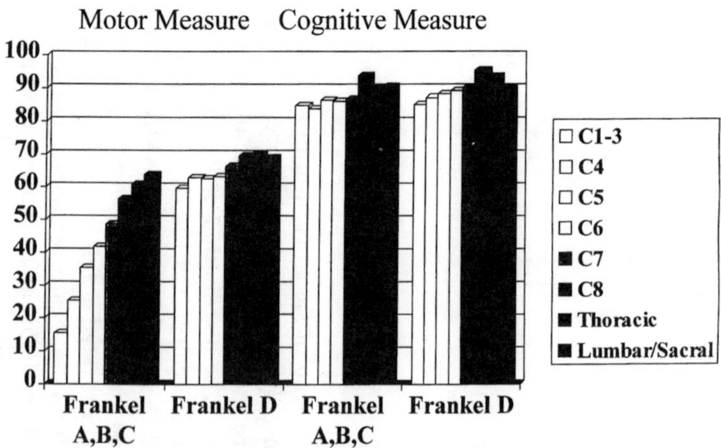

FIGURE 24.2 Discharge FIM™ motor and cognitive measures at discharge.

impairment, disability, and handicap were evaluated by Dijkers (1997). His meta-analysis of 22 studies found that quality of life, defined variably as happiness, psychological well-being, morale, and life satisfaction, tended to be lower in persons with SCI than for persons without disabilities. Overall, he found weak and statistically nonsignificant associations between quality of life and impairment, whereas disability correlations tended to be stronger (averaging −.21). Average handicap measure correlations were even stronger, averaging −.17 for aspects of handicap having to do with family role, −.30 with occupation; −.24 with mobility; −.45 with formal social integration; and −.29 with informal social integration. An important consequence of these observations is that persons with severe impairment and consequent disability can achieve a satisfactory quality of life. The psychological and vocational implications of SCI are reviewed in the next section of this chapter.

Psychological and Vocational Implications

Several recurring concerns have been the focus of rehabilitation professionals who work with persons who sustain SCI, reflecting increasing life expectancies and opportunities for employment and community living. Trieschmann (1992) listed several questions:

- "How do we teach people to cope more effectively with this disability?" (p. 58).
- "How can we facilitate better communication among professionals and people with SCI to enhance independent functioning within the hospital and community environment?" (p. 59).
- "What are the best methods of promoting wellness in the SCI community?" (p. 59).
- "How do we teach coping skills to [persons with] new SCI with a history of alcohol and drug abuse?" (p. 60).

Described below are the major themes in the psychological and vocational literature that help answer these questions.

Psychological Issues

Early theories drew on clinical experience and often focused on patients' emotional responses immediately after injury and the consequent life disruption (Hohmann, 1975; Mueller & Thompson, 1950; Shontz, 1965; Siller, 1969; Stewart, 1978). This focus reflected the fact that rehabilitation hospitalizations were long, life expectancies were shortened, and societal accommodation of persons with disabilities was minimal. The early work of Dembo, Leviton, and Wright (1956), which subsequently was elaborated by Wright (1983), has influenced greatly our thinking about post-SCI reactions. They defined a concept termed disability acceptance, which was defined by (1) the enlarging of one's scope of values, (2) containing disability effects, (3) emphasizing self-evaluation with asset values rather than deriving one's self-worth by comparing oneself with others, and (4) subordinating the importance of physique and physical appearance. These concepts build on Kurt Lewin's (1935) field-theoretic approach to personality and focus on intrapsychic processes.

Trieschmann (1988) described a spinal injury–specific model of adjustment built on a view that equates disability adjustment with balance in life, in which persons should be understood as integral mind-body systems. Her systems model describes behavior, health, and adjustment as being determined by psychological resources, biological-organic state, and environmental characteristics. She defined rehabilitation as "the process of teaching people to live with their disability in their own environment" (p. 26). Consequently, no specific end point of adjustment is possible or desirable.

Shontz (1982) describes the paradox resulting from psychological adaptation to an unchangeable condition, such as disability: the disability exists for the person with the condition only while adaptation is in process. Persons "outside" the disability still react to its visible aspects and may treat the person as "handicapped" when adaptation is complete. Shontz extended Dembo's (1969) distinction between insiders (those with a condition) and outsiders by noting that, from the perspective of the person who has dealt successfully with chronic illness or disability, one no longer adapts *to* illness or disability because the condition no longer exists. To quote,

> . . . like everyone else, [persons with disabilities] adapt to the full array of possibilities and limitations that are afforded by the complete panorama of their biological states and their social and physical environments. . . . The question [for rehabilitation professionals] is how they come to satisfactory and satisfying terms with the same world in which everyone lives. (p. 155)

From this perspective, the same evidence of psychological adjustment is used with people with disabilities as for everyone else. Satisfactory adaptation is evident when disability is no longer the dominant issue.

The psychological literature on post-SCI adaptation has been dominated by several topics. Livneh and Antonak (1997) summarize them as (1) disagreement about the nature and sequence of adaptation processes and (2) incomplete understanding as to the nature, severity and course of depression. More recently, substance abuse as a characteristic that affects rehabilitation processes and reflects preinjury behaviors has gained attention. This controversy and literature is summarized below.

Several clinicians and researchers have described the expectation that persons experience a more or less predictable sequence of reactions to loss accompanying injury (Elliott & Frank, 1996). The work of George Hohmann (1975), a psychologist who sustained SCI, described denial, withdrawal, hostility, and reactions against dependence similar to descriptions of reactions to terminal illness and chronic health conditions (Kübler-Ross, 1969; Parkes, 1972). The attractiveness of sequential phases of adaptation is reflected in care plans for nurses that incorporate stage model interventions (French & Phillips, 1991). Fink (1967) and Shontz (1965) described disability as a crisis-inducing event and posited four stages, beginning with shock, then defensive retreat, acknowledgment, and finally adaptation. The consequences of progressing or failing to progress through these hypothesized stages was examined by Heinemann and Shontz (1984, 1985), who found no single, common underlying process of adjustment. Instead, in their personological study of adjustment, they described how people find different solutions to life problems that seem similar because of the similar impairment. Symbolic integration of loss was more complete in a person who experienced a sequence of emotional reactions. We concluded that the meaning of the loss, the person's already established means of dealing with life disruption, and the context within which the person undergoes rehabilitation and community reentry affects the way in which emotional and behavioral reactions are experienced. On the basis of life narrative interviews with 50 adults who had lived with SCI for more than 22 years, Crewe (1997) reached a similar conclusion that the ways in which people cope with SCI reflects their global perspective on life.

Stage models of adjustment have been criticized for a lack of empirical evidence (Trieschmann, 1988) and for failing to account for variability in individuals' response to life disruption (Silver & Wortman, 1980). The opportunity for adjustment ought to be reflected in time since injury, a crude marker of adjustment. Krause and Crewe (1991) examined the effect of age, time since injury, and time of measurement on adjustment in two groups of renal clinic outpatients, recruited in 1974 and 1985. They divided participants into five cohorts, based on age and time since injury. The group originally recruited in 1974 was reassessed in 1985; both groups averaged nearly 10 years since injury. They derived indices of activity, medical stability, adjustment, interpersonal satisfaction, and economic satisfaction from a Life Satisfaction Questionnaire. The nature of SCI-related adjustment reflected the index used. Activities were more strongly related to chronological age; in contrast, medical problems were more strongly related to time since injury. Life satisfaction and self-rated adjustment were related to both age and time since injury. Older persons reported less activity, as reflected in sitting tolerance and frequency of leaving home, and less satisfying lives, as measured by number of visitors, sex life, and self-rated adjustment. Nonetheless, older participants were more satisfied with their living arrangements, had longer workweeks, and reported greater satisfaction with employment. Developmental evidence of adjustment was found in correlations between time since injury and enhanced psychological functioning, as measured by satisfaction with living arrangements and employment, self-rated adjustment, length of workweek, and medical adjustment. Their findings suggest that age and time since injury have different influences. Younger persons have greater opportunity to deal with consequences of their injury but often are dealing with different developmental issues. This study illustrates the outcomes of a developmental process, the stages or turning points of which are not evident in studies of group averages.

Antonak and Livneh (1991; Livneh & Antonak, 1997) view disability adaptation from a developmental perspective. They describe a hierarchy of reactions to disability using an ordering-theoretic data analysis procedure. Evidence for a nonlinear, multidimensional process was found in a sample of 118 adults who sustained SCI, stroke, myocardial infarction, amputation, sensory impairment, or degenerative conditions. Reactions to impairment and disability were categorized in eight emotional states: shock, anxiety, denial, depression, internalized anger, externalized hostility, acknowledgment, and adjustment. Their statistical method allows contingent relationships to be examined in a cross-sectional design. They reported a pattern of nonlinear, empirical contingencies in which five of the six nonadapted responses were prerequisites for the two adapted responses (acknowledgment and adjustment). Prerequisites to adaptation were anxiety, depression, internalized anger, and externalized hostility, though considerable variability in the sequence of these reactions was reported. This analytic approach allows us to characterize individual differences in the sequence of stages: people sometimes regress to earlier stages or bypass stages because of their life situation or capacity to cope effectively. Shock was often a prerequisite of depression and internalized anger, which in turn, were prerequisites of acknowledgment and adaptation. Only denial occurred independently of the two sets of reactions. This model allows for persons to acknowledge a disability but not attain a high level of adjustment. This developmental perspective, which considers an individual's life course, identity, and commitments before SCI, allows us to understand better how SCI affects psychological well-being.

Cognitive-phenomenological perspectives also have been used to inform our understanding of post-SCI adjustment processes. One widely adopted model was described by Lazarus and Folkman (1984); their stress and coping theory allows us to view adverse life events as experiences that tax adaptive resources, threaten well-being, and place individuals at risk for stress-related dysfunction and psychopathology. The effect of individual differences in coping styles on psychological distress and depression has been explored to clarify the process by which adaptation occurs. Frank, Umlauf, Wonderlich, and associates (1987) used cluster analysis to identify subgroups of persons with recent SCI based on scores from the Ways of Coping Checklist and the Millon Health Locus of Control Scale. One group more strongly endorsed all coping factors and relied less on internal attributions than did the second group. The two groups also differed on measures of depression, negative life events, and general distress. The group using more coping strategies also reported higher levels of depressive symptoms, more negative life stress, and more negative life events in the past year. The groups did not differ in severity of injury, age, time since injury, or positive life stressors during the past year. Although they used a cross-sectional design, the authors speculate that the coping efforts of persons in the first group were less effective because their external health locus of control is associated with greater distress and depression. They speculate that external events are important in affecting mood and attributional styles.

Subsequently, this group of investigators reported the relationship between coping styles and psychological distress in 57 inpatients with SCI who were undergoing initial rehabilitation (Buckelew, Baumstark, Frank, & Hewett, 1990). They divided their sample into three, equal-sized groups defined by distress level. Persons experiencing higher distress were also more likely to report using self-blame, wish-fulfilling fantasy, emotional expression, and threat minimization to cope, compared to persons with moderate and low levels of distress. While the groups did not differ in age, time since injury, gender, level of injury, or marital status, self-blame was strongly correlated with distress, revealing the maladaptive consequences of this coping strategy. Time since injury was not correlated with coping strategy. Relatedly, Frank and Elliott (1987) reported that psychological distress as measured by the SCI was related to life events independent of time since injury. External events disrupted well-being regardless of time since injury. Frequent use of coping strategies does not necessarily reflect success in managing psychological distress but rather ineffective efforts to deal with stress.

The relationship between coping strategies and adjustment 5 years after rehabilitation was investigated by Hanson, Buckelew, Hewett, and O'Neal (1993). Adjustment was assessed with measures of psychological distress, disability acceptance, hours working, and medical status. In a sample of 28 people who had completed an assessment during rehabilitation, they found modest correlations between coping strategies at the two assessments: people who coped by seeking information ($r = .39$), emotional expression (.49), and self-blame (.50) tended to do so at both assessments. They also reported that coping strategies employed during acute rehabilitation were not related to adjustment measured 5 years later. Coping strategies at the follow-up assessment were related to adjustment in that persons reporting greater use of cognitive restructuring and less use of wish-fulfilling fantasy experienced greater disability acceptance. Whereas self-blame was related to greater psychological distress during rehabilitation, there was no relationship 5 years later. These results support the notion that coping strategies are dynamic and reflect developmental experiences.

How people negotiate reality, particularly a reality that is threatening to the self, was the focus of work by Elliott, Witty, Herrick, and Hoffman (1991). In contrast to the traditional view that psychological health is characterized by accurate reality perceptions, an alternative perspective posits both protective (e.g., excuse making) and enhancing (e.g., hope) behaviors as useful in managing perceptions of disruptive events such as disability. Both agency, a person's determination to meet personal goals, and pathways, a sense of being able to achieve goals successfully, are viewed as components of hope and as being necessary for psychological adjustment. They found, in a sample of 57 adults who were interviewed an average of 5 years after SCI, that hope predicted both depression and psychosocial impairment; a greater sense of pathways was associated with less depressive symptoms and impairment (as measured by the Sickness Impact Profile) regardless of time since SCI. They also observed an interaction between agency and time since injury; persons with a higher sense of agency reported less psychosocial impairment shortly after injury. In contrast, level of agency was unrelated to psychosocial impairment in persons who had lived longer with SCI. These results provide evidence for a reality negotiation process by which individuals are able to make favorable self-presentations.

Changes in rehabilitation practices also may affect well-being in addition to individuals' coping efforts. Buckelew and associates (Buckelew, Frank, Elliott, Chaney, & Hewett, 1991) explored the effects of developmental factors and changes in rehabilitation practices on health locus of control and psychological distress in samples of 53 persons who sustained SCI between (1) 1981 and 1982 or (2) between 1984 and 1986, and who were an average of 3.6 and 1.7 years postinjury, respectively. The second group had earlier transfers to rehabilitation and shorter rehabilitation stays than did the first group. The investigators found that age and time since injury were unrelated to health beliefs and to psychological distress, though the second group experienced greater anxiety, phobic anxiety, psychoticism, and hostility. These results illustrate the important consequences of rehabilitation practices resulting from efforts to contain health care costs. Questions of who experiences greater well-being, how adaptation proceeds, and how adaptation can be supported become even more important in light of health care changes.

The effect of social support on long-term adjustment of persons with SCI also has been scrutinized. Schulz and Decker (1985) studied a group of 100 middle-aged and older community residents who had an average of 20 years of postinjury experience. Self-reported well-being was only slightly lower than that of peers without disabilities. In addition, well-being was associated with high levels of social support, satisfaction with social contacts, and perceived control over well-being after controlling statistically for health and income. They concluded that respondents attained favorable self-perceptions by selectively focusing on attributes in which they had an advantage, by ascribing meaning to injury, and by defining standards of adjustment in which they could excel. This coping process is congruent with Wright's (1983) model of value changes that defines how disability acceptance proceeds. Using Wright's terms, favorable coping outcomes were achieved by subordination of physique and employing asset values.

Rintala and associates (Rintala, Young, Hart, Clearman, & Fuhrer, 1992) also explored relationships between well-being and social support. They recruited a community sample, oversampled women, and measured health status and secondary medical complications objectively (e.g., urinary tract infections, pressure ulcers). Their sample of 140 persons averaged 10.6 years postinjury. They used Schulz and Decker's questionnaire and found, as expected, that greater levels of social support were associated with greater life satisfaction, better self-assessed physical health, and the absence of urinary tract infections. Satisfaction with social support was also associated with lower levels of depressive symptoms and greater life satisfaction. The secondary medical complications were unrelated to satisfaction with support, however. They found a gender difference in these associations: the association between social support and life satisfaction was about twice as strong for men as for women. Mechanisms that might account for these results include others' influence on health maintenance activities, social support serving to reduce stress, and others' provision of goods and services that enhance health. Given the correlational nature of the cross-sectional study, it may be that healthy persons attract the support of others and are more able to seek support from others.

Evidence for a relationship between social support, coping efforts, and long-term adjustment among veterans was reported by Coca (1991). Veterans perceiving greater support from family and friends reported greater disability acceptance and lower levels of psychological distress. The strongest predictors of disability acceptance were income and social support from friends. In turn, friends' support was positively correlated with planful problem solving and seeking social support and negatively correlated with self-controlling coping efforts and escape-avoidance.

Elliott, Herrick, Witty, Godshall, and Spruell (1992) investigated the relationship between social support and depression in a sample of 182 patients an average of 8 years after injury. Lower levels of depressive symptomatology were associated with stronger support in the form of relationships that reassured self-worth and a sense of social integration. Evidence of a developmental process was evident in a modest correlation between greater depression and less time since injury; time since injury was unrelated to any of the social support measures. Similarly, Elliott and associates (Elliott, Herrick, et al., 1991) reported in a sample of 156 persons with SCI that those with higher levels of support, that facilitated social integration and reassured personal worth, were less depressed; further, higher levels of assertiveness and social support were associated with lower levels of depression and psychosocial impairment as measured by the Sickness Impact Profile. Longitudinal designs would provide evidence of causal relationships; however, these results suggest that people who solicit social support and relate assertively experience better mental health.

A longitudinal perspective of social support and coping over 1 year was reported in a sample of 120 persons with SCI (McColl, Lei, & Skinner, 1995). Support and coping were assessed at 1, 4, and 12 months after rehabilitation discharge. The assessments of support distinguished instrumental, informational, and emotional components. Although results evaluating a structural model supported a single-factor construct of support and coping, the structure of support changed from a high level of informational support at 1 month to greater emotional support at the 4- and 12-month time points. The consistency of coping efforts by the sample suggests that their method elicited a dispositional tendency rather than a situational means of coping with SCI-related experience; 80% of the variance in coping at 12 months was explained by coping efforts at 4 months. Perceived availability of support had direct effects on later coping. Social support at 1 month had a positive effect on coping at 4 months. Support at 4 months, however, had a negative effect on coping at 12 months. The investigators speculated that change in the factor structure of social support might account for their results: changing perceptions of needs and circumstances may have influenced coping strategies. The possibility that continuing high levels of social support come to inhibit independent coping might guide rehabilitation professionals' efforts in helping families to develop effective caregiving roles. Evidence for the changing effects of support on coping strategies provided by this study underscores the need to consider the developmental and dynamic nature of adjustment.

The literature on adjustment processes following SCI is striking for the paucity of studies that assess interventions designed to improve mood and well-being. Glass (1994) describes issues in designing intervention studies for persons with SCI. Elliott and Frank (1996) note the lack of health services research studies that evaluate psychotherapeutic or pharmacological interventions for depression. They recommend that depression should be measured by using current diagnostic criteria and nomenclature, investigators should distinguish depression from other conditions, reliable and valid measures should be used, and self-report measures should be supplemented by interviewer-collected information. The benefits of differentially weighting symptoms was illustrated in their study of depression diagnosis (Clay, Hagglund, Frank, Elliott, & Chaney, 1995). They also urge that precursors of distress be identified in order to guide prevention and intervention strategies. A common sign of distress is abuse of alcohol and other drugs and misuse of prescription medications; the next section explores this topic.

The prevalence of substance abuse problems in persons who incur traumatic SCI has emerged as an important issue in rehabilitation settings (Heinemann, 1993; Radnitz & Tirch, 1995). Alcohol and other drug abuse can contribute to onset of disability when a person is intoxicated, limit rehabilitation gains by impairing learning, and hamper rehabilitation outcomes by contributing to increased morbidity and mortality. Intoxication is a frequent contributor to SCI onset; estimates of intoxication at injury onset vary from 17% to 68% (Frisbie & Tun, 1984; Fullerton, Harvey, Klein, & Howell, 1981; Galbraith, Murray, Patel, & Knitt-Jones, 1976; Gale, Dikmen, Wyler, Temkin, & McClean, 1983; Heinemann, Goranson, Ginsburg, & Schnoll, 1989; O'Donnell, Cooper, Gessner, Shehan, & Ashley, 1981–2). Staff at a Model SCI Systems facility investigated the prevalence of intoxication at SCI onset prospectively (Heinemann, Schnoll, Brandt, Maltz, & Keen, 1988). Serum ethanol greater than 50 mg/dl was observed in 40% of the cases, 35% of the sample had evidence of substances with abuse potential in their urine, and 62% had either serum ethanol greater than 50 mg/dl or a positive urine analysis. Although false-positive results may reflect occasional or low-dose use of substances that were detected by toxicology screens, these results highlight how often substance use is associated with SCI.

Some persons continue to use alcohol and other drugs after initial care for SCI. The rate of moderate and heavy drinking by vocational rehabilitation and independent living center clients with SCI was nearly twice the rate reported in the general population (46% vs. 25%) in one early study (Johnson, 1985). The rate of alcoholic symptoms varied from 49% of persons with recent SCI (Heinemann, Donohue, Keen, & Schnoll, 1988) to 62% of vocational rehabilitation facility clients (Rasmussen & DeBoer, 1980). We assessed chronicity of substance use in 103 persons with recent SCI (Heinemann, Donohue, et al., 1988), including those, described above, for whom toxicology screens were obtained. Lifetime exposure to and recent use of several substances with abuse potential were greater in this sample than in a national sample collected by the National Institute on Drug Abuse (1988). The 18–25-year-olds in the SCI sample reported significantly greater exposure to amphetamines, marijuana, cocaine, and hallucinogens, as well as recent use of alcohol, amphetamines, marijuana, cocaine, and hallucinogens. Those who were 26 years of age and older in the SCI group reported significantly greater exposure to narcotic analgesics and tranquilizers and recent use of tobacco, alcohol, amphetamines, and marijuana that was at least 10 percentage points greater than the national sample. Within the SCI sample, young adults (18–25 years) reported greater recent use of marijuana before injury and greater cocaine exposure than did the older group. In contrast, the older group reported greater tobacco exposure. Intoxication at time of injury was an important marker for prior substance use: 39% who reported being intoxicated at injury also reported greater exposure to tobacco, amphetamines, marijuana, hallucinogens, tranquilizers, and sedatives, as well as recent use of tobacco, alcohol, amphetamines, cocaine, and hallucinogens.

This literature demonstrates the need to screen for substance abuse in persons who incur traumatic injury. Clinical implications are clear; the lifetime exposure to and recent use of substances indicates that many persons with SCI are at risk for substance abuse. Although substance use is not necessarily substance abuse or dependence nor does use necessarily result in specific problems, it is important to understand the context, expectancies, and motives for use. For some persons, substance use may be a means of reestablishing social relationships. For others, it may mark an effort to manage stress. Yet for others it may reflect an escalating pattern of addiction. Clinicians should take note of substance use and inquire about its relationship with other problems.

Investigators have examined relationships between intoxication at injury and individual differences such as sensation seeking. Mawson, Jacobs, Winchester, and Biundo (1988) reported that persons who scored high on a measure of sensation seeking were younger and more likely to be using substances at the time of injury. In contrast, Rohe and Basford (1990) found that only the MacAndrew Alcoholism Scale of the Minnesota Multiphasic Personality Inventory distinguished patients with blood alcohol concentrations from patients without blood alcohol concentrations and a normative sample. Precursors, consequences, and associated features of substance use require further research to clarify these issues.

Hawkins and Heinemann (1998) examined relationships between medical complications resulting in hospital stays and the use of alcohol and illicit substances in 71 persons during their first 30 months after SCI. Medical records were reviewed for pressure ulcers and urinary tract infections, two common complication following SCI. They distinguished abstainers after injury who did or did not abuse alcohol before injury. Abstainers with histories of drinking problems before SCI were at greater risk for infections 7 to 12 months after injury and had longer hospital stays. We also found that preinjury illicit substance abuse was related to an increased risk of pressure ulcers 30 months after SCI. Perhaps lifestyle characteristics of postinjury abstainers, such as reduced attention to self-care, create specific risks that account for this finding. It may be that former drinkers have not implemented the self-care skills that were a focus during inpatient rehabilitation. Clinical implications are clear: rehabilitation professionals should inquire about substance use patterns, monitor psychological well-being, and explore the ways in which self-care habits are related to substance use.

In summary, rehabilitation professionals are coming to realize that the expectation that persons with SCI will experience predictable emotional reactions in a specific sequence or develop clinical depression are unsupported by the literature and potentially harmful (Frank, Elliott, Corcoran, & Wonderlich, 1987). Even though the rate of suicide may be two to six times greater for persons with SCI than for able-bodied peers (Charlifue & Gerhart, 1991), specific characteristics appear to place people at risk. These characteristics include pre- and postinjury despondency; a sense of shame, apathy, and hopelessness; family disruption before injury; alcohol abuse; active involvement in SCI etiology; and antisocial behavior. Based on a review of case histories, Judd and Brown (1992) add to this list schizoid, depressive, and narcissistic personality characteristics; postinjury depression; and the views of important others who see death as preferable to living with SCI. Depression, particularly severe depression (with suicide considered), may be an understandable but maladaptive reaction to crisis. The psychological structure and life experiences of some individuals may well place them at risk for negative reactions. Understanding these personal characteristics and the meaning individuals ascribe to the experience of injury is necessary before an intervention is made. The importance of this approach is illustrated by the observation that rehabilitation staff frequently overestimate the level of depression experienced by patients (Cushman & Dijkers, 1990).

This appreciation for individual differences in adaptation following SCI is reflected in Hammell's (1992) statement that

> the rehabilitation team will need to become more flexible in recognizing the heterogeneity of the life values of the individual. . . . The lifelong process of adjustment to disability and to interacting with society and the environment is not complete at discharge from an inpatient facility. Rather, this is when true adjustment and adaptation begins. (p. 324)

Livneh (1986) describes intervention strategies that reflect a sensitivity to individuals' experiences of coping with crisis. He proposes that the timing of psychotherapeutic strategies—supportive, insight-oriented, cognitive, and behavioral—consider the person's experience and needs.

In addition to psychological and social needs, substance abuse issues are often important during rehabilitation. Unfortunately, these issues have often been overlooked during rehabilitation. This oversight results from rehabilitation programs that do not recognize substance abuse treatment as part of their mission and from staff who do not know how to recognize substance abuse problems and consequently are unlikely to intervene in a timely and effective manner. However, it is clear that early identification of persons with SCI who abuse or are addicted to substances should minimize the incidence of secondary complications, decrease the cost of rehabilitation, and improve rehabilitation outcome. Specific suggestions regarding assessment and management of substance abuse also emerge from this literature review. Assessment of alcohol and other drug use should be a routine part of inpatient screenings in acute care and rehabilitation programs for persons incurring SCI. Professionals may need continuing education to recognize alcohol and other drug abuse; alcoholism and other drug abuse treatment professionals can be consulted to acquire this knowledge. Not only are disability-related issues such as architectural accessibility and functional abilities important to address, but so are attitudes toward persons with disabling conditions that may limit program access. In larger communities, chemical dependence treatment programs designed specifically for persons with physical disabilities are another treatment alternative (Anderson, 1980–1; Lowenthal & Anderson, 1980–1; Sweeney & Foote, 1982).

Vocational Issues

An important goal for many persons with SCI following medical rehabilitation is employment. For previously employed persons, return to work often serves as an important indicator of successful societal participation. Employment, although not the only goal sought by persons with SCI, requires not only individual skills and persistence but employer readiness to accommodate physical needs, co-worker sensitivity, and reduction of environmental barriers and economic disincentives. Dijkers, Abela, Gans, and Gordon (1995) summarized general observations about vocational issues from Model SCI Systems data:

- Greater impairment severity is associated with a lower post-SCI employment rate (e.g., post-SCI employment rates are greater among persons sustaining paraplegia than among those with quadriplegia and among persons with incomplete lesions than those with complete lesions).
- Employment is greater among younger adults, among those with greater educational attainment, and among those with pre-SCI employment experience.
- The rate of employment increases as persons live longer with SCI and for persons who complete vocational rehabilitation programs.
- Persons from minority backgrounds are less likely to obtain employment, even after considering age, education, gender, marital status, and severity of impairment.

The National SCI Database classifies vocational activities in terms of competitive employment, homemaking, receiving on-the-job training, working in a sheltered workshop, retired, studying, unemployed, and "other," which includes volunteering and receiving disability or medical leave payments. The first anniversary of SCI provides the earliest meaningful snapshot of how people use their time. Figure 24.3, drawing from Dijkers, Abela, Gans, and Gordon (1995), summarizes the primary vocational status at time of injury and 1 year later; a strong relationship is evident between activities at the two time points. Specifically, respondents were most likely to be engaged in the same activity 1 year after SCI as they were at time of injury. The group unemployed at injury was the only group most likely to report a different primary activity 1 year after SCI. Other than persons who were employed at the time of SCI, the group unemployed at SCI onset was the most likely to report employment after SCI. The primary vocational status of National Database respondents over time shows a steady increase in the proportion of persons working until 11 years post-SCI. For women, the proportion of National SCI Database respondents reporting homemaking and retirement remains fairly constant over the first 15 years after SCI. The proportion of women studying increases to about 3 years after SCI, then declines. The

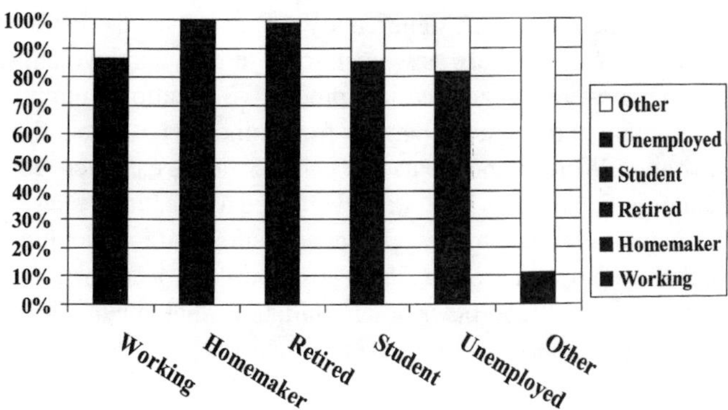

FIGURE 24.3 Vocational activity 1 year after SCI by preinjury vocational status.

Adapted from Dijkers, Abela, Gans, & Gordon (1995).

proportion reporting unemployment reaches a low point between 3 and 7 years after SCI, then increases. For men, the rate of employment increases steadily to about 10 years post-SCI, then declines slowly. The proportion reporting student status increases to about 3 years post-SCI, then declines slowly. The proportion of men who are retired remains relatively small and constant until nearly 15 years after SCI. The select nature of persons followed by Model Systems facilities and the difficulty in contacting people many years after SCI probably affects these observations. Nevertheless, these data describe general patterns of vocational participation that serve to guide our understanding of when and for whom various activities are likely.

James, DeVivo, and Richards (1993) examined the relationship between employment and demographic characteristics. They contrasted the postinjury employment status of persons enrolled in the National SCI Statistical Center database. They found that age, race, and education predicted employment status, with education being an especially strong predictor for African Americans. Gender was related to reemployment only for African Americans, and neurological level of injury was predictive only for Caucasians.

Young and associates (Young, Alfred, Rintala, Hart, & Fuhrer, 1994) examined the vocational status of persons with SCI living in the community. They examined a sample of 100 men and 40 women drawn randomly from a large community-based sample of 640 persons with SCI. They reported that 27% were employed, 35% were in unpaid productive activities, and 38% were unemployed. Whereas veteran status, vocational training, marital status, age, age at onset, and years since injury were not related to vocational status, gender, ethnicity, education, and disability severity were significantly correlated with vocational status. Though men were twice as likely as women to be in paid employment (30% vs. 15%), more women were categorized in a productive vocational mode (83% vs. 57%). The employment rate among persons from minority backgrounds was only one third the rate of White respondents (11% vs. 33%). As expected, educational attainment and functional status were strongly related to vocational status. Considered together in a multivariate model, greater education and functioning independently predicted employment. Such findings support the need for architectural, transportation, vocational, and other policy initiatives that enhance the employment opportunities for persons with severe disabilities and those from minority backgrounds.

Krause (1990) sought to identify common adjustment patterns among persons who achieved different levels of productivity following SCI. In a sample of 344 respondents, he reported that 45% were gainfully employed, 14% were engaged in unpaid productive activities (school, volunteering, or homemaking), and 41% were not engaged in any productive activities. Persons who were employed had the best overall adjustment, followed by persons engaged in unpaid productive activities and those who were unemployed. Contrary to expectations, injury level was not related to level of productive activity, although participants with tetraplegia reported working fewer hours per week. Krause (1992b) subsequently evaluated the relationship between work history and adjustment after SCI among 283 former clinic outpatients. He classified respondents as (1) currently employed, (2) currently unemployed but employed at some time since injury, and (3) never employed since injury. Persons reporting any employment tended to be younger at injury than were those never employed. Currently employed respondents had more years of education than the other two groups and reported more positive feelings about their lives.

More recently, Krause (1996) evaluated two competing hypotheses regarding employment and adjustment following SCI using a sample of 142 adults who completed questionnaires on two occasions, 11 years apart. He reported a relationship between adjustment and employment among persons who became employed. Greater social and educational activity were precursors to employment; however, employment appeared to have a greater impact in enhancing adjustment. As expected, becoming unemployed was associated with a decline in adjustment. He concluded that the results are consistent with a hypothesis that achieving employment leads to superior adjustment, rather than the reverse relationship.

Krause and Anson (1996) assessed attributions of unemployment among 231 persons with SCI who were between the ages of 18 and 59 years of age and had sustained SCI at least 2 years earlier. The majority of respondents attributed unemployment to the physical limitations resulting from SCI, but external factors, such as the job environment, inaccessible work settings, and potential loss of benefits, also were cited. Among Caucasian respondents, men were more likely to identify physical factors as a cause of unemployment, whereas women cited family reasons more often.

Krause (1997) examined the relationship between personality characteristics, employment, and productivity after SCI in 242 persons between the ages of 18 and 60 years. He distinguished respondents as (1) gainfully employed, (2) productive-unemployed (students, volunteers, homemakers), and (3) nonproductive-unemployed. Gainfully employed respondents had significantly higher scores than did the nonproductive-unemployed group on measures of achievement, control, positive affect, and constraint and lower scores on measures of alienation and aggression. The productive-unemployed group scored significantly higher than the nonproductive-unemployed group on measures of control and lower on stress, alienation, and negative affect; their stress scores also were lower than those of the employed group. He concluded that characteristics often associated with SCI onset are related to poor personal adjustment and nonproductivity after SCI rather than SCI per se.

Krause and Anson (1997) reported differences in life satisfaction, adjustment, and life problems in the same sample. Members of the employed group reported superior adjustment, compared with the unemployed and nonproductive-unemployed group on a majority of the scales, and superior scores to the productive-unemployed on only one measure of career satisfaction. They noted the strong association of both education and employment with quality of life after SCI.

McShane and Karp (1993) evaluated employment after SCI in 120 former patients of a rehabilitation center. Employment status was predicted by education, motivation to work, social support, and access to and ability to drive one's own car. Education and lesion level were associated with work motivation, and age at injury predicted education.

In summary, these studies provide a foundation for optimism in our view of vocational possibilities following SCI. Not only do people survive following SCI at a greater rate than in the past but new pharmaceuticals reduce the severity of neurological impairment if administered soon after injury. The functional status attained reflects the severity of residual impairment, but the development of vocational rehabilitation services, civil rights legislation such as the Americans with Disability Act, a growing activist and advocacy movement by persons with disabilities, and more accepting societal attitudes help assure growing vocational opportunities. Large barriers still remain for many persons who consider employment, including financial disincentives inherent in Social Security and private disability policies, inaccessible and poorly funded transportation systems, employer resistance, and psychological issues. New policy initiatives that address these barriers are needed to enhance further the quality of life and societal participation of persons with SCI.

REFERENCES

American Spinal Injury Association. (1992). *Standards for neurological and functional classification of spinal cord injury patients* (rev. ed.). Chicago: Author.

Anderson, P. (1980–1). Alcoholism and the spinal cord disabled: A model program. *Alcohol Health and Research World, 5*, 37–41.

Antonak, R. F., & Livneh, H. (1991). A hierarchy of reactions to disability. *International Journal of Rehabilitation Research, 14*, 13–24.

Bracken, M. B., Shepard, M. J., Collins, W. F., Holford, T. R., Young, W., Baskin, D. S., Eisenberg, H. M., Flamm, E., Leo-Sommers, L., Mawon, J., Marshall, L. F., Perot, P. L., Jr., Piepmeier, J., Sonntag, V. K. H., Wagner, F. C., Wilberger, J. E., & Winn, H. R. (1990). A randomized, controlled trial of methylprednisolone or naloxone in the treatment of acute spinal-cord injury. *New England Journal of Medicine, 322,* 1405–1411.

Buckelew, S. P., Baumstark, K. E., Frank, R. G., & Hewett, J. E. (1990). Adjustment following spinal cord injury. *Rehabilitation Psychology, 35*, 101–109.

Buckelew, S. P., Frank, R. G., Elliott, T. R., Chaney, M. A., & Hewett, J. (1991). Adjustment to spinal cord injury: Stage theory revisited. *Paraplegia, 29*, 125–130.

Buckelew, S. P., Hanson, S., & Frank, R. G. (1991). Psychological factors and adjustment to spinal cord injury. *NeuroRehabilitation, 1*(4), 36–45.

Charlifue, S. W., & Gerhart, K. A. (1991). Behavioral and demographic predictors of suicide after traumatic spinal cord injury. *Archives of Physical Medicine and Rehabilitation, 72*, 488–492.

Clay, D. L., Hagglund, K. J., Frank, R. G., Elliott, T. R., & Chaney, J. M. (1995). Enhancing the accuracy of depression diagnosis in patients with spinal cord injury using Bayesian analysis. *Rehabilitation Psychology, 40,* 171–180.

Coca, B. (1991, August). *Coping, social support and acceptance of disability among persons with SCI.* Paper presented at the 99th annual convention of the American Psychological Association, San Francisco.

Crewe, N. M. (1997). Life stories of people with long-term spinal cord injury. *Rehabilitation Counseling Bulletin, 41,* 26–42.

Cushman, L. A., & Dijkers, M. P. (1990). Depressed mood in spinal cord injured patients: Staff perceptions and patient realities. *Archives of Physical Medicine and Rehabilitation, 71*, 191–196.

Dembo, T. (1969). Rehabilitation psychology and its immediate future: A problem of utilization of psychological knowledge. *Rehabilitation Psychology (Psychological Aspects of Disability), 16*, 63–72.

Dembo, T., Leviton, G., & Wright, B. A. (1956). Adjustment to misfortune: A problem in social-psychological rehabilitation. *Artificial Limbs, 3*, 4–62.

Dijkers, M. (1997). Quality of life after spinal cord injury: A meta-analysis of the effects of disablement components. *Spinal Cord, 35,* 829–840.

Dijkers, M. P., Abela, M. B., Gans, B. M., & Gordon, W. A. (1995). The aftermath of spinal cord injury. In S. L. Stover, J. A. DeLisa, & G. G. Whiteneck (Eds.), *Spinal cord injury: Clinical outcomes from the Model Systems* (pp. 185–212). Gaithersburg, MD: Aspen.

Ditunno, J. F., Cohen, M. E., Formal, C., & Whiteneck, G. G. (1995). Functional outcomes. In S. L. Stover, J. A. DeLisa, & G. G. Whiteneck (Eds.), *Spinal cord injury: Clinical outcomes from the Model Systems* (pp. 170–184). Gaithersburg, MD: Aspen.

Donovan, W. H. (1981). Spinal cord injury. In W. C. Stolov & M. R. Clowers (Eds.), *Handbook of severe disability* (pp. 65–82). Washington, DC: U.S. Government Printing Office.

Elliott, T. R., & Frank, R. G. (1996). Depression following spinal cord injury. *Archives of Physical Medicine and Rehabilitation, 77,* 816–823.

Elliott, T. R., Herrick, S. M., Patti, A. M., Witty, T. E., Godshall, F., & Spruell, M. (1991). Assertiveness, social support and psychological adjustment following spinal cord injury. *Behavior Research and Therapy, 29,* 485–493.

Elliott, T. R., Herrick, S. M., Witty, T. E., Godshall, F., & Spruell, M. (1992). Social support and depression following spinal cord injury. *Rehabilitation Psychology, 37*, 37–48.

Elliott, T. R., Witty, T. E., Herrick, S. M., & Hoffman, J. T. (1991). Negotiating reality after physical loss: Hope, depression and disability. *Journal of Personality and Social Psychology, 61,* 608–613.

Fink, S. (1967). Crisis and motivation: A theoretical model. *Archives of Physical Medicine and Rehabilitation, 48*, 592–597.

Frank, R. G., & Elliott, T. R. (1987). Life stress and psychologic adjustment following spinal cord injury. *Archives of Physical Medicine and Rehabilitation, 68*, 344–347.

Frank, R. G., Elliott, T. R., Corcoran, J. R., & Wonderlich, S. A. (1987). Depression after spinal cord injury: Is it necessary? *Clinical Psychology Review, 7,* 611–630.

Frank, R. G., Umlauf, R. L., Wonderlich, S. A., Askanazi, G. S., Buckelew, S. P., & Elliott, T. R. (1987). Differences in coping styles among persons with spinal cord injury: A cluster-analytic approach. *Journal of Consulting and Clinical Psychology, 55*, 727–731.

French, J. K., & Phillips, J. A. (1991). Shattered images: Recovery for the SCI client. *Rehabilitation Nursing, 16*, 134–136.

Frisbie, J. H., & Tun, C. G. (1984). Drinking and spinal cord injury. *Journal of the American Paraplegia Society, 7*, 71–73.

Fullerton, D. T., Harvey, R. F., Klein, M. H., & Howell, T. (1981). Psychiatric disorders in patients with spinal cord injuries. *Archives of General Psychiatry, 38*, 1369–1371.

Galbraith, S., Murray, W. R., Patel, A. R., & Knitt-Jones, R. (1976). The relationship between alcohol and head injury and its effects on the conscious level. *British Journal of Surgery, 63*, 128–130.

Gale, J. L., Dikmen, S., Wyler, A., Temkin, N., & McClean, A. (1983). Head injury in the Pacific Northwest. *Neurosurgery, 12*, 487–491.

Glass, C. A. (1994). Psychological intervention in physical disability—with special reference to spinal cord injury. *Journal of Mental Health, 3,* 467–476.

Go, B. K., DeVivo, M. J., & Richards, J. S. (1995). The epidemiology of spinal cord injury. In S. L. Stover, J. A. DeLisa, & G. G. Whiteneck (Eds.), *Spinal cord injury: Clinical outcomes from the Model Systems* (pp. 185–212). Gaithersburg, MD: Aspen.

Hamilton, B. B., Granger, C. V., Sherwin, F. S., Zielezny, M., & Tashman, J. S. (1987). A Uniform National Data System for Medical Rehabilitation. In M. J. Fuhrer (Ed.), *Rehabilitation outcomes: Analysis and measurement.* Baltimore, MD: Brookes Publishing Co.

Hammel, K. R. W. (1992). Psychological and sociological theories concerning adjustment to traumatic spinal cord injury: The implications for rehabilitation. *Paraplegia, 30*, 317–326.

Hanson, S., Buckelew, S. P., Hewett, J., & O'Neal, G. (1993). The relationship between coping and adjustment after spinal cord injury: A 5-year follow-up study. *Rehabilitation Psychology, 38,* 41–52.

Harvey, R. F., & Jellinek, H. M. (1981). Functional performance assessment: A program approach. *Archives of Physical Medicine and Rehabilitation, 62*, 456–460.

Hawkins, D., & Heinemann, A. W. (1998). Substance abuse and medical complications following spinal cord injury. *Rehabilitation Psychology, 43,* 125–139.

Heinemann, A. W. (1993). *Substance abuse and physical disability*. New York: Haworth Press.

Heinemann, A. W., Donohue, R., Keen, M., & Schnoll, S. (1988). Alcohol use by persons with recent spinal cord injuries. *Archives of Physical Medicine and Rehabilitation, 69*, 619–624.

Heinemann, A. W., Goranson, N., Ginsburg, K., & Schnoll, S. (1989). Alcohol use and activity patterns following spinal cord injury. *Rehabilitation Psychology, 34*, 191–206.

Heinemann, A. W., Hamilton, B. B., & Johnston, M. V. (1998). *Relation of rehabilitation intervention to functional outcome: Final report.* State University of New York, Buffalo: Rehabilitation Research and Training Center on Functional Assessment and Evaluation of Rehabilitation Outcomes.

Heinemann, A. W., Kirk, P., Hastie, B. A., Semik, P., Hamilton, B. B., Linacre, J. M., Wright, B. D., & Granger, C. V. (1997). Relationships between disability measures and nursing effort during medical rehabilitation for patients with traumatic brain and spinal cord injury. *Archives of Physical Medicine and Rehabilitation, 78*, 143–149.

Heinemann, A. W., Linacre, J. M., Wright, B. D., Hamilton, B. B., & Granger, C. (1993). Relationships between impairment and disability as measured by the Functional Independence Measure. *Archives of Physical Medicine and Rehabilitation, 74,* 566–573.

Heinemann, A. W., Linacre, J. M., Wright, B. D., Hamilton, B. B., & Granger, C. V. (1994). Prediction of rehabilitation outcomes with disability measures. *Archives of Physical Medicine and Rehabilitation, 75,* 133–143.

Heinemann, A. W., Schnoll, S., Brandt, M., Maltz, R., & Keen, M. (1988). Toxicology screening in acute spinal cord injury. *Alcoholism: Clinical and Experimental Research, 12*, 815–819.

Heinemann, A. W., & Shontz, F. C. (1984). Adjustment following disability: Representative case studies. *Rehabilitation Counseling Bulletin, 28*, 3–14.

Heinemann, A. W., & Shontz, F. C. (1985). Methods of studying persons. *Counseling Psychologist, 13*, 111–125.

Hohmann, G. (1975). Psychological aspects of treatment and rehabilitation of the spinal injured person. *Clinical Orthopedics, 112*, 81–88.

James, M., DeVivo, M. J., & Richards, J. S. (1993). Postinjury employment outcomes among African-American and White persons with spinal cord injury. *Rehabilitation Psychology, 38,* 151–164.

Johnson, D. C. (1985). *Alcohol use by persons with disabilities*. Madison, WI: Wisconsin Department of Health and Social Services.

Judd, F. K., & Brown, D. J. (1992). Suicide following acute traumatic spinal cord injury. *Paraplegia, 30*, 173–177.

Krause, J. S. (1990). The relationship between productivity and adjustment following spinal cord injury. *Rehabilitation Counseling Bulletin, 33*, 188–199.

Krause, J. S. (1992a). Adjustment to life after spinal cord injury: A comparison among three participant groups based on employment status. *Rehabilitation Counseling Bulletin, 35,* 218–229.

Krause, J. S. (1992b). Employment after spinal cord injury. *Archives of Physical Medicine and Rehabilitation, 73*, 163–169.

Krause, J. S. (1996). Employment after spinal cord injury: Transition and life adjustment. *Rehabilitation Counseling Bulletin, 39,* 244–255.

Krause, J. S. (1997). Personality and traumatic spinal cord injury: Relationship to participation in productive activities. *Journal of Applied Rehabilitation Counseling, 28,* 15–20.

Krause, J. S., & Anson, C. A. (1996). Self-perceived reasons for unemployment cited by persons with spinal cord injury: Relationship to gender, race, age and level of injury. *Rehabilitation Counseling Bulletin, 39,* 217–227.

Krause, J. S., & Anson, C. A. (1997). Adjustment after spinal cord injury: Relationship to participation in employment or educational activities. *Rehabilitation Counseling Bulletin, 40,* 202–214.

Krause, J. S., & Crewe, N. M. (1991). Chronologic age, time since injury, and time of measurement: Effect on adjustment after spinal cord injury. *Archives of Physical Medicine and Rehabilitation, 72*, 91–100.

Kübler-Ross, E. (1969). *On death and dying*. New York: Macmillan.

Lazarus, R., & Folkman, S. (1984). *Stress, appraisal and coping*. New York: Springer Publishing Co.

Lewin, K. (1935). *A dynamic theory of personality*. New York: McGraw-Hill.

Linacre, J. M., Heinemann, A. W., Wright, B. D., Granger, C. V., & Hamilton, B. B. (1994). The structure and stability of the Functional Independence Measure. *Archives of Physical Medicine and Rehabilitation, 75,* 127–132.

Livneh, H. (1986). A unified approach to existing models of adaptation to disability: Part 2. Intervention strategies. *Journal of Applied Rehabilitation Counseling, 17*, 6–10.

Livneh, H., & Antonak, R. F. (1997). *Psychosocial adaptation to chronic illness and disability*. Gaithersburg, MD: Aspen.

Lowenthal, A., & Anderson, P. (1980–1). Network development: Linking the disabled community to alcoholism and drug abuse programs. *Alcohol Health and Research World, 5*, 16–19.

Matthews, P. J., & Carlson, C. E. (1987). *Spinal cord injury: A guide to rehabilitation nursing*. Rockville, MD: Aspen.

Mawson, A. R., Jacobs, K. W., Winchester, Y., & Biundo, J. J. (1988). Sensation-seeking and traumatic spinal cord injury: Case-control study. *Archives of Physical Medicine and Rehabilitation, 69*, 1039–1043.

McColl, M. A., Lei, H., & Skinner, H. (1995). Structural relationships between social support and coping. *Social Science and Medicine, 41,* 395–407.

McShane, S. L., & Karp, J. (1993). Employment following spinal cord injury: A covariance structure analysis. *Rehabilitation Psychology, 38,* 27–40.

Mueller, A., & Thompson, C. E. (1950). Personality problems of the spinal cord injured. *Journal of Consulting Psychology, 4*, 189–192.

National Institute on Drug Abuse. (1988). *National household survey on drug abuse: Main findings*. Rockville, MD: National Institute on Drug Abuse.

Nixon, V. (1985). *Spinal cord injury: A guide to functional outcomes in physical therapy management.* Rockville, MD: Aspen.

O'Donnell, J. J., Cooper, J. E., Gessner, J. E., Shehan, I., & Ashley, J. (1981–2). Alcohol, drugs and spinal cord injury. *Alcohol Health and Research World, 6,* 27–29.

Parkes, C. (1972). *Bereavement: Studies of grief in adult life.* New York: International University Press.

Pope, A., & Tarlov, A. R. (1991). *Disability in America.* Washington, DC: National Academy Press.

Radnitz, C. L., & Tirch, D. (1995). Substance misuse in individuals with spinal cord injury. *International Journal of the Addictions, 30,* 1117–1140.

Rasch, G. (1960). Probabilistic models for some intelligence and attainment tests. Copenhagen: Paedogogiske Institut (reprint, Chicago: University of Chicago Press, 1980).

Rasmussen, G. A., & DeBoer, R. P. (1980). Alcohol and drug use among clients at a residential vocational rehabilitation facility. *Alcohol Health and Research World, 5*, 48–56.

Rintala, D. H., Young, M. E., Hart, K. A., Clearman, R. R., & Fuhrer, M. J. (1992). Social support and the well-being of persons with spinal cord injury living in the community. *Rehabilitation Psychology, 37*, 155–164.

Rohe, D. E., & Basford, J. R. (1990). Traumatic spinal cord injury, alcohol, and the Minnesota Multiphasic Personality Inventory. *Rehabilitation Psychology, 34*, 25–32.

Scherer, M. J. (1988). Assistive device utilization and quality-of-life in adults with spinal cord injuries and cerebral palsy. *Journal of Applied Rehabilitation Counseling, 19,* 21–30.

Schulz, R., & Decker, S. (1985). Long-term adjustment to physical disability: The role of social support, perceived control and self-blame. *Journal of Personality and Social Psychology, 48*, 1162–1172.

Shontz, F. C. (1965). Reactions to crisis. *Volta Review, 67*, 364–370.

Shontz, F. C. (1982). Adaptation to chronic illness and disability. In T. Millon, C. Green, & R. Meagher (Eds.), *Handbook of clinical health psychology* (pp. 153–172). New York: Plenum.

Siller, J. (1969). Psychological situation of the disabled with spinal cord injuries. *Rehabilitation Literature, 30*, 290–296.

Silver, R., & Wortman, C. (1980). Coping with undesirable life events. In J. Garber & N. Seligman (Eds.), *Human helplessness: Theory and applications*. New York: Academic Press.

State University of New York at Buffalo. (1993). *Guide for the Uniform Data Set for Medical Rehabilitation.* Buffalo, NY: Uniform Data System for Medical Rehabilitation.

Stewart, T. D. (1978). Coping behavior and the moratorium following spinal cord injury. *Paraplegia, 15*, 338–342.

Stover, S. L., DeLisa, J. A., & Whiteneck, G. G. (1995). *Spinal cord injury: Clinical outcomes from the Model Systems* (pp. 185–212). Gaithersburg, MD: Aspen.

Sweeney, T. T., & Foote, J. E. (1982). Treatment of drug and alcohol abuse in spinal cord injury veterans. *International Journal of the Addictions, 17*, 897–904.

Trieschmann, R. B. (1988). *Spinal cord injuries: Psychological, social, and vocational rehabilitation* (2nd ed.). New York: Demos Publications.

Trieschmann, R. B. (1992). Psychosocial research in spinal cord injury: The state of the art. *Paraplegia, 30*, 58–60.

Whiteneck, G. G., Charlifue, S. W., Gerhart, K. A., Overholser, J. D., & Richardson, G. N. (1992). Quantifying handicap: A new measure of long-term rehabilitation outcomes. *Archives of Physical Medicine and Rehabilitation, 73,* 519–526.

World Health Organization. (1980). *Classification of impairments, disabilities, and handicaps.* Geneva, Switzerland: Author.

World Health Organization. (1993). Foreword. In *International classification of impairments, disabilities, and handicaps: A manual of classification relating to the consequences of disease.* Geneva, Switzerland: Author.

Wright, B. A. (1983). *Physical disability: A psychosocial approach.* New York: Harper and Row.

Young, M. E., Alfred, W. G., Rintala, D. H., Hart, K. A., & Fuhrer, J. J. (1994). Vocational status of persons with spinal cord injury living in the community. *Rehabilitation Counseling Bulletin, 37,* 229–243.

Chapter 25

Hemiplegia

Leonard Diller

MEDICAL BACKGROUND

Stroke is the third leading cause of death in the United States and the leading cause of disability. Approximately 550,000 people suffer strokes each year, and nearly one third die from them, whereas 3,000,000 people with various neurological impairments are alive following stroke. Stroke is the leading cause of focal neuropsychological impairment. The abrupt onset and devastating results convey the layman's description perhaps more accurately than the term *cerebrovascular accident* because the event may not be cerebrovascular nor accidental (Weibe-Velasquez & Hachinski, 1991). Strokes, marked by sudden paralysis and loss of consciousness have been noted since ancient times. Approximately three quarters of strokes are caused by cerebral infarct. Intracerebral or subarachnoid hemorrhages account for 15%. With newer developments in brain imaging, there has been a dramatic increase in understanding the chain of events that occur in stroke. Diagnostic investigation clarifies the area of brain damage as well as the underlying pathology that gave rise to the chain of events in a more precise way than previously had been possible. Even with laboratory studies the diagnosis may still reflect a "best guess."

The epidemiology of stroke is becoming clearer with detailed study. Risk factors for stroke can be divided into those that are modifiable such as transient ischemic attack (TIA), diabetes mellitus, hypertension, atrial fibrillation, substance abuse, and smoking. The major risk factor is hypertension. Among non-modifiable risk factors, the most important is age. Strokes increase dramatically with age and tend to double with each decade after age 55. First ever strokes account for 75% of the incidence, and recurrent strokes account for 25%. However, gender, race, and family history can contribute as etiologic factors. Strokes occur more often in males than in females and more often in African Americans than in Caucasians. In Western countries there appears to be a decline in stroke, perhaps because of public education with regard to the modifiable risk factors (Gresham et al., 1995).

Of those who survive the initial onset, the most frequent presenting problem is hemiplegia, or hemiparesis, which occurs in about 75%–88% of survivors at 30 days, with an equal occurrence of right and left hemiparesis. Generally, the paralysis occurs on the side of the body opposite the brain damage, so an individual with right brain damage (RBD) will sustain a paralysis or weakness on the left side of the body. An individual with left brain damage (LBD) will sustain a paralysis or weakness on the right side of the body. During the acute period there is a high incidence of associated neurological deficits, ranging from 12% to 56%. The deficits include ataxia (20%), hemianopsia (26%), visual-perceptual defects (32%), aphasia (30%), dysarthria (48%), sensory deficits (56%), cognitive deficits (36%), depression, bladder control (29%), and dysphagia (12%) (Gresham et al., 1995). The deficits often coexist, so management is complicated. On long-term follow-up 6 to 12 months later, there is a lower incidence of deficits in bladder control, dysarthria, aphasia, and dysphagia. The long-term cognitive and emotional sequelae will be discussed below. One important medical concern is the incidence of comorbidities that might affect management and rehabilitation potential. Among these are hypertensive heart disease, obesity, coronary heart disease, arthritis, diabetes mellitus, and congestive heart failure.

Tracking the course of recovery over time is an important consideration. Most recovery takes place within the first 1–3 months. Although recovery may continue, particularly with regard to language and visual perception, the pace of recovery slows. As rehabilitation, particularly at the inpatient level, usually takes place during the first 3 months, it is often difficult to tell whether gains are due to natural recovery or rehabilitation. Recent studies suggest that for patients undergoing rehabilitation, functional recovery of motoric independence can continue beyond 3 months despite the lack of gain in neurological markers. Furthermore, whereas rehabilitation in stroke may result in reduction of neurological impairment as well as of disability, disability is reduced even in those patients who show no change in impairment. This suggests that gains in disability do not stem from recovery alone but may be the result of interventions in rehabilitation (Roth et al., 1998).

FUNCTIONAL LIMITATIONS

Traditional medicine has been concerned with disease management and cure. Rehabilitation has moved beyond these concerns to issues in living with the effects of disease and trauma. Whereas neurological deficits are generally associated with impairments, rehabilitation is concerned with functional limitations and handicap. Functional limitations involve the quality of daily activities, commonly expressed by the degree of dependence in the physical, cognitive, social, emotional, and vocational domains. Instruments to assess functional limitations permit quantifiable observation that can be used to track outcomes, recovery, and individual and program differences. An indication of the rapid development in the field can be seen by examining the most common method of assessing functional limitations—the Functional Independence Measure (FIM). The FIM has been adopted by 1,300 participating facilities and 70,000 trained clinical raters. At the end of 1997, data have been collected on more than 3 million patients (Granger, 1998).

Studies in community-based samples of hemiparesis patients who have not undertaken formal rehabilitation indicate that although only 27% of survivors were independent in walking during the first week after stroke, 85% were independent at 6 months. In activities of daily living, help was needed for bowel and bladder incontinence, grooming, toileting, feeding, dressing, bathing, and/or transfers in 77%–88% of the cases at 3 weeks after onset (Dombovy, 1993; Wade & Hewer, 1987). On follow-up 6 months to 5 years later, help was needed in 24%–53% of the cases. In patients who have completed inpatient rehabilitation, FIM scores on motor activities improved by 38%, and cognitive scores improved by 11% at discharge. The benefits of these improvements have been translated into a reduction of caregiver hours (Roth et al., 1998).

Eighteen percent of stroke survivors participate in rehabilitation. The most prominent reason for rehabilitation in stroke is hemiplegia or hemiparesis. Of those patients who do not enter rehabilitation, the majority are discharged home with or without outpatient services or are discharged to nursing homes (10%–29%). Discharge destination depends in large part on the person's clinical status as well as social factors. For example, there is a higher incidence of discharge to nursing homes or sheltered dwellings among persons living alone at the time of the stroke than among those coming from intact families (Powell, Diller, & Grynbaum, 1976).

PSYCHOLOGICAL PROBLEMS

A psychological problem maybe defined as a difficulty in meeting the task demands in rehabilitation and/or in assuming the premorbid or normative role expectations following discharge because of a problem in the cognitive or emotional functioning of the person and/or an environmental problem. In this chapter we are largely concerned with the difficulties in the person; hence, we focus on the psychological problems. Psychological problems may be related to cultural or environmental circumstances and may be referred to as psychosocial problems. Psychological difficulties attributable to the environment during rehabilitation may require an examination of the attitudes of the rehabilitation team or of significant others. Two problems that tend to arise after inpatient rehabilitation is completed and that may be overlooked are sexual functioning (Monga, 1997) and driving (Fisk, Owsley, & Pulley, 1997; Galski, Bruno, Zorowitz, & Walker, 1993).

Psychological problems may be expressed as difficulties in learning, attitudes and/or behaviors that interfere with maximum utilization of the program, increasing length of stay, accidents, disturbance in patient well-being, problems in staff management, or difficulties in family relationships. The psychologist generally translates presenting problems into difficulties in cognition, emotion, and/or motivation as these interact with current circumstances. The translation also factors in premorbid personality, which might influence the response to the current situation (Langer, 1992). In a retrospective chart survey of 200 inpatients, approximately 13% had evidence of prior psychiatric histories (Padrone, 1995).

The proper diagnosis is important not only to facilitate the direction of therapy but also because patients, families, and even members of the rehabilitation team might misattribute the sources of a patient's problem. Misattribution might lead to unnecessary self-blame or anger on the part of a therapist or a family member.

Clinically, it might be useful to describe mental life in terms of cognition, affect, and motivation. This categorization permits the organization of a large body of psychological studies within a framework that is meaningful for rehabilitation. One can indicate the incidence of impairments, their relationship to rehabilitation, some common methods used in their assessment, and finally, treatment methods. This encompasses the historical emphasis of different professional approaches. Whereas psychologists have emphasized information processing and affective responses, other therapists in rehabilitation tend to use the label "lack of motivation" in describing a difficult patient.

Cognition is "the mental process or faculty by which knowledge is acquired, or that which comes to be known through perception, reasoning, or intuition" (*American Heritage Dictionary*). Cognitive changes may be end points of processes involving language, attention, perception, and memory. A diffuse or global decline in cognitive functioning yields the clinical picture of dementia.

Complex and specific patterns of cognitive dysfunction have been identified. Among the most prominent are apraxia, aphasia, and visual-perceptual deficits. Apraxia is a disorder of learned movement that can not be explained by the patient's deficits in strength, coordination, sensation, or lack of comprehension. Apraxias have been observed in both clinical testing and activities of daily living (ADLs). Aphasia is a disturbance in communication in language-related events, generally resulting from damage to the dominant hemisphere; it occurs more often in individuals with right hemiparesis than in those with left hemiparesis. Aphasia is manifested by problems in comprehension and expression including difficulties in reading and spelling. It is distinguished from the neuromotor components of language (e.g., dysarthria, where the difficulty may lie in executing a sequence of voluntary movements). Perceptual difficulties may appear in several ways, including visual field defects, color recognition, diplopia, visual gaze, and depth perception, that may affect rehabilitation. The most prominent problem is that of visual neglect or hemi-inattention. It occurs more often in RBD with left hemiparesis than in LBD with right hemiparesis. Hemi-inattention is a complex disorder, with diminished awareness of space on the side opposite to the damaged hemisphere. The diminished attention is manifested by errors of omission. It occurs with regard to location on the body (body image) as well as location external to the body (extrapersonal space). It can involve visual and tactile modalities and, to a lesser extent, auditory modalities. Hemi-inattention can be observed in clinical testing as well as in ADLs (Gordon & Diller, 1983).

Emotional reactions are generally divided into depression, anxiety, and hostility. Poststroke depression has been cited as the most common untreated disability secondary to stroke (Gordon & Hibbard, 1997). Although reported in the stroke literature since the turn of the century, it had not been regarded as a serious problem in rehabilitation settings until the 1980s. Earlier observers focused on denial of affective reactions in stroke patients. Depression has several features, including attitudes reflecting hopelessness and pessimism, nonverbal demeanor, and vegetative disturbances in eating and sleeping. Earlier observers attributed depression to a grieving response or a catastrophic response to frustrations and losses associated with stroke; however, recent observers have implicated biological factors via locus of brain damage (Starkstein & Robinson, 1990) and social factors via the social isolation following stroke. Depression in stroke has a high frequency of characteristics of anxiety (Starkstein & Robinson, 1990). Other psychiatric disturbances, such as hallucinations, mania, delusions, personality alterations, and obsessive-compulsive disorders, occur less often.

Motivation is an individual's response to a rehabilitation program in terms of participation or compliance with its task demands (Hyman, 1971; Thompson, 1991). Poor motivation can be attributed to many factors, but two stand out. First, there maybe a lack of congruence between the patient's goals and the goals of the rehabilitation team. For example, if the patient wants only a cure for his or her condition, anything less is viewed as a failure in treatment. The goals may be influenced by a number of circumstances, including retention of a premorbid self-concept, emotional flooding by anger or depression, cognitive incompetence related to neurologically based unawareness, pain, or cultural factors that influence the meaning of the occurrence of a stroke. Second, apathy or hypoarousal, which might be a direct consequence of the stroke, may be misconstrued as a lack of interest or depression rather than as a neurologically based problem (Diller, Goodgold, & Kay, 1988).

The cognitive, emotional, and motivational domains interact and influence each other. Although the domains may exist separately, a cognitive problem is likely to occur together with an emotional and/or motivational problem, and vice versa (Diller et al., 1988).

There are no formal data on actual psychological problems because their manifestations are diverse. An informal survey of the time spent by occupational and physical therapists indicates that in one large rehabilitation facility more than 40 hours of therapist time in a given week was taken up with the management of behavioral problems (Padrone, 1995). Despite the absence of documentation on the incidence of psychological problems, there is a great deal of information on cognitive, emotional, and motivational factors that play a role in rehabilitation, information that can be used to understand and help management of psychological problems.

Stroke patients perform more poorly on standard cognitive tests than do normal subjects (Egelko et al., 1989) and orthopedic patients (Osmon, Smet, Winegarden, & Ghandavadi, 1992). Cognitive performance is lower in patients after a stroke at 6-month follow-up in comparison with actual prestroke scores (Kase et al., 1987). Although cognitive disturbances are most acute at the time of onset, they may persist for longer periods (Egelko et al., 1989). For example, at 3 months, problems in memory still remain for 29% of a group that returned to the community (Wade, Parker, & Langton-Hewer, 1986). In another study, using a more functional test of memory, 49% were found to be below the lowest scores of non-brain-damaged persons at 7 months after onset (Lincoln & Tinson, 1989). Hemi-inattention is present in 72% of patients with RBD and 62% of those with LBD at 3 days after stroke. At 3 months it is still present in 75% of RBD patients who originally showed neglect and 33% of LBD patients who originally showed neglect (Stone et al., 1991). Wide variation in estimates occur in part because of the variation in tests that are used. It appears that the more extensive and inclusive the test battery, the higher the incidence (Schenkenberg, Bradford, & Ajax, 1980).

Affective disturbance places patients at risk and is clearly a problem. In comparison with a prestroke indicator of depression, at 6 months after stroke, patients are significantly depressed (Kase, 1993). However, it is difficult to draw firm conclusions regarding major issues. For example, estimates of depression vary from 11%–68% (Gordon & Hibbard, 1997), depending on the hemispheric and anatomic location but even more important, on methods of assessment. Assessment of depression in hemiparetic patients is difficult because instruments to assess depression involve self-report, which may be influenced by the presence of aphasia, lack of awareness, cognitive confusion, or somatic manifestations (which may be attributed to organic conditions such as lability) or by being in a hospital (which might influence eating and sleeping patterns) (Gordon & Hibbard, 1997). Time of assessment also may play a role (Schubert et al., 1992a). Depression is underreported in self-report or medical intake interview and is likely to decrease during a rehabilitation program (Schubert et al., 1992). Data are ambiguous with regard to long-term status (Gordon et al., 1985; Thompson, 1991). Some with earlier major depression still remain in this state at 2 years and even longer, and minor depression may get worse (Parikh et al., 1990).

With regard to motivation, a substantial number of stroke patients are unaware of various aspects of stroke. Unawareness tends to be greater in the acute phase (Hier, Mondlock, & Caplan, 1983). However, after the acute phase, unawareness is unrelated to time since onset (Hibbard, Gordon, & Stein, 1992). Unawareness is not a unitary phenomenon. More people are aware of physical impairments than of affective and cognitive impairments (Anderson & Tranel, 1989; Hibbard et al., 1992). Half of stroke patients are aware of memory and mood disorders, but patients tend to exaggerate memory problems (Tinson, 1987) and minimize self-report of perceptual problems (Diller & Weinberg, 1993) and depression (Hibbard et al., 1992). Patients may misattribute their problems. For example, an individual with a perceptual problem who denies it may, when pressed, state that a problem exists but it is a memory problem (Diller & Weinberg, 1993). There are differences between individuals who overtly deny a problem and those who passively acknowledge a problem but remain unresponsive. The level of denial is related to cognitive competence (Diller & Weinberg, 1993).

Although motivation may be affected by the neurobiology of stroke, cultural factors play a role. Stroke patients with similar neurological impairments but in different settings (i.e., a public vs. a private university medical rehabilitation program) differed in attitudes to authority and in feelings about controlling their health-related activities (Powell et al., 1976).

Another aspect of lack of motivation is that of hypoarousal. RBD stroke patients make fewer movements than do LBD patients in performing a block design task (Ben Yishay et al., 1974) even when solving a problem correctly. RBD and LBD patients are slower in reaction time tasks than normal subjects, and their response rate is slower (Egelko et al., 1989). Some find that reaction time improves during a rehabilitation program; others report that even with improvement it is a most persistent impairment at 1-year follow-up (Egelko et al., 1989). Prigitano and Wong (1997) note that speed of finger tapping but not grip strength is impaired in the hand that is ipsilateral to the side of brain damage in unilateral stroke patients. Theoretically, speed should be affected only on the side contralateral to the brain damage. They argue that the degree of impairment is an indicator of the degree of bilateral damage and that the task activates bilateral cerebral hemispheres.

Psychological Problems and Program Participation

Many aspects of ADL are related to perceptual and cognitive problems. Patients with spatial constructional problems perform poorly in dressing, eating, walking, and grooming (Warren, 1990). Patients with visual neglect have difficulty (Gordon & Diller, 1983) in academic tasks (reading, writing, written arithmetic), grooming (shaving in men, makeup in women), instrumental activities (reading a menu, using a telephone, household activities), driving, telling time from a clock (Titus, Gall, Yerxa, Robertson, & Mack, 1991). A given ADL task may depend on the integration of several abilities; therefore, failure may occur for different reasons by patients with different patterns of cognitive deficits. Thus, in learning to transfer to and from a wheelchair, overall gain is related to cognitive competency. In individuals with left hemiparesis, mastery is associated with errors on spatial tasks. In individuals with right hemiparesis mastery is associated with speed in processing information (Diller, Buxbaum, & Chiotelis, 1972). Similarly, with regard to the occurrence of accidents on a rehabilitation program, LBD patients with neglect on a visual cancellation test are more likely to have multiple accidents. RBD patients who are too slow on the same test are more likely to have accidents (Diller & Weinberg, 1970). A further example of a common path of difficulty due to different sources of dysfunction may be found in the observation that problems in recognizing affective dimensions of verbal expression (aprosodia) occur equally in RBD and LBD stroke patients.

Poor performance on cognitive tasks predicts outcome in inpatient rehabilitation (Ben Yishay, Gerstman, Diller, & Haas, 1970; Galski et al., 1993) and on long-term follow-up (Wade et al., 1986). Although different combinations of tests have been used, motor impersistence and logical memory have contributed to predictions (Ben Yishay, Gerstman, Diller, & Haas, 1968). Visual neglect in rehabilitation predicts poorer ADLs on long-term follow-up (Denes, Semenza, Stoppa, & Lis, 1982; Kinsella & Ford, 1980). Prigitano and Wong (1997) found that speed of reaction time using the hand ipsilateral to the brain damage predicts goal attainment in rehabilitation. They suggest that this is a behavioral marker of the integrity of the intact hemisphere, which could be used to predict rehabilitation outcome.

Depression has been shown to be related to increased length of stay on inpatient programs (Schubert, 1992b), lower ADL scores (Schubert, 1992c), discharge to a facility rather than to home (Cushman, 1987), and cognitive impairment (Starkstein & Robinson, 1990). Depression appears to become an increasingly potent factor with increasing time (Thompson, 1991). It is associated with decline in social (Parikh et al., 1990) and sexual activities (Monga et al., 1997). Although depression is not originally associated with severity of impairment, with time, depression becomes increasingly related to severity of impairment (Robinson, 1985; Thompson, 1991). In an outpatient sample, depression was associated with a lack of meaning in life and overprotection (Thompson, 1991). In a follow-up of patients 10 years postonset, Morris et al. (Morris, Robinson, Andrzejwski, Samuels, & Price, 1993) found that patients diagnosed as depressed on examination 1 to 3 weeks after a stroke had a mortality rate 3.4 times higher than nondepressed patients.

Motivation in outpatient treatment has been related to overprotection, lower cognitive functioning, lower sense of meaning, and less hope (Thompson, 1991). Those who held themselves responsible for the stroke had a poorer adjustment (Thompson, 1991).

Identifying Psychological Problems

Specific problems might be detected in initial clinical impression, the medical chart, reports by family or staff, or self-report. Because the incidence of cognitive and/or emotional impairments is high, routine screening is recommended to identify stroke patients at risk of not benefiting from a program or posing management problems. In initial medical screenings, chart reviews suggest that depression (Schubert et al., 1992d) and visual-perceptual problems (Weinberg & Diller, 1966) may be overlooked.

Although brief screening for psychosocial problems may be part of an initial medical examination, further levels of screening by a psychologist should be considered. An informal survey of consecutive admissions to an inpatient service of 200 patients, of whom 30% were stroke patients, found the presence of depression/anxiety in 63% (Padrone, 1995). With the scarcity of available time and the increasing trend toward curtailing lengths of stay in inpatient rehabilitation, psychologists are in the position of having to choose between concentrating their efforts on a few problem patients who may require extensive in-depth evaluations and many patients with different degrees of psychological problems. The former approach involves a few patients who might consume more team resources; the latter approach involves less in-depth contact and permits the psychologist to participate more actively in case management by the rehabilitation team. The psychologist in the latter approach samples in a more limited way domains of language, attention, perception, memory, and psychomotor proficiency as well as patient goals, concerns, and affective state. The psychologist is in a position to be more effective with a larger number of patients, although the diagnostic judgments are based on less fine-grained analysis of impairments. The former approach pursues the development of more refined test batteries to parse deficits; the latter seeks shorter batteries to deal with the logistics of decision making and management. Hajek et al. (1998) found that measures of disability that are designed to detect cognitive factors (e.g., FIM) are often insensitive to cognitive impairments. For example, stroke patients who perform well on the cognitive sections of the FIM may not do well on neuropsychological tests. A brief test that may be useful for screening purposes is the Neurobehavioral Cognitive Status Examination (Osmon et al., 1992). A more complete description of instruments that might be used for screening can be found in (Caplan & Schechter, 1995; Wagner, Nayak, & Fink, 1995).

To permit quantified measures of cognitive disability rather than impairments, functionally based measures of cognitive tasks that are useful for stroke patients have been introduced. The basic idea is to sample an area of cognitive function by using tasks from daily life (e.g., following a series of directions and then recalling the directions, reading a menu) rather than items derived from psychometric tasks with no intrinsic use in daily life. Such tasks are useful to assess visual neglect (Rivermead Behavioral Inattention Test [Wilson, Cockburn, & Halligan, 1987]) and memory (Rivermead Behavioural Memory Test [Wilson, Cockburn, & Baddley, 1989]). Subjective ratings of memory impairment by patients and by relatives are more related to the Rivermead Behavioral Memory Test than to conventional memory tests.

The assessment of emotional state utilizes information from history, clinical interview, and external observers. Methods include symptom checklists and formalized scales. Although formal scales (e.g., Zung [1965]), Beck Depression Inventory, Geriatric Depression Scale [Yesavage et al., 1982]) have been used in epidemiological and community-based studies (Kase, 1987) for clinical purposes they may not be useful. Toedter et al. (1995) found that stroke patients were unreliable reporters of their mood states. Changes in depression may not be detected by formal instruments but reported by observers (Diller, 1992). Biochemical markers such as the dexamethasone suppression test (DST) have yielded questionable results in detecting poststroke depression (Grober et al., 1991).

In the absence of standardized tests, assessment of motivational problems generally is based on history, interview, and clinical observation. Review of medical chart records suggests that motivational problems are the most frequently cited complaint. Whereas a patient whose goals deviate from those of the team might be at risk of poor cooperation, a modest degree of denial expressed as an optimistic outlook is a useful prognostic sign (Powell et al., 1976). Patients typically rate their progress at a higher level than therapists do and attribute their success to factors different from those their therapists cite (Tamerin, 1964). Caregivers typically attribute greater satisfaction to patients than patients do themselves (Heinemann, Cichowski, & Kan, 1997).

TREATMENT

The patient who refuses to go to classes, the patient who is depressed or angry, or the patient who is apathetic may have disturbances in perception, affect, and/or motivation. It is useful to consider a treatment plan that addresses all of the elements. For example, cognitive perceptual remediation is not effective if it is seen as a series of straightforward exercises without taking into account the fact the patient may be unaware of a problem or too upset to participate. Anger may be internally derived, but its management must take into account the staff's response.

Perceptual Cognitive Disorders

Hemi-inattention maybe a simple phenomenon to illustrate. For example, the patient omits drawings on the left side of the page. When one breaks down the responses for treatment purposes, there is a nest of behaviors that can be used as key points in therapy. Typically, one begins to scan the visual environment by starting from the left and directing the gaze to the right. Patients with hemi-inattention will have difficulty in finding a reference point or a starting point to anchor the beginning of a search for the stimulus; once the point is anchored, some patients will respond impulsively and skip important features of their environment; patients have problems in two-dimensional space, such as reading, as in well as three-dimensional space (locating the body in space) and may bump into objects or misreach objects set on a table; patients have difficulty in benefiting from feedback; patients may be unaware of specific difficulties, and out of a fear that they are losing their minds, they may try to cover up problems by denying their existence, or they may misattribute their errors to a memory problem. Each of these points can be incorporated into a strategy that combines arranging tasks with graded degrees of difficulty and relating them to problems in the environment outside the test room. For example, a patient in early stages of rehabilitation with major difficulties in neglect can be given simple bedside exercises: tracking pictures on the wall or squares on the hospital ceiling. Patients may be taught to slow impulsive responses by pacing, for example, pointing to and reciting targets aloud. A therapeutic concern is to maintain awareness of the problem while showing strategies to resolve it and its relevance for important features of daily living.

These points have been translated into specific techniques (Diller & Riley, 1993) in a series of controlled studies. Improvements were noted in academic skills (e.g., reading, written arithmetic, appreciation of space on and off the body, and perceptual organization). While the experimental group maintained the level of gain at 5-months' follow-up after discharge, the controls improved to the same level as the treated group, except for the fact that the treated patients spent more free time in reading (Gordon et al., 1985). In a study comparing the effectiveness of concentrated practice on a narrow range of tasks, a "depth" approach, versus practice over a wide range of tasks, a "broad" approach, both groups performed better than a control group. This suggested that a narrow focus, which involves repetitive practice with the same materials, is more helpful for severely impaired patients, whereas less intense exercise with a broader range of materials is more useful for patients with milder impairments. In addition, exercises to stimulate arousal made the program more effective (Diller, Goodgold, & Kay, 1988).

The basic strategy has also been applied to a patient with a mild neglect, which was presented as a problem in memory and losing track of conversations (Diller & Weinberg, 1986); to patients with severe neglect and underarousal (Diller & Weinberg, 1993); to a patient who had difficulty in recognizing faces (Weinberg & Diller, in press). Strategies have been elaborated to translate or modify the principles for use by a whole team, to be incorporated into ADL training, improving table-reaching behavior (Antonucci et al., 1995), and avoiding obstacles in wheelchair maneuvers (Rapport et al., 1993). In all of these applications, there is recognition of the difficulties in generalizing the effectiveness of the training into functional activities.

Alternative behavioral approaches with somewhat different emphases have been suggested. Three examples illustrate this:

1. Activation of movement on the impaired side of space to increase awareness has been shown to be effective. Thus, activation of the impaired limb yields improvement in personal space (hair combing), locomotor space (circuit walking), and reaching space behavior (placing buns in a tray), although only the gains in reaching space behavior were maintained on follow-up (Robertson, Hogg, & McMillan, 1998). The theory behind this approach is that stimuli from the intact hemisphere overwhelm stimuli from the impaired hemisphere to dampen activation in the impaired hemisphere. Attention to stimuli in the space opposite to the impaired hemisphere is impoverished. Activating the impaired hemisphere by movement of the opposite side of the body will offset the dominance of the intact hemisphere.

2. It might be argued that a major feature of the syndrome is the displacement of the normal body axis, which serves as a referent for egocentric or personal body space. This can easily be demonstrated by touching an RBD patient on the back along the shoulder blades and asking the patient to indicate when the "backbone," or midpoint, is reached. RBD patients displace the midline to the right, while LBD patients and normal subjects are accurate in locating the midline. Wiart et al. (1998) have been able to train patients to improve in definition of egocentric space by using trunk rotation to track a target.

3. Transcutaneous electrical stimulation on the impaired side of space may modulate higher cortical representations of space via the sensory systems (Vallar, Rusconi, & Bernardini, 1996).

Results of these studies indicate that psychologists can play a useful role with regard to the perceptual problems presented by RBD patients either by direct intervention programs or by serving as consultants to occupational and physical therapists.

Management of Emotional Problems

As with emotional problems in individuals who have not suffered a stroke, both psychopharmaceutical and psychotherapeutic methods are used. The pharmaceutical approach uses antidepression medication (e.g., nortriptyline (Lipsey, Robinson, Pearlson, Rao, & Price, 1984) or psychostimulants (e.g., methylphenidate). There are few controlled studies, with small numbers of patients, so results must be interpreted cautiously. Electroconvulsive therapy also has been used, but despite some reports of favorable outcomes, there are noticeable side effects in a significant number of cases; it should be considered only as a last resort (Gordon & Hibbard, 1997). A complication with all of the biological approaches can be a patient's unwillingness to consent to the treatments. In addition, pharmaceutical approaches require sophistication in managing polypharmacological reactions.

With regard to the psychotherapeutic treatment of depression in stroke, a variety of therapies are available. Perhaps the most common is supportive therapy. Psychodynamic (Langer, 1992) and cognitive behavioral approaches are clinically useful (Hibbard, 1990). Some modifications have to be made to take into account language and perceptual problems (Langer, 1992). Psychotherapists also must take into account cognitive limitations resulting from brain damage. In addition to limitations in processing information, there is a possibility of the patient's perseverating affective states as well as ideas and language. Thus, in response to the question "Why are you crying?" the patient responded, "Because my sister died two years ago."

There is only one formal clinical trial on the efficacy of psychotherapy up to this point. When depressed stroke patients were placed into groups that offered differing combinations of psychotherapeutic and pharmacological therapy and a no-therapy control, 74% of psychotherapy patients showed an elevation in mood, whereas only 36% of controls showed an elevation (Gordon, 1992). While results did not differ by hemispheric locus, patients with different-sided hemispheric lesions showed different correlates with improvement. One of the by-product findings was the refusal of patients to enlist in a psychopharmacological study. There are useful clinical case descriptions of psychodynamic (Langer, 1992; Langer & Padrone, 1992) as well as cognitive behavioral approaches (Hibbard et al., 1990).

In a novel approach, a paraprofessional coach, working under supervision, combined methods of perceptual remediation and applications of solution-focused therapy to family systems (DeShazer, 1988). An experimental group ($n = 10$) of outpatient hemiparetic patients, when compared with a control group ($n = 12$), showed an increase in instrumental ADLs (dressing/bathing), increased out-of-home visits, better caregiver mood, less report of worsening mood, and increased time in reading. The approach is promising because it is a service that can be delivered at home by a graduate student working under close supervision (Diller, 1992).

Group therapy approaches are useful, with modifications that take cognitive limitations into account. A variant is the psychoeducational group, where information is presented in a psychotherapeutic context. In inpatient settings the logistics can pose a problem because of the wide range of impairments and shortened lengths of stay. Sherr and Langenbahn (1992) describe an outpatient program emphasizing group approaches. They have developed a hierarchic model for teaching problem solving that provides a methodology for dealing with cognitive as well as emotional factors before training in logical thinking.

VOCATIONAL REHABILITATION

Although stroke is usually associated with old age, it has been estimated that 30% of strokes occur in people under 65. In a sample of more than 400 cases of hemiplegia due to stroke, where subjects engaged in inpatient rehabilitation over a 1-year period, 10% were between the ages of 45 and 54 (Diller, 1992). Thus, many of the survivors of stroke are of working age. Unfortunately, the public at large, physicians, families, and even professionals who work with patients have little hope for the patients' successful return to work. The stigma associated with stroke carries over to those who lose confidence in their abilities and give up hope. The estimates of return to work vary widely; however, in the largest follow-up study of patients aged 21–65 years, Black-Schaffer and Osberg (1990) found that, of 79 patients who were working at the time of stroke, 49% had returned to work 6 months after rehabilitation. The mean time to return to work was 3.1 months. Ninety percent returned to their old jobs, but only 23% were working the same number of hours. Other follow-up studies report lower figures (Zuger & Boehm, 1993).

It is apparent that physical factors play a role. The presence of aphasia adds complications in vocational planning; even those with aphasia who return to work take much longer (Weissberg, Esibell, & Zuger, 1971). Socioeconomic and family support play important parts. As might be expected, individuals with more education and greater prestroke job skills are more successful. Individuals without families and members of minority groups are less likely to return to work. Support from families and employers is very important. Clinically, the problem of too much support becomes an issue. The popular notion that stroke maybe caused by stress contributes to this idea (Zuger & Boehm, 1993).

It is important to have a proper vocational evaluation and access to a full range of vocational services, including a rehabilitation counselor, proper work sampling methods, counseling, and supportive employment, wherein support is rendered by a job coach who conducts in situ evaluations with action plans for all parties relevant to the employment process. All of these activities should occur only after a careful analysis of the patient's premorbid life style (Zuger & Boehm, 1993). In general, vocational rehabilitation must be rendered on a case-by-case basis.

CONCLUSIONS

The patient who has suffered a stroke usually is referred to rehabilitation with a primary presenting problem of hemiparesis or hemiplegia. However, because hemiplegia is associated with brain damage, this problem is often part of a larger symptom complex that involves sensory, linguistic, cognitive, and emotional factors. We have focused on the cognitive and emotional factors because they may interfere with the maximum utilization of rehabilitation and return to the normal role expectations. Psychologists have developed methods of assessment and treatment that can play an important role in rehabilitation.

REFERENCES

Antonucci, G., Guariglia, C., Judica, A., Magnotti, L., Paolucci, S., Pizzamiglio, L., & Zuccolotti, P. (1995). Effectiveness of neglect rehabilitation in a randomized group study. *Journal of Clinical Experimental Neuropsychology, 9,* 383–389.

Ben Yishay, Y., Gerstman, L. J., Diller, L., & Haas, A. (1970). Prediction of rehabilitation outcomes from psychometric parameter in left hemiplegia. *Journal of Consulting and Clinical Psychology, 34,* 36–41.

Ben Yishay, Y., Gerstman, L. J., Diller, L., & Haas, A. (1968). The relationship between impersistence, intellectual function, and outcome of rehabilitation in patients with left hemiplegia. *Neurology, 18,* 852–861.

Ben Yishay, Y. B., Diller, L., Mandleberg, I., Gordon, W. A., & Gerstman, L. J. (1974). Differences in matching persistence behavior during block design performance between older normal and brain damaged persons. *Cortex, 6.*

Black-Schaffer, R. M., & Osberg, J. S. (1990). Return to work after stroke: Development of a predictive model. *Archives of Physical Medicine and Rehabilitation, 71,* 285–290.

Caplan, B., & Schecter, J. (1995). The role of nonstandard neuropsychological assessment in rehabilitation: History, rationale, and examples. In L. A. Cushman & M. J. Sherer (Eds.), *Psychological assessment in medical rehabilitation.* Washington, DC:American Psychological Association.

Cushman, L. A. (1988). Secondary neuropsychiatric complications in stroke: Implications for acute care. *Archives of Physical Medicine and Rehabilitation, 69,* 877–879.

Denes, G., Semenza, C., Stoppa, E., & Lis, A. (1982). Unilateral spatial neglect and recovery from hemiplegia: A follow up study. *Brain, 105,* 543–552.

DeShazer, S. (1988). *Clues: Investigating solutions in brief therapy.* New York: W. W. Norton.

Diller, L., Goodgold, J., & Kay, T. (1988). *Final report to NIDRR–Research and Training Center*. New York: New York University Medical Center, Department of Rehabilitation Medicine.

Diller, L. (1992). *Psychological and social adjustment after stroke: Final report to NIDRR*. New York: New York University, Department of Rehabilitation Medicine.

Diller, L., Buxbaum, J., & Chiotelis, S. (1972). Relearning motor skills in hemiplegia: Error analysis. *Genetic Psychology Monographs, 85*, 249–286.

Diller, L., Goodgold, J. G., & Kay, T. (1988). *Rehabilitation of traumatic brain injury and stroke; final report*. Research & Training Center, Department of Rehabilitation Medicine, NYU School of Medicine. Washington, DC: NIDRR.

Diller, L., & Weinberg, J. (1970). Evidence for accident prone behavior in hemiplegic patients. *Archives of Physical Medicine and Rehabilitation, 51*, 358.

Diller, L., & Weinberg, J. (1985). Learning from failures in perceptual cognitive retraining in stroke. In B. Uzzell & Y. Gross (Eds.), *Clinical neuropsychology of intervention* (pp. 283–293). Boston: Martinus Nijhoff.

Diller, L., & Weinberg, J. (1993). Styles of response in perceptual retraining. In W. A. Gordon (Ed.), *Advances in stroke rehabilitation* (pp. 162–182). Andover, MA: Andover Medical Publishers.

Diller, L., & Riley, E. (1993). The behavioral management of neglect. In I. H. Robertson & J. C. Marshall (Eds.), *Unilateral neglect: Clinical and experimental studies*. Hove, UK: Erlbaum.

Dombovy, M. L. (1993). Rehabilitation and the course of recovery after stroke. In J. P. Wishnant (Ed.), *Stroke: Populations, cohorts, clinical trials*. Oxford, Boston: Butterworth-Heineman.

Egelko, S., Simon, D., Riley, E., Gordon, W., Ruckdeschel-Hibbard, & Diller, L. (1989). First year after stroke: Tracking cognitive and affective deficits. *Archives of Physical Medicine and Rehabilitation, 70*, 297–302.

Fisk, G. D., Owsley, C., & Pulley, L. V. (1997). Driving after stroke: Driving exposure, advice, evaluations. *Archives of Physical Medicine and Rehabilitation, 78*, 1338–1346.

Galski, T., Bruno, R. L., Zorowitz, R., & Walker, J. (1993). Predicting length of stay, functional outcome, and aftercare in the rehabilitation of stroke patients: The dominant role of higher cognition. *Stroke, 24*, 1794–2000.

Gordon, W. A. (1992). *The treatment of affective deficits in stroke population: Final report*. Unpublished manuscript. New York: Mt. Sinai School of Medicine, Department of Medical Rehabilitation.

Gordon, W. A., & Hibbard, M. R. (1997). Poststroke depression: An examination of the literature. *Archives of Physical Medicine and Rehabilitation, 78*, 658–663.

Gordon, W. A, Hibbard, M. R., Egelko, S., Diller, L., Shaver, M. S., Lieberman, A. L., & Ragnarsson, K. T. (1985). Perceptual remediation in patients with right brain damage: A comprehension program. *Archives of Physical Medicine and Rehabilitation, 66*, 353–364.

Gordon, W. A., Hibbard, M. R., Egelko, S., Riley, E., Simon, D., Diller, L., Ross, E. D., & Lieberman, A. (1991). Issues in the diagnosis of post-stroke depression. *Rehabilitation Psychology, 36*, 71–88.

Granger, C. V. (1998). The emerging science of functional assessment: Our tool for outcome analysis. *Archives of Physical Medicine and Rehabilitation, 79*, 235–242.

Gresham, G. E., Duncan, P. W., Stason, W. B., et al. (1995). *Post stroke rehabilitation* (Clinical Practice Guideline No. 16). Rockville, MD: Agency for Health Care Policy and Research, USPHS.

Grober, S. E., Gordon, W. A., Silwinski, M., Hibbard, M. R., Aletta, E. G., & Paddison, P. L. (1991). Utility of the Dexamethasone Test in the diagnosis of poststroke depression. *Archives of Physical Medicine and Rehabilitation, 72*, 1076–1079.

Hajek, V. E., Gagnon, S., & Ruderman, J. A. (1997). Cognitive and functional assessments of stroke patients: An analysis of their relation. *Archives of Physical Medicine and Rehabilitation, 78*, 1327–1331.

Heinemann, A. W., Cichowski, K., & Kan, E. (1997). Mapping differences in patient satisfaction. *Archives of Physical Medicine and Rehabilitation, 78,* 900.

Hibbard, M. R., Gordon, W. A., Stein, P., Grober, S., & Sliwinski, M. (1992). Awareness of disability in patients following stroke. *Rehabilitation Psychology, 37*, 103–119.

Hibbard, M. R., Grober, S. E., Gordon, W. A., Aletta, E. A., & Freeman, A. (1990). Cognitive therapy and the treatment of poststroke depression. *Topics in Geriatric Rehabilitation, 5,* 43–55.

Hier, D. B., Mondlock, J., & Caplan, L. (1983). Behavioral abnormalities after right hemisphere stroke. *Neurology, 33*, 337–344.

Hyman, D. M. (1971). The stigma of stroke. *Geriatrics*, 132–141.

Kase, C., Wolf, P. A., Kelly Hayes, M., Kannel, W. B., Bachman, D. L., & Linn, R. T. (1987). Intellectual decline following stroke: The Framingham study. *Neurology, 37*(Suppl. 1), 119.

Kinsella, G., & Ford, B. (1980). Acute recovery patterns in stroke patients. *Medical Journal of Australia, 2,* 663–666.

Langer, K. G. (1992). Psychotherapy with the neurologically impaired adult. *American Journal of Psychotherapy, 46.*

Langer, K. G., & Padrone, F. J. (1992). Psychotherapeutic treatment of awareness in acute rehabilitation in traumatic brain injury. *Neuropsychology Rehabilitation, 2*, 59–71.

Lipsey, R., Robinson, R. G., Pearlson, G. D., Rao, K., & Price, T. (1984). Nortriptyline treatment of post stroke depression: A double blind study. *Lancet, 11*, 297–300.

Monga, T. M. et al. (1997). Sexuality post stroke. *Physical medicine and rehabilitation. State of the art reviews*. Philadelphia: Hanley & Belfus.

Monga, T. N., Lawson, J. S., & Inglis, J. (1986). Sexual dysfunction in stroke patients. *Archives of Physical Medicine and Rehabilitation, 67*, 19–22.

Morris, P. L. P., Robinson, R. G., Andrzejwski, P., Samuels, J., & Price, T. R. (1993). Association of depression with 10-year mortality in stroke. *American Journal of Psychiatry, 150*, 124–129.

Osmon, D. C., Smet, I. C., Winegarden, B., & Ghandavadi, B. (1992). Neurobehavioral Cognitive Status Examination: Its use with unilateral stroke patients in a rehabilitation setting. *Archives of Physical Medicine and Rehabilitation, 73*, 414–418.

Padrone, F. (1995). *Review of inpatient psychological services at the Rusk Institute of Rehabilitation Medicine*. Unpublished manuscript, NYU Medical Center, Rusk Institute of Rehabilitation Medicine.

Parikh, R. M., Robinson, R. G., Lipsey, J. R., Starkstein, S. E., Federoff, J. P., & Price, T. E. (1990). The impact of post stroke depression on recovery of activities of daily living over a two year follow-up. *Archives of Neurology*, *47*, 785–790.

Powell, B., Diller, L., & Grynbaum, B. (1976). Rehabilitation performance and adjustment in stroke patients: A study of social class factors. *Genetic Psychology Monographs*, *93*, 287–352.

Prigitano, G. P., & Wong, J. L. (1997). Speed of finger tapping and goal attainment after unilateral cerebral accident. *Archives of Physical Medicine and Rehabilitation*, *78*, 847–852.

Robertson, I. H., Hogg, K., & McMillan, T. M. (1998). Rehabilitation of unilateral neglect: Improving function by contralateral limb activation. *Neuropsychological Rehabilitation*, *8*, 19–30.

Robinson, R. G., Bolduc, G. A., & Kubos, K. L. (1985). Social functioning assessment in stroke patients *Archives of Physical Medicine and Rehabilitation*, *66*, 498–500.

Roth, E. J., Heinemann, A. W., Lovell, L., Harvey, R. L., Mcguir, J. R., & Diaz, S. (1998). Impairment and disability: Their relation during stroke rehabilitation. *Archives of Physical Medicine and Rehabilitation*, *79*, 329–341.

Schenkenberg, T., Bradford, D. C., & Ajax, E. T. (1980). Line bisection and unilateral visual neglect in patients with visual impairment. *Neurology*, *30*, 509–517.

Schubert, D. S., Burns, R., Paras, W., & Sioson, E. (1992a). Decrease of depression during stroke and amputation rehabilitation. *General Hospital Psychiatry*, *14*, 135–141.

Schubert, D. S., Burns, R., Paras, W., & Sioson, E. (1992b). Increase of medical hospital length of stay by depression in stroke and amputation patients; a pilot study. *Psychotherapeutics and Psychosomatics*, *52*, 61–66.

Schubert, D. S., Taylor, C., Lee, S., Mentari, A., & Tamaklo, W. (1992c). Physical consequences of depression in the stroke patient. *General Hospital Psychiatry*, *14*, 69–76.

Schubert, D. S., Taylor, C., Lee, S., Mentari, A., & Tamaklo, W. (1992d). Detection of depression in the stroke patient. *Psychosomatics*, *33*, 290–294.

Sherr, R. L., & Langenbahn, D. M. (1992). An approach to a large scale outpatient neuropsychological rehabilitation. *Neuropsychology*, *6*, 417–426.

Starkstein, S. E., & Robinson, R. G. (1990). Neuropsychiatric aspects of stroke. In Coffey & J. L. Cummings (Eds.), *Textbook of geriatric psychiatry*. Washington, DC: American Psychiatric Press.

Stone, S. P., Wilson, B., Wroot, A., Halligan, P. W., Lange, S. L., Marshal, J. C., & Greenwood, R. J. (1991). The assessment of visual spatial neglect after acute stroke. *Journal of Neurology, Neurosurgery, and Psychiatry*, *54*, 345–350.

Tamerin, J. S. (1964). The perception of progress in rehabilitation. *Archives of Physical Medicine and Rehabilitation, 45,* 17–22.

Toedter, L. J., Schall, R., Reese, C. A. S., Hyland, D. T., Berk, S. N., & Dunn, D. S. (1995). Psychological measures: Reliability in the assessment of stroke patients. *Archives of Physical Medicine and Rehabilitation*, *76*, 719–725.

Thompson, S. C. (1991). The search for meaning following stroke. *Basic and Applied Social Psychology, 12,* 81–86.

Titus, M. N., Gall, N. G., Yerxa, E. J., Robertson, T. A., & Mack, W. (1991). Correlation of perceptual performance and activities of daily living in stroke patients. *American Journal of Occupational Therapy*, *45*, 510–518.

Vallar, G., Rusconi, M. L., & Bernardini, B. (1996). Modulation of neglect hemianesthesia by transcutaneous electrical stimulation. *Journal of the International Neuropsychology Society*, *2*, 452–459.

Wade, D. T., Parker, V., & Langton-Hewer, R. L. (1986). Memory losses after stroke: Frequency and associated losses. *International Rehabilitation Medicine*, *8*, 68–74.

Wade, D. T., & Hewer, R. L. (1987). Functional activities abilities stroke: Measurement, natural history, and prognosis. *Journal of Neurology, Neurosurgery, and Psychiatry*, *50*, 177–182.

Wagner, M. T., Nayak, M., & Fink, C. (1995). Bedside screening of neurocognitive function. In L. A. Cushman & M. J. Scherer (Eds.), *Psychological assessment in medical rehabilitation*. Washington, DC: American Psychological Association.

Warren, M. (1990). Identification of visual scanning deficits in adults after cerebrovascular accidents. *American Journal of Occupational Therapy*, *44*, 391–399.

Webster, J. S., Roades, L. A., Morrill, B., Rapport, L. J., Abadee, P. S., Sowa, M. V., Dutra, R., & Godlewski, C. (1995). Rightward orienting bias, wheelchair maneuvering, and fall risk. *Archives of Physical Medicine and Rehabilitation*, *76*, 924–928.

Webster, J. S., Jones, S., Blanton, P., Gross, R., Beissel, G., & Wofford, J. (1984). Visual training with stroke patients. *Behavior Therapy, 15*, 129–143.

Weinberg, J., & Diller, L. (1966). Denial of a reading disability. *American Psychology*, *74*.

Weinberg, J., & Diller, L. (1968). On reading newspapers by hemiplegics: Denial of visual disability. In *Proceedings of the 76th Annual Convention* (pp. 655–656). Washington, DC: American Psychiatric Association.

Weinberg, J., & Diller, L. (in press). Dealing with rationalization and unawareness in the treatment of visual inattention. In K. E. Langer, L. Laatsch, & L. Lewis (Eds.), *Psychotherapy in individuals with acquired brain injury*. New Haven, CT: International Universities Press.

Weinberg, J., Diller, L., Gordon, W. A., Gerstman, L. G., Lieberman, A., Lakin, P., Hodges, G., & Ezrachi, O. (1977). Visual scanning training effect on reading related tasks in acquired right brain damage. *Archives of Physical Medicine and Rehabilitation*, *58*, 479–487.

Weinberg, J., Diller, L., Gordon, W. A., Gerstman, L., Lieberman, A., Lakin, P., Hodges, G., & Ezrachi, O. (1979). Training sensory awareness and spatial organization in people with right brain damage. *Archives of Physical Medicine and Rehabilitation*, *60*, 491–496.

Weissberg, S., Esibell, N., & Zuger, R. R. (1971). Factors in the vocational success of hemiplegic patients. *Archives of Physical Medicine and Rehabilitation*, *52*, 441–447.

Wiart, L., Saint Come, A. B., Debelleix, X., Petit, H., Joseph, P. A., Mazaux, J. M., & Barat, M. (1997). Unilateral neglect syndrome rehabilitation by trunk rotation and scanning training. *Archives of Physical Medicine and Rehabilitation*, *78*, 424–436.

Wiebe-Valesquez, S., & Hachinski, V. (1991). Overview of clinical issues in stroke. In R. A. Bornstein & G. Brown (Eds.), *Neurobehavioral aspects of cerebrovascular disease* (pp. 111–130). New York, Oxford: Oxford University Press.

Wilson, B. A., Cockburn, J., & Halligan, P. (1987). *The Rivermead Behavioural Inattention Test*. Gaylord, MI: National Rehabilitation Service.

Wilson, B. A., Cockburn, J., & Baddley, A. (1989). *The Rivermead Behavioural Memory Test*. Gaylord, MI: National Rehabilitation Service.

Yesavage, J. A., Brink, T. L., Rose, T. L., Lum, O., Huang, V., & Adair, M. (1982). Development and validation of a geriatric rating scale: A preliminary report. *Journal of Psychiatric Research*, *17*, 37–49.

Zoccolotti, P., & Judica, A. (1991). Functional evaluation of hemineglect by means of a semistructures scale: Personal extrapersonal differentiation. *Neuropsychology Rehabilitation*, *1*, 29–44.

Zuger, R. R., & Boehm, M. (1993). Stroke: A new challenge for vocational rehabilitation. In W. A. Gordon (Ed.), *Advances in stroke rehabilitation*. Boston, New York: Andover Medical Publishers.

Zung, W. K. (1965). A self-rating scale of depression. *Archives of General Psychiatry*, *12*, 63–70.

Chapter 26

Substance Use Disorders

Constance Corley Saltz, Marcia Lawton, and Muriel Gray

The abuse of and dependence on recreational, medicinal, and otherwise harmful substances has been noted historically for centuries, accompanied by a wide range of explanations of causality. Although a discussion of etiology is beyond the scope of this chapter, awareness of the impact of harmful substances on persons presenting in health care settings (whether due to the consequences of one episode of using crack or a long-term addiction to tobacco) is essential for practitioners. The thrust of this chapter is to help those in a gatekeeper role to identify addiction and to know how to refer the client to an appropriate component of the continuum of care.

The chapter begins with an overview of the prevalence, cost, and consequences of chemical abuse and dependency, with a brief presentation of definitions and terminology. The chapter then focuses on addiction, using the substance of alcohol to explore the addiction process, screening, intervention, treatment, and recovery. Relevant considerations pertaining to several other major addictions (especially cocaine and nicotine) are addressed. Implications for treatment on both the practice and policy levels are discussed in the concluding section of the chapter.

PREVALENCE

The most recent national survey on drug abuse (Substance Abuse and Mental Health Services Administration [SAMHSA], 1996) found that overall drug use has leveled off since 1995. However, a substantial number of persons in the United States continue to abuse one or more of the following substances: alcohol, tobacco, marijuana, cocaine/crack, heroin, hallucinogens, inhalants, and psychotherapeutic drugs used for nonmedical purposes (e.g., sedatives, tranquilizers, stimulants, analgesics, and anabolic steroids).

According to the National Household Survey on Drug Abuse (SAMHSA, 1996), legal drugs are the most used and abused. Although per capita alcohol consumption has declined, alcohol continues to be the most commonly used and abused substance. It is used by approximately 51% of the U.S. population age 12 and older. Of those users, about 16% engaged in binge drinking, and 5.4% were heavy drinkers. An estimated 7% of adults have an alcohol use disorder (either abuse or dependence), and 45% of the traffic crash deaths in the United States are attributed to alcohol consumption (National Institute on Alcohol Abuse and Alcoholism [NIAAA], 1997). Alcohol in combination with other drugs was mentioned in 39% of deaths reported in medical examiner cases (SAMHSA, 1995). The prevalence of substance use disorders in general and alcohol use disorders in particular is difficult to determine. Data gathered from the National Hospital Discharge Surveys concluded that hospital discharge records may underrepresent the extent of disorders related to alcohol use. It found that, whereas 7.4% of hospital patients had an alcohol-related diagnosis, when screened specifically for alcohol problems, 22% screened positive (NIAAA, 1997). Substance use disorders also lead to myriad social, legal, and job-related problems.

Tobacco, like alcohol, is a highly addictive legal substance. It is used regularly by 29% of the U.S. population age 12 and older. According to the Monitoring the Future study (National Institute on Drug Abuse [NIDA], 1996), tobacco use was slightly down for adults, whereas use among adolescents increased.

Approximately 6% of the U.S. population 12 years of age and older reported current use of an illicit substance in the 1996 National Household Survey on Drug Abuse (NIDA, 1997). Marijuana is the most commonly used illicit substance. Of current illicit drug users, 77% reported marijuana use (SAMHSA, 1997). The director's report to the National Advisory Council on Drug Abuse (NIDA, 1997) reports a resurgence in marijuana use among adolescent emergency department mentions, treatment admissions, and arrests. The rate of marijuana initiation is at the highest level ever among U.S. youth between the ages of 12 and 17 (SAMHSA, 1997). Along with tobacco and alcohol, marijuana is considered to be a "gateway" substance to other drug use (NIDA, 1991).

The proportion of the population age 12 and older who are current cocaine users remains stable at approximately 0.8% (SAMHSA, 1997). However, cocaine was the most frequently reported substance in drug abuse deaths. According to data from the Drug Abuse Warning Network (SAMHSA, 1997), it was reported in 46% of drug-related deaths.

According to 1995 medical examiner data, heroin is the second most often mentioned substance in drug abuse deaths (SAMHSA, 1997). Preliminary results from the 1996 National Household Survey on Drug Abuse report decreasing overall heroin use but an increased number of new users between the ages of 12 and 17. They also show that most new heroin users are under the age of 26 (SAMHSA, 1997).

Despite the overall leveling of drug use in the United States, the 1996 National Household Survey found that new hallucinogens and inhalant use had increased among youth (ages 12–17) and among young adults (18–25) (SAMHSA, 1997).

CONSEQUENCES AND COSTS

Regular use of harmful drugs (and sometimes even a single incident of use of a drug such as crack) can have major adverse medical, psychological, psychiatric, economic, and social consequences. The medical complications resulting from alcoholism (Kinney & Leaton, 1991) perhaps best illustrate how one widely available substance can affect almost every body system: cardiovascular, gastrointestinal, genitourinary, endocrine, nervous, musculoskeletal, and immune systems. Major nutritional deficits can result from chronic alcoholism, as well as changes in the skin and hair (Kinney & Leaton, 1991). Hematological disorders are more common in alcoholics than in the population at large, and at least 10% of all cancers occur in sites affected by heavy drinking (Kinney & Leaton, 1991).

In terms of psychological/psychiatric consequences of misuse of alcohol and/or most other harmful substances, the following may result: intoxication, craving, depression/mood swings, anxiety, paranoia, hallucinations/delusions, organic brain syndromes (both acute and chronic), and flashbacks (Kinney & Leaton, 1991). Suicide is a major risk among alcoholics: an estimated 7%–21% of alcoholics commit suicide (Kinney & Leaton, 1991).

Although calculating the economic costs of substance abuse and dependence is more difficult than for other illnesses, the costs of alcohol, tobacco, and other drugs are estimated as close to or in excess of $400 billion (Center on Addiction and Substance Abuse [CASA], 1993). Although the primary costs are those of health care expenditures, such figures also take into account lost productivity from employee substance abuse and social losses from premature deaths, substance-induced psychiatric disorders, and family disruption. The impact of substance use disorders on the family will be further discussed below.

DEFINITIONS AND TERMINOLOGY

Several concepts are important in defining and identifying maladaptive effects of harmful substances. These include abuse, dependence, tolerance, withdrawal, and addiction.

Two diagnostic categories that broadly cover chemical misuse are included in the *Diagnostic and Statistical Manual of Mental Disorders* (4th edition; herein referred to as DSM-IV): psychoactive substance abuse and psychoactive substance dependence (American Psychiatric Association [APA], 1995).

CRITERIA FOR SUBSTANCE DEPENDENCE

A maladaptive pattern of substance use, leading to clinically significant impairment or distress, as manifested by three (or more) of the following, occurring at any time in the same 12-month period.

(1) tolerance, as defined by either of the following:

 (a) a need for markedly increased amounts of the substance to achieve intoxication or desired effect
 (b) markedly diminished effect with continued use of the same amount of the substance

(2) withdrawal, as manifested by either of the following:

 (a) the characteristic withdrawal syndrome for the substance (refer to Criteria A and B of the criteria sets for Withdrawal from the specific substances)
 (b) the same (or a closely related) substance is taken to relieve or avoid withdrawal symptoms

(3) the substance is often taken in larger amounts or over a longer period than was intended
(4) there is a persistent desire or unsuccessful efforts to cut down or control substance use
(5) a great deal of time is spent in activities necessary to obtain the substance (e.g., chain-smoking), or recover from its effects
(6) important social, occupational, or recreational activities are given up or reduced because of substance use
(7) the substance use is continued despite knowledge of having a persistent or recurrent physical or psychological problem that is likely to have been caused or exacerbated by the substance (e.g., current cocaine use despite recognition of cocaine-induced depression, or continued drinking despite recognition that an ulcer was made worse by alcohol consumption) (p. 181)

CRITERIA FOR SUBSTANCE ABUSE

A. A maladaptive pattern of substance use leading to clinically significant impairment or distress, as manifested by one (or more) of the following, occurring within a 12-month period:

(1) recurrent substance use resulting in a failure to fulfill major role obligations at work, school, or home (e.g., repeated absences or poor work performance

related to substance use; substance-related absences, suspensions, or expulsions from school; neglect of children or household)

(2) recurrent substance use in situations in which it is physically hazardous (e.g., driving an automobile or operating a machine when impaired by substance use)

(3) recurrent substance-related legal problems (e.g., arrests for substance-related disorderly conduct)

(4) continued substance use despite having persistent or recurrent social or interpersonal problems caused or exacerbated by the effects of the substance (e.g., arguments with spouse about consequences of intoxication, physical fights)

B. The symptoms have never met the criteria for Substance Dependence for this class of substance. (pp. 182–183)

Tolerance occurs with the regular consumption of a substance over an extended period and is one of the defining characteristics of alcohol addiction (Kinney & Leaton, 1995). Withdrawal results in the development of adverse physical symptoms when the use of a substance is stopped (Beasley, 1990).

Addiction, the primary emphasis of this chapter, is a physiological process in which the addicted person craves one or more substances, used the substance(s) compulsively (daily and/or in binges), and continues using the substance(s) despite a range of adverse consequences (Beasley, 1990). Tolerance and withdrawal occur with many forms of addiction (e.g., alcohol). Denial of the addiction itself is usually also a hallmark of addiction.

Given the multifactorial nature of addiction, the following factors must be taken into account during assessment, intervention, treatment, and recovery: biological, psychological, social/economic, and spiritual. This will be referred to as the biopsychosocial-spiritual approach. The process of addiction to alcohol through the steps to recovery is now presented to exemplify this approach.

ALCOHOLISM AS AN EXAMPLE OF ADDICTION

The nature of the addiction process has been most extensively studied and is best understood with alcoholism. Therefore, alcoholism is used here to demonstrate the highlights of the addiction process, screening, recovery, intervention, and treatment.

Addiction Process

Alcoholism has generally been accepted, since the American Medical Association (AMA) declaration in 1956, as a primary, chronic, progressive, fatal, family disease. The most notable aspect of alcoholism (or any addiction) is the development of the denial system. This is not simply a psychological defense used to cope with anxiety but a complex system composed of multiple mechanisms (blaming, minimizing, rationalizing, intellectualization, humor, and others, depending on the individual), which become an unconscious way to protect a lifestyle focused on alcohol. One of the best practical resources on understanding denial, from Hazelden ("Dealing with Denial," 1975), describes it as follows:

> The development of a denial system is a cardinal and integral feature of chemical dependency. It is one of the major symptoms of this disease and develops along with the more visible symptoms, i.e., harmful consequences. To a greater or lesser extent, it can be found in all chemically dependent persons. Denial is the fatal aspect of alcoholism and other drug dependencies. It impairs the judgment of affected individuals, and results in self-delusion which keeps them locked into an increasingly destructive pattern. It is the denial system which, for example, permits a chemically dependent person to ignore a physician's advice of "stop or you will die." (p. 9)

In addition to the denial system, alcoholism is characterized by certain predictable signs and symptoms that manifest themselves as the illness progresses. There are some discrepancies as to what constitutes alcoholism or at what point one crosses the imaginary line. There does appear to be fairly wide acceptance that once a person reaches a stage where there are physical consequences (tremors, liver damage, etc.) and loss of ordinary willpower, alcoholism is in the picture. Other consequences may occur earlier in the process: psychological (e.g., guilt), mental (e.g., preoccupation with alcohol), and spiritual (e.g., moral deterioration) signs; these deserve as much attention as do the physical consequences.

A very important aspect of this chronic illness is relapse; it is later addressed in more detail. What triggers this relapse or resumption of use varies. Gorski (Miller, Gorski, & Miller, 1982) and Marlatt (Marlatt & Gordon, 1985), coming from different philosophical orientations (the former, from a disease orientation, and the latter, from a learned-behavior one), both stress the significance of relapse in addiction. Among the 37 signs of relapse that Gorski lists are several indicating that the addiction is being activated even before the alcoholic resumes drinking: recurrence of the denial system, tendencies toward loneliness, a feeling that nothing can be solved, progressive loss of daily structure, thoughts of social drinking, and unreasonable resentments.

The role of the family in maintaining or returning to addiction to alcohol has been increasingly studied (Wegschneider, 1981). Alcoholism has been described as a hanging mobile: as one member changes, the others have to make adjustments to acquire an equilibrium. Jackson (1954) spells out the seven adjustment stages through which family members go as the alcoholic progresses in his or her disease: attempts to deny the problem, social isolation, disorganization of family structure, efforts to reorganize in spite of the problem, attempts to escape the problem, reorganization of part of the family, and finally, recovery and reorganization of the whole family.

In understanding the significance of the family it is important to address two concepts, enabling and codependency. Enabling is any behavior on the part of anyone that protects the alcoholic's denial system. Codependency is a term full of confusion in the addiction field today. It currently has a variety of meanings, many of which focus on it as an addiction in its own right, whereby the codependent is addicted to having someone else provide emotional support and in fact defines his or her own identity by that relationship. Probably the best and most useful definition of codependency is the following: "Codependency is a pattern of painful dependency upon compulsive behaviors and on approval from others in search for safety, self-worth and identity. Recovery is possible" (Lawson, 1990, p. 1).

Screening for Alcoholism

An overall recommendation is that the practitioner work with an individual to examine at a conscious level the client's relationship with alcohol. If the client is comfortable in that relationship and does not let alcohol control behavior and the ability to deal effectively with life stresses and problems, then he or she is probably not an alcoholic. To assist further in the decision about drinking behavior, Alcoholics Anonymous (AA) has prepared a brief pamphlet that includes questions such as (a) do you wish people would mind their own business about your drinking—stop telling you what to do? (b) have you ever switched from one kind of drink to another in hope that this would keep you from getting drunk? (Alcoholics Anonymous, 1973).

As a guideline, if the client answers yes to 4 or more of the 12 questions, then there is probably trouble with alcohol. The counselor can review this material with the client along with information on the progressive signs of alcoholism (e.g., using the chart developed by Glatt in 1957, based on Jellinek's research published in 1954). Additional tools are available in the form of the Trauma Scale (Skinner, Holt, Schuller, Roy, & Israel, 1984), the CAGE (Ewing, 1984), the Michigan Alcoholism Screening Test (MAST) (Seizer, 1971), and formalized interviews such as the Addictions Severity Index (ASI) (McLellan, Luborsky, Woody, & O'Brien, 1980).

The CAGE is composed of four simple questions:

1. Have you ever tried to cut down on your drinking?
2. Do you get annoyed when drinking is criticized?

3. Do you feel guilty about your drinking?
4. Do you use alcohol as an "eye-opener"?

A score of two yes answers constitutes concern. The MAST is a self-report test with 25 items regarding the consequences of problem drinking; a positive answer of 12 or 13 deserves taking some action. The ASI is a structured clinical interview suitable for use with both alcoholic and drug-addicted patients. It can be administered by a technician in about 20 to 30 minutes and provides a problem severity profile reflecting six areas: medical, psychological, legal, family/social, employment/support, and chemical abuse. Each area is measured independently, and the severity is derived from two kinds of information, the client's subjective judgment and objective data (e.g., lab reports).

There are some clinical lab tests available (serum γ-glutamyltransferase and aspartate amniotransferase) that can indicate an alcohol problem, but unfortunately they lack diagnostic specificity and are not positive until later stages of addiction when denial is strongest (NIAAA, 1990). Sometimes particular negative consequences of alcoholism (e.g., citations for driving under the influence) can be indicators of alcoholism; the helpful role these can play in presenting the reality of the illness will be discussed in the intervention section.

Recovery from Alcohol

On the Jellinek chart referred to earlier (Glatt, 1957), recovery is pictured as a mirror-image representation of the addiction process. However, more research, done by Brown (1985) on a dynamic, developmental model of recovery, belies this description. Brown discovered a process whereby the individual undergoes a second-order change regarding the ability to control drinking. The stages are (a) drinking: "I can control my drinking," "I am not an alcoholic"; (b) transition: "I cannot control my drinking," "I am an alcoholic"; (c) early recovery: same as transition but with a beginning awareness of the environment and a slight interpersonal focus; (d) ongoing recovery: same as transition but with increased awareness of environment and relationship between self and others.

Brown (1985) acknowledges the role of AA in accomplishing these changes. Since its inception in 1935, AA has been beneficial to many alcoholics as a support system that recognizes the internal healing that occurs in recovery. This self-help movement emphasizes self-responsibility and surrender to a higher power. The focus is on spirituality, the energy force within each one, rather than on religion, a manmade institution with a set of rules (Lawton, 1991a). This is the spiritual component mentioned in the biopsychosocial-spiritual approach discussed in the introduction and in Kuhn's (1988) article, which provides a spiritual inventory for the medically ill patient. It should be noted that recovery is an internal healing process with its own developmental stages and is distinct from the external treatment given to an individual.

Intervention with the Alcoholic

Because the denial system is the most crucial aspect of addiction, it is essential that it be addressed to stop the cycle and promote recovery. Johnson (1980) found that, by involving significant others (or concerned persons) in the planning part of the intervention and helping break through their denial, there was increased likelihood of reaching the alcoholic. A trained professional teaches the concerned persons about alcoholism as a disease, helps them collect factual data about the consequences of the alcoholic's drinking, and works through the concerned persons' anger and judgmental attitudes through attendance at counseling meetings and Al-Anon support groups. The group then formalizes a concrete plan with clear alternatives, such as "go to treatment" or "accept my having to leave the family."

Following a real crisis (such as arrest for driving under the influence), when the alcoholic's guilt is the highest and defenses are the weakest, the group meets with the alcoholic and presents the prepared choices. When done in a factual, nonjudgmental, caring manner that taps into the core being of the alcoholic, it is most likely to achieve changes.

Treatment for Alcoholism

Since its inception in 1948, the Minnesota Model (developed at Hazelden by Dan Anderson) has gained widespread recognition as the treatment of choice for the alcoholic and family. It focuses on the holistic nature of alcoholism and is best described as having the following components:

1. Philosophy of treatment: assumption that alcoholism/chemical dependency exists; it's a multiphasic illness; focus on the phenomenon of addiction as the major presenting problem; denial is part of the illness.
2. Goals of treatment: improved mental and physical health achieved through total abstinence.
3. Content of treatment: help people take better care of themselves by understanding chemical dependency as well as the strategies that will help maintain sobriety.
4. Quality of interdisciplinary staff: trained people who meet professional standards to address the physical, social, family, spiritual, and psychologi-

cal areas; important that recovering chemically dependent people are part of the staff.

5. Duration of treatment: length of stay based on the average time it takes a typical patient to complete primary care; treatment duration must remain individualized.
6. Intensity of treatment: living in a therapeutic community that includes lectures, group meetings, individual meetings with professionals as needed, aftercare planning.
7. Context of treatment: atmosphere conducive to self-evaluation; environment in which people are treated with dignity and respect by staff who are caring and concerned—a caring community.
8. Quality assurance measures: process and outcome quality measurements (Engelman, 1989).

Although the Minnesota Model focuses on a therapeutic community to provide services, earlier detection of alcoholism and limited insurance coverage for treatment have led to a broader and more varied choice of options, with emphasis on utilizing outpatient services initially if not exclusively in some instances. A diagram of the current continuum of care in the addiction field is depicted in Figure 26.1.

Although this picture appears somewhat confusing to the uninitiated, efforts are under way to help clarify placement criteria. In particular, the American Society of Addictive Medicine (ASAM) and the National Association of Alcohol Treatment Programs (NAATP) cooperated in developing a set of guidelines that has been well accepted by the field (Lawson, 1991b). Four different levels of care are highlighted: outpatient, outpatient with partial hospitalization, medically monitored intensive inpatient, and medically managed intensive inpatient. The assignments are not limited to "medical necessity" but include biopsychosocial considerations.

SPECIAL CONSIDERATIONS WITH OTHER ADDICTIONS

Cocaine

Although cocaine is a stimulant rather than a depressant, the cocaine addict (like the alcoholic) nevertheless manifests the characteristics common to addiction, such as the denial system, preoccupation, and loss of control. "Coke" addiction has its own distinctive signs and symptoms (e.g., weight loss, chronic runny nose, frequent upper respiratory infections, loss of interests, auditory hallucinations, and

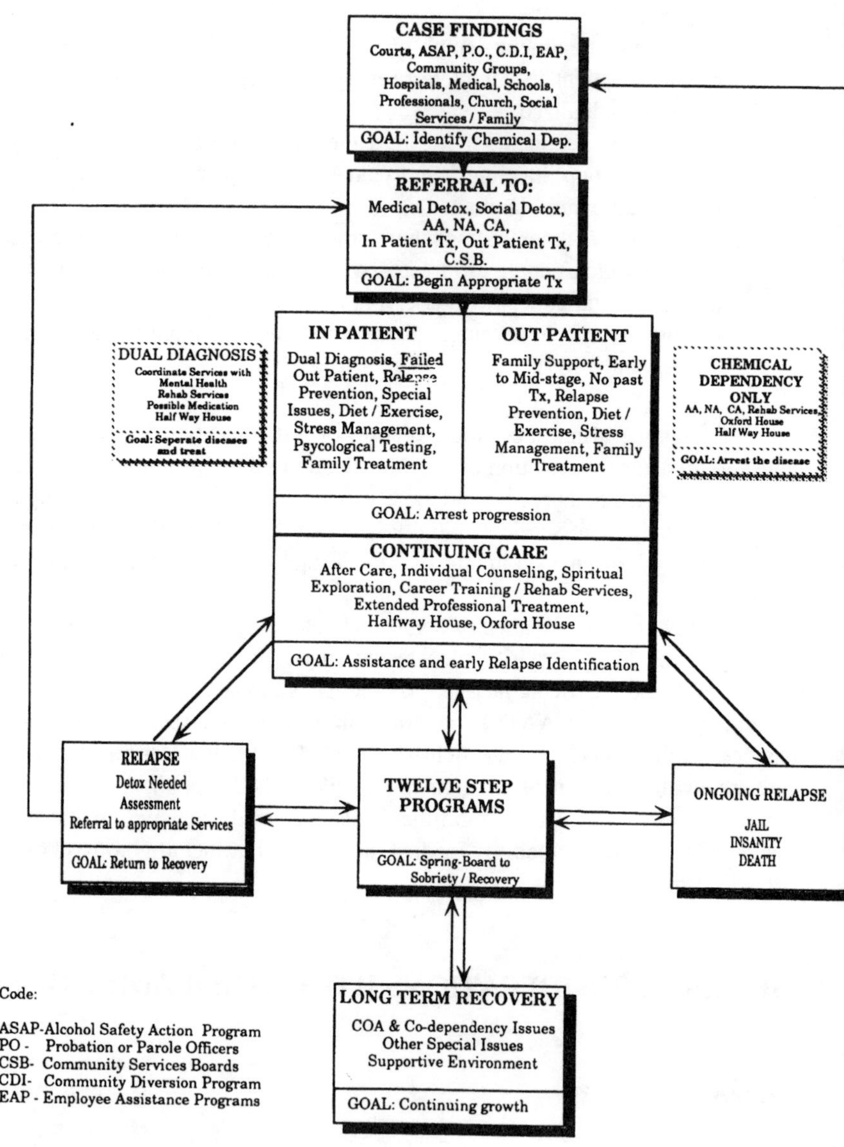

FIGURE 26.1 Current continuum of care.

repetitious compulsive acts such as tapping fingers or playing with hair). They occur in a sequence of three phases: crash, withdrawal, and extinction.

The fatal nature of cocaine may more likely be played out in heart failure rather than in liver or pancreatic diseases as seen in alcoholism (Nuckols, 1989). One substantial difference encountered in cocaine addiction is the problem of intense cravings, which serve to perpetuate the use of cocaine. This appears to be the result of the vivid euphoric memories associated with cocaine binges. Also, with cocaine addiction there is the issue of illegality, which can intensify the isolation because of the perceived need to keep the use secret for fear of the legal consequences. Finally, a further complication resulting from cocaine addiction is the situation in which intravenous needles are used, leading to an increased possibility of acquired immune deficiency syndrome (AIDS).

In treating cocaine addiction it appears that simply using the standard addiction approach of breaking denial is not sufficient. Additionally, pharmacological nonaddictive antidepressants (e.g., imipramine) are being tried, along with psychotherapeutic treatment focusing on the systematic desensitization of addicts to craving-loaded cues like razor blades or syringes (Gawin, 1990).

Nicotine

Although nicotine follows the benchmarks for addiction in its own right, it is mentioned here because of another interesting aspect: it can be a gateway and/or trigger to another addiction, especially alcohol. Evidence is mounting to suggest that it plays a part in preventing quality sobriety or in fact even abstinence from other substances. Treatment is increasingly moving away from dealing with one addiction at a time and including trigger addictions as part of the initial treatment. For example, hospital units use decaffeinated coffee and have "no smoking" rules (Henningfield, Clayton, & Pollin, 1990; Pletcher, Lysaght, & Human, 1990).

Other Addictions

So far, except for codependency, which appears to be in a class of its own, the discussion has been on drug addictions (primarily alcohol, cocaine, and nicotine). It is also possible to demonstrate the same major characteristics of addiction (denial system, loss of control, preoccupation, and moral deterioration) with other compulsive behaviors, such as overeating and gambling. It is not within the scope of this chapter to address the many details associated with a specific addiction. Two general resources that cover the substance addictions in more depth are *Concepts of Chemical Dependency* (Doweiko, 1996) and *Visions of Addiction* (Peele, 1988).

Misuse and abuse of prescription and over-the-counter medications also is receiving increased attention. Older persons "are at particularly high risk for addiction due to their more frequent use of medications to treat a variety of acute and chronic medical conditions, to economic stability for the majority, and to a high prevalence of depression and anxiety disorders" (Lowinson, Ruiz, Millman, & Langrod, 1992, p. 849). Polyaddiction among older persons may be masked by the greater prevalence of multiple medical conditions.

RELAPSE PREVENTION

Regardless of the substance, primary intensive treatment alone is not sufficient for these disorders. Relapse prevention as a biopsychosocial strategy to maintain abstinence and a healthy lifestyle is critical (Gray, 1993).

Although relapse prevention is individualized to address client needs, most such treatment plans include social support approaches, lifestyle change approaches, cognitive-behavioral approaches and pharmacological approaches (USDHHS, 1995; Wormer, 1995).

Research studies (NIAAA, 1997) cite that the availability of social resources following primary intensive inpatient treatment increased the rate of abstinence among patients. Social resources may include psychosocial therapy, relationship enhancement, aftercare groups, family networks, and many types of support groups. The most prevalent type of support groups associated with abstinence from substance use and the prevention of relapse are 12-step programs such as AA and Narcotics Anonymous. Rational Recovery, a support group using a cognitive approach based on rational-emotive therapy is a relatively new support group, offering an alternative to the spirituality-based 12-step programs. Other support groups, like Women for Sobriety, are population-specific; and still other approaches (e.g., One Church One Addict) are religion- and church-based.

Approaches addressing lifestyle changes focus on breaking ties with drug users and teaching ways of coping with negative behaviors while acquiring a new social identity as a non-substance-user. Many of these approaches utilize a cognitive-behavioral approach to teach self-efficacy and avoidance skills, using such instruments as Situational Confidence Questionnaire (Annis & Graham, 1988) and workbooks such as the *Staying Sober Workbook* (Gorski, 1989) to identify warning signs and internal and external cues associated with cravings.

According to *Effectiveness of Substance Abuse Treatment* (USDHHS, 1995), many pharmacotherapies are now available for the treatment of substance use disorders and the prevention of relapse. For opiate addiction such drugs as buprenorphine, clonidine, methadone, naltrexone, and LAAM (levo-alpha-acetyl methanol) are approved as opiate-craving blockers. Some of these also have been found effective in the treatment of alcohol use disorders: specifically, disulfiram

(Antabuse), an alcohol-sensitizing agent for avoidance of alcohol consumption, and naltrexone for alcohol craving and opiate addiction. Some antidepressant medication trials have found mixed results in reducing cocaine abuse. The efficacy of these therapies continues to be studied.

IMPLICATIONS

Greater societal awareness of the multidimensional impact of chemical abuse and dependency has led to increased prevention efforts as well as awareness of the need for early recognition and treatment. Health care professionals are in a critical position (as gatekeepers to a range of services and programs) to provide and/or refer those at risk to educational, diagnostic, intervention, and treatment options. Addiction per se must be considered a primary illness in health care settings. If overlooked or inadequately treated, it will continue to take its toll on individuals, their families, and society at large. Identifying and managing triggers (e.g., caffeine and nicotine) for other chemical use and addiction, especially among young persons and those who are compromised by health problems or are otherwise vulnerable because of changes in social status (such as unemployment or homelessness) are essential. Building support for persons at risk may require community-based treatment and referral, with long-term follow-up and services to pertinent family members and significant others. Although they are beyond the scope of this chapter, there are additional considerations in working with persons who abuse or are addicted to multiple substances and in addressing those persons who may also have a psychiatric history. Access to care and follow-up for those with multiple treatment needs is often inadequate and sometimes inappropriately provided.

Addiction, like other chronic disorders, is a lifelong illness requiring a comprehensive approach. Given the rapid and confusing changes in the organization and financing of health care services, treatment for addicted persons and/or their families may be compromised. This is particularly evident with the introduction of managed care and cost-containment approaches intended to control costs in the traditional medical acute-care setting, where treatment is based on medical necessity and physician's orders. These same criteria are not always applicable to the rehabilitation model needed for addiction, a chronic, multidimensional illness for which family support and aftercare services are critical (Spicer, 1991). Managed care will undoubtedly have an impact on the current role of employee assistance programs (EAPs), which serve as an identification/referral arm for industry in the area of chemical abuse and dependency. EAPs could be considered as duplication of, replacement for, and/or supplements to managed care programs. In any event, the trend is toward reduced reimbursement of fewer services, which will profoundly affect access to essential treatment and follow-up for addicted persons and their families.

In spite of the negative aspects of addiction, with its stigma and pervasive prevalence, there is a very positive aspect to be considered. Since the beginning of AA in 1935 there has emerged increasing hope for converting the crisis of addiction into an opportunity to improve the overall quality of one's life. With the advent of the Hughes Act in 1970, the chances to capitalize on these opportunities were enhanced as the stigma was decreased and appropriate resources were developed. Although currently there seems to be a loss of momentum and a shift backward toward an emphasis on controlling drug use through supply and/or punishment, the progress and gains of the past several decades are still available for those who have the motivation and access to services. Using the biopsychosocial–spiritual approach, it is the professional's role to identify the addiction, challenge the denial system of the patient, and work with the patient and his or her family to find the resources necessary for treatment and recovery. With appropriate and adequate care, persons who abuse or are addicted to harmful substances can return to and/or maintain healthy and productive lives.

REFERENCES

Alcoholics Anonymous. (1973). *Is AA enough?* New York: Alcoholics Anonymous World Services.

American Psychiatric Association. (1995). *Diagnostic and statistical manual of mental disorders* (4th ed., rev.). Washington, DC: Author.

Annis, H., & Graham, J. (1988). *Situational Confidence Questionnaire (SCQ-39) user's guide*. Toronto: Addiction Research Foundation.

Beasley, J. (1990). *Diagnosing and managing chemical dependency*. Durant, OK: Essential Medical Information Systems.

Brown, S. (1985). *Treating the alcoholic: A developmental model of recovery*. New York: John Wiley and Sons.

Caring Community Series. (1975). *Dealing with denial*. Center City, MN: Hazelden.

Center on Addiction and Substance Abuse. (1993). *The cost of substance abuse to America's health care system: Report 1. Medicaid hospital costs*. New York: Columbia University Press.

Doweiko, H. (1996). *Concepts of chemical dependency*. Pacific Grove, CA: Brooks/Cole.

Dube, C. E., Goldstein, M. G., Lewis, D. L., Myers, E. R., & Zwick, W. R. (Eds.). (1989). *Project ADEPT: Curriculum for primary care physician training*. Providence, RI: Brown University, Center for Alcohol and Addiction Studies.

Ewing, J. A. (1984). Detecting alcoholism: The CAGE questionnaire. *Journal of the American Medical Association, 252,* 1905–1907.

Gawin, F. (1990). Cocaine addiction: Psychology and neurophysiology. *Science, 251,* 1580–1585.

Glatt, M. M. (1957). Group therapy in alcoholism. *British Journal of Addiction, 54,* 21–28.

Gorski, T. (1989). *The staying sober workbook*. Independence, MO: Herald House Press.

Gray, M. (1993). *Relapse prevention*. In L. Straussner (Ed.), *Clinical work with substance abusing clients*. New York: Guilford Press.

Haverkos, H., Genser, S., Grace, W., & Smeriglio, V. (1991). Complications of drug misuse. *Current Opinion in Psychiatry, 4,* 454–459.

Henningfield, J., Clayton, R., & Pollin, W. (1990). Involvement of tobacco in alcoholism and illicit drug use. *British Journal of Addiction*, *85*, 279–292.

Jackson, J. K. (1954). The adjustment of the family to the crisis of alcoholism. *Quarterly Journal of Studies on Alcoholism*, *15*, 562–586.

Jans, P. (1991). *Delivery of services: Continuum of care*. Unpublished manuscript, Virginia Commonwealth University, Richmond.

Jellinek, J. K. (1954). *The disease concept of alcoholism*. New Haven, CT: College and University Press.

Johnson, V. E. (1980). *I'll quit tomorrow*. New York: Harper & Row.

Kinney, J., & Leaton, G. (1995). *Loosening the grip: A handbook of alcohol information*. St Louis: Mosby-Year Book.

Kuhn, C. C. (1988). A spiritual inventory of the medically ill patient. *Psychiatric Medicine*, *6*(2), 87–100.

Lawton, M. J. (Ed.). (1990). Codependency: The search for definition. *Addiction Letter*, *6*(8), 1.

Lawton, M. J. (Ed.). (1991a). A thread in the tapestry of life. *Addiction Letter*, *7*(11), 8.

Lawton, M. J. (Ed.). (1991b). Two provider groups propose patient placement criteria. *Addiction Letter, 7*(2), 3.

Lowinson, J., Ruiz, P., Millman, R., & Langrod, J. (1992). *Substance abuse: A comprehensive textbook* (2nd ed.). Baltimore: Williams and Wilkins.

Marlatt, G., & Gordon, J. (1985). *Relapse prevention*. New York: Guilford Press.

McLellan, A. T., Luborsky, L., Woody, G., & O'Brien, C. (1980). An improved diagnostic evaluation instrument for substance abuse patients: The Addiction Severity Index. *Journal of Nervous and Mental Diseases*, *168*, 26–33.

Miller, M., Gorski, T., & Miller, D. (1982). *Learning to live again*. Independence, MO: Independence Press.

National Institute on Alcohol Abuse and Alcoholism. (1990). *Alcohol and health*. Washington, DC: U.S. Government Printing Office.

National Institute on Alcohol Abuse and Alcoholism. (1997). *Alcohol and health*. Washington, DC: U.S. Government Printing Office.

National Institute on Drug Abuse. (1991). *Drug abuse and drug abuse research*. Washington, DC: U.S. Government Printing Office.

National Institute on Drug Abuse. (1996). *The Monitoring the Future Study, 1975–1995*. Washington, DC: U.S. Government Printing Office.

National Institute on Drug Abuse. (1997). *Epidemiologic trends in drug abuse*, Vol. 1 (NIH Publication No. 97-4204). Rockville, MD: National Institutes of Health.

Nuckols, C. C. (1989). *Cocaine: From dependency to recovery*. Blue Ridge Summit, PA: TAB Books.

Peele, S. (Ed.). (1988). *Visions of addiction: Major contemporary perspectives on addiction and alcoholism*. Lexington, KY: Lexington Press.

Pletcher, V., Lysaght, L., & Human, V. (1990). *Treating nicotine addiction.* Center City, MN: Hazelden.

Selzer, M. L. (1971). The Michigan Alcoholism Screening Test: The quest for a new diagnostic instrument. *American Journal of Psychiatry, 127*(12), 89–94.

Skinner, H., Holt, S., Schuller, R., Roy, J., & Israel, Y. (1984). Identification of alcohol abuse using laboratory tests and history of trauma. *Annals of Internal Medicine, 101*, 847–851.

Spicer, J. (1991, May). The rehabilitation concept and managed care: Uneasy partners. *Professional Update*, p. 3.

Substance Abuse and Mental Health Services Administration. (1995). *Drug Abuse Warning Network annual medical examiner data 1995.* Washington, DC: U.S. Government Printing Office.

Substance Abuse and Mental Health Services Administration. (1996). *National household survey on drug abuse: Main findings, 1995.* Washington, DC: U.S. Government Printing Office.

Substance Abuse and Mental Health Services Administration. (1997). *Preliminary results from the 1996 national household survey on drug abuse.* Washington, DC: U.S. Government Printing Office.

U.S. Department of Health and Human Services. (1995). *Effectiveness of substance abuse treatment* (DHHS Publication No. SMA 95-3067). Washington, DC: U.S. Government Printing Office.

Wegschneider, S. (1981). *Another chance: Hope and health for the alcoholic family.* Palo Alto, CA: Science and Behavior Books.

Wormer, K. (1995). *Alcoholism treatment: A social work perspective.* Chicago: Nelson-Hall Publishers.

Chapter 27

Visual Impairments

Bruce P. Rosenthal and Roy Gordon Cole

Vision impairment affects a significant proportion of middle-aged and older Americans. One in six adults (17%), age 45 and older, representing 13.5 million Americans, reports some form of vision impairment even when wearing glasses or contact lenses (The Lighthouse National Survey on Vision Loss, 1995). The prevalence of visual impairment increases with age and is estimated as follows:

1. 15% of Americans age 45–64, representing 7.2 million persons.
2. 17% of Americans age 65–74 years and older, representing 3.1 million persons.
3. 26% of Americans age 75 years and older, representing 3.5 million persons (Robinson, Acorn, Miller, & Lyle, 1997; The Lighthouse National Survey on Vision Loss, 1995).

According to a Gallup poll, blindness is "the worst thing that can happen" to 42% of the Americans polled (Research to Prevent Blindness, 1989). It has also been reported that 71% of Americans age 45 and older fear being blind more than being deaf, and 76% fear being blind more than having to use a wheelchair (The Lighthouse, 1995). Fortunately, the blindness that people often think of (cannot see light, needs a guide dog, has to learn braille) rarely occurs. It is not uncommon, however, to have a loss of vision to the point that one has a significant problem in maintaining a satisfactory quality of life. What this means can vary from individual to individual, so a careful evaluation of the patient's abilities and needs is required before attempting to implement a rehabilitation program.

FACTORS AFFECTING VISUAL FUNCTION AND THEIR TREATMENT

The main impairments affecting visual function are reduced visual acuity, visual field loss, poor contrast sensitivity, and lighting and glare problems. These factors and their treatment are discussed below.

Visual Acuity

Based on 1990 estimates, approximately 2.3 million Americans aged 40 years and older have a best corrected visual acuity of worse than 20/40 but better than 20/200 in the better eye, and 912,000 individuals are legally blind (Prevent Blindness America, 1994).

Measured visual acuity gives us an indication of the patient's ability to resolve detail. "Normal" acuity (e.g., 20/20) is based on the assumption that an individual should be able to separate objects that are 1 minute apart in visual angle. People can have better vision (20/15 and even 20/10). The limitation on acuity level is generally determined by the spacing of the cones. Cone spacing predicts that the smallest features of the acuity target should be about half a minute apart corresponding to a Snellen acuity of 20/10 (Arditi, 1997). Visual acuity is generally written as a fraction, the numerator of which represents the test distance and the denominator of which represents the letter size.

$$\text{visual acuity} = \frac{\text{testing distance}}{\text{letter size}}$$

The letter size is actually a distance measurement: the distance at which the letter must be held to subtend a visual angle of 5 minutes at the eye. When test distances in feet are used, we see acuities such as 20/20 or 20/200. When metric distances are used, these acuities become 6/6 and 6/60. All acuities can be represented as decimal acuities, and this is done by "dividing out the fraction"; that is, 20/20 becomes 1.0; 20/200 becomes 0.1. Another way that visual acuity can be defined is as follows:

$$\text{visual acuity} = \frac{\text{distance at which letter was read}}{\text{distance at which letter subtends 5' of arc}}$$

When working with people whose vision is significantly reduced, the acuity can still be measured accurately. One technique simply involves walking the patient up to the test chart, thus reducing the test distance and increasing the sensitivity of the chart. Another technique is to use a test chart with larger letters or numbers and a larger selection of intermediate sizes. In this case, very low levels of vision can still be measured, even worse than 20/2000.

A patient with reduced visual acuity is unable to resolve detail. In some cases, all that is needed is an up-to-date refraction, resulting in a new pair of glasses for general wear. When glasses by themselves are not adequate, additional treatment must be initiated. This is generally accomplished by making the image on the retina larger, that is, using some form of magnification. Magnification can be provided in one of three ways: making the object larger (e.g., large-print books), moving the object closer (e.g., sitting closer to the television), or using some optical device to make the object look bigger (e.g., a telescope to see distant objects better or a magnifier for reading). One of the goals of the low-vision examination (discussed below) is to determine and prescribe the appropriate level and type of magnification.

Visual Field

Whereas visual acuity gives us an indication of the patient's ability to resolve detail, the visual field gives us information regarding the patency of the whole retina (the central and the peripheral retina). When we test the visual field, we are generally, but not exclusively, evaluating "peripheral vision." This is important for the patient to detect objects around him. Once the individual detects an object, he can look at it and identify it (using visual acuity). The visual field becomes an important factor when discussing and considering training for mobility problems.

Perimetry, which is the technique of measuring the visual fields, employs a variety of techniques. These may include manual as well as automated evaluation of the entire visual field with kinetic or static stimuli. The automated perimeter has paved the way for more standardized and accurate visual field testing in all types of patients, including those with low vision (Bass & Sherman, 1996).

There are different ways that the visual field can be affected. A loss of vision in an area is referred to as a scotoma. It should be noted that scotomas in the visual field can have almost any size and shape, and the number of scotomas a patient has can also vary significantly. Scotomas can be located in the center of the macula (referred to as a central scotoma), affecting straight-ahead vision with a concurrent reduction in visual acuity. The magnification principles discussed above would apply. Scotomas also can be located adjacent to the central area (paracentral scotoma). In this case, acuity is usually not affected; interference comes from the scotoma's closeness to what is being viewed.

An overall peripheral field defect can interfere with mobility. This is the situation when only a small central part of the visual field remains. Mobility problems generally occur when the overall remaining central field subtends an angle of about 5 degrees. Scotomas also can be limited to one side of the visual field (hemianopia). These can be very detrimental to patient function because the patient cannot see objects to that side. This can interfere significantly with general mobility, as well as with near tasks like reading and writing.

In some cases, scotomas are caused by the treatment the patient receives, for example, the multiple small scotomas that occur following laser photocoagulation for conditions such as macular degeneration and diabetic retinopathy. The treatment of a visual field defect will vary, depending on the size, location, number, and severity of the scotomas. Generally, there is no good treatment available, and the patient must learn to live with and compensate for the defect. In some cases, optical intervention (prisms or mirrors) will help.

Contrast

Visual acuity charts measure high-contrast vision (very black letters on very light backgrounds). Most of the world, however, is not high-contrast, and this can explain some situations in which patients feel their vision has worsened although the measured acuity is the same. If tested on a contrast sensitivity chart, the doctor might find that the contrast sensitivity of the patient has changed; this would then account for the subjective change in perceived vision.

The benefit of contrast sensitivity testing is that it often gives us an indication of who will respond poorly to standard magnification levels or who will need higher levels of lighting to perform their desired tasks. It is not unusual, in fact, to see patients function with significantly weaker lenses when very bright light (e.g., using a halogen bulb) is incorporated into the task (along with appropriate glare-control techniques).

Lighting and Glare

It is often impossible to predict how much light a patient needs. Often, too much can be as detrimental as not enough. The best way to test for lighting level is to see how the patient responds to different light levels and note the effect of the light levels on patient performance. Patients also complain about glare. One broad definition of glare is "light that does not contribute to retinal imagery but has an adverse effect on visual efficiency, visual comfort, or resolution" (Waiss & Cohen, 1991, p. 436). Intraocular glare problems can sometimes be solved by removing the source of the glare (e.g., cataracts) or by modifying the light coming into the eye (e.g., use of special filters, such as yellow lenses, or visors). If the glare is external in source, one can either modify the environment or filter out the distracting wavelengths causing the glare problem.

DEFINITIONS AND STATISTICS

Legal Blindness

Probably the most common definition of blindness states that an individual is legally blind if either the best corrected visual acuity (with standard lenses) is 20/200 (6/60) or worse in the better eye or if the peripheral visual field is restricted to 20 degrees or less in the widest meridian of the better eye.

The leading causes of new cases of legal blindness according to the National Society to Prevent Blindness (1980) are the following:

1. glaucoma (12.5%)
2. macular degeneration (11.7%)
3. senile cataract (8.3%)
4. optic nerve atrophy (7.0%)
5. diabetic retinopathy (6.6%)
6. retinitis pigmentosa (4.7%)
7. myopia
8. all others

The acuity part of this definition dates back to 1935, when the Social Security Act, with its benefits to the blind, was passed. The visual field part was added as an amendment the following year (Simons, 1991). This definition has been adopted widely by federal, state, and local agencies throughout the United States. It is even used by the Internal Revenue Service to determine tax benefits.

The problem with this definition of legal blindness is that it has little or no experimental basis. Anyone working in the field has had patients with relatively poor visual acuity or visual field (considered legally blind) who functioned very well and other patients, with relatively good visual acuity and fields (not legally blind) who could barely do anything for themselves. Thus, from a rehabilitation point of view, it makes more sense to talk in terms of visual disability.

Disorder, Impairment, Disability, and Handicap

There have been many attempts at defining visual impairment. The World Health Organization (WHO, 1993) devised a classification of impairments, disabilities, and handicaps that has been applied to vision. This *International Classification of Impairments, Disabilities and Handicaps* (ICIDH) is a classification system that distinguishes between the consequences of diseases, accidents and disorders on these three different levels (Visio, 1993).

A visual impairment can be defined generally as any loss or abnormality of an anatomical structure or a physiological or psychological function. The visual impairment may be categorized as normal, near-normal, moderate, severe, profound, near total, or total vision loss, depending on the visual acuity or the visual field. Some examples of visual impairments would be reduced acuity, loss of contrast, and visual field loss.

There is a continuum in the classification of visual performance. Individuals classified with low vision may have visual acuity ranging between 20/30 and 20/40 to 20/1000, with the term *blindness* applied to all categories with performance worse than this (hand motion, light perception, no light perception) (WHO, 1977).

Another classification system, developed by August Colenbrander (1977), shows how *impairment* relates to *disorder* and *disability*. A disorder may be defined as "any deviation from normal structure and or function of the body or parts thereof" (e.g., a cataract). A disorder can lead to an impairment, which is "a disorder interfering with an organ function" (e.g., reduced visual acuity, reduced visual field, reduced contrast sensitivity). An impairment can lead to a disability, which is "the lack, loss, or reduction of an individual's ability to perform certain tasks" (e.g., cannot read a newspaper). It should be noted that *impairment* refers to the basic functions performed by a part of the body, whereas *disability* refers to tasks performed by a person.

A handicap is "a disadvantage for a given individual, resulting from an impairment or a disability, that limits or prevents the fulfillment of a role that is normal (depending on age, sex and social-cultural factors) for that individual" (Visio, 1993). A patient could be considered *handicapped* if reading the newspaper is an activity that is important in this person's life. Individuals who do not need to read the newspaper and do not want to should not be considered handicapped by this disability.

Arditi and Rosenthal (1996) defined visual impairment as a significant limitation of visual capability resulting from disease, trauma, or congenital condition that cannot be fully ameliorated by standard refractive correction, medication, or surgery. An impairment is manifested by one or more of the following:

1. Insufficient visual resolution (worse than 20/60 in the better eye with best correction of ametropia).
2. Inadequate field of vision (worse than 20 degrees along the widest meridian in the eye, with the more intact central field, or homonymous hemianopsia).
3. Reduced peak contrast sensitivity (<1.7 log CS binocularly).

OVERVIEW OF TOTAL VISION REHABILITATION

Before any type of visual rehabilitation is considered, the patient must have a thorough medical eye evaluation, along with the initiation of any medical and/or surgical interventions. The ultimate goal in the rehabilitation of a visually impaired person is to maximize the use of any residual vision and compensate for vision loss.

Maximizing the Use of Residual Vision (Low Vision/Low Vision Rehabilitation)

Before any type of general rehabilitation services are recommended and implemented, it is important that a low-vision evaluation be done. The low-vision evaluation will identify the patient's functional goals (visual), assess the patient's current level of visual functioning, and determine whether any modifications can be made to attain these goals. As mentioned, the objective of the low-vision evaluation is to maximize the use of the residual vision. Based on the results of this evaluation, the patient will be categorized as either "sighted" or "blind" and will be guided into the appropriate rehabilitation model. Thus, the low-vision evaluation is the key component tying together the medical model and the rehabilitation model and making certain that patients are channeled into the correct programs.

In January 1990, a conference was held at which 14 vision rehabilitation agencies from around the country collaborated on the growing problem of age-related vision loss (Lighthouse, 1990a). During this conference, there was discussion of low-vision as the core service, particularly the evaluation component of the examination. The low-vision evaluation provides older persons their first opportunity to work with a low-vision clinician who will assess their residual vision, detail how the vision loss has personally affected their functional abilities, and explore in a receptive environment ways in which that vision may be enhanced or maximized. This is a unique service that is only carried out by either a low-vision practitioner, a free-standing low-vision service, or a vision rehabilitation agency. The expertise that exists among low-vision specialists and vision rehabilitation agencies should be developed and marketed because it is this service that most responds to the chief complaint of older persons with vision loss (Lighthouse, 1990b, p. 3). The chief complaint of a majority of older persons was previously identified (in this same reference) as "I want to see better."

Compensating for Vision Loss (General Vision Rehabilitation Care)

Once the vision rehabilitation care (low-vision care) has been completed or at least initiated to the point that current functional levels and desired goals have been determined, the general rehabilitation of the patient can be initiated. (It should be noted that there are occasions when the entry point for the patient into rehabilitation services occurs in the agencies providing general vision rehabilitation care. However, a low-vision evaluation must be an essential component of any of the rehabilitation services described below.) The rehabilitation can include but is not necessarily limited to the following:

Activities of daily living training, to enable the patient to perform satisfactorily those activities that are commonly needed in one's day-to-day living style. These include such things as food preparation and consumption ("seeing" the food on the plate), personal grooming techniques (applying makeup, shaving, etc.), selecting the appropriate clothing (coordination of colors, etc.), and general house maintenance and cleaning.

Communications skills training, to develop the ability of the patient to handle the common interactions with other individuals. This includes both direct verbal communication between individuals and use of the telephone, special hearing amplifying devices, and the like.

Orientation and mobility training, to enable the patient to navigate safely both indoors and outside. Travel training stresses safe travel and teaches techniques that include detecting obstacles ahead, crossing the street, locating the destination, and using public transportation.

Educational and vocational training, to provide the patient with an educational background (possibly including college and graduate school), at a minimum, the educational experience needed to attain a minimal level of competency. Then, with vocational training, the patient can learn the work skills necessary to be employed and to maintain a certain degree of independence. Included in this is the provision of any special optical devices needed for the specific task being performed, as well as any special equipment (e.g., special computer systems) needed by the patient.

Psychological and social counseling, to help the patient deal with problems in acknowledging and accepting the loss of vision and interacting with other people.

Family and peer counseling, to help family and friends understand and deal with the problems the patient is having. Support groups may also provide help for adjusting to vision loss.

Other needed services: Some patients have very specific and unusual needs. It is important that the patient be carefully questioned as to the problems and needs to be addressed and that the patient be referred to the appropriate individual or agency to receive the necessary services.

Note that these descriptions and definitions can vary from one agency or organization to another and should be taken only as guidelines. It is important to contact the local agencies in your area to find out the specific programs that are offered, how to refer patients, and other information.

THE ROLE OF PATHOLOGY IN VISUAL IMPAIRMENT

One of the ways to understand the various pathologies that result in a visual impairment is to understand how light travels through the eye.

The cornea and the lens, which are the primary refracting structures of the eye, are the main systems that focus images onto the retina, which is located at the back of the eye. After passing through the lens, the light must travel through the vitreous, which is a clear, jellylike material that fills the interior of the eye. Problems such as cataracts and corneal disease affect these systems and generally result in the patient's experiencing an overall blurred image (reduced visual acuity), decreased contrast, and glare.

Eventually, the light will fall on the retina, a structure that is, in effect, a dual image-processing system. The central portion of the retina (macular area) is associated with straight-ahead vision, color, and detail discrimination. The macular area plays a major role in such functions as reading, facial discrimination, and object identification. Problems in the macular area can cause a reduction in visual acuity or a loss of central visual field (a central scotoma, or blind spot). Some of the common conditions in which the macular region is affected include albinism, macular degeneration, and diabetic retinopathy.

The second portion of the retina, the peripheral retina, is associated with object awareness and motion detection. Its function is to allow one to become aware of objects to the side (peripherally, i.e., up, down, right, left, etc.), and it plays a major role in mobility (i.e., one's ability to navigate around objects and people without bumping into them). Conditions that affect the peripheral retina result in a loss of side vision, with or without a concurrent reduction in visual acuity. Some of these conditions are glaucoma, retinitis pigmentosa, strokes, or tumors.

Cataract

Description of Medical Condition. The lens is composed of three layers: the nucleus (center), the cortex, and the capsule. It is clear at birth, but throughout life the lens continues to produce cells that become increasingly yellow with age. A cataract (opacity or clouding of the lens) may develop as a result of aging, trauma, hereditary factors, birth defects, or a systemic condition such as diabetes.

Cataracts are a normal part of aging. Approximately 50% of Americans between 65 and 74 and 70% over age 75 have cataracts (Faye, Rosenthal, & Sussman-Skalka, 1995). Caucasians are three times as likely as Blacks to develop cataracts, smokers have a 60% increase, and those taking medication for gout are twice as likely to develop cataracts.

Functional Presentation of Medical Condition. The greater the progression of the cataract, the greater the visual impairment from the effects of glare, loss of contrast, and decreased visual acuity.

Treatment and Prognosis. Normally, cataracts can be treated very simply: surgical excision and replacement of the cataract with an intraocular lens (IOL). Cataract extraction, which is sometimes done on an outpatient basis, is considered one of the safest surgical procedures. Assuming a healthy retina, the prognosis for functional cure of any patient problems is high. There is a problem, however, that an underlying ocular pathology such as macular degeneration has been difficult to detect because the opaqueness of the cataract prevents a good look at the inside of the eye. If another condition exists, it must be dealt with in its own regard.

Cataract surgery is indicated when (1) visual function is impaired and it becomes difficult to pursue normal activities such as reading or independent travel or (2) there are medical complications occurring from very advanced cataracts.

Two types of cataract surgery are generally performed. Extracapsular extraction involves the removal of the lens nucleus in one piece from the capsular bag. An IOL is then inserted in the posterior chamber of the eye (behind the iris) during surgery to replace the lens that has been removed.

A second procedure, more commonly implemented in developing countries, is an intracapsular extraction, in which the entire contents (lens and capsule) are removed during surgery. The surgical removal of the lens is then followed by an optical correction with an aphakic spectacle correction or contact lenses.

Psychological and Vocational Implications. Assuming no complications, there should be no psychological or vocational implications following cataract surgery. In fact, many individuals are amazed that the visual acuity and color vision is so improved with surgery and that the glare disability has disappeared.

Corneal Disease

Description of Medical Condition. It has been reported that diseases of the cornea are the leading cause of visits to physicians for medical eye care in the United States (Leonard, 1996; National Eye Institute, 1993). Composed of three layers and two membranes, the cornea is normally clear, but changes in any of the corneal layers can cause the retinal image to be blurred. The cornea is a structure that is prone to dystrophies, deposition, noninflammatory progressive thinning (keratoconus), infection, viral diseases, and trauma. It can sometimes be restored with medical treatment but may require either laser treatment or a corneal transplant.

Functional Presentation of Medical Condition. Interference with corneal integrity can result in a blurred or distorted image on the retina. A totally opaque cornea can prevent light from reaching the retina altogether. Patients with corneal disease may experience severe glare, cloudy vision, and also problems with reduced visual acuity.

Treatment and Prognosis. Keratoplasty is the primary method of restoring vision for an individual with a diseased, irregular, or scarred cornea. The procedure involves transplanting a healthy cornea from a compatible donor. It is done to improve the visual acuity as well as preserve the anatomy and physiology of the cornea, remove active disease tissue, and improve the cosmetic appearance of the cornea. The four leading indications for corneal transplantation in the United States are keratoconus, corneal edema after cataract surgery, corneal scarring, and Fuch's dystrophy (Krachmer & Palay, 1991; Lindquist, McGlothan, Rotkis, & Chandler, 1991). Recently, lasers have been used to treat some corneal problems. Where surgery is contraindicated, a scarred or disfigured cornea can be cosmetically "corrected" with a contact lens to match the fellow eye.

Psychological and Vocational Implications. In addition to improving visual function with corneal surgery, a cosmetic contact lens or prosthetic shell should be considered when the cosmetic appearance will enhance professional or personal goals. Consultations with a prosthetic specialist should be considered as early as possible. Vocational goals will be dependent on the degree to which the retinal image is compromised.

Macular Degeneration

Description of Medical Condition. Macular degeneration is considered one of the leading causes of visual impairment in older adults. Figures for 1990 show an estimated 13.2 million Americans (Caucasian) age 40 and over (15%) who have signs of macular degeneration.

As previously noted, the light-sensitive tissue of the eye, the retina, is composed of a central and peripheral system of receptors. The macula is centrally located in the retina and analogous to the film in a camera. It is the area where most of the color photoreceptors (the cones), which specialize in daylight vision, acuity (resolution, letter reading), and color perception are concentrated and tightly packed. The peripheral retina contains the majority of the rods, which are specialized for night vision as well as motion detection.

The macula is composed of the fovea (the area having the highest resolution and best visual acuity), the parafovea, and the perifoveal areas. Most frequently associated with the aging process, age-related maculopathy is categorized as either the "dry" or "wet" (exudative) type. It is caused by degenerative changes that can result in atrophy, hemorrhage, exudates, fibrovascular scars, or cyst formation of the macular and paramacular areas.

Risk factors associated with macular degeneration include White race, family history, high blood pressure or a history of hypertension, and light iris color (Maguire, 1997). Another risk factor associated with macular degeneration is smoking. There appears to be an incidence of macular degeneration in smokers that is two to four times the rate of the nonsmoker. It is still too early to determine whether supplementing the diet with antioxidant vitamins, such as C and E, and selenium, along with the beta carotenoids, such as lutein and zeaxanthin, will have any effect on the reduction of macular disease.

Functional Presentation of Medical Condition. The effect of structural changes in the macula may be visually manifested as distortions, a decrease in the visual acuity, a decrease in color recognition, a loss of contrast, or an absolute or relative area of no vision (scotoma). Reading also may become progressively more difficult as the disease progresses, driving may have to be discontinued, and employment may be impossible without special low-vision intervention. In addition, macular degeneration has been linked with depression.

Treatment and Prognosis. Fluorescein angiography and indocyanine green (ICG) (Guyer, Yannuzzi, & Slakter, 1994) are two of the diagnostic procedures that are used to evaluate the proliferative angiogenic processes of macular degeneration and determine whether laser treatment might be indicated to slow the progression of the disease. Laser photocoagulation may be indicated to slow down the exudative or hemorrhagic (wet) type of macular disease if detected in the early stages. Patients are also able to monitor the course of the disease with the Amsler grid to determine whether there is a change in the macular area. Any sudden change of the grid (such as waviness or distortion) may be indicative of a leaking retina that might be amenable to laser treatment. Additional treatments that have been investigated for macular degeneration include the use of radiation therapy, laser treatment of drusen, photodynamic therapy, submacular surgery, retinal cell transplantation, and the use of vascular endothelial growth factor (VEGF). The effectiveness of these treatments has not yet been established.

A low-vision evaluation is recommended to determine which lenses are of value for distant, intermediate, and near tasks. The power and type of magnification is determined by the extent of the visual loss. Except in a minority of cases, functional ability is generally retained to the end, with the use of low-vision devices such as microscopic and telescopic lens systems and absorptive lenses. Talking books are available, free of charge, from the local library system through the federal government. Bold felt-tip pens, talking clocks, and checkbook stencils are some other nonoptical devices that are available for the person with macular disease and low vision. Through the use of low-vision devices, individuals are often able to function with visual acuity as low as 20/1000.

Psychological and Vocational Implications. As with most visual losses, individuals are most concerned that the condition will progress to complete blindness. Where possible, the eye care provider and low-vision specialist must reassure the patient that low-vision devices will generally permit the patient to return to normal activities of daily living, such as reading, maintaining a checkbook, or going to museums and the theater. If necessary, other rehabilitation services, such as training in orientation and mobility and activities of daily living, should be advised.

Diabetic Retinopathy

Description of Medical Condition. It is estimated that 16 million people in the United States have diabetes, of which more that one half are not aware that they have the disease (American Diabetes Association, 1995; Leonard, 1996). Late-onset diabetes is the most common form and accounts for 90% of all persons with diabetes (American Diabetes Association, 1988; Flom, 1992). In this country, diabetes accounts for about 5,000 new cases of blindness each year, and diabetic individuals have a 25 times greater risk for blindness than the general population (Flom, 1992). Approximately 40% of persons with diabetes have diabetic retinopathy, one of the most devastating conditions affecting the eye. The early, or background, stage manifests itself with small hemorrhages in the eye. This eventually may lead to the more serious proliferative type, which can cause retinal scarring, hemorrhaging into the vitreous, and even retinal detachment.

Functional Presentation of Medical Condition. Diabetic individuals often experience fluctuating or severely decreased visual acuity, which in turn may cause difficulty in reading and seeing the markings on a syringe. They also may experience problems due to glare, reduced contrast sensitivity, and various types of visual field problems. In addition, diabetic individuals can even have transient episodes of diplopia.

Treatment and Prognosis. The Diabetes Control and Complications Trial (DCCT) study showed that strict control of blood sugar is required to reduce the incidence of complications once considered an inevitable result of diabetes (DCCT Research Group, 1995; Fuchs, 1996). Despite regulation of the condition with diet, oral medication, or insulin, however, many individuals still continue to have progressive visual loss. Photocoagulation may be indicated when there is leaking of the blood vessels. In addition, panretinal photocoagulation of the peripheral retina may be indicated to preserve remaining vision, and a cataract may have to be removed.

Despite continued vision loss, low-vision devices will often be of value in enabling an individual to maintain everyday activities. Prisms also have been used to correct for the transitory diplopia. Prognosis, however, must remain guarded.

Psychological and Vocational Implications. Individuals are often depressed and should be directed to a social worker, psychiatrist, psychologist, or discussion group for support. Rehabilitation considerations must include not only vision but also the effect of this debilitating disease on other systems.

Glaucoma

Description of Medical Condition. Glaucoma is a disease that, if left untreated, results in the destruction of the peripheral retina. The causes of glaucoma are varied and may be congenital, hereditary, systemic, traumatic, secondary, drug-induced, neoplastic, or surgically induced.

The philosophy of the etiology of glaucoma has been changing. There are basically three types of glaucoma that affect the eye: (1) chronic open-angle glaucoma, in which elevated pressure over time eventually affects the optic nerve and visual field; (2) acute (closed-angle) glaucoma, in which there is a rapid increase or spiking of the intraocular pressure that may be accompanied by intense pain and even nausea or vomiting; and (3) low-tension glaucoma, which may be caused by a decrease in blood flow to the optic nerve.

Functional Presentation of Medical Condition. Over a period of time, especially if left untreated, irreversible optic nerve and visual field damage will take place, impairing night vision, visual acuity, mobility, and even the reading skills of the patient. In addition, glare and light sensitivity are also prevalent in individuals with glaucoma.

Treatment and Prognosis. Medications that decrease production of aqueous humor or facilitate outflow of fluid through the trabecular meshwork are generally the first treatments instituted with the glaucoma patient. Some of the drugs used to reduce the IOP are the anticholinergic drugs, beta-blocking agents, carbachol, carbonic anhydrase inhibitors, epinephrine, and pilocarpine. Argon laser trabeculoplasty (ALT), in use since 1979, relieves buildup of pressure by creating drainage holes. Another procedure is a trabeculectomy, which is designed to lower pressure by cutting out a small section of the drainage system (Harrison, 1996).

Low-vision devices, including spectacles, hand and stand magnifiers, closed circuit television (CCTV), lighting, and nonoptical devices are used to return an individual with glaucoma to normal visual function. Absorptive lenses, especially those that transmit in the yellow visible portion of the spectrum seem to be especially beneficial for outdoor as well as indoor wear. The lenses enhance the apparent brightness of the scene and often aid in mobility.

Psychological and Vocational Implications. Progressive loss of vision, even with the most rigid compliance, may result in difficulty in performing one's job or pursuing normal activities. Modifications in the work space may be required, with high technology, including voice-output devices. Intervention and support groups also should be considered, along with orientation and mobility training for independent travel.

Albinism

Description of Medical Condition/Disability Condition. Albinism is a trait that is inherited through autosomal recessive or sex-linked transmission and results in characteristics that affect the pigmentation of the skin and hair as well as the iris and retina. In addition, nystagmus and a significant refractive error are also generally associated with albinism. There is a lack of the pigment in the body and the eye in the tyrosinase-negative (ty-neg oculocutaneous) form of albinism. This "typical" person with albinism has white or platinum hair and irises that appear to be pink. In the tyrosinase positive (ty-positive-oculocutaneous) type of albinism there is some degree of pigmentation in the eye and skin. The ocular albino, however, is distinctive in the lack of pigmentation in the eye only.

Functional Presentation of Medical Condition/Disability Condition. Photophobia varies with the type of albinism. For example, the ty-negative albino is characteristically more sensitive to light than the ty-positive or ocular albino. Nystagmus is also more noticeable in the ty-neg albino than in the ocular albino.

Persons with albinism have a decrease in visual acuity due to macular aplasia, but, as mentioned, the severity of the visual decrease varies with the type of albinism. With regard to visual acuity, the ty-neg albino has the severest visual impairment, and the ocular albino has the least.

Treatment and Prognosis. Because refractive errors are generally significant, the albino should be evaluated for corrective spectacle lenses as early as possible, as well as for absorptive lenses to reduce light sensitivity. The individual with albinism also responds favorably to low-vision devices, including strong microscopic reading lenses, magnifiers, absorptive lenses, and telescopic lenses and should be referred to a specialist in low vision prior to entry into school.

Psychological and Vocational Implications. The individual with albinism is generally singled out early in life by her or his peers as being different because of physical appearance. Parents and children should have family counseling by a individual familiar with visual disabilities. Vocational implications have changed dramatically during the past decade, with the acceptance of persons having albinism into most occupations, including medicine.

Retinitis Pigmentosa

Description of Medical Condition/Disability Condition. Retinitis pigmentosa (RP), which is a progressive eye disease that affects the pigmentary layer of the retina, is the most common cause of inherited blindness (National Eye Institute, 1993). In addition, approximately 30% of people with RP report some degree of hearing loss (National RP Foundation, 1995). Though there are many variants of RP, it most commonly affects the periphery or midperiphery of the retina.

The speed of the progression of visual field loss varies with each individual; some progress to a significant loss of functional visual field.

The electroretinogram (ERG) is essential in differential diagnosis of RP. The ERG will typically reveal a decreased or absent scotopic response and a reduction in the photopic response as the condition progresses. The visual field is also diagnostically significant in recording the progression of the visual field loss. It is impossible, however, to predict whether an individual diagnosed in the early stages will rapidly progress to a loss of functional vision.

Functional Presentation of Medical Condition/Disability. Night vision and peripheral vision loss go hand in hand. The more advanced the RP, the greater the loss of peripheral vision and the more difficult it is to travel. Legal blindness, as previously noted, is 20 degrees or less in the better eye. Mobility, however, does not generally become a significant problem until the visual loss is 5 degrees or less. Reading also becomes progressively more difficult as the visual field becomes small.

Glare or light sensitivity is frequently associated with RP, especially when a small posterior subcapsular cataract is associated with the condition.

Treatment and Prognosis. At present no medical or surgical treatments are known to stop or decrease the progression of RP. Periodic eye examinations are essential in monitoring the progression of the condition. Refractive corrections are necessary, along with absorptive lenses to cut down on glare or light sensitivity. In addition, contrast-enhancing lenses such as the NOIR or Corning CPF series may be very beneficial in enhancing performance and reducing adaptation times between outdoors and indoors.

CCTV is also indicated when reading becomes too difficult with optical devices. CCTV provides the ability to reverse polarity so that white letters can be placed on a black background, and it enables one to regulate the brightness and contrast of the image viewed. Special prism lenses have been used in the later stages of RP to increase the awareness of the periphery. The Nightscope, which was intended to be used for mobility under dim illumination by individuals with RP, has been found to have very limited use.

As the progression continues, so will the loss in mobility. A traveling cane, special laser cane, sensory device, or Seeing Eye dog may be indicated to assist in independent travel.

Psychological and Vocational Implications. The fear of total blindness and loss of independence is uppermost in the minds of most individuals with RP. Psychological and family counseling are indicated, as well as genetic counseling for persons contemplating having children.

In accordance with motor vehicle laws, individuals with serious progressive visual field loss should not contemplate occupations that will necessitate driving.

Peripheral Visual Field Loss from Strokes or Tumors

Description of Medical Condition. Peripheral visual field loss can be the result of inflammatory, vascular, congenital, toxic, or degenerative changes. A person who has a stroke or tumor can be left with a resultant visual field loss that may be partial, bilateral, unilateral, homonymous, eccentric, bitemporal, superior, inferior, or nasal. This problem may be compounded by the cognitive, motor, and language disorders that may result from stroke or head trauma (Cohen & Waiss, 1994). In addition there are more complex aspects of the visual process that can be affected. These include perception of visual form, color, object meaning, recognition, and attention. There also may be disorders of the visual system such as hallucinations (Brown & Murphy, 1992).

Functional Presentation of Medical Condition. A complete bilateral loss of the left or right side of vision (homonymous hemianopia) is often the result of a vascular accident. Reading disability is greater when the defect falls in the right visual field. The strategy behind the treatment of hemianopsia is to take the visual information present in the nonseeing portion of the field and transfer it for processing in the functioning area of the field (Cohen & Waiss, 1996). Optical treatment generally involves the use of prisms and mirrors. Mobility and night vision may be impaired when there is an overall peripheral field loss, and losing one's place while reading is often the result if there is a loss in the left visual field.

Treatment and Prognosis. Generally, visual field loss is accompanied by "spatial neglect" in the area of the field loss. Prisms have been used to enhance rather than expand spatial awareness when there is a loss in the peripheral visual field. Also, mirrors have been placed on glasses, with less success than prisms, to facilitate peripheral field awareness. Low-vision devices, including CCTV, have also been of value in reading and vocational pursuits.

Psychological and Vocational Implications. Individuals with peripheral field loss may need counseling to understand the extent of the loss. Driving, though legal, may be dangerous when there is a significant peripheral loss, especially to one side. Individuals with this condition should therefore be discouraged from driving.

REFERENCES

American Diabetes Association. (1988). *Physician's guide to non-insulin dependent (Type II) diabetes: Diagnosis and treatment* (2nd ed.). Alexandria, VA: Diabetes Association.

American Diabetes Association. (1995). *Diabetes facts and figures* [On-line]. Available: http://www.diabetes.org/ada/c20f.html

Arditi, A. (1997). The macula's role in the acuities. *Aging and Vision News, 9*(2), 3.

Arditi, A., & Rosenthal, B. (1996, July). *Developing an objective definition of visual impairment.* Paper presented at the VISION 96 International Conference on Low-Vision Proceedings, Madrid, Book 1.

Bass, S. J., & Sherman, J. (1996). Visual field testing in the low vision patient. In. B. P. Rosenthal & R. G. Cole (Eds.), *Functional assessment of low vision.* St. Louis: C. V. Mosby.

Brown, G. C., & Murphy, R. P. (1992). Visual symptoms associated with choroidal neovascularization: Photopsias and the Charles Bonnet Syndrome. *Archives of Ophthalmology, 110,* 1251.

Cohen, J. M., & Waiss, B. M. (1994). An overview of visual rehabilitation for stroke and head trauma patients. *Aging and Vision News, 6,* 3, 11.

Cohen, J. M., & Waiss, B. M. (1996). Visual field remediation. In R. G. Cole, & B. P., Rosenthal (Eds.), *Remediation and management of low vision* (pp. 1–126). St. Louis: C. V. Mosby.

Colenbrander, A. (1977). Dimensions of visual performance. *Transactions of the American Academy of Ophthalmology and Otolaryngology, 83,* 322.

The DCCT Research Group. (1995). *Ophthalmology, 102,* 647–661.

Faye, E. E., Rosenthal, B. P., & Sussman-Skalka, C. J. (1995). *Cataract and the aging eye.* New York: The Lighthouse.

Flom, R. (1992). Low vision management of the diabetic patient. *Problems in Optometry, 4,* 2–3.

Fuchs, W. (1996). Preventing diabetic vision loss. *Aging and Vision News, 8*(1), 6–7.

Guyer, D. R., Yannuzzi, L. A., Slakter, J. S., et al. (1994). Digital indocyanine green videoangiography of central serous chorioretiopathy. *Archives of Ophthalmology, 112,* 1057–1062.

Harrison, R. (1996). Glaucoma: New concepts, new treatments. *Aging and Vision News, 8*(1).

Krachmer, J., & Palay, D. (1991). Corneal disease. *New England Journal of Medicine, 325,* 1805–1806.

Leonard, R. (1996). *Statistics on vision impairment: A resource manual.* New York: The Lighthouse Inc., Arlene R. Gordon Research Institute.

The Lighthouse. (1990a). *Proceedings of the Lighthouse National Center for Vision and Aging, Miami Conference, January 13–14, 1990.* New York: Authors.

The Lighthouse. (1990b). *Statistics on blindness and vision impairment: A resource manual.* New York: Author.

The Lighthouse. (1995). *The Lighthouse National Survey on Vision Loss: The experience, attitudes, and knowledge of middle-aged and older Americans.* New York: Author.

Lindquist, T. D., McGlothan, J. S., Rotkis, W. M., & Chandler, J. W. (1991). Indications for penetrating keratoplasty 1980–1988. *Cornea, 110,* 210–216.

Maguire, M. (1997). Who is at risk? *Aging and Vision News, 9*(2), 5.

National Eye Institute. (1993). Vision research: A national plan 1994–1998 (NIH Publication No. 95-3186). Bethesda, MD: National Eye Institute.

National RP Foundation. (1995). *Fact sheets: Information about retinitis pigmentosa.*

National Society to Prevent Blindness (Prevent Blindness American). (1980). Visual problems in the U.S.

Research to Prevent Blindness. (1989). *Fear of blindness: Progress report.* New York: Author.

Robinson, B., Acorn, C. J. M., Millar, C. C., & Lyle, W. M. (1977). The prevalence of selected ocular diseases and conditions. *Optometry and Vision Science, 74*(2), 91.

Simons, K. (1991). Visual acuity and the functional definition of blindness. In W. Tasman & E. A. Jaeger (Eds.), *Duane's clinical ophthalmology* (Vol. 5, rev. ed., pp. 1–21). Philadelphia: J. B. Lippincott.

U.S. Agency for Health Care Policy and Research. (1993). *Cataract in adults: Management of functional impairment.* Rockville, MD: Author.

Visio. (1993). *Interdisciplinary model for the rehabilitation of visual impaired and blind people* (Report No 93-2, English version). Huizen, the Netherlands.

Waiss, B., & Cohen, J. (1991). Glare end contrast sensitivity for low vision practitioners. *Problems in Optometry, 3,* 433–448.

World Health Organization. (1977). *International classification of diseases* (ICD-9; 9th revision). Geneva: Author.

World Health Organization. (1993). International classification of impairments, disabilities, and handicaps. A manual of classification relating to the consequences of disease (new ed.). Geneva: Author.

PART III

SPECIAL TOPICS

Chapter 28

Alternative Medicine and Its Relationship to Rehabilitation

Mary F. Bezkor and Mathew H. M. Lee

Health or wellness is a dynamic and constantly evolving process. It can be encompassed in the ancient symbol of yin-yang (see Figure 28.1). The symbol contains two equal forces in perpetual motion. Each contains an element of the other and exists in an interrelated fashion. Yang is often depicted as day, brightness, heaven, sun, and male. Yin is often depicted as night, darkness, earth,

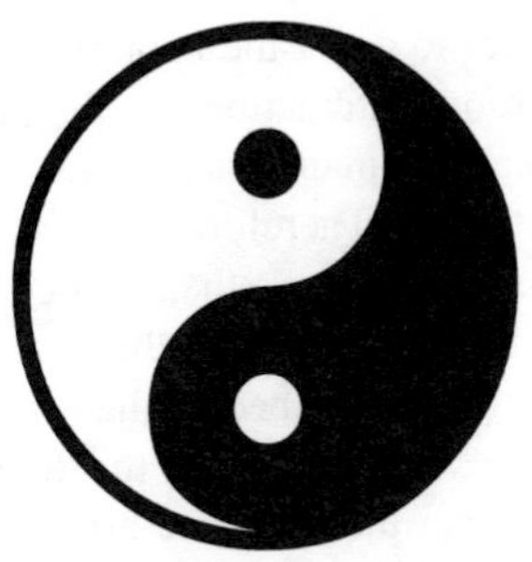

FIGURE 28.1 Yin–yang symbol.

moon, and female. Their harmonious balance is used to represent the cosmos. It is an excellent symbol to represent the body in balance, or homeostasis, free of turmoil or dis-ease (disease). Many alternative therapies are based on flow of vital energy (*chi*) and homeostasis, or holistic (whole body) balance. This symbol of beautiful simplicity may be used to understand the process of feeling well by attaining equilibrium.

Practitioners of traditional Western medicine are familiar with the techniques of specialization, exacting precision and detail. Preservation of a whole picture or a holistic quality may often be lost. Whole-body issues deal with function, a subjective sense of wellness, and interrelation of coexisting body states. Often the healer and sufferer may be at odds in attaining a "cure." By aligning what the two are seeking, a more effective combined result is often achieved. Open communication between practitioner and patient is a key element in the healing process. It may account for an expanding role and demand for alternative healing therapies.

Alternative routes may sometimes surprise the traditional practitioner. Often old remedies, consisting of plant life (belladonna/atropine) or practical manual application (compression/massage), have later led to traditional technical-medical practice. Sometimes ancient remedies are looked at with fresh eyes and new applications (e.g., acupuncture) are found. The modern person, who is looking at a longer lifespan and possibly facing risks of associated disability, pain, or dysfunction, may feel that traditional avenues have not completely answered his or her needs. A natural tendency is to explore alternative solutions. This process will begin with or without the knowledge or consent of the practitioner. If an open line of communication is preserved, a more harmonious balance can be expected.

The practitioner can assist in educating, screening, and interrelating alternative and traditional selections. The traditional practitioner need not necessarily advocate nor practice alternative arts. By simply being aware of the risks and potential benefits involved in alternative practices the traditional practitioner can better integrate these therapies to assist the patient. An important role would be to warn the patient of hazardous interactions. If the practitioner is open to new ideas, patients are more likely to maintain an open dialogue about alternative therapies they are participating in. Therefore, any treatment interactions can be more successfully anticipated. Alternative therapies can be easily and effectively used as an adjuvant to traditional care. Often they are a needed source of hopefulness when traditional methods have been exhausted.

Alternative therapies are often based on the five senses (vision, hearing, touch, smell, taste). Some visual therapies are art therapy and certain hypnotic techniques. Music therapy involves the auditory system; chanting, singing, primal scream, and vocalization also involve auditory responses. Reiki, touch therapy, pet therapy, and massage all use tactile qualities. Aroma therapy uses the sense of smell. Taste is very important in the successful incorporation of diet and herbal therapy to seek harmonious balance. The five senses are, in fact, the basis of the traditional review of systems for health maintenance. The addition of movement and mechanical principles, such as active exercise, postural exercise, movement therapy, kinesiology, yoga, tai chi, dance therapy and many other disciplines, is the very basis of rehabilitation.

Health is a dynamic and flowing energy system. The therapeutic environment is another essential feature in alternative healing. Older arts, such as *feng shui* (wind and water), focus on the arrangement of the home and work environment to create a peaceful and harmonious atmosphere. This is said to be achieved through the use of texture, color, sound, and light, as well as other qualities, to allow free energy flow within a specific environment. Horticultural therapy makes use of plants and a quiet healing atmosphere to help promote feelings of wellness, productivity, and self-esteem. It is often the description or definition of these techniques that makes traditional practitioners either comfortable or uneasy with the solution. Proper lighting, noise level, and visual stimulation in work and home environments have often been studied in industry and architecture to shape productivity and task performance. They are also used to enhance tranquillity, relaxation, and healing in hospital environments.

Alternative solutions often call for an environment free of the hospital structure, and this has long been a source of conflict between patient and practitioner. Now, as patients are facing shorter and shorter periods of hospitalization, healing environments outside the traditional hospital setting are not only necessary but much sought after. More of the recuperative process occurs outside the traditional structure. The sufferer or recovering person is also allowed a more active and more effective role in his or her health recovery, becoming a more dynamic element in the solution.

CRITIQUING AND ASSESSMENT OF ALTERNATIVE TREATMENTS

It is difficult for the practitioner to assess the wide range of alternative therapies available. The absence of regulation, double-blind studies, and other traditional avenues of exploration or scientific method make the situation more confusing. Again the need for openness and communication is stressed. If a method is reliable, it should therefore be reproducible. A safe, effective, and beneficial treatment should not crumble in the light of examination.

The following may help the clinician to evaluate some of the proposed methods and therapies: a number of therapies that differ widely in acceptance, efficacy, and traditional foundation. They may stimulate the reader to further knowledge, exploration, and examination of the roots of so-called traditional methods.

Acupuncture

Acupuncture is an ancient healing Chinese art that has been available and growing in increased acceptance in the United States since the 1970s. Thin, sterile, stainless steel needles are inserted into the body in precisely mapped acupuncture points. There is minimal skin penetration, and no chemicals are injected. There is usually no bleeding. Pain relief can be variable. There are reports of pain reduction, relaxation, a sense of drowsiness, or even euphoria. One hypothetical model for acupuncture efficacy is the release of endorphins, the natural morphine-like substance that occurs in the body.

The principles of acupuncture are often extended into such techniques as acupressure, Shiatsu, acupoint massage, and trigger points. The ancient art describes the enhancement or flow of Chi (life energy). Precise mapping of acupuncture points encompasses almost all bodily functions. However, in Western adaptations the most reliable applications seem to be in pain relief and analgesia. Precautions include strict observation of sterile technique and universal precautions for care of needles.

Biofeedback

Biofeedback utilizes the electrical and other natural signals generated by the body to promote the retraining of functions that may elude traditional voluntary training methods. Electromyography (EMG), electroencephalography (EEG), and electrocardiography (ECG) may all be used. Self-regulation of biological functions can be used for relaxation, pain reduction, and anxiety relief. A training effect often requires several sessions. Sometimes follow-up sessions are required to attain a sustained effect.

Hypnosis and Other Techniques

The use of hypnosis, guided imagery, and other such techniques can be effective in controlling an individual's reaction to life events and can aid in pain reduction and relief of anxiety. Often, positive images are used to alleviate otherwise stressful situations and circumstances. The subject is engaged in a number of treatment and training sessions and is then encouraged to use the process in an independent setting. This is a more self-directed solution, and there is better control of one's symptoms because the treatment can be done in an independent setting.

Music Therapy

Music therapy can involve the production of or the appreciation of music. Playing an instrument or singing requires the subject to take part in an active process and also creates vibratory and auditory feedback. Production of music on a performance level can integrate the subject into a communal surround and deal with issues of self-esteem and self-actualization.

The appreciation of or listening to music can produce relaxation and pain reduction, as well as enhance knowledge and information. Communal participation is again involved when music appreciation occurs in a group setting. Music therapy is often involved in reducing the pain and anxiety involved in medical testing, stressful situations, and ongoing chronic pain and disability.

Horticultural Therapy

Horticultural therapy advocates the concept of the healing environment and active participation in the growth process. Live plants in a quiet and serene environment that incorporates the principles of planting, growing, and ultimately healing aid in producing a therapeutic effect. Horticultural therapy may be used to deal with healing, renewing, and coping with loss. When done in a therapeutic setting, communal interaction may be another beneficial element.

Pet Therapy

In pet therapy live animals are used to encourage contact, positive expression, and companionship. This therapy is often practiced in therapeutic settings and geriatric centers, and reporting of results has been generally positive. Proper supervision, with attention to the health and care of both people and animals is most important. Screening for health-related issues is always essential. Some positive aspects may be the opportunity to express closeness, friendship, and love in settings where these important elements of life have been severely diminished. Reports of lowered blood pressure, increased energy, relaxation, and possible longevity in people who have positive interactions with animals may be upheld by further study.

Art Therapy

Art therapy may be used for the production or the appreciation of various forms of art. Materials such as paint, pencils, and clay can enhance manual dexterity. The active process of creation encourages expression. A subject too difficult or complex to verbalize may be portrayed in an artistic form. Art encompasses painting, sculpture, pottery, drawing, and other creative forms. It offers an outlet for visual and tactile expression.

Dance Therapy

Dance therapy incorporates movement, contact, and auditory appreciation and may be used as a source of nonverbal personal expression. The capacity for individualization and personal styling is infinite, and dance is often more engaging than repetitive routine exercise. Music appreciation is an incorporated feature.

Aroma Therapy

Olfactory sensation is used to promote a therapeutic effect through the use of sprays, scents, or essential oils. Aromatic substances are used on the body, fabric, or in a soothing bath to promote various responses such as relaxation, sleep enhancement, energy promotion, revitalization, or stress relief. This is one of the few therapies to center on the importance of olfactory input. The sense of smell is often intimately linked to taste. It may have key emotional triggers and associations. It is interesting that this area is now attaining some renewed interest.

Feng Shui

This ancient Eastern art that translates as "wind and water" stresses the importance of a suitable home and work environment for proper energy flow, or *chi* (life flow). Although the importance of mirrors, water, furniture, color, or fabric within the home or work environment is stressed, there are other things to be considered. The patient/sufferer may spend many hours in a home or therapeutic setting. The amount of light, noise, temperature, and stimulation may be an essential factor in promoting or detracting from a healing environment. The traditional practitioner may wish to consider this ancient Chinese art as a tool in understanding the effect of environment.

Crystal Healing

The use of precious and semiprecious stones and crystals to promote a therapeutic effect involves holding and applying these objects to the body. A stone may have certain attributes associated with it, for example, amethyst (healing powers) and rose quartz (attraction for universal love). These claims have yet to be proved, but there is something to be said for the association of an object and a positive wish or image for an individual. The simple use of quartz in an ultrasound or Doppler machine makes us traditionally comfortable.

Diet

The use of diet and nutrition is sometimes viewed as an alternative practice. A good nutritional state is the very basis of sound medical practice. Often the patient requires guidance from the practitioner to make sound assessments. Hypertension and diabetes are often managed by the patient's nutritional state. Proper balance of food groups, essential amino acids, vitamins, and minerals is necessary. Many times a person must be cautioned of health risks associated with extreme dietary plans. This particularly applies to diets that incorporate periods of fasting. Proper intake of water also should be stressed. It is beneficial for the practitioner to participate in the educational process associated with sound nutritional health.

Yoga

Yoga as a form of exercise and movement therapy may be beneficial in some conditions (pain, muscle stiffness, stress). The practitioner should be aware of certain positions that may stress underlying lumbar conditions. Persons inexperienced in yoga may experience peroneal nerve stress during lotus positioning. Yoga provides an additional element of relaxation that may be of some benefit for chronic pain sufferers.

Tai Chi

Tai chi is an Eastern martial art that may also serve as a form of movement therapy. In fact it is practiced by the elderly in China as a type of maintenance exercise. The art involves various positions or forms and is often compared to shadow boxing. Combining the effect of movement and posturing, tai chi translates as "supreme ultimate."

Water Therapy and Massage Therapy

Water and massage therapies are traditional mainstays of rehabilitation practice and may be seen in various interpretations among alternative treatments. The use of a soothing bath in aroma therapy may have positive therapeutic qualities. Sometimes it is our explanation of the mechanism of benefit that differs. Massage may be practiced by a traditional physical therapist as well as by one who is aware of the arts of shiatsu and acupoint. It is of interest that many aspects of the effects of water and massage and the resultant systemic response can still benefit from further exploration. At times nontraditional therapies may have a very similar treatment or practice but their beneficial effects are attributed to different mechanisms.

Reiki

Reiki is a system of touch therapy that promotes balance and harmony of the body energy flow; it has both Tibetan and Japanese origins. The translation is "universal life force." Light touch of the hands is applied to the body of the subject to promote the free flow of life energy. The energy fields of both the subject and the healer are important. Physical contact, stress relief, and interpersonal relatedness may be some of the essential features of this therapy. It is good to consider one of the five spiritual principles of *reiki*: "Just for today I shall not worry."

Homeopathic and Herbal Therapy

Homeopathy is the use of small amounts of a substance that would normally produce a symptom in order to potentiate a systemic effect and allow the body to combat the symptom or disease state. Essentially, this means stimulating the body response or immune system. Although many traditional practitioners may be uncomfortable with the term *homeopathy*, there is complete ease with the principle of immunology.

Homepathy is based on the principle of Hahnemann's law of similars, which states that "like cures like," and the law of infinitesimals, which notes that the lower the dose of the remedy, the greater the potential for efficacy. Those suffering from cancer, HIV-associated disease, and chronic pain, as well as the severely disabled, are often interested in the possibilities offered by homeopathic solutions. Homeopathy is often classified as a New Age solution.

Efficacy or failure of homeopathic remedies may lie in the proposed amounts or purity of the product used to produce the so-called immune effects. Another argument in efficacy may be the chosen routes of administration. Many of the remedies are orally delivered.

The National Center for Homeopathy states that practitioners include physicians, osteopaths, naturopaths, nurse practitioners, physician assistants, dentists, and others. The practitioner is advised to be aware of the effects, claimed benefits, and potential risks of homeopathic and herbal products, as noted in the following:

Ginseng claims are for vitalization, energy boost, sexual stamina, and stimulation of the immune system. There is a potential risk of increasing hypertension and a caution for pregnant women and nursing mothers. Some extracts may contain significant levels of alcohol.

Ginkgo biloba is claimed to lessen the effects of memory loss, of interest to persons affected by Alzheimer's disease. To date its efficacy is not proven but may merit further research.

DHEA (dehydroepiandrosterone) is claimed to boost energy and immune qualities as a "fountain of youth," but its effects have yet to be proved. It is a naturally occurring substance in the body produced by the adrenal gland.

Ma huang is claimed to enhance energy and sport performance, as well as aiding in weight loss. It contains ephedrine and has been associated with heart attack, stroke, seizure, dizziness, and arrhythmias.

Echinacea is essentially an extract from the sunflower, reportedly enhancing immune qualities and often used as a cold remedy. Definitive proof of its efficacy is still pending, but it may merit further investigation.

Ionic zinc is claimed to reduce the duration and symptoms associated with the common cold. Double-blind study results have been reported.

St. John's wort is claimed to alleviate symptoms of depression. In considering possible side effects of this substance, of note are the many associated side effects reported in standard antidepressant medications.

Other Therapies

It may be difficult for the practitioner to review and critique the entire range of alternative approaches. The following are examples:

Iridology: mapping of the iris as a gauge of physical wellness.

Electromagnetic therapy: magnet application (often worn within garments) to enhance energy flow.

Reflexology: stimulation and mapping of the points of the feet to reflect total body health.

If the practitioner is unfamiliar with what the patient may be engaged in it is best to simply listen to a technique as described. It may not be possible to comment on efficacy, but it may be very simple to caution regarding hazards and conflicting health risks.

REGULATION, LICENSING, CERTIFICATION

Some alternative therapies offer their own process of credentialing. It is possible for a *reiki* healer to be certified and ultimately become a *reiki* master. There are two fully accredited naturopathic medical schools in Seattle, Washington, and Portland, Oregon. A Washington law required insurers to cover services from licensed providers of the state, including alternative therapies such as massage, acupuncture, and naturopath; but the law was invalidated at a federal judge level.

Levels of credentialing, training, testing, regulation, double-blind experimentation, and research may vary widely among the alternative therapies. Reimbursement is often not available for such therapies, necessitating a significant personal expenditure on the part of the patient. Alternative therapies are demanding acceptance and availability. One positive aspect of this movement is the open assessment and disclosure of alternative practices. Perhaps an improved system of supervision and investigation may provide a safer and higher quality product for the general public. If the practices are sound and safe, further disclosure and inquiry should uphold their potential for efficacy.

Trust is an important factor in the choice of nontraditional solutions. The simple distrust of the traditional approach does not guarantee the safety or efficacy of a nontraditional route. Lack of traditional recognition does not invalidate a particular approach; for example, acupuncture is gaining greater acceptance and availability. This result was furthered by expansion of knowledge and investigation. Communication and cultural exchange may contribute to harmony and life flow.

SUGGESTED READINGS

Bezkor, M. F., & Lee, M. H. M. (1997). Noninvasive techniques for managing pain. In *Expert pain management* (p. 179). Springhouse, PA: Springhouse Corp.

Dossey, B. M., Keegan, L., Guzzetta, C. E., & Kolkmeier, L. G. (1995). *Holistic nursing: A handbook for practice* (2nd ed.). Gaithersburg, MD: Aspen.

Henig, R. M. (1997, April–May). Medicine's new age. *Civilization*, p. 42.

Holman, J. R. (1997, July). Can these pills make you live longer? *Reader's Digest*, pp. 81–86.

It's magic! The Alzheimer's dog. (1997, Winter). *Vim and Vigor*, p. 4.

Lee, M. H. M. (1989). *Rehabilitation, music and human well-being*. St. Louis: MMB Music.

Liao, S. J., Lee, M. H. M., & Ng, L. K. (1994). *Principles and practice of contemporary acupuncture*. New York: Marcel Dekker.

Page, L. (1997). Demand for alternative care not quashed by Washington ruling. *American Medical News, 40*(22), 3.

Rand, W. L. (1995). *Reiki, the healing touch: First and second degree manual*. Southfield, MI: Vision Publications.

Stewart, J. C. (1993). *The reiki touch*. Houston, TX: The Reiki Touch.

Wolf, S. L., Coogler, C., & Tingsem, Y. (1997). Exploring the basis for tai chi chuan as a therapeutic exercise approach. *Archives of Physical Medicine and Rehabilitation, 78,* 886–892.

Chapter 29

Rehabilitation Nursing: Educating Patients Toward Independence

Jeanne Dzurenko

Managed rehabilitation care is rapidly changing the face of traditional rehabilitative services, with many implications for patient education as a result. Patients now transfer to rehabilitation facilities hampered by their acute medical processes. The rehabilitation unit must learn to incorporate these sicker patients and begin restoration to optimal functioning in less time. Seven-day-a-week therapy services are being sought by managed care companies in an effort to minimize inpatient days.

Home care and outpatient rehabilitative services have expanded in an effort to continue patient therapies in lower cost environments. Thus, patients are required to learn without the round-the-clock presence of professionals. The family becomes an essential member of the rehabilitative team, to support and reinforce those self-care techniques taught by the professional staff.

The goals of any rehabilitation program are to maximize independence and minimize the effects of a chronic illness or acute traumatic injury. In addition to treating the physical disability, the therapeutic philosophy of rehabilitation addresses the emotional, social, and psychological problems of patients. Existing rehabilitation programs are based on the pioneering efforts of Dr. Howard A. Rusk, which were developed in 1942 to assist injured World War II personnel. Today, the American Rehabilitation Association (ARA) recognizes that rehabilitation services restore quality of life as well as reduce health care costs.

Rehabilitation nursing encompasses caring for a variety of disabilities. The case mix may be composed of individuals who have had amputations, joint replacements, strokes, spinal cord injuries, and cardiac events that require rehabilitation. Whether adult or pediatric, inpatient or outpatient, education is a key component of any comprehensive rehabilitation program. Rehabilitation nurses are essential providers of that education.

Following traumatic injury or chronic illness, restorative therapy teaches patients to bathe, dress, and feed themselves. The ultimate goal is to enable the individual to perform activities of daily living (ADL) independently. Measuring functional ability after setting realistic, attainable goals will foster success (Williams, 1994).

The approach to rehabilitation should be interdisciplinary as well as multidisciplinary. Physical therapy, occupational therapy, speech therapy, vocational rehabilitation, therapeutic recreation, psychology, social services, and nursing are the disciplines involved. This approach allows each specialty to focus on the individual's affected function that its department aims to maximize. Depending upon the person's age, the goals of the rehabilitation program may vary. In the elderly, vocational training may not be relevant, as retirement may have occurred prior to the onset of disability; therefore, functional independence is the highest achievable goal. On the other hand, a young individual may require functional retraining as well as educational and vocational programs because both goals are important.

As an interdisciplinary model, the ability of the nurse to understand the other professionals' techniques and focus on a common goal allows for a comprehensive integrated program. Effective group interaction, cohesive working relationships, and mutual evaluation will produce greater results than when each discipline functions independently (Melvin, 1980). The education component is at the core of every rehabilitation program. The sections that follow describe prevalent diagnoses found in dedicated rehabilitation hospitals and the roles of the nurse in educating individuals with these disabilities.

WHAT IS STROKE?

Stroke affects 550,000 people each year. It is the third leading cause of death in the United States, according to the Agency for Health Care Policy and Research (AHCPR). Although the majority of stroke victims are elderly, stroke can affect middle-aged individuals as well. Some patients may recover from this event with little residual dysfunction; however, many patients demonstrate physical and behavioral changes. An educational program about stroke should include the following:

- definition of stroke
- risk factors

- functional changes
- behavioral changes
- visual changes
- cognitive changes
- communication deficits
- sensory changes
- complications of stroke

Because of the varying levels of injury, the nursing care should include both group and individual teaching. Group sessions can be utilized to cover the definition of stroke, associated risk factors, and prevention; individual sessions will help patients and their caregivers to better understand specifically what has happened to them. Combining both methods with frequent reinforcement and clear, concise audiovisual aids and handouts will improve the patient's ability to cope with the changes associated with stroke.

The AHCPR has developed clinical practice guidelines for health care professionals on the subject of poststroke rehabilitation (Gresham et al., 1995). Consumer guidelines about stroke care also have been published by the agency. The following discussion highlights key points of the seven subcategories recommended for inclusion in a stroke program.

A stroke results from a blockage (cerebral thrombosis) or a ruptured blood vessel (cerebral hemorrhage). The severity of this event, which occurs in the brain, determines how bodily functions are affected. Depending on which side of the brain the stroke occurs in, stroke patients will present with different disabilities. Audiovisual aids describing blood flow to the brain and pictorials demonstrating a thrombosis versus a hemorrhage should be available. Risk factors can be grouped into two categories, those that can be controlled and those that cannot. Discussing risk factors according to these categories is essential for patients and families to better understand why strokes occur. High blood pressure, heart disease, and transient ischemic attacks are medical problems that increase a person's risk for a stroke. Cigarette smoking also has been demonstrated to be a cause of stroke. Medical management of the first three and abstinence from the fourth risk factor should be reinforced.

The noncontrollable risk factors include age (older people at greater risk), being male, being of African-American heritage, having a history of a prior stroke, and having a family history of stroke.

THE EFFECTS OF STROKE

A left cerebrovascular accident (CVA) results in right hemiparesis. Nursing care objectives for patients in this group are an understanding of right-sided paralysis, speech-language deficits such as aphasia and dysarthria, behavioral changes manifested by slow, disorganized movements, and memory deficits associated with a left CVA. For a right CVA, paralysis on the left side of the body, spatial-perceptual deficits, impulsive behavior, and memory deficits should be the topics of learning. Descriptive examples of behavioral changes and expected responses will assist patients and families to adjust to the cognitive changes associated with stroke.

After the general explanation of the two types of strokes, the nurse's focus must be centered on routine care and management. Prevention of blood clots and pressure ulcers due to immobility are important aspects of care.

Safe transfers and mobility to prevent falls and related injuries should be addressed. Toileting routines can be difficult and frustrating for both patient and family. Incontinence, although usually temporary in stroke patients, must be controlled to maintain personal hygiene and the dignity of the patient. Teaching the family to use external or indwelling catheters, incontinence briefs, and enemas routinely facilitates coping with this sequelae. To achieve a return to self-management, stroke rehabilitation often involves repetitive therapy. Because the patient may present with cognitive and perceptual deficits, this retraining may seem nonpurposeful. Assisting patients and family members to understand the meaning of repetition and how it relates to their personal goals can restore confidence and reduce anxiety (Folden, 1994).

Communicating with a stroke victim also requires educational objectives. Encouraging caregivers to speak slowly, avoid talking loudly, and remain calm while awaiting a response can optimize effective communication. Aphasia and dysarthria are common in stroke patients, and speech-language pathologists routinely involve family members in therapy sessions. Acquiring the ability to communicate with a stroke victim requires an understanding of the effects of a CVA on language.

Educating family members about stroke is an active process. Group instruction is not sufficient; instead, active participation during therapy sessions and at the bedside will foster independence and help patients to achieve their goals. Within the therapeutic milieu, opportunities to attend stroke classes will reinforce individualized learning and provide a supportive environment.

As with any other disabilities, health care professionals must attend to the educational and supportive needs of families. Combined education and counseling has been demonstrated to be more beneficial to both patient and family than education alone (Folden, 1994).

In addition to psychological support, the interdisciplinary team must be sensitive to role changes that occur as a result of chronic illness. Entenlante and Kern (1995) found that wives' roles are altered significantly following their husbands' stroke. Assessment of the wife's ability to act as economic provider, financier, and homemaker must be completed during the inpatient hospitalization.

Adults are able to identify their own learning needs; therefore, it is crucial to include them in the educational plan of care. A study that compared the educational wants of male and female family members assessed the importance of four categories: assisting disabled adults, maintaining their own well-being, maintaining family well-being, and learning about health and human resources (Vanetzian & Corregun, 1995). According to the results, male family members rated learning to assist disabled adults highest, whereas female family members prioritized learning about health and human resources. This study reinforces the need for careful assessment and planning of any educational program.

SPINAL CORD

Spinal cord injuries (SCI) occur from falls, sports, or motor vehicle–related trauma. Impairments result in varying degrees of disability, depending on the location of the injury. SCI rehabilitation can be grouped into five general categories, which can be addressed by nursing care:

- Effects of SCI on mobility.
- Effects of SCI on bladder function.
- Effects of SCI on bowel function.
- Sexuality.
- Discharge planning.

In order for patients to better understand the nature of their disability, a discussion about the anatomy and physiology of the nervous system, types of injuries and levels of impairments should be the introductory phase of the program. Paraplegia versus quadriplegia, complete versus incomplete injuries, and functional levels will demonstrate to patients the variation within spinal cord impairment.

Utilization of audiovisual aids to define the central nervous system function and differentiate between the types of injuries is essential. Reinforcement of learning through pictorials will foster a better understanding of what has happened. There are various videos currently available that will assist the nurse in explaining spinal cord function and the effects of injuries.

Bladder Management

Bladder management is an important focus of SCI care. The use of indwelling catheters and their care should be discussed. Patients must have an understanding of catheter care, whether suprapubic or urethral. If the patient requires intermittent catheterization, the procedure and care of the catheters (cleaning, storage) must be taught. A study survey of 175 rehabilitation facilities found that, although health care professionals use sterile catheters and gloves in the hospital setting, patients are taught to cleanse and reuse catheters in the home setting (Rainville, 1994). Soap and water are the most popular cleansing agents for home use. Bladder management should focus on preventing urinary tract infections; therefore, catheter care is an integral part of the program.

Patients should be taught signs and symptoms of infection. Complications related to altered bladder function, such as reflux, bladder or kidney stones, infections, and signs and symptoms of these complications, also should be reviewed.

Bowel Management

Bowel management is another area that requires attention in SCI patients. A successful bowel routine should be completed within 45 minutes to minimize complications and avoid accidents. Components of a bowel management education program may vary depending on whether the bowel is spastic or flaccid. Medications for the neurogenic bowel include laxatives, stool softeners, and suppositories. Proper dosing and scheduling enhance the development of a routine.

Potential problems associated with a neurogenic bowel include constipation and impaction, diarrhea, and autonomic dysreflexia. Maximizing independence with bowel routine is achieved through detection of these complications and early intervention. Coping with bowel incontinence is attainable through education.

A spastic bowel results from upper motor neuron disease. It is demonstrated by the presence of anal tone on examination. Diet, stool softeners, laxatives, and a suppository will regulate a spastic bowel. A bowel routine might include medications, digital stimulation, and the Valsalva maneuver. In patients with autonomic hyperreflexia, stimulation should be minimized with the use of a topical anesthetic jelly. In a flaccid bowel with absent anal tone, bulk formation rather than stool softening is indicated.

The nurse should facilitate an understanding of the need for a bowel routine and hopefully foster compliance. Individuals with SCI may take weeks or even months to establish a routine. In any case, the combination of one-to-one instruction and attendance at SCI group sessions should be encouraged. While individual instruction addresses each person's own situation, group instruction for SCI has the advantages of motivation, sharing of experience, and peer support. Research has demonstrated that SCI patients respond positively to group instruction (Payne, 1993).

Sexuality

Sexuality is a topic that should be raised with all SCI patients and their partners. Whether they are young or old, this population requires assistance in expressing their fears about sexuality as well as in learning alternatives to genital intercourse.

Depending on the level of SCI, a patient may experience altered physical sensation. The SCI patient should be made to realize that sexuality is not merely physical but rather part of the emotional being of the individual.

Sex education has two elements: cognitive and personal application (Leyson, 1991). The first element includes watching videos and reading; the personal application is more individualized.

In both cases, the nurse must have competence about the topic and feel comfortable discussing issues of sex and sexuality. Leyson (1991) describes competence as including knowledge about sexual responses of males and females, dysfunctions and their treatment, and the ability of the counselor to encourage experimentation while minimizing feelings of embarrassment. Comfort with the topic is equally important. Many health care professionals have difficulty discussing sexuality issues because of the sensitivity of the content. As with any other education program, repetition will increase comfort because each session will build on previous knowledge and experience.

Sexuality covers a broad range of issues. The concerns of women are different from those of men. The focus of sex education programs should be on addressing sexual behavior, desire, orgasms, erection, and infertility. Volumes have been written on these topics. Whatever an individual's education need, it is essential that the learning process preserve his or her dignity.

Sexual behavior in our society usually is associated with the act of sexual intercourse. Our emotions and the center of the brain control sexuality. Pleasure results from all forms of intimacy, and SCI individuals must be allowed to explore "de-genitalized" sexual behavior to meet their needs and desires (Stien, 1995).

Personal expectations must be a focus of education. For example, the nurse should not minimize a man's need to experience an erection if that is what is important to him. For that person, therapeutic rehabilitation may include review of technical and pharmacological aids or penile implants.

In any case, SCI patients should have the opportunity to discuss and learn about options. Focusing on receiving pleasure as well as giving it will boost confidence. Adapting to SCI will include taking responsibility for one's own sexual pleasure. Often the focus lies in pleasing the partner, or "performing." Effective education in this area will redirect the individual to explore his or her own sexuality and discover that the only difference between SCI patients and others is the interrupted connection between the higher centers of the brain and the lower body. As our ability to experience sexual pleasure is located in the brain, SCI individuals are no different from the rest of us (Stien, 1992).

CARDIAC REHABILITATION

Cardiac rehabilitation employs the utilization of a multidisciplinary program to maximize activity tolerance following an acute cardiac event. Since 1980 cardiac rehabilitation has been a standard inpatient therapy, having evolved from progressive ambulation following an acute myocardial infarction in the early 1900s. Currently, various models are utilized in both inpatient and outpatient settings. Overall, research has demonstrated that the implementation of cardiac rehabilitation programs has brought about a 20% reduction in cardiovascular deaths and a 37% reduction in sudden death within the first year following an acute myocardial infarction (Pashkow, 1993).

This secondary prevention will minimize the risk for further injury through a combined program of education and therapy. Medication compliance to control hypertension, weight management, and dietary modification can decrease the complications associated with coronary artery disease (Mullinax, 1995). Regardless of the treatment arena, nursing care is a key component in the cardiac rehabilitation plan of care. The following components should be considered.

Medication compliance during the recovery phase of an acute cardiac episode provides patients with the pharmacotherapeutical support necessary to stabilize heart function. Reinjury to the heart is potentiated by noncompliance; therefore, instruction on dosing, drug actions, side effects, and how to manage missed doses is of paramount importance. Daily reinforcement by the nursing staff complements any formalized medication instruction. In addition, patient involvement in a self-administered medication program is encouraged. Because the goal of any rehabilitation program is to foster independence, self-medicating while still in a hospital setting reassures the patient and caregiver. The support offered by members of the interdisciplinary team can lead to confident self-management of the medication regimen. The self-medication concept and program implementation have been discussed at length in a previous chapter.

Management of hypertension, dietary modification, and weight control are additional topics that should be incorporated into the overall cardiac rehabilitation program. Minimizing risk through education about salt intake, dietary cholesterol, and obesity and its effect on heart function can increase both patient and caregivers knowledge. Written materials about these topics should be utilized to reinforce teaching postdischarge. Organizations such as the American Heart Association (1994) produce comprehensive "Recovery Kits" that are informational and easy to understand. As with any educational tool, be sure that the content fits your institutional philosophy, serves as a supplement to your educational process, and is appropriate for the intended audience.

The age of your patient should be considered when planning an individualized program. An acute cardiovascular event may change your patient's lifestyle, role, or disposition. Psychosocial support should be offered to all cardiac rehabilitation patients. When activity tolerance and endurance is altered, the patient's life can dramatically change. Addressing these issues with patients as individuals or in groups will promote healing. For the elderly, psychosocial functioning was demonstrated to be significantly better in patients who participated in self-management education following the onset of cardiovascular disease (Clark et al., 1992).

Involving all members of the rehabilitation team can improve the overall health status of this patient population. While therapists focus on ADL and endurance, nutritionists help promote proper dietary modification. Social workers and psychologists help patients to cope with altered lifestyles and family roles. Nurses assess progress and reinforce the goals of the program. With physician guidance, the team ultimately maximizes the patient's functional ability postinjury.

AMPUTEES

Amputees require a comprehensive rehabilitation program. The loss of a limb is devastating to both patient and family. In addition to being disabled, the patient has to cope with an altered body image. The nursing care plan should include psychological support, and education focusing on stump care, phantom pain, prostheses, and mobility are key components.

Having identified the need for a national movement to address amputation rehabilitation, the Veterans Administration has developed the Special Team for Amputation, Mobility and Prosthetics/Orthotics (STAMP). This multidisciplinary approach includes guidelines for care of the residual limb, limb wrapping, phantom pain, transfer techniques, and prosthetic care (Heafy, Golden-Baker, & Mahoney, 1994).

Nursing care will include skin care of the residual limb, such as assessment of the suture line for signs of infection and methods to prevent skin breakdown. Limb wrapping is generally taught early in the postoperative phase to minimize edema and prepare the stump for prosthesis. Safe transfer training and mobility must be taught. Adaptive equipment needs also should be assessed and education about safe use implemented.

Advanced prosthetics technology has allowed for lighter and more comfortably fitting artificial limbs. Care and maintenance of the prosthetic socket and knowledge about proper donning and doffing will help the patient to manage independently (Yetzer, Kauffman, Sopp, & Talley, 1994).

Finally, the need for psychological support should not go unnoticed. The grieving process should be encouraged as a normal reaction for both patient and family members. Learning to verbalize the feelings associated with a loss may be difficult; therefore, nurses must teach the involved parties what to expect and how to cope. Depending on the existing coping skills, support groups or individualized psychotherapy may be appropriate. The involvement of a social worker and psychologist will help the patient to adjust to the anticipated lifestyle changes.

OTHER NURSING CARE ISSUES

Although nursing care can be disability-focused, general plans of care are common to all rehabilitation patients. Pressure ulcer prevention for any patient with limited mobility should be incorporated into the nursing care plans. Frequent position change, skin care, and adequate nutritional intake should be addressed. The AHCPR has developed clinical practice guidelines for pressure ulcer prevention. Proper wheelchair positioning to minimize pressure over bony prominences through the use of cushions and other devices can be beneficial to any rehabilitation candidate with limited mobility. Keeping skin clean and dry and the inclusion of moisturizers and barrier creams for patients with incontinence may be added to this daily routine. Finally, adequate nutrition intake, particularly for a patient susceptible to skin breakdown, will minimize the adverse effects to the skin.

Foot care is another focus of education for rehabilitation candidates. Self-assessment of toes and feet, cleansing, and gentle care will minimize the complications that can develop.

Discharge planning can never be discussed too much. Although patients are interviewed about the discharge plan early in the hospitalization and the discussion continues until the actual discharge, there should be a formal class in which to discuss options and have a question-and-answer period. Opening the class to all patients and families at any point in their rehabilitation stay can reflect positively on the outcome of the class. By listening to other peoples' fears and concerns, patients and families are able to encourage and support one another. A camaraderie develops as each patient sees that he or she really is not alone when planning to reenter the community. Common topics included in the program are equipment and its uses, community referrals, follow-up visits, and medication regimens.

This type of program also allows family members who may have missed some of the one-to-one meetings with the social workers or discharge planner to seek answers and reassurance from the rehabilitative staff.

SELF-CARE DAYS AND INDEPENDENT LIVING EXPERIENCE

After the individual disciplines have completed their therapeutic regimens, patients begin a series of self-care days accompanied by a family member. With the assistance of the interdisciplinary team, the patient progresses toward a higher level of independence, and family members observe the patient as he or she completes the tasks of self-care. The interdisciplinary team also evaluates the patient's readiness for an independent living experience (ILE). Once the patient has mastered self-care, the ILE is arranged.

The ILE is the final step in the rehabilitation continuum prior to discharge. Its objectives are fourfold:

1. to promote a realistic experience,
2. to provide an opportunity to apply newly learned ADL skills,
3. to develop confidence, and
4. to develop abilities to manage community living.

The patient and caregiver are invited to this "day at home" simulation in an apartment-like setting. A nurse will observe and supervise the patient through all of the activities learned during the hospitalization. Proper transfer techniques, bathing, showering, dressing, and meal preparation will be performed. This program facilitates the experience of a postdischarge routine for patient and caregiver while they are still in the supportive environment of the hospital. Patients and their families are offered this "trial and error day" to experience their anticipated challenges of living at home and to allay their fears.

Often, patients are able to perform ADLs in the rehabilitation setting, but the techniques learned are forgotten because of the stress of being home alone or because of the changed environment. For example, a patient may have mastered bathing independently in the roll-in shower at the rehabilitation facility; however, once home, showering requires the additional step of transferring to a tub chair. Because of the extra energy and step involved, the patient may become discouraged and never attempt to shower. The ILE will occur in a similar home environment and permit the patient to practice the activity. This process can be individualized to mimic the barriers of the permanent home. Through a thorough home assessment, the nurse or therapist can re-create the setting and foster independence within the home constraints.

Families are encouraged to participate, share their concerns, discuss fears, and ask questions. Their involvement in the ILE will offer insight to the future patient living at home. The goal and plan that have been set from admission can be demonstrated with confidence. Depending on individual needs, patient and family may grocery-shop, prepare a meal, or launder clothes. The choice of activities is left to patient and family, but patients are encouraged to select the tasks they feel most unsure performing. Ultimately, the ILE will restore the patient's ability to function within the community.

COMMUNITY REFERRALS

The transition from hospital to home requires additional support to patients and their families. An efficient discharge plan from a rehabilitation setting includes referrals to community agencies. Various disease-related organizations offer comprehensive services to their members. Support groups for both patients and family members can be found for diseases such as stroke, SCI, and multiple sclerosis. The Center for Independent Living of the Disabled in New York (CIDNY) offers counseling, equipment loan, entitlement advice, and housing information. Other agencies may offer transportation, recreational activities, and respite care. Early assessment of individual patients' communities will enable the interdisciplinary team to incorporate the services of community agencies into the discharge plan.

SUMMARY

As the health care industry moves toward managed care, the ways in which rehabilitative services are provided will change. As lengths of stay shorten, it will become even more imperative that health care professionals perform accurate evaluations and begin therapy immediately.

Patient and family education is the backbone of every rehabilitation plan of care and helps to facilitate a smooth transition from hospital to home. Individual and group classes reinforce the accomplishments achieved in physical, occupational, and speech therapy. Motivation and progress are fostered through an interdisciplinary approach that includes the patient and family as integral participants in the process. To do this effectively, goals must be individualized, mutual, and realistic. No matter how small the gains may seem to others, it is these small achievements that produce the larger and ultimate goal of independence. The nurse plays a key role in delivering care that ultimately enhances the quality of life for those affected by disability or chronic illness (Association of Rehabilitation Nurses, 1995).

REFERENCES

American Heart Association. (1994). *Recovering from a stroke.* Dallas, TX: Author.

Association of Rehabilitation Nurses. (1995). *ARN purpose.* Glenview, IL: Author.

Clark, N. M., Janz, N. K., Becker, M. H., Schork, M. A., Wheeler, J., Liang, J., Dodge, J. A., Keteyian, S., Rhands, K. L., & Santinga, J. T. (1992). Impact of self-management education on the functional health status of older adults with heart disease. *Gerontologist, 32,* 438–443.

Entenlante, T., & Kern. J. (1995). Wives' report role changes following a husband's stroke: A pilot study. *Rehabilitation Nursing, 20,* 155–160.

Folden, S. (1994). Effect of a supportive educative nursing intervention on older adults perceptions of self-care after a stroke. *Rehabilitation Nursing, 19,* 163–168.

Galarneau, L. (1993). An interdisciplinary approach to mobility and safety education for caregivers and stroke patients. *Rehabilitation Nursing, 18,* 395–398.

Gresham, G. E., Duncan, P. W., Stason, W. B., Adams, H. P., Jr., Adelman, A. M., Alexander, D. N., Bishop, D. S., Diller, L., Donaldson, N. E., Granger, C. V., Holland, A. L., Kelly-Hayes, M., et al. (1995). *Post-stroke rehabilitation: Assessment, referral, and patient management.* Clinical Practice Guideline No. 16. Rockville, MD: U.S. Department of Health and Human Services, Public Health Service, Agency for Health Care Policy and Research.

Heafy, M., Golden-Baker, S., & Mahoney, D. (1994). Using nursing diagnoses and interventions in an inpatient amputee program. *Rehabilitation Nursing, 19,* 163–168.

Leyson, J. (Ed.). (1991). *Sexual rehabilitation of the spinal cord injured.* Clifton, NJ: Human Press.

Melvin, J. (1980). Commentary: Interdisciplinary and multidisciplinary activities and the ACRM. *Archives of Physical Medicine and Rehabilitation, 61.*

Mullinax, C. (1995). Cardiac rehabilitation programs and the problem of patient dropout. *Rehabilitation Nursing, 20*(2) 90–92.

Pashkow, F. (1993). Issues in contemporary rehabilitation: A historical perspective. *Journal of the American College of Cardiology, 21,* 822–834.

Payne, J. (1993). The contribution of group learning to the rehabilitation of spinal cord injured adults. *Rehabilitation Nursing, 18*, 375–379.

Rainville, N. C. (1994). The current nursing procedure for intermittent urinary catheterization in rehabilitation facilities. *Rehabilitation Nursing, 19,* 330–333.

Stien, R. (1995). Sexual dysfunctions in the spinal cord injured. *Paraplegia, 30*(1), 54–57.

Vanetzian, E., & Corregun, B. (1995). A comparison of the educational wants of family caregivers of patients with stroke. *Rehabilitation Nursing, 20,* 149–154.

Williams, J. (1994). The rehabilitation process for older people and their careers. *Nursing Times, 90*(15), 32–34.

Yetzer, E. A., Kauffman, G., Sopp, F., & Talley, L. (1994). Development of a patient education program for new amputees. *Rehabilitation Nursing, 19,* 163–168.

Chapter 30

Social Work and Rehabilitation

Esther Chachkes

HISTORY OF MEDICAL SOCIAL WORK

Social work in a rehabilitation setting extends the role of the social worker in a medical setting. Medical social work is a professional discipline with skills and knowledge that facilitate realistic treatment planning and patient management of illness and disability.

Medical social work has a long history, beginning at the turn of the century. At the end of the 19th century, concerns were being raised about the living conditions of the medically ill and the connection between social conditions and the delivery of medical care. Dr. Richard Cabot (1915), a physician at the Massachusetts General Hospital in Boston, has been credited with founding the first department of hospital-based social work in 1905, influenced by a program developed by Johns Hopkins College in which medical students made home visits to learn about the social and family problems of patients. Dr. Cabot believed that the root causes of illness were found in social conditions as well as in physiological ones and thus saw collaboration with social services as essential. He advocated an approach that supported social, educational, and preventive activities. Working from a public health perspective, he understood the role of community organization and patient advocacy and identified functions of the social worker, including those of teacher, interpreter, referee, and investigator. Cabot knew the difference between neighborliness, charity, and professional intervention (Cabot, 1915).

Cabot's view of social work profoundly influenced the development of the profession in medical care. The specialization grew, and in 1918 the American Association of Hospital Social Workers was founded (Sites, 1955). During the Depression era, social work in public hospitals expanded, and a social work component was introduced to public relief agencies. In the 1950s through the 1970s, hospitals expanded. This was the result of the shift from a chronic care focus to an acute care focus; the new treatments, including antibiotics, and new technologies that were developed after World War II made major strides in the rehabilitation of patients and in survival rates of acutely ill patients. Departments of Social Work grew, as well, in response to increases in the numbers of beds and of patients served and to the subsequent demands for more support services.

In the 1960s and 1970s, hospitals as medical centers incorporated a community perspective that emphasized the importance of social work, with its knowledge of social welfare issues and community resources and fostered its growth. The social work role expanded to include advocacy, outreach, case finding, and information and referral (Bartlett, 1961; Bracht, 1978; Carlton, 1984; Chachkes, 1994; Rehr, 1985).

In more recent years, with changes in the direction of hospital organization and administration, the profession has maintained several important functions, primarily discharge planning and psychosocial counseling to facilitate coping and adaptation to illness and disability. Currently, social work has joined in the efforts to reduce length of hospital stay and minimize unnecessary patient use of hospital resources.

When rehabilitation centers were developed, social work was incorporated into the multidisciplinary approach to care that is the hallmark of the rehabilitation setting. Social work training in providing assistance to patients and families who must make quick decisions and solve problems in the life-changing crises that characterize disability is consistent with rehabilitation goals. In addition, social workers mobilize community resources and help patients and families identify inner strengths and utilize the resources of the family support system—critical aspects in enhancing adaptation and managing the disability postdischarge.

SOCIAL WORK IN REHABILITATION

Illness and disability can result in intense psychosocial and emotional turmoil as the patient and family try to cope with often drastic changes in their lives. For the patient and the patient's family, many elements of a supportive plan of care must be put into place to enable the patient to organize his or her life to manage the impact of the disability and to restore as much functioning and quality of life as is possible. The patient is called on to tolerate the limitations of the disability, to adapt to these limitations by acceptance, to develop compensatory defenses, and to organize the psychosocial environment to facilitate adjustment. This includes rethinking aspirations, goals, and expectations and accepting changes in interpersonal relationships as well as managing the physical environment. Coping, adaptation, and adjustment are the major emotional strategies that must be employed (Russell, 1988).

In the rehabilitation setting, social work focuses on patient and family understanding of the nature and level of disability, adjustment to the disability, and assessment of motivation, expectations, and goals for rehabilitation and plans for discharge and community reintegration. The social worker is a member of the rehabilitation team and is the link between the inpatient setting and community resources, providing for the patient's safe transition back into the community. The National Association of Social Workers (NASW; 1996) states that no other profession or occupational group has this focus on the utilization of resources on behalf of people.

Because the team is a critical aspect of treatment planning in rehabilitation, team skills such as the ability to collaborate and to advocate for the patient are important to how effective the social worker will be. Russell (1988, p. 944) emphasizes that "the rehabilitation team is the core of the diagnosis, treatment, and follow-up care for the patient who is disabled or handicapped. The elusive quality of the team interaction must be blended with the individual professional expertise of the clinical social worker to work out the best possible outcomes for the patient and for family members." He adds that the social worker must approach the team with a "sense of competence while contributing toward the combined competence of all team members involved."

As part of the team, the social worker brings information gathered from a psychosocial assessment to the treatment planning discussion. A psychosocial assessment includes information about the total social and emotional environment of the patient, from the physical layout of the home to the nature of the patient's informal support system and ego strengths, the past history of the patient and family that is pertinent to the current plan of care, and other factors. Basically, a psychosocial assessment identifies strengths and resources that can be mobilized to assist the patient in the process of coping, adaptation, and adjustment and the barriers to this process, whether psychological, environmental, or interpersonal (Carlton, 1984; Compton & Galaway, 1989).

One of the challenges for social workers in rehabilitation is helping the patient and the family come to terms with the permanence of the disability and the expectations that may be held regarding outcome and future functioning. Helping people to deal with this information about prognosis demands that the social worker establish a trusting and supportive relationship and assess the strengths, capacities, and vulnerabilities of the patient/family. The intervention most needed is helping the patient/family to obtain information about the disability, the anticipated treatment plan, and the prognosis and to help them process and integrate this information so that they can make appropriate decisions and problem-solve in an effective manner. As family needs compete, decisions must be made as to which needs will hold priority and in what time frame. This involves thought and discussion, which leads to negotiation, compromise, and planning. Honest communication between family members is essential. These situations are not short-term, and they will not generally resolve quickly or easily. Therefore, problem solving is an ongoing effort, and the family must learn to view this as a constant element in their lives.

The major processes for accomplishing social work goals and the scope of practice in the rehabilitation setting are discharge planning, psychosocial counseling, psychosocial health education, and case management. The focus of practice includes the patient and the patient's family and significant others who will carry caregiving responsibilities.

DISCHARGE PLANNING

Discharge planning is a major social work function in the rehabilitation setting. Although discharge planning is a multidisciplinary effort, the social worker generally takes the lead in developing and coordinating the plan. The discharge plan provides for the transition from the acute rehabilitation setting to the community or to an alternative level of care. Most disabled patients, however, are not institutionalized and can go home. Increased availability of transportation, assistive devices, and outpatient services provide previously homebound patients with access to the community and allow them to participate in community and work more easily. Linkage to appropriate resources in the community is essential to ensure a safe discharge plan and to promote the patient's reentry into community life.

Discharge planning is a complex process. The plan must match individual and family needs and must include resources that are both available and affordable. Many discharge plans are relatively easy to arrange, particularly when informal support systems are available and finances are not a problem. However, in many cases planning is more complicated. Home care needs that require the services of professionals in the home or custodial care for patients who cannot be left alone, assistive devices and equipment not covered by insurance policies, and specialized programs for ongoing care may be difficult to arrange. Even more difficult may be the organization of a caregiving system that will be available to the patient. The social worker often must help families negotiate the availability of family members for caregiving tasks and the sharing of caregiving burdens. Issues of dependency and emotional reactions such as anger, anxiety, and depression must be identified, explored, and dealt with in order for the discharge plan to be appropriate and realistic (Brashler, 1994; Kadushin & Kulys, 1993; Volland, 1988; Young, 1994).

Discharge planning, then, demands a combination of skills, from psychosocial counseling and advocacy to knowledge of community resources and the ability to negotiate bureaucratic systems to obtain them. Currently, this extends to dealing with managed care companies and the structures developed to manage cost and utilization of medical resources (Byrne & Sauselein, 1994).

Young (1994) warns that managed care and capitation may drive patients through the system faster, with subacute and step-down care offered in another setting. The demand for reduced acute care stays impacts on the consistent caregiving that a longer stay and stable environment provide. Discharge planning must help patients and families to understand these quicker transitions, and the discharge planner must be the guide to helping them prepare for and anticipate the impact of changing venues of care (Young, 1994).

Brashler (1994) believes that decreasing lengths of stay leave some patients and families unprepared to leave the hospital, and their anger is displaced onto the social worker as the discharge planner. Families have less time to participate in community reentry activities or practice new skills at home on therapeutic passes. Their confidence level is lower, and their anxiety levels are higher. They are often less sure of their abilities to manage what is needed (Brashler, 1994).

It is essential, therefore, that the rehabilitation team help patients and families to understand what and how care will continue to be provided and to assess the appropriateness of care in the home, in outpatient programs, or in residential placements. This is a considerable challenge for the discharge planner. If resources appear to be inadequate for the family, the social worker is often called on to advocate with the managed care case manager and other third-party payers to expand on limited benefits and resources. Success in obtaining these expansions of services is often not possible.

Although the linkage with community resources after discharge is a basic focus of the discharge plan, counseling is the essential aspect and core of the process. Engaging patients and families who are experiencing crises and helping them identify needs and resources in order to make dramatic and critical life decisions is a challenge to even the most skilled professional. Patients and families need real control over their lives and the decision-making process. They must understand the full range of choices that are realistic and available to them, and they must be able to deal with the limitations that the disability imposes. The involvement of the patient and family in the discharge planning process can provide an opportunity for education and support that is significant in facilitating control, understanding, and coping (Lawrence, 1988). In the following situation, the difficult decision about planning for discharge is illustrated:

> Dr. Jones, a 75-year-old married physician sustained a severe stroke, resulting in hemiplegia and aphasia. He was wheelchair-bound and incontinent of urine.

The patient and his wife had been married for 40 years, and his wife was the office manager for the patient's medical practice. She was accustomed to spending all her time with him. After the stroke she felt helpless, unable to care for his physical needs, and extremely distressed over the aphasia. The patient was always the strong figure in the family and now was extremely physically dependent and depressed. Experiencing his impairments as a loss, his wife had difficulty accepting his limitations and pushed him to do more than he could. The social worker met with her and her children to help them understand the patient's ongoing care needs and facilitate a decision-making process. The process entailed weighing realistic options and mourning the loss of the husband and father that they knew and of future retirement plans together. It was very difficult for the wife to admit that she could not manage him at home, and she saw herself as a failure and as disloyal. With the social worker's help she was able to define a new role for herself and deal with her feelings about being unable to care for her husband. This allowed the family to speak more openly with the patient and to pursue a more realistic discharge plan. The patient was discharged to a skilled nursing facility.

PSYCHOSOCIAL COUNSELING

Social work counseling is centered on the identification of individual and environmental strengths. Social work values are based on the belief that therapeutic interventions should focus on releasing individual capacities and enhancing the environment in which these can be best mobilized and put to use (Compton & Galaway, 1989; Loewenberg & Dolgoff, 1992). These values are also congruent with recent changes in the view of disabled individuals, as a result of the disability movement and the Americans with Disabilities Act of 1990. The view of disability as "sickness" and of disabled people as unable to work or participate in a range of social activities has changed. As such, interventions that help to identify and capture the capacity for adaptation, change, and growth and that involve the patient as an active and responsible partner in care have gained prominence (Mackelprang & Salsgiver, 1996). Social work values fit easily with the goals of rehabilitation, which are to facilitate maximum functioning and quality of life, encouraging independence and patient involvement.

Social work counseling techniques rely more on interventions that characterize shorter term treatments and crisis intervention than on those associated with longer term psychotherapeutic techniques. These are by necessity time-limited and solution-focused, encouraging problem solving around concrete goals and active dynamic involvement of the patient and family (Reiss, Steinglass, & Howe, 1993; Steinglass, 1992; Steinglass & Horan, 1988).

The social work perspective is a person-in-environment one that focuses on the individual in his or her social and interpersonal world. This involves assessments that extend from a review of the physical arrangement of living quarters to strategies that strengthen family cohesiveness and support. A critical element in the process is helping the individual to focus on ego strengths and to enhance decision-making capacities, self-image, and skills to maximize independence and self-sufficiency. A major aspect of this approach is the focus on the caregiving and support network that will surround the patient in the community (Gitterman & Germain, 1980; Lawrence, 1988). Because the family usually provides most of the caregiving to the patient, it is a primary focus for social work intervention.

FOCUS ON FAMILIES

Most families do not abandon their loved ones, and historically, the sick have been cared for within the locus of family. Only in the past two centuries or so has health care been professionalized, and even during most of this period, family members have continued to take a leading role in caring for the sick. Today's changing health care delivery system has imposed renewed responsibilities on the family to augment care provided by professionals. In particular, the trend toward managed care and concomitant pressures to lower costs have resulted in a shift of the service site from inpatient to ambulatory care settings or the home and a reduced length of hospital stay. If the family is well prepared and able to support the patient during the hospital stay and after discharge, the result may be more efficient use of medical resources and more effective caregiving. To do so, however, many families will need the education, psychosocial counseling, and support that take into account the unique complexities of each family's set of relationships and that can assist families in garnering resources, strengthening kinship ties, negotiating the web of familial relationships, making difficult decisions and adapting problem-solving approaches.

The family's capacity to respond to the patient's needs is shaped by the many unique features of every family system. Families are dynamic, interactional entities that are embedded in their social context and culture. They actively respond to events over time and are themselves constantly evolving. However, there are certain elements that characterize the family in our culture that significantly affect their capacity or will to manage the role of caregiver. These include the interrelationship or fit of illness-patient-family; family structure; family health beliefs and ethnicity; the stage in the family life cycle; family history of illness, loss, and adversity; and the ethical issues surrounding patient rights (Chachkes & Christ, 1996).

Families both affect and are affected by a patient's disability. More important is what has been termed the fit or lack of fit between the triad of (1) the needs, demands, and challenges of the disability; (2) the family members affected; and (3) the family's characteristics and coping abilities (Gitterman & Germain, 1980;

Rolland, 1994). In this context, the goal of social work practice is to improve the fit by increasing the family's capacity to respond to the patient's needs and reducing unnecessary or ineffective efforts.

Families respond differently to different types of disabilities or stages of a particular disability and course of recovery. For example, some families have a more fatalistic approach to life and a limited sense of their own internal control over events, including illness and disability, and may not have sufficient determination or optimism to manage today's complex treatment protocols or to wholeheartedly believe in the efficacy of current treatment. Conversely, some families have a strong sense of their ability to control events, have experienced many life successes, and believe in the effectiveness of modern medical practices. They may function quite well with demanding treatment protocols during crises as well as with the rigorous demands of chronic illness and disability. Understanding these different responses is essential in providing appropriate help. The social worker must account for the unique constellation of strengths and vulnerabilities of families confronted with these increased and newer responsibilities.

Furthermore, family structures have changed in a number of ways that affect their capacity to cope with the illness of an individual member. For example, today's working women may have less time and emotional and financial resources available to fulfill their traditional caregiving role. The result may be difficulty in balancing multiple roles, work role strains, and work disruptions (Kramer & Kipnis, 1995).

At the same time, the extended family has become fragmented because of economic shifts, job reallocations, patterns of divorce and remarriage, and for other social reasons. In addition, certain family structures have become much more prevalent in American society. These structures include those of the stepfamily, or "blended family"; domestic partnership; the geriatric family; the single-parent family; and in higher concentrations in some areas of the country, the immigrant family. Families with these special structures tend to have particular vulnerabilities that influence their ability to cope with illness, especially if it is chronic or prolonged. Their unique characteristics often require that professionals develop inventive ways of assisting them in network building and providing them with effective educational strategies to accommodate their special needs (McGoldrick, Anderson, & Walsh, 1989; McGoldrick, Pearce, & Giordano, 1982).

The family's beliefs about disability, their familiarity with modern medicine, their existing relationships with health care systems, their education, and their general characteristics of resilience all have an effect on their capacity to understand, integrate, and utilize education and support. The impact of these beliefs is most vividly demonstrated in families that have recently emigrated from other countries. Language differences also can be a major barrier to compliance with today's sophisticated and complex treatment regimes.

The needs of the patient and family also are shaped by the stage of development of the family in the family life cycle. Carter and McGoldrick (1989) have developed a framework for understanding the family life cycle based on life stages that define predictable developmental tasks and life challenges. For example, if the mother of young children is the patient confronting a chronic disability, being able to identify ways of fulfilling her parenting role may be critical to her ability to utilize timely and effective treatment. She may deny her illness and postpone treatment if she fears that separation from her children will have destructive effects. A 17-year-old young adult with a recent spinal cord injury that has rendered him quadriplegic will be dealing with increased dependency in managing bathing, dressing, and bowel and bladder care when maturational tasks should be centered on separation from family and establishing greater independence. Choosing a college and dealing with sexual and social relationships—critical issues in young adulthood—are disrupted by this injury and must be redefined within the context of greater physical dependency and emotional crisis (Carter & McGoldrick, 1989).

The patient's and family's ability to understand information about the disability and to follow treatment plans can be significantly affected by prior experiences of illness and loss. If the experience was negative, there can be an unrealistic pessimism and hopelessness even in the face of more optimistic treatment results. Or conversely, a good prior experience may make realistic acceptance of the limitations of functioning more difficult.

Realities of family function and family structures raise interesting questions about the ability of some families to participate in these added responsibilities for caregiving. First of all, familial relationships are complicated. Traditional moral obligations to assume the burden of care have weakened and can break down under the pressures of extensive caregiving. This has become more problematic as societal resources are less available. In addition, there are multiple family needs competing for attention. The needs of the disabled person must be weighed alongside the needs of the family unit. How much should families be expected to bear—how much is too much, and how much is too little? The ethical issues surrounding these concerns are a current topic of debate (Nelson & Nelson, 1995). Should families be forced to make extraordinary sacrifices or do they have the right to appeal? Should the health care system be held accountable and responsible when families cannot and should not shoulder these burdens?

Although the course of treatment and the crisis points of an illness have a significant impact on the family's capacity to manage effectively, sufficient attention often has not been given to defining the trajectory of a disability for families and for patients. Families need to know the dimension of time and prognosis—that is, the duration and course of the disability and predicted outcome—and the phases, including the coping tasks they present (Aadalen & Kahn-

Stroebel, 1981; Christ & Siegel, 1990; Rolland, 1994). This information is often not sufficiently communicated to families.

There are certain times when patients and families have more difficulty coping and around which supportive interventions can be particularly helpful. Some important phases of the rehabilitation process are the first months after onset of the disability, when survival issues may be paramount and shock, panic, and denial prevail; the immediate postacute phase as the patient and family begin to recognize and understand the extent and limitations of the disability; the defining moments when certain treatments are discontinued, with accompanying patient/family anxiety (e.g., weaning from respirators and when the patient has plateaued and further progress is not anticipated) (Aadalen & Kahn-Stroebel, 1981).

Another critical aspect of helping the family of the rehabilitation patient is the acknowledgment that life does not return to normal but normal becomes redefined as the family struggles to integrate changed roles and dramatic alterations in functioning. Family caregiving, then, is not sporadic. Families must juggle trying to coordinate the patient's care, maintaining jobs and other responsibilities, and organizing the tasks of daily living. Some families handle this with a minimum of stress; for others the experience is overwhelming, confusing, and troublesome.

It is critical not to downplay the essential contribution of family care and the level of expertise and commitment required to perform many of its most complex and demanding tasks (Levine, 1996). The family's enhanced role in health care must be acknowledged and legitimized. The social worker should be proactive in family intervention and not rely solely on the family to identify problems, locate the professionals who could give information, determine the timing for consultation, and formulate relevant questions. A proactive approach recognizes the family's role and responsibility, includes education and support as early as possible, and provides for follow-up monitoring of the family as well as the patient's functioning (Christ & Siegal, 1990; Fawzy, Fawzy, Arndt, & Pasnau, 1995).

Effective family interventions must also consider cultural issues. A patient/family must be understood within the context of cultural background and ethnicity. Cultural factors play an important role in how a patient maintains healthy behaviors, complies with medical regimens, and copes with the course of the disability.

All cultures and ethnic groups have systems of health beliefs: ways of explaining how illness occurs, how it can be cured or treated, and who should be involved in doing this. Culturally based notions about family roles, gender issues, communication patterns, religious beliefs, and a range of other factors also influence how information is understood and processed.

Whatever cultural differences exist among peoples, cross-cultural variations also exist within cultures. Discussions about culture are generalizations, whereas individual behaviors are influenced by a variety of issues that include personality, temperament, and individual experiences. Differences in social classes within a country, which may reflect profound financial, educational, religious, and cultural influences, may be even more significant. Other influencing factors include the degree of mainstream cultural assimilation and acquisition of language.

The ability to provide appropriate care to culturally diverse populations demands an understanding of how these differences impact on the ways in which people use health care, respond to the health care system, and are able to adapt and conform to the expectations and values of mainstream American medical care (Chachkes & Christ, 1996). Understanding cultural values is an important part of the psychosocial assessment, and social workers are trained to identify relevant issues. Social work values promote respectful, culturally sensitive, and effective approaches to patient care and the enhancement of strengths in different cultures rather than being critical of them or labeling them as pathological.

EDUCATIONAL INTERVENTIONS

A major aspect of social work practice is psychosocial education, helping the patient and family to understand, integrate, and use information about diagnosis, the course of treatment, the expected outcomes, and factors related to self-care. This is a multidisciplinary function that has long been recognized as a critical element in the patient's recovery and the family's ability to cope successfully. In today's health care environment, with shortened lengths of stay and health care delivery taking place increasingly in the outpatient setting, there is a greater emphasis on patient preparation for care at home. In addition, biomedical advances have brought new treatments and new technologies into the health care arena. Managing these newer and more complex treatments at home without professional assistance creates a challenge even for the most competent and resourceful patients.

Most of us do better when we are prepared. Knowing what to expect helps us to formulate the coping strategies that will support us in the face of impending crises. Sometimes it is necessary to learn new ways of doing things, which often means unlearning old ways that have been entrenched in our daily approach to situations. How patients integrate knowledge and change behaviors is complicated at best, and it is the focus of much professional attention. Although good communication skills are imperative, it often is not enough to communicate well. Patients and families need time and repeated education to truly understand and integrate the information. This is particularly so because patients and families are being asked to integrate information at a time of vulnerability, when they are in crisis and anxious or afraid. Motivation, language skills, intelligence, comfort in asking questions, dealing with authority, and readiness to listen to information that may be new or anxiety-provoking are all influenced by individual reactions to events taking place.

To make patient education relevant to a patient's life, it is important to understand the range of psychosocial and emotional issues that must be dealt with, including cultural perspectives and norms. To be truly patient-centered, all educational efforts must include the patient's family, care partners, or others who are significant in the patient's daily life. Principles of adult learning and the skills needed for effective pedagogic communication are critical if health care providers are to be effective. Social work can play a critical role in identifying psychosocial barriers and facilitating the integration of knowledge. In many cases, the social worker is the educator, particularly when the information deals with psychosocial issues. The social worker provides the family with information about psychosocial processes, the predictable human experience of the disability, typical emotional reactions to phases of treatment and recovery, and typical crises and emergencies and strategies for their management (Vanetzian & Corrigan, 1995).

CASE MANAGEMENT

It is often difficult to distinguish between the case management role and the traditional social work discharge-planning role as there is necessarily some overlap in professional activities. Both include psychosocial assessment, establishment of a care plan, coordination of activities related to the implementation of the plan, documentation, and referrals to community resources. However, case management, in many settings, is an attempt to provide some continuity of care, allowing one professional to follow a patient throughout the stay in the particular setting as well as postdischarge. Currently, a number of disciplines have been designated as case managers, but notably they are most often social work and nursing. Frequently, the two disciplines share this function. Case management also has been used as utilization management in an effort to monitor and ensure the appropriate use of medical resources and inpatient days. Counseling of the patient and family has generally remained separate from the case management role, with its emphasis on reimbursement issues, insurance contracts, and the intricacies of capitated benefits (Opper, 1996).

SUMMARY

Social work interventions in rehabilitation focus on the person in his or her environment. As such, psychosocial counseling, education, discharge planning, and case management all involve assisting patients and families to identify and mobilize both personal and interpersonal strengths in order to more successfully cope with and manage the impact of illness and disability on their lives. In addition, the social worker helps to strengthen the environment of care by identifying and linking people to community resources and protective support systems.

REFERENCES

Aadalen, S., & Kahn-Stroebel, F. (1981). Coping with quadriplegia. *American Journal of Nursing, 81,* 1471–1477.

Bartlett, H. (1961). *Social work in the health field.* Washington, DC: NASW.

Bracht, N. (1978). *Social work in health care.* New York: Haworth Press.

Brashler, R. (1994). Changes in practice intensify need to engage families in discharge planning. *Discharge Planning Update, 14*(3), 7–11.

Byrne, D., & Sauselein, G. (1994). Utilization review and discharge planning: Integration maximizes benefits. *Discharge Planning Update, 14*(3), 12–15.

Cabot, R. (1915). *Social service and the art of healing.* New York: Moffat, Yard and Co.

Carlton, T. (1984). *Clinical social work in health care settings.* New York: Springer Publishing Co.

Carter, B., & McGoldrick, M. (1989). Overview. In B. Carter & M. McGoldrick (Eds.), *The changing family cycle: A framework for family therapy* (pp. 3–28). Needham Heights, MA: Allyn & Bacon.

Chachkes, E. (1994). *A study of job satisfaction and turnover among hospital social worker.* Unpublished doctoral dissertation, Wurzweiler School of Social Work, Yeshiva University.

Chachkes, E., & Christ, G. (1996). Cross cultural issues in patient education. *Patient Education and Counseling, 27,* 13–21.

Christ, G., & Siegel, K. (1990). Monitoring the quality of life needs of cancer patients. *Cancer, 65,* 760–765.

Compton, B., & Galaway, B. (1989). *Social work processes.* Belmont, CA: Wadsworth Publishing.

Fawzy, F., Fawzy, N., Arndt, L., & Pasnau, R. (1995). Critical review of psychosocial interventions in cancer care. *Archives of General Psychiatry, 52,* 100–113.

Gitterman, A., & Germain, C. (1980). *The life model of social work practice.* New York: Columbia University Press.

Kadushin, G., & Kulys, R. (1993). Discharge planning revisited: What do social workers actually do in discharge planning? *Social Work, 38,* 713–726.

Kramer, J., & Kipnis, S. (1995). Eldercare and work-role conflict: Toward an understanding of gender differences in caregiver burden. *Gerontologist, 35,* 340–359.

Lawrence, F. (1988). Discharge planning: Social work focus. In P. Volland (Ed.), *Discharge planning: An interdisciplinary approach to continuity of care* (pp. 119–152). Owings Mills, MD: National Health Publishing.

Levine, C. (1996). *Family caregiving in an era of change.* Background paper. New York: Nathan Cummings Foundation.

Loewenberg, F., & Dolgoff, R. (1992). *Ethical decisions for social work practice.* Itasca, IL: F. E. Peacock.

Mackelprang, R., & Salsgiver, R. (1996). People with disabilities and social work: Historical and contemporary issues. *Social Work, 41*(1), 7–14.

McGoldrick, M., Anderson, C., & Walsh, F. (1989). *Women in families: A framework for family therapy.* New York: W. W. Norton.

McGoldrick, M., Pearce, J., & Giordano, J. (Eds.). (1982). *Ethnicity and family therapy.* New York: Guilford Press.

National Association of Social Workers, New York City Chapter. (1996). *Social work: A unique profession vital to life and safety.* Unpublished manuscript.

Nelson, H., & Nelson, J. (1995). *The patient in the family: An ethics of medicine and families.* New York: Routledge Kegan-Paul.

Opper, R. (1996). Case management in rehabilitation: A logical transition for social work? *Continuum, 16*(6), 3–5.

Rehr, H. (1985). Medical care organizations and the social service connection. *Health and Social Work, 10,* 245–257.

Reiss, D., Steinglass, P., & Howe, G. (1993). The family's organization around the illness. In R. R. Cole & D. Reiss (Eds.), *How do families cope with chronic illness?* (pp. 173–213). Hillsdale, NJ: Lawrence Erlbaum.

Rolland, J. (1994). *Families, illness, and disability.* New York: Basic Books.

Russell, M. (1988). Clinical social work. In J. Goodgold (Ed.), *Rehabilitation medicine* (pp. 942–950). St. Louis: C. V. Mosby.

Sites, M. (1955). *History of the American Association of Medical Social Workers.* Washington, DC: American Association of Medical Social Workers.

Steinglass, P. (1992). Family systems theory and medical illness. In R. J. Sawa (Ed.), *Family health care* (pp. 18–29). Newbury Park, CA: Sage.

Steinglass, P., & Horan, M. E. (1988). Families and chronic medical illness. In F. Walsh & C. Anderson (Eds.), *Chronic disorders and the family* (pp. 127–141). New York: Haworth Press.

Vanetzian, E., & Corrigan, B. (1995). A comparison of the educational wants of family caregivers of patients with stroke. *Rehabilitation Nursing, 20,* 149–154.

Volland, P. (1988). *Discharge planning: An interdisciplinary approach to continuity of care.* Owings Mills, MD: National Health Publishing.

Young, R. (1994). Evolution of discharge planning in rehabilitation: A perspective. *Discharge Planning Update, 14*(3), 3–5.

Chapter 31

Telehealth: Emerging Technology in Rehabilitation and Health Care

Robert L. Glueckauf, Brad Hufford, Jeff Whitton, Jeff Baxter, Paul Schneider, Janet Kain, and Susan Vogelgesang

OVERVIEW

Over the past 10 years, telecommunications-mediated health care services (also known as telehealth and telemedicine) have grown substantially across the United States and other developed countries (Nickelson, 1996). There are currently over 25 telehealth centers across the United States and Canada. Several proponents have argued that telehealth may resolve pressing national health problems such as the high costs of specialty services in rural areas, prison systems, and the armed services.

Although telecommunications-mediated health services (TMHS) have expanded at a rapid pace, there is currently a significant gap between demand for TMHS and scientific knowledge. We currently have only limited information about how and under what conditions telehealth leads to positive health outcomes. Furthermore, research on consumer perceptions about the desirability of telehealth services and their cost-effectiveness only recently has been undertaken. This is especially true for applications to the field of rehabilitation and health psychology.

In the first portion of this chapter we will define the field of telehealth and provide a framework for categorizing the technologies used to deliver telehealth services. In the second section we will delineate the historical background of telehealth and the rationale for the acceptance of telehealth as a vehicle for the delivery of health care services. Third, we will review pertinent outcome research on telecommunication-mediated interventions in rehabilitation and health psychology, particularly E-mail, telephone, and closed-circuit television (CCTV) videoconferencing studies. Fourth, we will describe our current research program examining the differential effects of home-based videoconferencing versus speakerphone versus traditional office-based therapy for at-risk rural teens with epilepsy and their families. Finally, future directions for research and practice in the use of telecommunication-mediated interventions in rehabilitation and health psychology will be proposed.

DEFINITION OF TELEHEALTH AND TYPES OF SERVICES

Telehealth refers to the use of electronic information and communications technologies to provide health services when participants are geographically separated (cf., Field, 1996). The range of telehealth services includes but is not limited to initial screenings, diagnostic exams, consultations, and short-term interventions. These services are performed by several different types of professionals, including radiologists, pediatricians, orthopedic surgeons, psychiatrists, social workers, and more recently, rehabilitation and health psychologists (e.g., Allen & Allen, 1994; Baer, Cukor, & Coyle, 1997; Glueckauf, 1996; Glueckauf et al., 1998a, 1998b).

The types of communication technologies used to provide telehealth services fall into two major categories: asynchronous and synchronous. *Asynchronous* communication refers to information transactions that occur among two or more persons at different points in time. Electronic mail (E-mail) is the most common form of asynchronous communication and has been used in the delivery of a variety of health care services. For example, as part of Gustafson and associates' (1993, 1994) Comprehensive Health Enhancement Support System (CHESS), women with breast cancer and persons with HIV/AIDS shared information about recent medical advances and offered emotional support. The primary mode of communication used by CHESS participants was E-mail.

Synchronous communication refers to information transactions that occur simultaneously among two or more persons. Synchronous telecommunications include computer-synchronous chat systems, telecommunications devices for the deaf, telephone, and more recently, videoconferencing. Chat systems permit users to communicate instantly with one another through typed messages. Users can "chat" in two different ways: (1) through channels, or "chat rooms," in which several individuals communicate simultaneously, or (2) through a direct connection in which two persons hold a private conversation. During chat room discussions, each person's contribution is displayed on-screen in the order of its receipt and is read by all participants in the "room" (Howe, 1997).

Telecommunication devices for the deaf, or telecommunication display devices (TDD), are instruments that facilitate text-based conversations through standard telephone lines. TDDs typically consist of a touch-typing keyboard, a single-line, moving-LED screen, text buffer, memory, and a signal light. The entire unit is approximately the size of a laptop computer. In 1993 there were approximately 175,000 TDDs in use across the United States (Harkins, 1993).

The most common form of synchronous communication is the telephone. The major advantage of telephone communication is its widespread availability and ease of access. The telephone has become the standard mode of communication in psychological practice for conducting preliminary screening interviews and follow-up sessions as well as for crisis intervention (Haas, Benedict, & Kobos, 1996).

Although the telephone is at present the most accessible form of communication technology, desktop videoconferencing may well become the modality of choice for delivering telehealth services in the 21st century. The typical desktop videoconferencing unit consists of a standard desktop computer (e.g., Compaq EP with a 400-MHz CPU, 64-Mb RAM, 10-Gb hard drive), a videoconferencing software kit (e.g., PicTel 100 or VTel Smart Station), camera, speakerphone, 17-inch monitor, and a digital network interface (e.g., telesync or ISDN). Transmission of simultaneous audio and video signals is accomplished through the use of integrated service delivery networks (ISDN) and, in certain cases, Switch 56 service.

The prediction of a boom in desktop telehealth applications is based on market trajectories that show increased penetration of ISDN services into the telecommunication marketplace, with a concomitant reduction in ISDN installation and user fees. Finnerman (1996) reported that primary ISDN installations expanded 250% per year during the period between 1993 and 1995; basic rate interface (BRI) installations (i.e., typical household ISDN service) expanded 35% for 1995 and are expected to increase at a rate of 50% or more thereafter (Webster, 1995).

According to Davey (1996), telecommunications companies recently have highlighted their capacity to provide differentiated services such as ISDN in appealing to new and old customers. More and more, consumers are demanding services that require greater bandwidth than plain old telephone lines (POTs), in combination with a modem, can accommodate. What makes ISDN services especially attractive is the ability to transmit data in digital format at speeds up to 1.54 Mb per second, facilitating sharp video quality and smooth data transfer operations.

The standard BRI ISDN system includes two B-channels that transmit dial-up voice and digital data information and one D-channel. The primary purpose of the D-channel is to provide call set-up information and signaling. The major differences between POTs and ISDN is that the former requires conversion of digital data to analog signal format for transmission via modem and then conversion back to digital format at the receiving end. In contrast, ISDN uses existing POTs wiring and switching systems to code, send, and receive in an all-digital format. As a result, transmission of voice, data, studio-quality sound, and moving images can be performed through a single service (i.e., ISDN).

BACKGROUND AND RATIONALE FOR THE GROWTH OF TELEHEALTH

The first telehealth application was carried out by a team of investigators at the Nebraska Psychiatric Institute (NPI; Wittson & Dutton, 1956). They established a video connection between the NPI and one of its satellites, state mental hospitals. Using closed-circuit TV, NPI psychiatrists provided neuropsychiatric assessments, consultations, and didactic information to state hospital staff.

Since the development of the NPI outreach project, the field of telehealth has expanded significantly across a variety of service domains and populations. The 1990s have been the banner decade for promotion of telehealth. According to Nickelson (1996), approximately 30% of rural hospitals currently employ some form of telehealth technology. More than 40% of telehealth programs have been in operation for fewer than 2 years. The most common clinical uses of telehealth are diagnostic consults, medical information transmissions, and management of chronic medical conditions. According to a recent *American Medical News* report ("Telemedicine activity triples," 1997), mental health consultation represented 20% of the total of telehealth services, rendering it the most frequently used telehealth care activity.

The impetus for the rapid growth of telehealth stems in large part from recent national and state legislation. From 1994 to 1995 federal and state budget allocations exceeded $100 million for telehealth programs. In the 104th Congress, 15 articles of legislation focused on the provision of telehealth services. The 1997 telehealth reimbursement provisions of the Balanced Budget Act authorized the reimbursement of telehealth services funded under Medicare. Telehealth services also are covered under Medicaid through innovative programs in certain states. Radiology and interactive video consultations are the most frequent uses of telehealth under Medicaid. For example, the Montana Medicaid program provides mental health and substance abuse services to clients who are frequently more than 100 miles away from their nearest practitioners. In 1996, California passed California State Bill 1665, requiring private managed care plans to cover telehealth services. Louisiana recently passed legislation endorsing telemedicine coverage. The new Louisiana law specifies reimbursement rates for physicians at the originating site and also includes language prohibiting insurance carriers from discriminating against telemedicine as a medium for delivering health care services (DeLeon, 1997a).

Three pervasive problems in our nation's health care system have significantly contributed to the growth of telehealth: (1) uneven geographic distribution of health care resources, including health care facilities and health manpower, (2) inadequate access to health care for certain segments of the population, including persons in rural areas, those who are geographically isolated and those who are physically confined, and (3) unswerving rise in the cost of health care, including the costs borne by public and private payers.

First, most health care services in the United States are centralized in metropolitan statistical areas. This has left a sizable segment of the population without adequate access to health services. Although a variety of outreach programs have been implemented, they have not succeeded in closing this resource gap. One of the most underserved constituencies are those in rural areas. More than 60 million persons, approximately 25% of the U.S. population, are living in rural areas (Office of Technology Assessment, 1990). For these individuals, travel to health services, particularly specialty services, may require several hours and attendant financial loss.

Second, several populations have inadequate access to health care, primarily as a result of geographic isolation or physical confinement. Native Americans often reside in geographic areas isolated from adequate health services. Military personnel have access to adequate health services while on base, but this situation can change dramatically when they are abroad. As a result of confinement, prison inmates may not obtain adequate health care services. In 1994, over 1,500,000 men and women were incarcerated in various prisons across the United States. This population is particularly at risk for health problems, especially infectious diseases and psychiatric disorders.

Groups who are homebound, such as geriatric populations with severe neurological and mobility disorders, older persons living in high-crime areas, and those with psychiatric disorders such as agoraphobia, may encounter difficulties in obtaining adequate health care. Their medical problems make it difficult to travel even short distances. In all these cases telehealth may offer a means for closing the gap between limited provider resources and the health care needs of the population.

Third, one of the most pressing problems in health care is the escalating cost of specialty services. This is particularly the case for persons in rural areas who may require treatment by specialists located in major metropolitan areas. Clients in rural areas frequently experience high transportation costs and concomitant loss of wages to obtain specialty health care unavailable in the rural areas.

Telecommunication-mediated specialty services delivered in the home or at a local medical facility have the potential of significantly reducing the economic hardship of rural citizens. However, the key question is whether such services can be provided without significant reduction in quality of care. A recent report by Nancy Ellery, administrator of the Health Policy and Services Administration of Montana, offered preliminary support for the cost-effectiveness of telehealth. Ellery estimated that their telehealth network saved rural mental health patients $65,000 in travel time, lost wages, food, and lodging in fiscal year 1995 (De-Leon, 1997b).

Health care providers also may benefit from the implementation of telehealth networks. Although the start-up costs of telehealth systems may be high, primarily as a result of equipment purchase and installation fees, provider organizations may ultimately show higher profit margins. Such profits are likely to accrue from lower overhead costs (e.g., reduced space requirements) and fewer client no-shows.

Further, client flow (i.e., the number of client appointments per unit of time) and providers' overall client base may increase. Currently, one of the most formidable economic challenges to rehabilitation professionals is the problem of insufficient access to clients in need of services. Telehealth has the potential of substantially expanding access to persons from rural areas and to homebound populations who require psychological services.

TELEHEALTH OUTCOME RESEARCH

Although telehealth holds considerable promise as a tool for reducing inequities in the allocation of health resources, access limitations, and escalating costs, evaluation of the benefits of telehealth has only recently begun. In keeping with the rehabilitation focus of the current text, we have restricted our review of telehealth research to studies involving persons with chronic disabilities, for which at least pre-post group evaluations were performed. This body of research can be divided into four categories of investigations: E-mail, telephone, CCTV videoconferencing, and comparative studies across telecommunication modalities.

E-mail Studies

David Gustafson and colleagues at the University of Wisconsin have conducted several investigations (Gustafson et al., 1993, 1994) of the effects of E-mail interventions for adults with chronic illnesses. Their work has focused on the development and evaluation of the Comprehensive Health Enhancement Support

System (CHESS), a home-based computer system that provides a variety of interactive services to individuals with life-threatening conditions, such as women with breast cancer and persons with HIV/AIDS. CHESS users are able to communicate with others via typed messages in a discussion or chat group, type in questions for experts to answer, read articles about others with similar health concerns, monitor their health status, and gain information about coping techniques. Of the multiple CHESS options, Gustafson et al. reported that the E-mail discussion group was used most often. It accounted for approximately 60% of uses in both their 1993 and 1994 investigations.

To date, Gustafson et al.'s most comprehensive outcome study (1994) is a quasi-experiment in which 104 persons with HIV/AIDS received CHESS in their homes for 3 to 6 months, compared to 97 controls with HIV/AIDS who were not offered CHESS or other additional support services. Participants with HIV/AIDS selected the E-mail discussion option for 73% of the total number of CHESS uses. At 2-month follow-up, Gustafson et al. found that CHESS participants rated their perceptions of quality of life (QOL) significantly higher on 5 of 8 QOL measures (e.g., increased participation in their own health care and increased cognitive functioning) than the 97 controls who did not receive CHESS services.

Telephone Studies

Evans and colleagues have performed the majority of home-based telephone evaluation studies (e.g., Evans, Fox, Pritzl, & Halar, 1984; Evans & Jaureguy, 1982; Evans, Smith, Werkhoven, Fox, & Pritzl, 1986). In the only controlled telephone study to date, Evans and Jaureguy (1982) provided group counseling services to 12 male veterans with visual disabilities. They found significantly lower levels of depression and loneliness and higher participation in social activities for counseling participants than for no-treatment controls (n = 12), who showed no change over time. The veterans' positive response to telephone-mediated counseling was consistent with findings from similar studies that relied on uncontrolled, single-group designs (Evans et al., 1984, 1986; Stein, Rothman, & Nakanishi, 1993).

Several investigators have assessed the impact of collecting psychological assessment data through face-to-face interviews versus telephone communication. For example, Aneshensel, Frerichs, Clark, and Yokopenic (1982) recruited 832 homes for participation in a community depression study. Respondents were randomly assigned to one of two conditions: face-to-face or telephone interviews in which they were administered the Center for Epidemiological Studies–Depression scale (CES-D). They found no differences between the two methods in nonresponse to symptom items, preference for specific response categories, internal consistency, mean depression scores, or proportion classified as depressed.

A similar pattern of findings was found by Baer, Cukor, and Coyle (1997), who compared administrations of the Yale–Brown Obsessive Compulsive Scale and the Clinical Global Improvement Scale over three different assessment modes: telephone administration, telephone administration via computer, and paper-and-pencil self-administration. No differences in mean scale scores were found across the three modes.

CCTV Studies

Two types of closed-circuit TV studies have been performed: (1) satisfaction and (2) video-assessment studies. In the only controlled CCTV satisfaction study to date, Dongier, Tempier, Lalinec-Michaud, and Meuneir (1986) assessed the perceptions of 50 clients with psychiatric problems who received CCTV interviews versus 35 matched controls who received the standard, face-to-face approach. All interviewees were asked to rate various aspects of the interview, such as feeling of ease during the interview, ability to express oneself, feelings of ease following the interview, the quality of the interpersonal relationship, and the utility of the assessment interview in guiding treatment. In addition, the psychiatrists and other team members involved in the interviews were asked to rate the quality of the patient-consultant relationship and the quality of written conclusions for diagnosis, management, and treatment and provide a global evaluation of the usefulness of the interview.

Dongier et al. (1986) found no significant differences in clients' satisfaction ratings between the CCTV and face-to-face conditions. In contrast, psychiatrists and team members rated CCTV as significantly inferior to face-to-face on written conclusions for diagnosis and global evaluations of the usefulness of the interview. Although the authors tended to minimize the psychiatrists' and the team's dissatisfaction with CCTV interviews as a result of small effect sizes, it is possible that professionals may be more skeptical about the validity of conclusions of audiovisual-based modalities. They may tend to emphasize the importance of direct "social presence" in obtaining good interview data.

Note, however, that this discrepancy may not generalize to interviews using structured inventories. Ball, Scott, McLaren, and Watson (1993) and Baer et al. (1995) found no significant differences on the Folstein Mini-Mental Status Examination, the Yale–Brown Obsessive Compulsive scale, and the Hamilton Depression and Anxiety Rating scales between CCTV and face-to-face administration. In addition, Baer et al. found that both clients and raters shared similar positive perceptions of the comfort, ease of self-expression, quality of the relationship, and helpfulness of the interview.

COMPARATIVE STUDIES OF TELECOMMUNICATION TECHNOLOGIES

Glueckauf and colleagues (Glueckauf, 1996; Glueckauf et al., 1998a, 1998b; Hufford, Glueckauf, & Webb, in press) are the first research group to perform a randomized, controlled study on the differential effects of videoconferencing versus speakerphone versus traditional, face-to-face psychological counseling. They are currently in the second year of their telehealth investigation and have accrued approximately 40% of their participant sample. Over a period of 4 years, 75 at-risk adolescents with epilepsy, ages 12 to 19, and their parents from the rural Midwest and Southeast will be randomly assigned to one of three conditions: (a) home-based (HB) family videocounseling ($n = 25$), (b) office-based family counseling ($n = 25$), and (c) a waiting list ($n = 25$). In addition, families in the HB videocounseling condition who do not have access to ISDN or Switch 56 service (anticipated $n = 25$) will be offered HB speakerphone counseling as an alternative. The differential effects of these counseling interventions on outcome will be assessed 1 week after the six-session counseling program and 6 months following treatment.

Purpose

The overall purpose of Glueckauf and colleagues' 4-year National Institute on Disability and Rehabilitation Research (NIDRR) project is to evaluate the impact of telecommunications-mediated therapy on the psychosocial and educational functioning of rural teens with epilepsy and their parents. The specific objectives of the study are to assess:

1. the differential impact of HB video, speakerphone, and office-based counseling on the level of improvement, severity, and frequency of specific problems identified by at-risk teens with epilepsy and their parents;
2. the differential effects of HB video, speakerphone, and traditional office-based family counseling on the therapeutic relationship between family member and counselor and on overall consumer satisfaction;
3. differences in adherence to intervention and attrition across the three counseling conditions; and
4. the cost-effectiveness of HB-video versus speakerphone versus office-based counseling.

The primary rationale for the NIDRR telehealth study stems from previous research comparing the effects of issue-specific, single family versus traditional multigroup psychoeducational therapy for at-risk teens with epilepsy and their parents (Carter, 1996; Glueckauf, 1992; McQuillen, Glueckauf, Webb, & Dairaghi, 1998). *Twenty-four of the 50 families (48%) who expressed a sincere interest in the study withdrew before the initial assessment interview.* Approximately 40% of these prospective participants reported that the primary reason they withdrew was the time and cost of long-distance travel. The average distance from home to our family intervention office in downtown Indianapolis for those who withdrew before initial assessment was 50 miles. In contrast, the mean travel distance for families who did not withdraw before assessment ($n = 26$) was 19 miles. These results suggested that at-risk teens with seizures who live in rural areas 1 to 2 hours outside metropolitan cities may be less likely to receive adequate counseling services. The time and costs of long-distance travel appear to preclude the opportunity for epilepsy-related family counseling. Of course, this finding is not unique to rural adolescents with epilepsy and their families. Counseling services for children and adults with disabilities in rural America are at best inadequate and in most cases nonexistent (Murray & Keller, 1991).

Although it is premature to report the results of the ongoing NIDRR telehealth project by Glueckauf et al., we do have preliminary findings from a pilot study on the differential effects of HB video versus speakerphone versus face-to-face office therapy for adolescents with epilepsy (Hufford et al., in press).

Initial Study

The primary objective of the study by Hufford et al. was to examine how adolescents with epilepsy and their parents differed in perceptions of comfort, distraction, and the quality of therapeutic relationship with counselors across three different modalities: (a) HB videosystem therapy, (b) HB speakerphone therapy, and (c) videotaped, office-based therapy. Three adolescents with epilepsy and their mothers participated in six family therapy sessions using Glueckauf's issue-specific family counseling model (see Glueckauf et al., 1998a, 1998b). The design of the study was a repeated-measures case study approach, specifically an A-B-C-B-C-A design with A standing for office therapy; B, for HB speakerphone therapy; and C, for HB videosystem therapy. Office therapy was followed by HB speakerphone and subsequently by HB videosystem therapy, then speakerphone, videosystem, and finally, office-based therapy.

AT&T's Vistium Model 70 was used to provide two-way audiovisual communication between counselors and the family in the videosystem condition. The Model 70 included an AT&T 8501 computer, a BRI interface for linkage with ISDN service, a CCD fixed-focus camera mounted on top of a 15-inch monitor, a built-in speakerphone, and TeleMedia Connection video-communication software. The speakerphone component of the Vistium 70 system provided the audio-only linkage for the speakerphone condition. The equipment used in the office-based sessions consisted of two videocameras mounted 6 inches below the ceiling of the family intervention room.

Overall, families reported moderately high levels of comfort and therapeutic alliance and low levels of distraction across the three treatment modalities. There were, however, notable differences *between conditions* on comfort with the technology and in-session distraction. Families reported lower comfort with the speakerphone technology than with interactive video and office-based therapy. The absence of visual input in the speakerphone condition and periodic difficulties hearing the specific wording of responses were major sources of discomfort for family members, particularly mothers. Families also endorsed higher levels of distraction using both speakerphone and interactive video than in face-to-face office therapy. The sources of distraction in the speakerphone and videosystem conditions centered on factors unique to home contact, such as telephone calls, pets disrupting the session, and neighbors visiting during the session.

Finally, adolescents indicated that they were more comfortable and less distracted than their mothers, particularly in the videosystem and speakerphone conditions. One possible explanation for the differences between adolescents' and mothers' comfort may be located in the use of computers for recreation. The adolescents reported that they enjoyed using the telecommunications equipment between therapy sessions. Two of the three adolescents specifically stated that they "liked playing games on the videosystem after the session." This natural association with recreation may have rendered the audiovisual conditions more attractive to adolescents than to their mothers, who had little contact with the computer between sessions.

In regard to distraction, mothers were substantially more distracted by internal states (e.g., fatigue) and by the responses of others (e.g., their child's behavior) than their adolescents were. The possibility that mothers may have shown a heightened vigilance and sensitivity to their child's behavior was consistent with earlier theorizing on mothers of children with epilepsy. Ziegler (1981) conjectured that mothers of children with epilepsy may engage in high levels of protective and monitoring behaviors to maximize their sense of control over an intermittent and often unpredictable disorder. Further research is needed to assess whether mothers of adolescents with epilepsy are more sensitive to distractions in therapy sessions than mothers of adolescents without a neurological disorder.

FUTURE DIRECTIONS FOR TELEHEALTH IN REHABILITATION AND HEALTH CARE SETTINGS

Outcome and Cost-Effectiveness Studies

As discussed previously, telehealth holds considerable promise for resolving the access barriers of persons in rural areas and homebound populations who require psychological services. However, we continue to lack basic information about how and under what conditions telecommunication-mediated services lead to positive psychological and health care outcomes. We also have limited information about the cost-effectiveness of telehealth services. This is especially true for cost-effectiveness of telehealth applications in rehabilitation and health psychology.

It is imperative that large-scale evaluations of the differential effects of telecommunications-mediated interventions become a funding priority for federal health care agencies, such as the National Institutes of Health, the Rehabilitation Services Administration, the Department of Defense, and the Office of Rural Health Policy. Although a substantial number of demonstration grants have been awarded over the past 5 years, funding for randomized clinical trials of the benefits of telehealth with chronic medical populations (e.g., persons with traumatic brain injuries and dementing disorders) has been slow to emerge. We can no longer tout the benefits of telehealth services for persons with chronic medical conditions without solid empirical evidence of their effectiveness. If we are to advance as a responsible scientific enterprise, we must begin to subject our basic assumptions about what works in telecommunications with our clients to scientific scrutiny.

Cost-effectiveness studies are also an integral component of the acceptance of large-scale telehealth interventions. To become a viable health service option, telehealth networks must show that the costs of treatment are at least equal to or less than those of alternative approaches that produce similar outcomes. Although several studies have documented the cost-effectiveness of psychotherapeutic interventions for psychiatric, substance abuse, and geriatric populations (see Glen, Lazar, Hornberger, & Spiegel, 1997; Krupnick & Pincus, 1992), there has been no published research, to date, on the cost-effectiveness of telecommunication-mediated psychological interventions for persons with chronic disabilities.

Process Studies

Although randomized, controlled field studies are the litmus test of the effectiveness of telehealth, it is essential to understand the social-psychological mechanisms that link intervention and outcome. We currently lack basic information about the factors that both enhance and reduce the quality (clarity, ease of use, distractibility, and comfort) of telehealth communications across modalities, age groups, minorities, and ethnic groups, and, in turn, their relationship with treatment outcome. We also have only limited knowledge about the impact of different telecommunication modalities (e.g., home-based videoconferencing vs. E-mail) on adherence to intervention, attendance, and attrition.

Practice Guidelines and Client Training Material

Practice guidelines are potentially powerful tools to enhance quality control. Guidelines provide a method of determining the most effective treatment of a disorder and establish accepted treatment approaches and duration of treatment modalities. They are likely to be critical to the broad-based acceptance of telehealth interventions and may help to establish the appropriate level of expertise of telehealth providers (cf., DeLeon, Frank, & Wedding, 1995). In fact, the Joint Working Group on Telemedicine (see National Telecommunications and Information Administration, 1997) has recently called for the development of practice guidelines in the delivery of telehealth services. The time is ripe for developing and evaluating the use of practice guidelines in the delivery of telecommunication-mediated psychological services to persons with chronic disabilities and their families. Furthermore, we also must create training materials for consumers of telehealth services. At present, the lay public has little guidance about how to purchase, install, and effectively use home-based telecommunications services.

REFERENCES

Allen, D., & Allen, A. (1994). Teleradiology 1994. *Telemedicine Today, 2,* 21–23.

Aneshensel, C. S., Frerichs, R. R., Clark, V. A., & Yokopenic, P. A. (1982). Measuring depression in the community: A comparison of telephone and personal interviews. *Public Opinion Quarterly, 46,* 110–121.

Baer, L., Cukor, P., & Coyle, J. T. (1997). Telepsychiatry: Application of telemedicine. In R. L. Bashshur, J. H. Sanders, & G. W. Shannon (Eds.), *Telemedicine: Theory and practice* (pp. 265–290). Springfield, IL: Charles C Thomas.

Baer, L., Cukor, P., Jenike, M. A., Leahy, L., O'Laughlen, J., & Coyle, J. T. (1995). Pilot studies of telemedicine for patients with obsessive-compulsive disorder. *American Journal of Psychiatry, 152,* 1383–1385.

Ball, C. J., Scott, N., McLaren, P. M., & Watson, J. P. (1993). Preliminary evaluation of a low-cost videoconferencing (LCVC) system for remote cognitive testing of adult psychiatric patients. *British Journal of Clinical Psychology, 32,* 303–307.

Carter, C. (1996). *Generalization across modalities, measures, and participants in family therapy for teens with epilepsy and their parents.* Unpublished master's thesis, Indiana University Purdue University, Indianapolis.

Davey, T. (1996). Telcos feel the heat, set to roll out new services. *PC Week, 13*(38), 1–3.

DeLeon, P. (1997a). *The 105th Congress evolves—quieter times.* [Available E-mail: federal-ppp@lists.apa.org. Subject: Division 18 column—October 1997.]

DeLeon, P. (1997b). *Steadily evolving into the 21st century—telehealth.* [Available E-mail: federal-ppp@lists.apa.org. Subject: Division 29 column—December, 1997.]

DeLeon, P. H., Frank, R. G., & Wedding, D. (1995). Health psychology and public policy: The political press. *Health Psychology, 14,* 493–499.

Dongier, M., Tempier, R., Lalinec-Michaud, M., & Meuneir, D. (1986). Telepsychiatry: Psychiatric consultation through two-way television, a controlled study. *Canadian Journal of Psychiatry, 31,* 32–34.

Evans, R. L., Fox, H. R., Pritzl, D. O., & Halar, E. M. (1984). Group treatment of physically disabled adults by telephone. *Social Work in Health Care, 9*(3), 77–84.

Evans, R. L., & Jaureguy, B. M. (1982). Group therapy by phone: A cognitive behavioral program for visually impaired elderly. *Social Work in Health Care, 7*(2), 79–90.

Evans, R. L., Smith, K. M., Werkhoven, W. S., Fox, H. R., & Pritzl, D. O. (1986). Cognitive telephone group therapy with physically disabled elderly persons. *Gerontologist, 26*(1), 8–10.

Field, M. J. (1996). *Telemedicine: A guide to assessing telecommunications in health care*. Washington, DC: National Academy Press.

Finnerman, M. F. (1996). Sizing up the ISDN market. *Business Communications Review, 26*(11), 81–85.

Glen, G. O., Lazar, S. G., Hornberger, J., & Spiegel, D. (1997). The economic impact of psychotherapy: A review. *American Journal of Psychiatry, 154,* 147–155.

Glueckauf, R. L. (1992). *Examining the links among the problem behaviors of at-risk adolescents with epilepsy, family and community processes, and intervention.* Innovation Grant (H133C20035), National Institute on Disability and Rehabilitation Research, USDE.

Glueckauf, R. L. (1996). *Home-based videocounseling for at-risk rural teens with epilepsy and their parents: An accessibility and outcome analysis.* Field-Initiated Grant (H133G60087), National Institute on Disability and Rehabilitation Research, USDE.

Glueckauf, R., Whitton, J., Kain, J., Vogelgesang, S., Hudson, M., Hufford, B., Baxter, J., Garg, B., & Herndon, M. (1998a). Home-based, videocounseling for families of rural teens with epilepsy: Program rationale and objectives. *Telehealth News* [On-line journal], *2*(1), 3–5. Available: World Wide Web URL: http//cybertowers.com/ct/telehealth/

Glueckauf, R., Whitton, J., Baxter, J., Kain, J., Vogelgesang, S., Hudson, M., & Wright, D. (1998b). Videocounseling for families of rural teens with epilepsy: Project update. *Telehealth News* [On-line journal], *2*(2), 2–4.

Gustafson, D. H., Hawkins, R. P., Boberg, E. W., Bricker, E., Pingree, S., & Chan, C. (1994). *The use and impact of a computer-based support system for people living with AIDS and HIV infection.* Unpublished manuscript, University of Wisconsin at Madison.

Gustafson, D. H., Wise, M., McTavish, F., Taylor, J. O., Wolberg, W., Stewart, J., Smalley, R. V., & Bosworth, K. (1993). Development and pilot evaluation of a computer-based support system for women with breast cancer. *Journal of Psychosocial Oncology, 11*(4), 69–93.

Haas, L. J., Benedict, J. G., & Kobos, J. C. (1996). Psychotherapy by telephone: Risks and benefits for psychologists and consumers. *Professional Psychology: Research and Practice, 27,* 154–160.

Harkins, J. E. (1993). Ergonomic considerations for communication technologies for deaf and hard-of-hearing people. In M. J. Smith & G. Salvendy (Eds.), *Human-computer interaction: Application and case studies.* New York: Elsevier.

Howe, D. (1997). *Free on-line dictionary of computing* [On-line]. [Available: World Wide Web URL: http://wombat.doc.ic.ac.uk/]

Hufford, B. J., Glueckauf, R. L., & Webb, P. M. (in press). *Rehabilitation Psychology.*

Krupnick, J. L., & Pincus, H. A. (1992). The cost-effectiveness of psychotherapy: A plan for research. *American Journal of Psychiatry, 149,* 1295–1305.

McQuillen, D., Glueckauf, R. L., Webb, P. M., & Dairaghi, J. E. (1998). *The development of therapeutic alliance in family therapy: The effects of therapy type, phase of life span, and stage of therapy.* Manuscript submitted for publication.

Murray, D. J., & Keller, P. A. (1991). Psychology and rural America: Current status and future directions. *American Psychologist, 46,* 220–231.

National Telecommunications and Information Administration. (1997, January 31). *Telemedicine report to Congress* [On-line]. [Available: World Wide Web URL: http://www.ntia.doc.gov/reports/telemed/]

Nickelson, D. W. (1996). Behavioral telehealth: Emerging practice, research and policy opportunities. *Behavioral Sciences and the Law, 14,* 443–457.

Office of Technological Assessment. (1990). *Health care in rural America* (OTA-H-434). Washington, DC: Government Printing Office.

Stein, L., Rothman, B., & Nakanishi, M. (1993). The telephone group: Accessing group service to the homebound. *Social Work with Groups, 16*(1–2), 203–215.

Telemedicine activity triples in one year, survey says. (1997, November 10). *American Medical News, 40*(42), 17.

Webster, J. (1995). ISDN update. *Telecommunications, 29*(9), 101–103.

Wittson, C. L., & Dutton, R. (1956). A new tool in psychiatric education. *Mental Hospitals, 7,* 11–14.

Ziegler, R. G. (1981). Impairments of control and competence in epileptic children and their families. *Epilepsia, 22,* 339–346.

Chapter 32

The Computer Revolution and Assistive Technology

Leonard Holmes

The computer revolution has accelerated the pace of change in many fields. Many conveniences that we now take for granted did not exist 20 years ago. The field of assistive technology in rehabilitation has benefited greatly from this revolution. In chapter 31 of this volume Robert Glueckauf and colleagues discuss the field of telehealth and the rapid changes that we have seen in this field. This chapter will focus on assistive technologies, the remarkable changes that have occurred in the past two decades. We will also get a glimpse of what the future holds.

Resources that may be found online will be highlighted whenever possible, to enhance the availability of this material. Online locations are subject to change, however. If you cannot find the material at the location specified, try using only the root domain (such as http://www.abledata.com without any additional directory information) or try searching with one of the major search engines.

The Americans with Disabilities Act (ADA; 1990) requires employers to make reasonable accommodation for employees with disabilities. The act states in part:

> No covered entity shall discriminate against a qualified individual with a disability because of the disability of such individual in regard to job application procedures, the hiring, advancement, or discharge of employees, employee compensation, job training, and other terms, conditions, and privileges of employment. (Sec. 102, Discrimination, 42 U.S.C. 12112(a), General Rule, 1990)

This legislation has had an important influence on the development of assistive technology. Employers now have a strong incentive to hire persons with disabilities and to ensure their continued employment.

ASSISTIVE DEVICES FOR PHYSICAL DISABILITIES

Assistive technology is not a new field. The technology of the time has been used for centuries to assist persons who are handicapped to live more normal lives. Prostheses and assistive devices have existed since the beginning of recorded history. Canes, crutches, and peg legs are a part of our history. Antique manual wheelchairs still work, and they still provide improved mobility for persons with disabilities. The future promises wheelchairs that warn the user before hitting an object and even models that shut down power to prevent the user from driving into objects (Kolar, 1996).

The 1990 U.S. census reported that more than 13.1 million people in the United States (over 5% of the population) used assistive technologies (Scherer & Galvin, 1996). This is more than double the 1969 figure of 6.2 million. The authors attribute this increase to three factors: longer lives resulting from greater rates of survival from trauma or disease, advances in microelectronics and computers, and the passing of legislation (such as the ADA) mandating assistive technology for persons with disabilities.

The relationship between the ADA and assistive technologies is actually even more complex. The rapid developments in assistive technology have allowed persons with severe handicaps to enter the workforce and participate more actively in society. Their participation was initially hindered by curbs, stairways, and employer attitudes. The ADA was needed as a response to these obstacles.

The pace of most technology has accelerated in recent years, and assistive technologies are no exception. Physical medicine and rehabilitation professionals now have a broad range of devices to choose from when working with a patient. This broad availability raises some interesting issues.

Surveys have found that around one third of assistive devices are abandoned and not used after a period of time (Phillips & Zhao, 1993). This finding has led to an increased emphasis on carefully matching the person with the proper assistive device. Galvin and Scherer (1996) edited an excellent volume reviewing all of the issues involved in this matching.

COMPUTERS AND DISABILITY

One device that has revolutionized the lives of people with disabilities is the personal computer. Computers allow people to be gainfully employed without requiring them to be physically fit. Many assistive devices have been developed specifically to allow even persons with severe disabilities to use computers.

A computer was once a closet-sized machine kept in a climate-controlled room in a research facility. Since the 1970s, computers have become smaller and smaller, and they have become more accessible to the population. Whole industries and career fields have been revolutionized by this rapidly changing technology. In addition to their integration into assistive devices, computers themselves have opened doors to persons with disabilities. Computers can assist an individual with a disability to perform a job that formerly required an able-bodied person. Computer skills have also become necessary in many jobs. This has resulted in a new generation of assistive devices that allow persons with disabilities to use computers.

Computers perform extremely rapid numeric calculations based on ones and zeros (on and off). All of a computer's other abilities are based on this simple core ability. Humans have to get data into and out of a computer in some manner. The devices that allow such interactions are known as input devices and output devices. The keyboard and the mouse are examples of input devices, and monitors are examples of output devices. Persons with disabilities are often able to use computers with only these common input and output devices, but some disabilities necessitate other methods of input and output.

Most personal computers use keyboards as input devices. Modern computers often use a mouse, trackball, or other point-and-click device in addition to a keyboard. This creates obvious problems for persons with many different disabilities.

Persons who are visually impaired are able to use large monitors that project text and graphics onto a much larger screen. Many computer manufacturers now include monitors 19 inches and larger as options with the purchase of a new personal computer. Apple Computer has included a screen magnification program with its operating systems since 1989. IBM's OS/2 and Microsoft's Windows 95 and Windows 98 include similar programs. Braille output devices also are available, although they are generally limited to text output. Some newer devices allow graphics to be displayed by producing raised tactile images of line drawings on a special touch tablet. Text-to-speech software also is useful for this population.

The most common specialized input device for this population has been the braille keyboard. Voice recognition software is developing quickly, however. It is finally sophisticated enough to convert fluent speech into text without requiring regular pauses. The rate of change in some of these areas is so fast that this chapter will probably be out-of-date before it is printed.

Persons with physical disabilities are able to take advantage of a wide range of input and output devices. Individuals unable to use a standard keyboard have a variety of options available to them. Keyboard-emulating devices take input from an alternative device and make it look as if it came from a keyboard. In this manner persons with disabilities can operate "keyboards" by pointing their heads in a certain direction, moving their eyes in a certain direction, using a mouth stick, sipping and puffing on a straw, or speaking commands. There are also special keyboards that include all keys in an arrangement for use by one hand, and there are versions of these devices that include the emulation of mouse movements and clicks. Many physically disabled persons use voice recognition software.

Computers can be integrated into mechanical devices and environmental control systems. Cheatham and Magee (1997) review the devices that allow persons with disabilities to adjust room lighting, temperature, and entertainment equipment. In a similar manner computers are becoming integrated into devices that aid in driving a car. These advances will someday allow the safe operation of a motor vehicle by people who cannot use the traditional hand and foot controls. Hearing aids are benefiting from digital signal processing based on computer technology. We have reached the point where it is difficult to identify where the computer ends and the assistive device begins.

It is easy to become overwhelmed by these computerized devices as they become more and more complex. The multidisciplinary team approach is essential in addressing this complexity. Each member of the team will be able to address different needs of the patient to assure that the technology is actually used.

ASSISTING MOBILITY

Wheelchairs and Scooters

When many of us think of assistive devices, we think of wheelchairs. Perry (1991) traces the history of wheelchairs to two-wheeled carts that were known in Sumeria and Assyria in 3500 BC. He reports that actual wheelchairs were not invented until the 5th century AD in China. By the 12th century they had been imported to Europe, where they gained acceptance. Perry notes that the first motorized wheelchair was developed in 1912 and that commercial production of motorized chairs began in 1916. Manual wheelchairs are still useful for many persons with disabilities, but high-tech wheelchairs and scooters, many of which incorporate computer technology, are increasingly extending the mobility of patients.

Cutter and Blake (1997) review the factors to consider in making a decision concerning the prescription of a wheelchair. Manual wheelchairs should be both lightweight and durable. Nonfolding wheelchairs are generally stronger, but they are less easily transported. A wheelchair athlete needs an entirely different type of manual wheelchair from that required by a severely disabled person. Newer wheelchair models allow flexible placement of leg rests, arms, seats, wheels, and other parts. This allows the chair to change with the patient as rehabilitation progresses. Variables such as the distance between the axles, height, width, and wheel type affect the balance and stability of the chair. Many wheelchairs now allow the adjustment of rear wheel camber (which allows the top of the rear wheels to be closer together than the bottom). Trudel et al. (Trudel, Kirby, Ackroyd-Stolarz, & Kirkland, 1997) state that users of adjustable camber chairs report significantly higher incidents of instability than do other users. Even the type of seat cushion used can be critical for the comfort and health of the user (Rosenthal et al., 1996).

Reclining wheelchairs are needed by some persons who have poor trunk stability or little ability to shift their weight. These chairs are heavier and bulkier than others. Computerized switches and controls have resulted in less bulk. The weight and bulk of any transportation device is important when community mobility is considered. A bulky scooter or reclining wheelchair is useful in a shopping mall only if you can transport it to the mall. Because of the ADA most communities in the United States provide public transportation for persons with disabilities. There are also funds available for some people who have to modify a van or automobile in order to transport a wheelchair or scooter.

Electrically powered wheelchairs and scooters sometimes incorporate some of the same assistive technology used in personal computer input devices. These chairs are less portable than manual chairs, but they can be operated by a much wider variety of persons. Joysticks are often used as the steering and acceleration mechanism on electric wheelchairs and scooters. If the person does not have the manual dexterity needed for such a control, a tongue control or a sip-and-puff system controls pneumatic switches that serve the same purpose. Voice-activated controls also exist, but they have not been widely used. Recent advances in speech recognition promise increasingly usable voice-activated controls. Scooters are useful for persons with limited endurance, but they are seldom adequate if there is significant neuromuscular dysfunction. Letts (1991) wrote an excellent review of the state of power wheelchairs in 1991.

ORTHOTICS AND PROSTHETICS

Orthotics is a term for applying something (an orthosis) to the outside of the body to straighten it or improve its function. These devices are usually considered independently of assistive devices, although the distinction is often blurred. Static orthoses are designed to immobilize a body part or to support it in a static position. Splints and casts that facilitate healing are examples. Dynamic orthoses are designed to assist joint mobility and paralyzed or weak muscles. Traditionally, levers, pulleys, springs, elastics, and mobile power sources have been used.

Computerization has resulted in the miniaturization of some of these components. J. F. Lehmann (1992) edited an excellent volume of articles that summarizes the state of orthotics research and practice at that time.

Prosthetic devices are designed to aid persons who have lost a major limb. Prosthesis use has been recorded as far back in history as India's Rig-Veda period (3500–1800 BC) (Saunders, 1986). Although the exact number of amputations performed in the United States is unknown, the Amputee Coalition of America (1997) estimated that there were 400,000 Americans who had lost or were missing one or more limbs. They estimated that 100,000 amputations were performed every year. Over half of all lower-limb amputations occur in individuals with diabetes, and 60% of all amputations are due to some form of vascular disease.

Artificial limbs have become much more sophisticated, and microelectronic advances in computer technology allow some advanced prostheses to be controlled by muscles that remain above the site of the amputation, allowing improved mobility. Such myoelectric prostheses are becoming much more popular. A set of electrodes in the prosthesis socket detects electrical signals from a voluntarily contracting muscle in the stump or residual limb. The signals are amplified and used to control an electric motor in the prosthesis. The Utah Elbow is an advanced example of such a prosthesis. It utilizes two sets of electrodes along with microprocessor technology to provide elbow function and "terminal device operation" (Leonard & Meier, 1993). The terminal device on this prosthesis can be either a myoelectric artificial hand or a voluntarily opening metal hook.

Research is progressing on allowing direct nervous system control of prostheses. This is another rapidly moving area of technology and one that will certainly have progressed even further by the time you read this. As with other assistive devices, the physician and patient have difficult decisions to make concerning which type of prosthesis to use. Sears (1991) provides some guidance in this area.

Computers are increasingly used in the design and manufacture of prosthetic devices (Lim, 1997). These methods reduce the problems of human error and accuracy loss in order to obtain a more perfect fit.

After an injury or amputation a patient usually is fitted with a temporary or preparatory prosthesis. This allows the patient to become accustomed to such a device at the same time as a customized permanent prosthesis is being prepared. The residual limb needs time to stabilize before a final, definitive prosthesis can be fitted. As with other assistive devices, prostheses are sometimes abandoned by their users. Advanced myoelectric prostheses are often quite heavy and can become uncomfortable after a time. Lighter devices are more comfortable but more limited in function. Matching the patient with the proper prosthesis is critical.

ASSISTIVE DEVICES FOR COGNITIVE IMPAIRMENTS

The ADA affects more than employers. Colleges and universities also have been required to make accommodations for students under the ADA. Learning disabilities and attention deficit disorder are examples of cognitive disabilities that often require accommodation, but more severe cognitive impairments, such as mental retardation, can also benefit from assistive devices. Computers with spell-checkers were among the first assistive devices to be used with these populations. Other general software, such as memory aids, reference software, and word-prediction software, is also useful for some members of these populations.

In addition to the use of these general population software packages, special software has been written especially for these populations. Brain-injured patients often need extensive cognitive retraining. This process can be repetitive and tedious, and computers are being used increasingly to assist. An example of these uses is a software program called Brain Train (Falconer, 1998), which is used by institutions as well as by patients and families. It consists of a set of 55 subprograms designed to assist in rehabilitation of cognitive and behavioral deficits in brain-injured persons. It is claimed that the software can also assist persons who are developmentally disabled or have learning disabilities. A second Brain Train volume focuses on vocational readiness. More information is available at http://www.brain-train.com.

Vanderheiden (1996) describes a hypothetical device called the Companion, which would incorporate many different functions into a true assistive device. He envisions this device as a combination of a calendar reminder system, cueing system, artificial intelligence system, global positioning system (GPS), mapping system, infrared link to communicate with computers and automatic teller machines (ATMs) and smart card/debit card, and communications link to a central resource service. He described the use of this hypothetical device with the following scenario:

> Tim is awakened in the morning by his Companion which reminds him what day it is and what he needs to do first. It also reminds him that he has a meeting tonight with his counselor and that he is supposed to appear at the alternate worksite this morning. Tim has worked out a routine with his Companion in which he sort of mumbles what he is doing as he is going through his morning routine, and the Companion notes whether any important activity seems to be missing or out of order and asks him simple questions as reminders. Tim walks out to the bus stop. As the buses pull up, he aims the Companion at the name on the bus windshield display and pushes the trigger; the Companion reads the name of the bus to Tim and also tells him whether the buses seem to be ahead of or behind schedule. Tim's Companion also knows exactly which bus stop they are standing at (from the satellite GPS), whether Tim is where he should be, what time it is, and when to expect the bus.
>
> When the correct bus arrives, Tim gets on board, authorizes his smart card by voice to transfer the proper fare to the bus, and takes his seat.
>
> On his way home from the meeting with his counselor, Tim is very tired, falls asleep on the bus, and rides past his normal transfer stop. The Companion

> detects this and tries to wake him; it is tucked between Tim and the side of the bus, however, so it is muffled and Tim does not hear the signal over the noise of street construction. When Tim wakes up, he finds himself in an unfamiliar neighborhood. He panics and gets off the bus, which drives away. He further panics and presses the Help button on his Companion. The Companion runs through a standard set of questions and comments to calm Tim and help him apply his own problem-solving skills. Tim aims the Companion at a number of street signs, pushing the button to have them read to him. The Companion realizes where they are, but does not have any information about the safety or potential resources for Tim in this neighborhood. It advises Tim to call in, so Tim pushes the button to contact the central resource point. A specially trained resource person appears on the Companion's screen; by using the Companion's camera, the resource person can also see Tim. All of Tim's information is displayed directly on the screen in front of the resource person, along with whatever information the Companion can provide on the situation, including Tim's exact location. The resource person directs Tim to a local building that will be safe and calls a cab, since there are no buses that will easily get Tim back home from that location at this time of night.

Although the Companion is a hypothetical device, it illustrates the potential of computer technology to revolutionize assistive devices for cognitive impairments.

THE INTERNET AND CONNECTIVITY

Another chapter in this book covers advances in telehealth and telemedicine. Most telehealth projects use high-speed networks that allow full-motion video and high-quality audio to connect underserved health care populations with urban medical centers. A slower network, the Internet, connects people all over the world. This network allows people with disabilities to connect with each other and to obtain information that would otherwise require traveling to a library. In that sense the Internet is an assistive device.

Persons with disabilities are now able to communicate easily with each other across long distances. They are also able to access information that was once available only in libraries. Because the Internet is simply a large network of computers, its document locations are subject to change. A few of the more stable Internet resources related to disabilities are listed here, but there is no guarantee that they will still be at these locations when you read this.

- http://www.usdoj.gov/crt/ada/—Americans with Disabilities Act Information on the Web. This site, sponsored by the U.S. Department of Justice, provides links to the text of the ADA, along with various explanatory documents and technical manuals.

- http://www.abledata.com/—the web address for the Abledata database of assistive technologies (an alternate address is http://trace.wisc.edu/tcel/abledata/). This database exists in various forms, but the on-line version is usually one of the most current. It was developed by The National Institute on Disability and Rehabilitation Research of the U.S. Department of Education.
- http://codi.buffalo.edu/—Cornucopia of Disability Information is a site at the State University of New York at Buffalo that provides disability resources for consumers and professionals.
- http://www.naric.com/naric/—The National Rehabilitation Information Center (NARIC) is a federally funded library and information center on disability and rehabilitation. NARIC collects and disseminates the results of federally funded research projects. Check http://www.cais.com/naric/search/ for other resources located at NARIC's Instant Disability Center.
- http://www.healthfinder.gov/—Healthfinder is the U.S. government's consumer gateway site for health information on the World Wide Web.

THE FUTURE?

There is a scene in one of the *Star Trek* movies in which Mr. Scott attempts to talk to a 20th-century computer. Nothing happens, of course. He then picks up the mouse and talks to the mouse. Again nothing happens. When he realizes that he must use his fingers to input information, he grumbles about the antiquated technology.

In the near future we will all talk to our computers. Speech recognition has just progressed to the point (in 1998) where it is truly useful. It will undoubtedly play a much greater role in the assistive devices of the future. The Internet and similar networks also will revolutionize access to information. Wireless modems already allow connection to the Internet. This capability may be built into future assistive devices. Will the wheelchair of the future come with built-in E-mail? Database capability and GPS also will be integrated into future devices. Enhanced speech synthesis will allow much more lifelike speech for those who can't speak on their own. Artificial limbs will likely become even more capable than natural limbs, realizing the dream of the "Six Million Dollar Man" and the "Bionic Woman" of television fame.

Vanderheiden's (1996) previously cited description of "the Companion" is a brave prediction of the future of assistive devices for cognitive impairments. Devices like the Companion will integrate old and new technology in a comprehensive way and will allow a severely disabled person to lead a much more normal life.

As computer technology gets faster, smaller, and lighter, the most sophisticated assistive devices will get smaller, lighter, and more capable. Space age polymers are replacing metal in many devices, and this also helps them lose weight. Someday we may no longer be required to trade the portability of a manual wheelchair for the improved mobility of a motorized wheelchair.

The best that we can really do is to predict the direction of things to come. If change continues at its current pace, this chapter will be obsolete before this book is revised. You, the reader, live in the future. You can see the future much more clearly than I.

REFERENCES

Americans with Disabilities Act. (1990). [Online]. Available: http://www.usdoj.gov/crt/ada/statute.html

Amputee Coalition of America. (1997). Causes and prevalence of limb loss. [Online]. Available: http://www.cdc.gov/nceh/programs/disabil/limb.htm

Cheatham, J., & Magee, K. (1997). Rehabilitation robotics and environmental control systems. *Physical Medicine and Rehabilitation: State of the Art Reviews, 11*(1), 133–150.

Cutter, N., & Blake, D. (1997). Wheelchair and seating systems: Clinical applications. *Physical Medicine and Rehabilitation: State of the Art Reviews, 11*(1), 107–132.

Falconer, J. (1998). Computers and brain injury: Some guidelines for rehabilitation [Online]. Available: http://www.brain-train.com/articles/computer.htm

Galvin, J., & Scherer, M. (Eds.). (1996). *Evaluating, selecting, and using appropriate assistive technology.* Gaithersburg, MD: Aspen.

Kolar, K. (1996). Seating and wheeled mobility aids. In J. C. Galvin & M. J. Scherer (Eds.), *Evaluating, selecting, and using appropriate assistive technology* (pp. 61–76). Gaithersburg, MD: Aspen.

Lehmann, J. F. (Ed.). (1992). Orthotics. *Physical Medicine and Rehabilitation Clinics of North America, 3,* 1.

Leonard, J., & Meier, R. (1993). Upper and lower extremity prosthetics. In J. DeLisa (Ed.), *Rehabilitative medicine principles and practice* (2nd ed., pp. 507–525). New York: J. B. Lippincott.

Letts, R. (1991). Power wheelchairs and other mobility aids. In R. M. Letts (Ed.), *Principles of seating the disabled* (pp. 263–286). Boca Raton, FL: CRC Press.

Lim, P. (1997). Advances in prosthetics: A clinical perspective. *Physical Medicine and Rehabilitation: State of the Art Reviews, 11*(1), 13–38.

Perry, A. (1991). The history of wheelchairs. In R. M. Letts (Ed.), *Principles of seating the disabled* (pp. 331–337). Boca Raton, FL: CRC Press.

Phillips, B., & Zhao, H. (1993). Predictors of assistive technology abandonment. *Assistive Technologies, 5,* 36–45.

Rosenthal, M., Felton, R., Hilean, D., Lee, M., Friedman, M., & Navach, J. (1996). A wheelchair cushion designed to redistribute sites of sitting pressure. *Archives of Physical Medicine and Rehabilitation, 77,* 278–282.

Saunders, G. T. (1986). *Lower limb amputations: A guide to rehabilitation.* Philadelphia: F. A. Davis.

Scherer, M., & Galvin, J. (1996). An outcomes perspective of quality pathways to the most appropriate technology. In J. C. Galvin & M. J. Scherer (Eds.), *Evaluating, selecting, and using appropriate assistive technology* (pp. 1–26). Gaithersburg, MD: Aspen.

Sears, H. (1991). Approaches to prescription of body-powered and myoelectric prostheses. *Physical Medicine and Rehabilitation Clinics of North America, 2*(2), 361–371.

Trudel, M., Kirby, R., Ackroyd-Stolarz, S., & Kirkland, S. (1997). Effects of rear-wheel camber on wheelchair stability. *Archives of Physical Medicine and Rehabilitation, 78,* 78–81.

U.S. Department of Health and Human Services. Prevalence of selected chronic conditions—United States, 1979–1981. (1986). *Vital and health statistics*, Series 10, (155), 29–32. Washington, DC: U.S. Government Printing Office.

Vanderheiden, G. (1996). Computer access and use by people with disabilities. In J. C. Galvin & M. J.Scherer (Eds.), *Evaluating, selecting, and using appropriate assistive technology* (pp. 237–276). Gaithersburg, MD: Aspen.

Chapter 33

Trends in Medical Rehabilitation Delivery and Payment Systems

Donald G. Kewman, Kristofer J. Hagglund, and Nancy E. Wirth

In the past 20 years, the U.S. health care system has been buffeted by explosive growth followed by massive pressures to contain costs. Medical rehabilitation was initially protected from cost-containment forces but is now undergoing significant transformation. This chapter will focus on the current status and trends in the payment for and delivery of medical rehabilitation services in the United States. It is possible to understand the current rehabilitation delivery system only within the context of health economic forces that are shaping its evolution.

The average annual per capita cost of health care in 1965 was $202, and total health costs consumed 5.7% of the U.S. gross domestic product (GDP). In 1994 the cost was $3,510, and total health costs consumed 13.7% of the GDP, or nearly 14 cents of every dollar spent (Health Care Financing Administration [HCFA], 1998). This growth in the proportion of the GDP consumed by health care has alarmed citizens and other payers of health care benefits, such as employers and government policymakers.

Growth in overall health care expenditures has been reflected in the growth of the rehabilitation field. For instance, during the period between 1990 and 1993, HCFA reported that payments for rehabilitation therapy in all settings increased 167%, to $10.4 billion (Shriver, 1996). The number of free-standing rehabilitation hospitals increased from 68 to 195 between 1965 and 1993, and the number of skilled nursing facilities (SNFs) increased from 8,200 to 10,400 between 1989 and 1995 (Frederickson & Cannon, 1995; HCFA, 1998).

Various factors have contributed to the tremendous growth in rehabilitation services. Advances in medical care have allowed more people to survive disabling conditions, thus increasing demand for services over longer periods of time. Buchanan, Rumpel, and Hoenig (1996) described an additional dynamic. They found that among Medicare recipients, growth in outpatient services from 1987 to 1990 was related to the availability of reimbursable services. Their analysis suggested that this growth was more likely attributable to good reimbursement to providers for their services and to provider decision making than to changes in demographics.

CONTINUUM OF REHABILITATION CARE

Inpatient Care

Rehabilitation services are delivered in a variety of settings, including intensive or critical care units, acute hospital units, inpatient rehabilitation programs, outpatient clinics, and home care. A common entry point for patients into the rehabilitation settings is from acute inpatient medical settings. In fact, 90% of patients admitted to inpatient rehabilitation settings are from acute hospital care. Eighty-two percent of patients are discharged from inpatient rehabilitation to the community; only 10% are discharged to nursing homes, and 6% return to acute care settings (Wolk & Blair, 1994).

Patients sometimes receive rehabilitation services from part or all of the rehabilitation team when they are in an intensive care or acute medical unit. If they transfer to a rehabilitation unit or facility, the services will consume a significant portion of the patient's day. In the case of Medicare patients, this constitutes a minimum of 3 hours per day. Typically, the interdisciplinary rehabilitation team will meet on a regular basis in "staffings" or patient care conferences to discuss each patient's progress and to refine goals and treatment strategies to ensure that services are delivered in a coordinated and efficient fashion.

Although the demand for inpatient rehabilitation services has remained strong, cost-containment efforts have put pressure on providers to reduce the length of rehabilitation hospitalization. This has created an increased need for rehabilitation services following hospital discharge and has been one reason for an increase in growth of subacute rehabilitation programs, home care services, and outpatient programs.

Subacute Rehabilitation, Skilled Nursing Facilities, and Residential Programs

Patients who can be safely discharged from the hospital but are not ready to return home may go to a subacute program, which is often part of an SNF. Alternatively, they may go to a regular nursing unit at an SNF or be admitted to a residential treatment program (often licensed as an adult foster care facility). Medicare recipients were more than three times more likely to be admitted to an SNF in 1994 compared to 1982 (HCFA, 1998a). Careful consideration of potential medical risks and patient safety in posthospital placement decisions is an important part of discharge planning (Wright, Rao, Smith, & Harvey, 1996).

Toward the end of the continuum of residential care are supervised living situations where a person may live in an apartment alone or with a roommate. These persons may function independently in the community but require some assistance or supervision by a rehabilitation provider, who may have contact with them once or several times a day. A new and growing living option, especially for the elderly, is an assisted living facility. Individuals usually live in apartment-like accommodations with assistance in homemaking chores and the availability of some supervision and personal assistance. These facilities are not regular venues for the delivery of rehabilitation services but constitute a major growth market in housing options for elderly persons with disabilities who do not have significant nursing care needs.

Home Care

The final step in the continuum of care is living at home with services provided either in an outpatient clinic or by home care providers. These community-based services may include personal assistance services, skilled nursing, and/or other services, such as occupational or physical therapy. The likelihood of a Medicare recipient receiving contracted services from a home health agency doubled between 1982 and 1994 (HCFA, 1998a). These home-based services may be combined with outpatient services from a rehabilitation clinic.

Personal assistance services are often a critical part of home care for persons with severe disabilities. Such services usually include help with activities of daily living (ADLs), such as eating, bathing, and grooming as well as mobility. The availability of personal care assistance has been shown to have a positive relationship with physical and mental health for persons with stroke, spinal cord injury, or traumatic brain injury. The provider is typically a nonprofessional, although there exist a handful of certification programs. These services are often provided by family members. When personal assistance is provided only by family members, the interpersonal relationships may become strained or distorted. Combining the assistance of unrelated persons with family members seems to be associated with the best health outcomes (Nosek, 1993). The need to improve funding for such services in order to avoid unnecessary institutionalization has been a major goal of public policy activism by consumer groups of disabled persons.

Outpatient Care

Outpatient rehabilitation clinics may be hospital-based or free-standing. Free-standing clinics may be privately owned by the providers working in the clinic (e.g., private practice clinic) or owned by a hospital, health system, or corporation that specializes in providing rehabilitative care. Some clinics may contain just one rehabilitation discipline, such as physiatry or physical therapy. Other clinics may provide a range of rehabilitative services. The Medicare designation for the latter is a comprehensive outpatient rehabilitation facility (CORF). Some outpatient facilities contain programs that treat specialized groups of patients, such as those with sports injuries, chronic musculoskeletal pain, traumatic brain injuries, work-related injuries, or those in need of vocational rehabilitation services. In some cases, the patient may attend a day treatment program at such a facility and receive a highly interdisciplinary and integrated care program of a specialized nature. In other cases, a periodic appointment with a single provider may meet the patient's needs.

In recent years, rapid growth has occurred in the number of specialized outpatient programs, such as day treatment or day hospital programs, in which patients can receive intensive and comprehensive services from an interdisciplinary team of rehabilitation professionals. These settings are appropriate for patients who no longer require the same level of physician and/or skilled nursing support available in a hospital or subacute facility but need extensive therapy to improve functioning. Many of these specialized outpatient day treatment programs have focused on caring for persons with brain injuries or patients with disabling musculoskeletal pain problems, including persons with work-related injuries. In the case of persons with musculoskeletal pain, sometimes the treatment venue has been the work site, where individuals receive therapy and resume their previous duties guided by the rehabilitation staff.

Telehealth

With many rehabilitation centers and specialty programs residing in large metropolitan areas and few programs in smaller cities and rural areas, accessibility to services remains a problem (see Glueckauf et al., chapter 31, this volume). The transmission of voice, data, and images to remote locations by using telecommunications techniques has given rise to increased opportunities for rehabilitation providers to offer some specialized information and services to remote locations, such as the offices of less specialized rural providers or the homes of patients (Temkin, Ulicny, & Vesmarovich, 1996). Various challenges remain to be overcome, such as reimbursement, licensing requirements in different states, privacy, and confidentiality. An American Psychological Association report raises concern that adoption of behavioral telehealth technology could force practitioners to see people online in order to reduce costs, without attention paid to the benefits of face-to-face interactions (Nickelson, 1997).

Vertically Integrated Continuum of Rehabilitation Care

Another major dynamic shaping the delivery system is the effort of hospitals and health care systems, including rehabilitation providers, to develop a vertically integrated continuum of rehabilitation care. The health system will own or contract with each component in the care continuum, including emergency transport, hospitals, rehabilitation facilities, subacute units, SNFs, outpatient clinics, and home care agencies (Shortell, Gillies, Anderson, Erickson, & Mitchell, 1996). In the past, outpatient rehabilitation therapy services and physician clinics tended to be practitioner-owned, private practice settings. Increasingly, such practices are being acquired by or are affiliating with a larger network. Many of these networks are publicly traded companies that are attempting to achieve sufficient geographic coverage to dominate a market, thereby reducing opportunity for small independent providers (Gill, 1995).

INTERDISCIPLINARY REHABILITATION CARE

As described in chapter 1, patients receive services from a variety of therapists to improve cognitive, behavioral, and physical functioning. The core rehabilitation team typically includes a physician (often a physiatrist, who is a physician practicing the specialty of physical medicine and rehabilitation), rehabilitation psychologist or neuropsychologist, social worker, nurse, physical therapist, occupational therapist, and speech/language pathologist. This team may be supplemented by various other professionals, including case managers, orthotists, prosthetists, recreation therapists, dietitians, rehabilitation engineers, vocational rehabilitation counselors, chaplains, teachers, and others.

In some inpatient programs, the patient may be treated by a team that specializes in a particular diagnosis, such as spinal cord injury or brain injury. Specialized teams have been shown to reduce length of stay (e.g., see Tator,

Duncan, Edmonds, Lapczak, & Andrews, 1993) with equal or better outcomes, presumably through greater efficiencies in patient care. The goal of therapeutic intervention is maximal independence and discharge to the "least restrictive" and usually least costly environment. Rehabilitation has been quite successful in this endeavor. Using spinal cord injury (SCI) as an example, 92% of individuals reside in private residences in the community following discharge and only 4% of persons with SCI are transferred to nursing homes (Dijkers, Buda Abela, Gans, & Gordon, 1995).

Technological aids that can assist persons with disability are a promising and increasingly important component of rehabilitative care (Symington, 1994). Rehabilitation engineers are sometimes involved in the evaluation and consideration of such equipment, as well as the customization of this equipment to meet the unique needs of users. However, funding to purchase this assistive technology remains out of reach for many consumers.

Over the past 20 years rehabilitation case managers have become a more significant part of the rehabilitation team. The role of case manager is often multifaceted and may be carried out by individuals with specific treatment roles on the team, such as a physician, nurse, psychologist, or social worker. However, in recent years, this role often has been assumed by an individual who specializes in this activity and is not a direct treatment provider. Most commonly, this person is either employed by the rehabilitation provider, the managed care organization (MCO), or the patient's insurance company. In some cases, there may be separate case managers associated with each of these interests.

Increasingly, these case managers play a pivotal role in recommending and arranging for the provision of needed care for the patient through the rehabilitation continuum. Also, this person may recommend against the approval or payment of services. This decision may be based on lack of insurance coverage for these benefits, lack of perceived need for the service, or the availability of a more cost-effective alternative. This role sometimes has led to friction between case managers and providers, who see their professional judgment challenged, and patients who resent being denied benefits to which they feel entitled.

Economic pressures to streamline the rehabilitation team have continued to mount, taking several forms. Some providers have made an effort to rely more heavily on technicians or aides to supply a range of rehabilitation services. Sometimes referred to as multiskilling, this mode of service provision often crosses traditional disciplinary lines; for example, a technician or unlicensed assistant may supply services usually provided by an occupational therapist and a physical therapist. Multiskilling has been criticized frequently because it was developed as a cost-containment method and may lead to the provision of service by unqualified providers, resulting in poorer rehabilitation outcomes.

FUNDING SOURCES FOR MEDICAL REHABILITATION

Private Payers

Employers pay for or subsidize health care coverage for the majority of working Americans and their families. Over the past two decades, private-sector MCOs have been "transforming the American health care system" (Tannenbaum & Hurley, 1995, p. 213). Nearly three quarters of the U.S. workforce with health insurance is enrolled in a managed care plan (Jensen, Morrisey, Gaffney, & Liston, 1997). The rapid conversion from fee-for-service to managed care in the private sector of health care is largely attributable to its cost-containment attributes. In 1995 health insurance premiums increased only 2.3%, a growth rate less than the rate of inflation (Jensen et al., 1997). Many believe that this slowed growth rate is a result of the growth of managed care, although there are insufficient data to make this causal conclusion (Jensen et al., 1997). Nevertheless, employers are pleased with the results, and managed care is likely to continue to remain the primary health care system for the private sector in the near future.

The most common types of managed care plans are health maintenance organizations (HMOs), preferred provider organizations (PPOs), and point-of-service plans (POSs). Although thorough descriptions of these types of managed care plans are beyond the scope of this chapter, the following summarizes the key differences.

HMOs are the oldest type of managed care plan, the most famous of which is Kaiser-Permanente, which began its public operation in 1945 and now has approximately 9.2 million enrollees (Iglehart, 1994). HMOs accept a capitation payment from the employer (or other payer) to deliver all the care necessary for its employees and their covered dependents. In a capitated contract, the HMO is paid a fixed sum of dollars for each member or enrollee of a plan, usually on a "per person per month" basis. The plan must meet the medical needs of all covered persons, using the aggregate of this fixed dollar amount. Typically, each enrollee in an HMO selects a primary care provider, who coordinates all care and who authorizes all care that he or she doesn't provide, including specialty care, hospitalization, and so on. The HMO may directly employ all, some, or none of the health care providers on its panel. If they are not employees of the HMO, the providers will usually have a contract with the HMO and share in the financial risks associated with the provision of care.

PPOs are plans created by an MCO to develop and contract with groups of providers, who agree to accept the plans' payment rates. The enrollee has a financial incentive to seek out the "preferred providers" because there may be no or lower co-payments. PPOs do not always have an assigned/selected primary care provider who authorizes services. Enrollees in POS plans have direct access to both preferred (or in-network) providers and out-of-network providers. Usually, enrollees select or are assigned a primary care provider who coordinates and authorizes care (often including out-of-network services). Again, the enrollee has a financial incentive to seek in-network services because the payment coverage is better.

Government Programs

Publicly financed health care programs accounted for nearly 47% of total national health care expenditures in 1998 ($540 billion of $1,147 billion). Medicare and Medicaid account for most of this spending, much of it directed to rehabilitation and other services for the elderly and people with disabilities. Patient populations at some rehabilitation facilities are composed primarily of Medicare and Medicaid recipients. Since their inception, both Medicare and Medicaid expenditures have consistently outpaced the rate of inflation and the rate of growth in expenditures of private funds. Federal and state legislative bodies have acted to slow this rapid growth rate through regulatory legislation and by encouraging experimentation in health care delivery models (Levit, Lazenby, & Braden, 1998). Health care delivery is being rapidly converted from fee-for-service reimbursement to managed care, especially capitated contracts with commercial MCOs.

Medicare

Title XVIII of the Social Security Act of 1965, otherwise known as Medicare, is the largest public payer of health care (Levit et al., 1998). Medicare is a social insurance program for persons over 65 years old and for people with disabilities who have a sufficient work history to qualify for Social Security disability insurance (SSDI) for 24 consecutive months. As of 1995, approximately 12% of Medicare beneficiaries (4.4 million) had a disability and were younger than 65 (Davis & O'Brien, 1996).

Part A of Medicare covers inpatient hospitalization, SNF care, home health care, and hospice care. Supplemental medical insurance (Part B) of Medicare is optional coverage that pays for physician and psychological services and other services, such as durable medical equipment, laboratory tests, medical supplies, and therapies (HCFA, 1998c). Contrary to popular belief, Medicare Part A expenditures are derived from mandatory payroll deductions from *current* wage earners. As health care costs rise and the population ages, Medicare Part A increasingly grows closer to financial insolvency. Depending on legislative action, Medicare Part A could exhaust its funds within the next few years. To slow down Medicare's cost inflation, federal legislation has encouraged experimental health care delivery programs and use of voluntary enrollment in managed care programs.

Medicaid

Medicaid (Title XIX of the Social Security Act) is a program jointly sponsored by the federal government and the states or territories. Within broad federal guidelines, each state establishes its own eligibility rules, determines the type and amount of services, sets provider payment rates, and administers its own program (HCFA, 1998b). States receive "matching" funds from the federal government to help offset the costs of care. The matching formula is based on the per capita income of each state or territory. Medicaid is the largest purchaser of health care services for the neediest and poorest people in the United States. In 1997, Medicaid covered approximately 40 million individuals, making it the most significant component of the "safety net." Medicaid's 1996 expenditures were $147.7 billion, representing 30.6% of government expenditures for health care in the United States (HCFA, 1998b).

Approximately 6.6 million, or 17%, of Medicaid recipients have a cognitive, psychiatric, or physical disability; and a significant portion of Medicaid beneficiaries have multiple disabilities, further complicating health care service delivery. Furthermore, the elderly or disabled with low incomes who are eligible for Medicare are also eligible for supplemental Medicaid coverage. As of 1995 there were approximately 5.9 million people who were dually enrolled as qualified medicare beneficiaries. Among those eligible for Medicaid because of a disability, the number of children has grown from 14% in 1987 to 22% in 1994. The most common diagnosis is mental retardation or developmental disability (44%), with psychiatric disorders being the next most common (23%) (HCFA, 1998b). This percentage is likely to grow substantially with the implementation of the Children's Health Insurance Program (CHIP) that is described below (Rosenbaum, Johnson, Sonosky, Markus, & DeGraw, 1998). In contrast, 32% of adults with disabilities have diseases of the musculoskeletal system, and 25% have diseases of the nervous system or sense organs. In this era of cost containment and experimentation with health care delivery, it is important to remember that people under 65 with disabilities comprise 17% of the enrollees in Medicaid, but spending for this group accounted for 41% of the costs in 1995 (HCFA, 1998a).

As with Medicare, basic medical services are covered by Medicaid. The states, however, have wide discretion in providing optional services, such as outpatient clinic services, diagnostic services, optometry, psychological care, rehabilitation, and physical therapy. Also like Medicare, fee-for-service reimbursement is the traditional payment system in Medicaid. Medicaid costs have been rising dramatically over the past decade, and state legislatures and governors, working with the HCFA, have been rapidly converting their Medicaid systems from fee-for-service to managed care. Both reimbursement/payment methodologies have created problems for obtaining health care for people with disabilities.

Common Deficiencies of Primary Care for Persons with a Disability

People receiving health care services from Medicaid and/or Medicare because of a disability typically have chronic and complex health problems. The complexity of their health care problems and their frequent need for a wide variety of services and specialized providers makes efficient delivery of health care services critical to preventing secondary conditions and maintaining the best quality of life. Unfortunately, access to health care services, especially primary care, has been a deficiency in the health care system (Burns, Batavia, Smith, & DeJong, 1990), including Medicare and Medicaid. For example, although the ADA requires clinics to be accessible, people with mobility impairments continue to have difficulties finding accessible clinics. Many clinic staff members are insufficiently trained to assist persons with mobility impairments or do not have access to the appropriate equipment needed for transfers to the examination table. In addition, this patient population frequently requires more time for their clinic appointments, needing additional assistance and time to undress. History taking is often lengthy because of a history of numerous hospitalizations and complications (Burns et al., 1990) as well as communication impairments. The office visit needs of people with disabilities combined with the low reimbursement from Medicaid contribute to the decision of many providers not to accept Medicaid patients.

Furthermore, different modes of treatment for primary care problems are frequently required because of the nature of the disability. Primary care physicians receive limited training in rehabilitation, and consumers report that primary care physicians sometimes confuse "normal" aspects of a chronic disabling condition with an urgent health care need. In general, people with disabilities often have difficulty finding primary care physicians who are knowledgeable about their disabilities (Francisco, Chae, & DeLisa, 1995; Gans, Mann, & Becker, 1993). They often must choose between attempting to educate their physicians or delaying/resisting seeking medical treatment (Burns et al., 1990).

Shortcomings of the Medicare and Medicaid System for Persons with Disabilities

The fee-for-service systems of Medicare and Medicaid have exacerbated some problems for persons with disabilities. Low reimbursement rates, limitations in coverage, and poor coordination of services place people with disabilities in a confusing and unfriendly health care maze. Furthermore, many people with disabilities have concomitant psychological and social problems, including affective and anxiety disorders, substance abuse or dependence, and social isolation (e.g., see Heinemann, Keen, Donohue, & Schnoll, 1988). For many, behavioral difficulties such as poor adherence to treatment regimens result in costly complications and secondary disabilities. These problems are exacerbated by low income and difficulties in meeting everyday basic living needs (Blendon et al., 1993). When psychological, social, and daily living needs go unmet, quality of life and medical status are worsened and health care costs are significantly increased (Friedman, Sobel, Myers, Caudill, & Benson, 1995).

The limited available research supports these impressions. For example, Rosenbach (1995) found that among nonelderly disabled Medicare beneficiaries, approximately 25% reported at least one unmet need resulting from a serious health problem. Despite the complex health care problems of this population, 9% reported no usual source of medical care, and an additional 9.4% had a usual source of care but no regular physician. The most common barrier to care was lack of or limited coverage for needed services and inability to pay (Rosenbach, 1995). These results were consistent with previous research demonstrating that 23% of nonelderly Medicare beneficiaries with disabilities had experienced a serious health problem over the course of a year but were unable to obtain the needed care. Financial barriers were again the most significant impediment to access (Rosenbach & Huber, 1993). A 1994 analysis of the Medicare Current Beneficiary Survey (MCBS) found that 26% of disabled Medicare beneficiaries delayed care because of costs, even though they were experiencing a serious health problem (Gold et al., 1997). These authors also found also that 14% reported problems obtaining care over the previous year, compared with only 3% of elderly Medicare beneficiaries.

Managed Care Models in Government-Funded Programs

Both Medicaid and Medicare have been experimenting with health care delivery models that provide an alternative to the fee-for-services system. Medicaid's conversion to managed care has been much more rapid than that of Medicare. Further legislation will be required to make such a dramatic shift in Medicare. Additionally, the Medicare program is exclusively administered through the federal government, whereas Medicaid is essentially 53 separate programs. This creates numerous obstacles to developing and implementing model managed care programs for Medicare recipients with disabilities compared to Medicaid, where each state government has some latitude in experimenting with alternative delivery systems.

Although most states began converting fee-for-service Medicaid to managed care with the use of a primary care case management model, there has been rapid growth in risk-based managed care contracting since 1994. In this situation a Medicaid agency contracts with an MCO to provide an agreed on set of services in exchange for a preset capitated payment for the entire health care needs of a patient. Payment is not contingent on the level of service provided unless special services or programs (i.e., transplant services) are exempted from the contract and paid by Medicaid on a fee-for-service basis. In many Medicaid programs, mental health services also are "carved out," creating a separate subcapitation despite the fact that most policy analysts recommend complete integration of mental health services. For rehabilitation clients this can result in a subcontract with a separate set of mental health providers that may not be a part of the rehabilitation team and lack specialized knowledge of the role of the person's disability. Also, savings incurred by this integration are not available to fund non-mental-health care. Until such services are integrated, the false distinction between mind and body will be perpetuated, and health care delivery will continue to be uncoordinated and ineffective. In addition, Medicaid plans often do not include people who receive both Medicare and Medicaid ("Qualified Medicare Beneficiaries"). The regulations of the two programs are frequently incompatible, thereby complicating the coordination of health care services and financing. States can apply to HCFA to obtain waivers to combine the funding streams of these two programs in order to develop innovative health care delivery programs.

Theoretically, managed care has the potential to improve care for medically complex, high-cost populations, such as people with disabilities (Reilly, Coburn, & Kilbreth, 1990) by employing organized delivery systems that emphasize timely, comprehensive, and community-based services. However, concerns have been raised about Medicaid's contracting with commercial MCOs to provide care for its beneficiaries with disabilities (e.g., Mitchell & Riley, 1997; Tannenbaum & Hurley, 1995). The complexity of the health care needs and the costs of care for people with disabilities may overwhelm an unprepared managed care system. Inadequate provider networks, lack of ancillary services, or inadequate capitation may result in clinical and financial disaster (Tannenbaum & Hurley, 1995). MCOs have traditionally avoided complex, high-cost populations and therefore have limited experience in implementing effective programs. MCOs that choose to serve people with disabilities will have to address these issues.

Research on the impact of managed Medicaid and Medicare has demonstrated mixed results. For example, a large 1996 national survey (Gold et al., 1997) of elderly and nonelderly individuals with disabilities compared the performance of Medicaid fee-for-service systems to managed care plans. People with disabilities experienced difficulty with obtaining needed services in both managed care and fee-for-service systems. The nonelderly disabled Medicare beneficiaries in managed care plans reported more frequently that they could not obtain a referral to a specialist from their primary care physician than did elderly who were in managed care. The former also reported unmet needs for hospitalization and home health care. They were more likely to experience delays in obtaining services while waiting for approval from their managed care plan. Furthermore, compared to the data from the fee-for-service survey and the elderly in managed care plans, people with disabilities had more trouble with access to care, especially specialty services (Gold et al., 1997).

Not all of the public sector managed care efforts have failed people with disabilities. In their review of five states that have implemented such programs, Gold, Sparer, and Chu (1996) highlight some programmatic aspects that have resulted in improved access and care. Overall, however, they concluded that people with chronic illness or disabilities are more vulnerable to problems in health care delivery. They noted also that most states had minimal baseline data on access to care and few quality assurance monitors to evaluate the specific problems that might be encountered by people with disabilities. They concluded that there is a need to develop new systems specifically for vulnerable populations. Rehabilitation models of care, described below, emphasize integrated and interdisciplinary methods and focus on long-term functional outcomes and reducing handicaps. Such models must be effectively integrated into managed care for people with disabilities.

Catastrophic Insurance

Little is known about how health care changes will affect the delivery of rehabilitation services paid for by other forms of disability insurance, such as no-fault automobile catastrophic insurance, long-term disability insurance, and workers' compensation. Workers' compensation is different from most health programs because it provides for income replacement for injured workers as well as medical care. The significant costs associated with these benefits have led to tremendous efforts to rehabilitate workers and return them to work. Medical case management has been used for many years by workers' compensation carriers in an attempt to control excessive costs secondary to overutilization of services. Prolonged disability is responsible for the greatest costs and involves medical, psychological, and socioecological issues that are best addressed by a multidisciplinary team. It is not clear, however, how often a rehabilitation model has been used effectively for temporarily or permanently disabled workers despite its proven efficacy with some groups of disabled persons.

Over the past two decades workers' compensation costs rapidly rose to become a substantial business expense. Dembe and colleagues (Dembe, Himmelstein, Stevens, & Beachler, 1997) reported that workers' compensation costs rose 64% from 1984 to 1993, after adjusting for inflation, and made up 2.4% of the private sector payroll in 1991. Medical care costs overtook income replacement in total workers' compensation costs, something that had not happened in many years. Also, market competition among workers' compensation carriers, workers' demands for improved care, and employers' efforts to reduce costs and streamline administration have contributed to reform efforts. With these concerns in mind, more than 25 states have begun to enact legislation to reform workers' compensation, most of them authorizing or mandating managed care health delivery (Dembe et al., 1997). Also, efforts have increased to link workers' compensation and general health care to reduce administrative costs, control cost shifting, and increase coordination of care, financing, and administration (Dembe et al., 1997).

Only a few studies have examined either the short-term or long-term outcomes among people with disabilities using payer source (e.g., workers' compensation) as a variable. Tate et al. (1994), for example, examined the effects of payer type (Medicaid, catastrophic insurance, and private payer), extent of benefits, and independent living resources on functional, psychological, and social outcomes among 111 individuals with SCI. All participants were at least 2 years postdischarge from acute rehabilitation. Among the most significant findings, people who had private insurance reported greater work and school activities compared to those with Medicaid or catastrophic no-fault insurance. Transportation benefits also were positively related to participation in work and school activities. Surprisingly, there was an inverse relationship between the extent of benefits and psychological and social outcome. The authors caution that the type of payment system and rules may foster dependency and poorer psychosocial outcome. Persons receiving catastrophic insurance benefits continually are forced to dramatize their needs to the insurance carrier or case manager in order to obtain benefits, sometimes creating a disincentive to increase independence. They suggested that a voucher system that allows personal choice of health care benefits may facilitate less dependency, improve psychological and social outcomes, and increase participation in functional activities, including work and school. The voucher system could be accompanied by an educational program to help individuals make choices of benefits that would maximize their independence and fit their unique situation.

FUNDING OF HEALTH CARE FOR CHILDREN WITH DISABILITIES

Approximately 5% of U.S. children and adolescents have a chronic health condition that interferes with one or more major life activities. Less than 1% of children have three or more chronic conditions, but developmental delays, learning disabilities, and emotional and behavioral problems are much more prevalent among this group of children with multiple chronic conditions (Newacheck & Stoddard, 1994). In general, children with chronic disabling conditions require coordinated specialized services, including occupational therapy, physical therapy, psychological and social services, speech and language therapy, and home care. As with adults, children with chronic disabling conditions are a relatively small percentage of children but utilize a large percentage of health care services (Newacheck & Taylor, 1992). Medicaid, which covers approximately 1 million children with physical or mental disabilities, spent $7.1 billion on health care for those children in 1995 (The Kaiser Commission on the Future of Medicaid, 1997). Also, children with chronic disabling conditions receive services funded by Title V programs (Social Security Act) such as the Bureau of Maternal and Child Health, state health care programs, and school systems.

In addition to federal- and state-funded health care programs, approximately 60% of children with chronic disabling conditions receive services funded by private insurance. Often, these policies have restrictions on the types and scope of services, especially ancillary services and home care (Shonkoff et al., 1994), and many have annual or lifetime caps on benefits and/or cover only part of the costs of health care services. The children receiving health care through Medicaid and private insurance are rapidly being enrolled into managed care programs. The implications of these changes have yet to be fully realized, but many children's health care advocates have expressed concerns similar to those stated about the limitations of managed care for adults with disabilities.

Research has revealed mixed results on the effects of managed care on the outcomes of children with chronic disabling conditions. For example, Horwitz and Stein (1990) compared benefits for a sample of HMOs with traditional indemnity insurers in Connecticut paying for services to children on a fee-for-service basis. HMOs were found to offer more preventive care and increased access to care. However, both plans tended to have restrictions on services most commonly used by these children (mental health services and durable medical equipment). Case managers from both plans focused more on controlling costs than coordinating care. The study concluded that neither organization offered a comprehensive system of care to children with special health care needs.

Fox and Wicks (1993) conducted a cross-sectional survey of almost 700,000 children with disabilities resulting from chronic conditions. HMOs typically approved specialty care only when significant improvement could be documented within a short time. Other identified problems included difficulty in accessing specialists, along with an insufficient number of specialists to provide consumer choice. Another survey (Fox, Wicks, & Newacheck, 1993) of state Medicaid offices documented that some HMOs were resistant to providing necessary mental health, speech, and occupational therapy services to children with special health care needs.

Children's Health Insurance Program

The Children's Health Insurance Program, codified as Title XXI of the Social Security Act, was enacted as part of the Balanced Budget Act of 1997. The purpose of this law was to extend insurance and health care to uninsured children. As a federal grant-in-aid program, this law encourages states to extend health care coverage either through Medicaid or through an alternative program to low-income, uninsured children. In return, the states may receive matching funds from the federal government. The Congressional Budget Office (CBO) projects that CHIP will significantly increase coverage for previously uninsured children (as many as 2.8 million) while leading to enrollment of another 660,000 already eligible for Medicaid under current regulations (Rosenbaum et al., 1998). An important regulation of CHIP for children with disabilities is that states may not deny enrollment or coverage because of preexisting conditions (Rosenbaum et al., 1998).

MANAGED CARE FOR PERSONS WITH DISABILITIES

The literature is nearly devoid of studies that evaluate private sector managed care programs for people with disabilities. Evaluation studies of managed care performance in the general population have focused on utilization of services and costs. Rarely are these measures of performance paired with analyses of the health status of the population. The results of the performance of managed care on health outcomes have been mixed, and there are virtually no data on functional health-related quality of life (Miller & Luft, 1994).

Three managed care programs designed specifically for people with disabilities have been evaluated and described in the literature. Wayne State University has utilized the rehabilitation model to develop a primary care system for Medicaid recipients with disabilities. This program has combined a rehabilitation hospital and a physiatry practice to provide a smooth transition from a comprehensive inpatient rehabilitation program to an outpatient program emphasizing a primary care system for adults with disabilities. The types of disabilities seen are varied but include traumatic brain injury, SCI, and stroke. In collaboration with Michigan's Medicaid agency, the program was able to improve access to care through funding of transportation; but after the Medicaid agency discontinued its support of this aspect of the program, the rate of "did not keep appointments" rapidly increased. This program provides a 24-hour on-call access to urgent medical service, and patients can be seen on an urgent basis in clinics during the work week. The program has developed close relationships with the emergency department and urgent care center to control unnecessary use of emergency services. Focusing on prevention and health maintenance, the program shows promise for achieving its goals of improved functioning, community reintegration, and reduction in unnecessary, high-cost treatment (Gans et al., 1993).

Similarly, Shepherd Rehabilitation Center of Atlanta has developed the Shepherd Care Network. Shepard is designing a primary care system for people with spinal cord dysfunction, brain injury, multiple sclerosis, and related disorders. The Shepherd Care Network will utilize nurse practitioners in collaboration with physiatrists to provide primary care around the Atlanta area. This program has been working with Medicaid to develop a contracted managed care arrangement to provide primary and rehabilitation care (DeJong, 1997).

Boston's Community Medical Group has been providing services to the severely disabled and people with AIDS since 1982 but began delivering care under a prepaid, capitated reimbursement system in 1992. The HMO that is responsible for the capitated contracting was the allied organization (Community Medical Alliance [CMA]), now part of Neighborhood Health Plan. Boston Community Medical Group has a reputation for emphasizing consumer autonomy in living and health care decisions. They have maintained a commitment to socially responsible, cost-effective care. This program has enjoyed great success because it utilizes providers knowledgeable about disability and has given them flexibility in ordering health care services. Providers and consumers work together in choosing the least restrictive but most effective health care service. This program achieved a decrease in medical costs of up to 35% in persons with SCIs, including fewer skin graft operations for pressure ulcers and fewer respiratory infections. Also, a CMA telephone survey found that 89% of respondents were satisfied with the program and 95% would recommend the program to others (Master et al., 1996).

FOR-PROFIT VERSUS NOT-FOR-PROFIT SECTORS IN THE DELIVERY OF REHABILITATION CARE

Many rehabilitation clinics and hospital services are for-profit taxpaying businesses with accountability to owners or stockholders for profitability. This means that the less income that is paid out for patient care and administrative expenses, the more money there is to invest in the growth of the company or to pay owners or stockholders. A study of the impact of the ownership arrangement and profitability in outpatient physical therapy clinics found that clinics jointly owned by physicians and physical therapists saw patients for 39%–45% more visits than in non-physician-owned comprehensive rehabilitation facilities providing services, and concomitantly, their revenue per patient was 30%–40% higher (Mitchell & Scott, 1992). Furthermore, it appeared that more care was delivered by unlicensed personnel in the physician-owned practices. Such findings have contributed to the regulations concerning physician referrals to rehabilitation facilities that they own. A study of home health agencies found that care was four times more expensive in for-profit proprietary agencies than in public agencies (Williams, 1994). When comparisons were made between for-profit and not-for-profit rehabilitation hospitals, for-profit hospitals showed higher net revenue and profits and employed fewer people than nonprofit hospitals did (McCue & Thompson, 1995). A large part of the growth in outpatient programs has been in for-profit corporations. Clearly, the potential for profit and growth has been recognized by these companies.

Nonprofit entities do not pay dividends on profits and do not answer to shareholders but still face pressures to hold down costs and realize a positive financial margin to reinvest in the organization's future. Some health care systems are owned and operated by local or state governments or the federal government. This includes city, county, and state health facilities and agencies as well as most public university medical centers. In addition, the military and Veterans Administration are among the largest providers of rehabilitation services (Wilson & Kizer, 1997). The Veterans Administration Medical Centers (VAMC) rehabilitation departments are particularly well known for work with military service veterans with stroke, SCI, and amputations. VAMCs offer comprehensive care, including some options for care in nursing homes, residential placements, and home care. Coverage and benefits are dependent on several factors, such as whether the health problem was incurred during or is related to service in the military (i.e., service-connected) and financial resources of the veteran.

SPECIFIC COST-CONTAINMENT STRATEGIES

Prospective Payment Systems

As mentioned earlier, much of the expansion in the continuum of rehabilitation care can be credited to a stable source of funding through Medicare and Medicaid recipients who comprise approximately half of patients seeking rehabilitation services (Aitchison, 1993). A second funding boon was the adoption of the Tax Equity and Fiscal Responsibility Act (TEFRA) in 1982, which allowed many rehabilitation hospitals and units to be reimbursed by Medicare on the basis of the hospital's cost per discharge, rather than on a less lucrative prospective payment system (PPS), under which facilities are reimbursed a predetermined fee for hospitalization according to the patient's diagnosis or diagnostic related groups (DRGs).

Exemption from prospective payment for rehabilitation facilities was made because DRGs did not account well for the high variability in hospital resource utilization for rehabilitation patients. Various shortcomings of this system are evident, and modifications are likely to occur (Wynn, 1997). Recently, an analysis by Schneider, Cromwell, and McGuire (1993) found that TEFRA limits have been insufficient to account for increases in costs of care provision by rehabilitation facilities. However, the TEFRA payment system has provided a financial incentive for rehabilitation hospitals to discharge patients quickly (Chan et al., 1997). The hospital can collect incentive payments from Medicare for reducing its per-patient charge up to 10% compared to a "base year," which can be accomplished by reducing length of patient stay. This has caused the number of discharges from rehabilitation hospitals to SNFs to increase 48% from 1992 to 1994 (Wynn, 1997). It also has caused facilities to try to admit fewer complex and severely disabled patients. In response to these issues, Congress passed a provision in the Balanced Budget Act of 1997 that mandated that a PPS be implemented on October 1, 2000. This means that some kind of PPS that pays for hospitalization based on characteristics of the patients will be adopted.

One PPS that has been considered in the past would have reimbursed facilities largely on the basis of a patient's level of physical and cognitive functioning. Harada, Kominski, and Sofaer (1993) developed one example of a system for classifying rehabilitation patients that would lend itself to a PPS. Patients are grouped into one of 33 functional-related groupings (FRGs) composed of patients with similar diagnostic characteristics and use of clinical resources. Sutton, DeJong, Song, and Wilkerson (1997) have concluded that such a model would do better to link resource utilization with reimbursement, resulting in greater equity for inpatient reimbursement. However, Sutton, DeJong, and Wilkerson (1996) indicated that an FRG-based reimbursement system must find a mechanism to make sure that there are financial incentives to providers for obtaining good functionally based outcomes. Stineman, Goin, Granger, Fiedler, and Williams (1997) proposed such an outcome-based payment system for rehabilitation, using comparisons with discharge expectancies for functional outcomes derived from large numbers of people classified according to FRGs.

Instead of the above models, the PPS currently being developed by HCFA will most likely use a reimbursement system for treatment of Medicare patients in hospital rehabilitation units similar to the one that has been developed for use by SNFs. This system uses information from a modified version of the Minimum Data Set (MDS) and resource utilization groups (RUGs). RUGs categorize patients according to typical patterns of utilization of staff time, effort, supplies, and equipment as well as certain functional characteristics of the patient (Fries et al., 1994; "What You Can Expect," 1998). Patients with greater needs are in a higher payment category. This system also would pay for patient care based on the number of days that it is delivered, unlike the current system or some of the proposed FRG-based systems in which the hospital receives a set amount regardless of the actual resources used. For non-Medicare patients, care may continue to be reimbursed at the lowest rate that a payer can negotiate. In this payment model, hospital stays and services are rationed through intensive case management or other incentives to the provider to contain costs. This is currently the case for many patients under managed care plans.

Increased Use of Nonprofessional Staff to Contain Costs

Reducing the number of highly compensated licensed professionals, such as physical therapists, who give direct care also would help to reduce costs. In this model of care, the licensed professional evaluates the patient and develops a treatment plan that is carried out under the professional's supervision by less trained staff. On the inpatient side, a similar evolution is taking place. Registered nurses are being replaced by a higher proportion of less-trained nursing personnel. Physician assistants and nurse practitioners are providing, at a lower cost, more of the daily care previously handled by physicians.

Accreditation agencies and professional organizations have traditionally been resistant to changes that dilute the use of highly credentialed professionals on the treatment team. In part this represented fear of reduced reimbursement for services, as well as concerns about decreased quality of care. Unfortunately, little research has been conducted to compare changes in quality of care caused by using less-trained personnel. Payers and many managed health organizations, as well as other health systems, are increasingly taking the stance that unless these less costly models of care can be proved less effective, they will proceed with the changes (Gill, 1995). An alternative view is that the current model of using primarily licensed and professional providers has proven efficacy and safety; therefore, reducing the training and certification level of providers without research demonstrating comparable safety and efficacy is an unacceptable risk. However, payers and managed health companies are not always accountable or legally liable for the decisions they make about service delivery that affects care because federal and state laws prevent bringing negligence cases by employees of companies that "self-insure" health coverage for their employees.

Accreditation agencies, such as the Commission for the Accreditation of Rehabilitation Facilities (CARF), also are responding to cost-containment pressures by considering modifications in accreditation guidelines that do not specify the professional disciplines needed to deliver rehabilitation services. Such changes are part of the ongoing evolution of the delivery of rehabilitation services but are often driven by economic considerations without research evidence demonstrating that such changes will not erode the quality or overall lifetime cost of care.

Decreased Hospitalization

With the increased penetration of managed care and the specter of additional cost-containment methodologies, traditional, institutionally based rehabilitation is undergoing significant changes in service delivery. Lengths of stay already have been severely shortened. From 1986 to 1992, rehabilitation inpatient days declined by 3 to 4 days, or about 15% of the total rehabilitation stay (Wolk &

Blair, 1994). This has resulted in a shorter time to reach rehabilitation goals. At the same time, occupancy rates have shown only slight changes, reflecting the increased number of patients admitted to most inpatient rehabilitation facilities even in the face of an increase in the number of inpatient programs. In the 3-year period from 1990 to 1992, decreased length of hospitalization resulted in improved efficiency in the average patient's gains in functional status per week, with little negative effect on the total level of functional gain achieved during the rehabilitation stay (Granger & Hamilton, 1994).

Most rehabilitation providers, however, are poised to move toward alternative rehabilitation settings such as subacute, outpatient, or home care, which are likely to continue to grow (DeJong, 1997). Lower overhead and costs of providing services on an outpatient basis has undoubtedly contributed to the growth of this sector of rehabilitation providers. The hope of payers such as insurance companies was that if patients could be provided services in these lower cost settings (compared to inpatient hospitals), then overall savings in health care costs could be attained. Efforts to contain costs by managed health organizations involve controlling utilization of expensive services, such as hospitalization and use of costly procedures. In the outpatient sector this takes the form of reducing the length and number of treatment sessions, as well as using more technicians rather than more costly licensed professionals, in the provision of hands-on treatment (Gill, 1995).

Treatment Guidelines

Increasingly, care is being provided according to guidelines or critical paths of care. This is an effort to provide cost-effective quality care by reducing variability in clinical practice by providers. In some settings, deviations from such guidelines must be justified by providers. This use of clinical guidelines increasingly involves the types of cases seen in rehabilitation, such as back pain (Low Back Pain Guideline Team, 1997) and SCI (Consortium for Spinal Cord Medicine, 1997), and home care (Gingerich & Ondeck, 1995).

CONSUMER PROTECTION/RIGHTS

In the past, consumers have generally viewed their health provider as an advocate for their obtaining the best care possible. It has been understood by consumers that most providers were paid under a fee-for-service arrangement in which the more service they delivered, the more money they were paid, and they profited from caring for the patient. There was little reason to doubt that everything that was medically necessary for the patient's care would be ordered by the provider.

Furthermore, because the providers made the decisions regarding care, they were legally liable for mistakes in decision making or service delivery. At times this led to the provision of excessive care and unnecessary health care costs for payers.

Now, the concern is the opposite. In a prepaid or capitated system the provider of services may receive a fixed amount based on diagnosis or have decisions regarding the kind or amount of treatment reviewed by payers or based on guidelines determined by others. In these managed health plans, the provider may be subject to strong financial incentives to limit care or provide less expensive care. In this case, the health care consumer can be less certain regarding the degree to which a treatment decision is motivated more by cost savings than by optimal care. In a poll commissioned by the American Psychological Association, 81% of adults sampled were very concerned about changes in the health care system. Thirty-six percent indicated that their main concern was quality of care, 25% indicated access or availability of care, and 21% were most concerned about cost (Newman, 1997). Nonelderly sick persons with managed health plans are significantly more likely than those with traditional fee-for-service insurance to complain of problems in obtaining treatment or diagnostic tests and uncaring physicians (Donelan, Blendon, Benson, Leitman, & Taylor, 1996).

These concerns have led to state and federal legislative and regulatory initiatives to safeguard consumer rights in key aspects of health care. In his 1998 State of the Union Address to Congress, President Clinton stated that medical decisions should be made by physicians and not health plan "accountants." He called on Congress to pass a patients' Bill of Rights that includes many patient protections, including regulations that would require sponsors of managed health plans to provide prompt local access to a sufficient number and mix of health professionals and facilities. In addition, they would be required to offer a "point of service" plan that allows access to out-of-network providers, including rehabilitation providers that the patients may not have access to among the closed panel of providers for their health plan. Regulations are being proposed that would require due process for patient grievances and permit patients to hold managed health plans liable for negligent decisions that affect their care. Other regulations have been proposed that would prohibit managed health plans from discriminating against providers based solely on their state licensure or certification. Insurance companies and managed health organizations are leading the charge to head off such regulation for fear that it will drive up health care costs and reduce profitability.

Coalitions representing business and insurance interests assert that such regulation is not needed because consumers have the option of changing health plans or providers if they are not satisfied with the care that they receive. In a perfect market system, this may be true, but this assertion ignores several important points. First, consumers may not always be able to judge when they are receiving inferior care or be in a position to change health plan or provider when they experience poor care. Second, consumers who receive their health benefits through an employer may be at the mercy of the limited options the employer offers. Third, many persons receiving rehabilitative care require services that are very costly to managed health plans. Those plans may not have a financial incentive to keep such patients as part of their plan and may actually benefit if the patient chooses another health plan.

Concern has been expressed about the lack of consumer ability to influence factors that would allow marketplace forces to operate in an efficient manner in health care (Bingaman, Frank, & Billy, 1993). Kuttner (1997) indicates that consumers lack the "symmetrical" market power with providers of health care that would allow self-correcting for exploitative practices. Various solutions to rectifying this inequity have been proposed, such as publication of "report cards" on health plans and hospitals. Another suggestion is to establish consumer councils elected by consumers who work with the managers of health care plans to improve service (Rodwin, 1997).

SINGLE PAYER SYSTEM

It is anticipated that the United states will spend $2.1 trillion or 16% of it gross national product on health care in the year 2007, more than any other country. The United States spends approximately 25% more per person than does Canada, a country that insures each citizen through government-administered provincial health plans. Government-administered health plans such as Medicare and Medicaid are touted as costing less in administrative expenses than private health plans. The goal of universal health coverage for all Americans has yet to be achieved, with about 15% of Americans going without health insurance at any one time. U.S. citizens are more likely than Canadians or Germans to report problems in obtaining and paying for health services (Donelan et al., 1996).

Perhaps the greatest threat to any market-based system is lack of access to benefits because of reductions in employer-subsidized health insurance (Bingaman et al., 1993). Incremental efforts to increase coverage, such as CHIP, passed by Congress in 1997, have made progress toward achieving this goal, but many have pointed to government-administered "single-payer" programs such as those in Canada as being a more viable model (Bennett & Adams, 1993; Norato, 1997).

Legislation is regularly introduced in Congress that would establish a single-payer system, but it has not yet received serious consideration. It is estimated that a single-payer plan would have lower administrative costs and untangle perverse financial incentives to physicians to ration care (McDermott, 1994).

THE FUTURE: A CONSUMER-DRIVEN SYSTEM OF HEALTH CARE

People with disabilities require health delivery systems designed specifically for their complex health care needs. As DeJong (1997) points out, people with disabilities have a "thinner margin of health" and need unique programs to engage in preventive and health maintenance practices. Also, they are more likely to acquire secondary conditions and have greater need for access to specialists and ancillary services, such as durable medical equipment and assistive technologies (DeJong, 1997). The field of rehabilitation is uniquely suited to the needs of people with disabilities because of its focus on long-term outcomes.

However, traditional rehabilitation needs restructuring. Rehabilitation providers and institutions are beginning to consider delivering comprehensive services under capitated, full-risk payment systems. The implications of these changes for people with disabilities and for the provision of rehabilitation services are profound and not yet fully understood. Initial evidence suggests that managed health models designed specifically to meet the highly variable and complete health care needs of people with disabilities can successfully enhance long-term outcome and be cost-effective. This requires understanding the long-term needs and costs of people with disabilities and delivering rehabilitation services in a cost-efficient but high-quality manner.

Community-based programs emphasizing preventive and health promotion intervention will be integral to high-quality care that maximizes long-term outcomes and cost control. Additionally, the independent living movement has become more sophisticated and is making headway in convincing policymakers that a consumer-driven health care system is not only appropriate to promote independent living but is likely to be cost-effective. For example, consumer-driven personal assistance programs are gaining popularity. A voucher system in which consumers exert greater control as to where health care dollars are spent may be the next shift in reimbursement systems. This would force providers and MCOs to compete for limited dollars by improving services and emphasizing outcomes. Information and marketing will be a major component of health delivery systems, but it will have to be supported by research on the long-term success of interventions and organized delivery systems.

REFERENCES

Aitchison, K. W. (1993). Rehabilitation at the crossroads: Financial and other considerations. *American Journal of Physical Medicine and Rehabilitation, 72,* 405–407.

Bennett, A., & Adams, O. (Eds.). (1993). *Looking north for health: What we can learn from Canada's health care system.* San Francisco: Josey-Bass.

Bingaman, J., Frank, R. G., & Billy, C. L. (1993). Combining a global health budget with a market-driven delivery system. Can it be done? *American Psychologist, 48,* 270–276.

Blendon, R. J., Donelan, K., Hill, C., Scheck, A., Carter, W., Beatrice, D., & Altman, D. (1993). Medicaid beneficiaries and health reform. *Health Affairs, 12*(1), 132–143.

Buchanan, J. L., Rumple, J. D., & Hoenig, H. (1996). Changes for outpatient rehabilitation: Growth and differences in provider types. *Archives of Physical Medicine and Rehabilitation, 77*(4), 320–328.

Burns, T. J., Batavia, A. I., Smith, Q. W., & DeJong, G. (1990). Primary health care needs of persons with physical disabilities: What are the research and service priorities? *Archives of Physical Medicine and Rehabilitation, 71,* 138–145.

Chan, L., Koepsell, T. D., Deyo, R. A., Esselman, P. C., Haselkorn, J. K., Lowery, J. K., & Stolov, W. C. (1997). The effects of Medicare's payment system for rehabilitation hospitals on length of stay, charges, and total payments. *New England Journal of Medicine, 337,* 978–985.

Consortium for Spinal Cord Medicine. (1997). *Acute management of autonomic dysreflexia: Adults with spinal cord injury presenting to health-care facilities.* Washington, DC: Paralyzed Veterans of America.

Davis, M. H., & O'Brien, E. (1996). Profile of persons with disabilities in Medicare and Medicaid. *Health Care Financing Review, 17,* 179–211.

DeJong, G. (1997). Primary care for persons with disabilities. *American Journal of Physical Medicine and Rehabilitation, 76*(3)(Suppl.), s2–s8.

Dembe, A. E., Himmelstein, J. S., Stevens, B. A., & Beachler, M. P. (1997). Improving workers' compensation health care. *Health Affairs, 16,* 253–257.

Dijkers, M. P., Buda Abela, M., Gans, B. M., & Gordon, W. A. (1995). The aftermath of spinal cord injury. In S. L. Stover, J. A. DeLisa, & G. G. Whiteneck (Eds.), *Spinal cord injury: Clinical outcomes from the model systems* (pp. 183–212). Gaithersburg, MD: Aspen.

Donelan, K., Blendon, R. J., Benson, J., Leitman, R., & Taylor, H. (1996). All payer, single payer, managed care, no payer: Patients' perspectives in three nations. *Health Affairs, 15,* 254–265.

Fox, H. B., & Wicks, L. B. (1993). Health maintenance organizations and children with special health needs: A suitable match? *American Journal of Diseases of Children, 147,* 546–552.

Fox, H. B., Wicks, L. B., & Newacheck, P. W. (1993). State Medicaid health maintenance organization policies and special needs children. *HealthCare Financing Review, 15*(1), 25–37.

Francisco, G. E., Chae, J. C., & DeLisa, J. A. (1995). Physiatry as a primary care specialty. *American Journal of Physical Medicine and Rehabilitation, 74,* 186–192.

Frederickson, M., & Cannon, N. L. (1995). The role of the rehabilitation physician in the postacute continuum. *Archives of Physical Medicine and Rehabilitation, 66*(Suppl. 12-S), SC 5–9.

Friedman, R., Sobel, D., Myers, P., Caudill, M., & Benson, H. (1995). Behavioral medicine, clinical health psychology, and cost offset. *Health Psychology, 14,* 509–518.

Fries, B. E., Schneider, D. P., Foley, W. J., Gavazzi, M., Burke, R., & Cornelius, E. (1994). Refining a case-mix measure for nursing homes: Resource Utilization Groups (RUG-III). *Medical Care, 32,* 668–685.

Gans, B. M., Mann, N. R., & Becker, B. E. (1993). Delivery of primary care to the physically challenged. *Archives of Physical Medicine and Rehabilitation, 74*(Suppl.), 515–519.

Gill, H. S. (1995). The changing nature of ambulatory rehabilitation programs and services in a managed care environment. *Archives of Physical Medicine and Rehabilitation, 76*(Suppl. 12), SC10–15.

Gingerich, B. S., & Ondeck, D. A. (1995). *Clinical pathways for the multidisciplinary home care team.* Gaithersburg, MD: Aspen.

Gold, M., Nelson, L., Brown, R., Ciemnecki, A., Aizer, A., & Docteur, E. (1997). Disabled Medicare beneficiaries in HMOs. *Health Affairs, 16*, 149–162.

Gold, M., Sparer, M., & Chu, K. (1996). Medicaid managed care: Lessons from five states. *Health Affairs, 15*, 153–166.

Granger, C. V., & Hamilton, B. B. (1994). The Uniform Data System for medical rehabilitation: Report of first admissions for 1992. *American Journal of Physical Medicine and Rehabilitation, 73*(1), 51–55.

Harada, N., Kominski, G., & Sofaer, S. (1993). Development of a resource-based patient classification scheme for rehabilitation. *Inquiry, 30*(1), 54–63.

Health Care Financing Administration. (1998a). *HCFA Statistics 1996 Expenditures Health Care Financing Administration* [On-line]. Available: http://www.hcfa.gov/stats/hstats96/

Health Care Financing Administration. (1998b). *Overview of the Medicaid Program* [On-line]. Available: http://www.hcfa.gov/Medicaid/mover.htm

Health Care Financing Administration. (1998c). *Overview of the Medicare Program* [On-line]. Available: http://www.hcfa.gov/Medicare/careoer.htm

Heinemann, A., Keen, M., Donohue, R., & Schnoll, S. (1988). Alcohol use in persons with recent spinal cord injuries. *Archives of Physical Medicine and Rehabilitation, 69,* 619–624.

Horwitz, S. M., & Stein, R. E. (1990). Health maintenance organizations versus indemnity insurance for children with chronic illness: Trading gaps in coverage. *American Journal of Diseases of Children, 144*, 581–586.

Iglehart, J. K. (1994). Changing course in turbulent times: An interview with David Lawrence. *Health Affairs, 13*(5), 65–77.

Jenson, G. A., Morrisey, M. A., Gaffney, S., & Liston, D. K. (1997). The new dominance of managed care: Insurance trends in the 1990s. *Health Affairs, 16*(1), 125–136.

Kaiser Commission on the Future of Medicaid. (1997). *Medicaid facts: Medicaid role for children*. Washington, DC: Author.

Kuttner, R. (1997). *Everything for sale: The virtue and limits of markets*. New York: Alfred A. Knopf.

Levit, K. R., Lazenby, H. C., & Braden, B. R. (1998). National health spending trends in 1996. *Health Affairs, 17*(1), 35–51.

Low Back Pain Guideline Team. (1997). *Guidelines for clinical care: Acute low back pain* [On-line]. Available: http://www.med.umich.edu/i/oca/practiceguides/index.htm

Master, R., Dreyfus, T., Connors, S., Tobias, C., Zhou, A., & Kronick, R. (1996). The Community Medical Alliance: An integrated system of care in greater Boston for people with severe disability and AIDS. *Managed Care Quarterly, 4*(2), 26–37.

McCue, M. J., & Thompson, J. M. (1995). The ownership difference in relative performance of rehabilitation specialty hospitals. *Archives of Physical Medicine and Rehabilitation, 76*, 413–418.

McDermott, J. (1994). Evaluating health system reform: The case for a single-payor approach. *Journal of the American Medical Association, 271,* 782–784.

Miller, R., & Luft, H. (1994). Managed care plan performance since 1980: A literature analysis. *Journal of the American Medical Association, 271*, 1512–1519.

Mitchell, E., & Riley, T. (Eds.). (1997). *Spotlight. How is Medicaid managed care serving people with disabilities?* Portland, ME: Center for Vulnerable Populations, National Academy for State Health Policy.

Mitchell, J. M., & Scott, E. (1992). Physician ownership of physical therapy services: Effects on charges, utilization, profits, and service characteristics. *Journal of the American Medical Association, 268,* 2055–2059.

Newacheck, P. W., & Stoddard, J. J. (1994). Prevalence and impact of multiple childhood chronic illnesses. *Journal of Pediatrics, 124*(1), 40–48.

Newacheck, P. W., & Taylor, W. R. (1992). Childhood chronic illness: Prevalence, severity, and impact. *American Journal of Public Health, 82,* 364–371.

Newman, R. (1997, March). *Keynote address.* Paper presented at the meeting of the American Psychological Association State Leadership Conference, Washington, DC.

Nickelson, D. (1997). Telehealth poses opportunities and challenges for psychology. *Practitioner Focus, 10*(2), 12.

Norato, J. F. (1997). National health care reform and a single-payer system: Messiah or pariah? *Journal of Health and Human Services Administration, 19,* 341–356.

Nosek, M. A. (1993). Personal assistance: Its effect on the long-term health of a rehabilitation hospital population. *Archives of Physical Medicine and Rehabilitation, 74,* 127–132.

Reilly, P., Coburn, A. F., & Kilbreth, E. H. (1990). *Medicaid managed care: The state of the art.* Portland, ME: National Academy for State Health Policy.

Rodwin, M. A. (1997). The neglected remedy: Strengthening consumer voice in managed care. *American Prospect, 34,* 45–50.

Rosenbach, M., & Huber, J. (1993). Utilization, access, and satisfaction with care among noninstitutionalized Medicare beneficiaries: A baseline analysis. In Health Care Financing Administration (Ed.), *Third annual report to Congress on monitoring utilization of and access to services for medicare beneficiaries under physician payment reform.* Washington, DC: Health Care Financing Administration.

Rosenbach, M. L. (1995). Access and satisfaction within the disabled Medicare population. *Health Care Financing Review, 17,* 147–167.

Rosenbaum, S., Johnson, K., Sonosky, C., Markus, A., & DeGraw, C. (1998). The children's hour: The State Children's Health Insurance Program. *Health Affairs, 17*(1), 75–89.

Schneider, J. E., Cromwell, J., & McGuire, T. P. (1993). Excluded facility financial status and options for payment system modification. *Health Care Financing Review, 15*(2), 7–30.

Shonkoff, J., Sweeney, M., McManus, M., Corro, D., Skubel, E., & McPherson, M. (1994). *Meeting the needs of chronically disabled children in a changing health care system* (Issue Brief No. 651). Washington, DC: George Washington University, National Health Policy Forum.

Shortell, S. M., Gillies, R. R., Anderson, D. A., Erickson, K. M., & Mitchell, J. B. (1996). *Remaking health care in America.* San Francisco: Jossey-Bass.

Shriver, K. (1996). Rehab providers fight HCFA data. *Modern Health Care, 26*(10), 130–132.

Stineman, M. G., Goin, J. E., Granger, C. V., Fiedler, R., & Williams, S. V. (1997). Discharge motor FIM-function related groups. *Archives of Physical Medicine and Rehabilitation, 78,* 980–985.

Sutton, J. P., DeJong, G., Song, H., & Wilkerson, D. (1997). Impact of a function-based payment model on the financial performance of acute inpatient medical rehabilitation providers: A simulation analysis. *Archives of Physical Medicine and Rehabilitation, 78*, 1290–1297.

Sutton, J. P., DeJong, G., & Wilkerson, D. (1996). Function-based payment model for inpatient medical rehabilitation: An evaluation. *Archives of Physical Medicine and Rehabilitation, 77,* 693–701.

Symington, D. C. (1994). Megatrends in rehabilitation: A Canadian perspective. *International Journal of Rehabilitation Research, 17*(1), 1–14.

Tannenbaum, S. J., & Hurley, R. E. (1995). Disability and the managed care frenzy: A cautionary note. *Health Affairs, 14*, 213–219.

Tate, D. G., Stiers, W., Daugherty, J., Forchheimer, M., Cohen, E., & Hansen, N. (1994). The effects of insurance benefits coverage on functional and psychosocial outcomes after spinal cord injury. *Archives of Physical Medicine and Rehabilitation, 75,* 407–414.

Tator, C. H., Duncan, E. G., Edmonds, V. E., Lapczak, L. I., & Andrews, D. F. (1993). Neurological recovery, mortality and length of stay after acute spinal cord injury associated with changes in management. *Paraplegia, 33*, 254–262.

Temkin, A. J., Ulicny, G. R., & Vesmarovich, S. H. (1996). Telerehab: A perspective of the way technology is going to change the future of patient treatment. *Rehab Management, 9*(2), 28–30.

What you can expect from a RUGs-based PPS. (1998, January). *Rehab Continuum Report, 7*(1), 3.

Williams, B. (1994). Comparison of services among different types of home health agencies. *Medical Care, 32,* 1134–1152.

Wilson, N. J., & Kizer, K. W. (1997). The VA health care system: An unrecognized national safety net. *Health Affairs, 16*, 200–204.

Wolk, S., & Blair, T. (1994). *Trends in medical rehabilitation.* Reston, VA: American Rehabilitation Association.

Wright, R. E., Rao, N., Smith, R. M., & Harvey, R. F. (1996). Risk factors for death and emergency transfer in acute and subacute inpatient rehabilitation. *Archives of Physical Medicine and Rehabilitation, 77,* 1049–1055.

Wynn, B. (1997). *Statement of Barbara Wynn, acting director, Bureau of Policy Development, Health Care Financing Administration, on rehabilitation and long-term care hospital payments: Hearing before the Subcommittee on Health, Committee on Ways and Means, U.S. House of Representatives,* 105th Congress, 1st sess.

Chapter 34

Legislation and Rehabilitation Service Delivery

Susanne M. Bruyère and
Rebecca K. DeMarinis

Over the course of the past 25 years, the field of rehabilitation has seen sweeping changes legislatively, as laws have been enacted that support the rights of individuals with disabilities and subsequently the efforts of the professionals who provide services to them. These legislative mandates have provided rights to persons with disabilities in accessibility of goods and services, transportation, telecommunications, housing, and employment (U.S. Department of Justice, 1997).[1] Although each of these areas is critically important for accessing a good and full life as an American citizen, it is the area of employment that we will be focusing on in this chapter. Not only rehabilitation legislation and legislation specifically targeted to persons with disabilities but also other pieces of employment legislation provide protections for persons with disabilities, and as such affect the functioning of rehabilitation professionals. For the purposes of this discussion, the laws that will be focused on are as follows: Titles I and V of the Rehabilitation Act of 1973 as amended, the employment provisions of the Americans with Disabilities Act (ADA) of 1990, the Family Medical Leave Act (FMLA), the Occupational Safety and Health Act (OSHA), the National Labor Relations Act (NLRA), and state workers' compensation laws.

Because rehabilitation professionals often come from varied backgrounds—rehabilitation psychologists, rehabilitation counselors or case managers, social workers working with persons with disabilities, or other rehabilitation professionals—their exposure to legislation affecting the rights of persons with disabilities will subsequently be varied. Those of us who come from a psychology background may have had exposure to health or confidentiality regulatory requirements; those who have had rehabilitation counseling training should have had exposure to the Rehabilitation Act, the Individuals with Disabilities Education Act (IDEA), the ADA, and other pieces of legislation targeting the rights of persons with disabilities, such as the Fair Housing Act, the Architectural Barriers Act, and the Air Carrier Access Act. Those who come from an industrial, organizational, human resource, labor relations, or employment services background may have had exposure to employment and labor law regulations. It is the purpose of this chapter to provide a common experience across several of these pieces of legislation, particularly as it relates to the employment or return-to-work process, for rehabilitation professionals who function with persons with disabilities.

This chapter provides a brief overview of each of the pieces of legislation, with an explanation of what issues, questions of concern, or critical areas in service delivery may arise from each. These are issues that have been of significant concern to employers who are attempting to fulfill their responsibilities under several—at times seemingly conflicting—pieces of disability and employment legislation (Gault & Kinnane, 1996). They are therefore of concern to the individual with a disability who is trying to either gain or maintain employment, as well as to the rehabilitation professionals who serve people with disabilities. The intent of this chapter is to contribute to the ability of rehabilitation professionals to assist employers and individuals with disabilities to navigate this maze. The authors offer a summary of some key factors in operating effectively within this regulatory environment, which rehabilitation professionals can use either in coaching individuals about their rights or in providing consultation to employers about their responsibilities to persons with disabilities to lessen or eliminate discrimination in the employment process.

EMPLOYMENT LEGISLATION AFFECTING REHABILITATION SERVICE DELIVERY

The Rehabilitation Act of 1973 As Amended

Two titles of the Rehabilitation Act will be discussed here: Title I, which deals with employment and related support services available to persons with disability as provided by the state-federal vocational rehabilitation system, and Title V, which prohibits discrimination on the basis of disability in programs conducted by federal agencies, in programs receiving federal financial assistance, in federal employment, and in the employment practices of federal contractors.

Title I of the Vocational Rehabilitation Act of 1973, as modified by the Rehabilitation Act amendments of 1992, has as its purpose

> to assist States in operating a comprehensive, coordinated, effective, efficient, and accountable program of vocational rehabilitation that is designed to assess, plan, develop, and provide vocational rehabilitation services for individuals with disabilities, consistent with their strengths, resources, priorities, concerns, abilities, and capabilities, so that such individuals may prepare for and engage in gainful employment. (Sec. 100(a)(2)

Some of the earliest legislative roots for the current vocational rehabilitation service delivery system as we know it today in the United States emerged over 75 years ago with the 1920 Civilian Rehabilitation (Smith-Fess) Act, Public Law 66-236 (Wright, 1980). The Rehabilitation Act has provided funds on a formula basis to states since that time. In the years following this legislation, vocational rehabilitation services have evolved and greatly expanded to provide an extensive array of both public- and private-sector services to address the employment and independent living needs of persons with disabilities.

Federal funding for the vocational rehabilitation service delivery system during 1996 was over $2 billion.[2] The state vocational rehabilitation system is made up of 82 agencies nationally, designated for both general rehabilitation services and for specific services to the blind and visually impaired in 25 states and territories. Thirty-two agencies offer combined services;[3] these are reportedly staffed nationally by approximately 15,000 personnel. Examples of the services that can be provided to persons with disabilities, as authorized under the legislation, are as follows: vocational assessment, career counseling, vocational training, job development and job placement, assistive technology, supported employment, and follow-along services. The legislative mandate requires that the order of selection for the provision of vocational rehabilitation services shall be determined on the basis of serving first those individuals with the most severe disabilities. Individuals with disabilities, including individuals with the most severe disabilities, are generally presumed to be capable of engaging in gainful employment, and the provision of individualized rehabilitation services is designed to improve their ability to become gainfully employed. A successful outcome is considered placement in an integrated employment setting at a prevailing wage, for a minimum of 60 days, although other vocational outcomes, such as homemaker or sheltered employment, are accepted as legitimate closures for certain individuals who are deemed unable to seek competitive employment. During fiscal year 1996, 1.36 million individuals received services from state vocational rehabilitation agencies, with 213,000 closed as successfully rehabilitated.[4]

The following are the provisions covered by Title V of the Rehabilitation Act, which deals with prohibitions in discrimination against persons with disabilities. Section 501 requires affirmative action and nondiscrimination in employment by federal agencies of the executive branch.[5] Section 503 requires affirmative action and prohibits employment discrimination by federal government contractors and subcontractors with contracts of more than $10,000.[6] Section 504 states that "no qualified individual with a disability in the United States shall be excluded from, denied the benefits of, or be subjected to discrimination under" any program or activity that either receives federal financial assistance or is conducted by any executive agency or the U.S. Postal Service. Requirements include reasonable accommodation for employees with disabilities, program accessibility, effective communication with people who have hearing or vision disabilities, and accessible new construction and alterations.[7]

The standards for determining employment discrimination under the Rehabilitation Act are the same as those used in Title I of the ADA, and therefore the issues for rehabilitation professionals in dealing with how these rights play out in the workplace are similar. The implications for rehabilitation professionals are discussed in greater detail under the presentation of issues around implementation of Title I of the ADA, which follows.

The Americans with Disabilities Act of 1990

The ADA is a landmark piece of civil rights legislation that extends the prohibitions against discrimination on the basis of race, sex, religion, and national origin to persons with disabilities. Individuals may have both rights and responsibilities under the law according to the many different roles they assume: as employers or consultants to employers, as practitioners providing health services to the public, or as individuals who today or in the future may be protected by the ADA (O'Keeffe, 1994). Title I, the employment provisions of the ADA, applies to private employers with at least 15 employees and to state and local government employers. The ADA protects qualified individuals with disabilities from discrimination. A qualified individual with a disability is a person who meets the necessary prerequisites for a job and can perform the essential functions with or without reasonable accommodation. A reasonable accommodation is any modification or adjustment to a job, an employment practice, or the work environment that makes it possible for a qualified individual with a disability to participate in the job application process, perform the essential functions of a job, and/or enjoy benefits and privileges of employment equal to those enjoyed by employees without disabilities.

The ADA employment provisions make it unlawful to discriminate on the basis of disability in a wide range of employment-related actions, including recruitment, job application, hiring, advancement, compensation, benefits, training, and discharge. Title I prohibits both intentional discrimination and employment practices with discriminatory effect. Additionally, Title I limits the use of both preemployment and postemployment medical examinations and inquiries. An individual with a disability may be subjected to a preemployment medical examination and inquiry only after a conditional offer of employment has been made and only if all entering employees in the job category are subjected to such an examination or inquiry regardless of disability. Postemployment medical examinations and inquiries must be job-related and consistent with business necessity. Employee medical information is to be maintained separately from other personnel information, treated in a confidential manner, and shared only with supervisors and managers who need to know about necessary restrictions on the work duties of the employee and necessary accommodations. First aid and safety personnel also can be given selected information if the disability might require emergency medical treatment, as can government officials investigating compliance with the ADA.

The reasonable accommodation requirement is central to the mandate of nondiscrimination against people with disabilities. Reasonable accommodation is not an entirely new concept. Reasonable accommodation is required under the Rehabilitation Act with respect to the employment and participation of individuals with disabilities under federal contracts and programs and under Title VII of the Civil Rights Act with respect to religious observances of employees. The ADA provides the following examples of reasonable accommodations: job restructuring; part-time or modified work hours; reassignment to a vacant position; acquisition or modification of equipment or services; appropriate adjustment or modifications of examinations, training materials, or policies; and provision of qualified readers or interpreters. Over the past 5 years, questions and concerns about accommodations for persons with psychiatric disabilities have been voiced by employers and their legal representatives (Pechman, 1995). In response to these concerns, the Equal Employment Opportunity Commission (EEOC) issued enforcement guidance on the ADA as it applies to persons with psychiatric disabilities (U.S. EEOC, 1997). This publication provides useful information, both to persons with disabilities and to the rehabilitation practitioners who provide services to them, about the rights of persons with disabilities to accommodation and disclosure of disability under the ADA.

Employers are not, under the ADA, required to hire employees who may pose a "direct threat" to the workplace safety or health environment (U.S. EEOC, 1992). The statutory definition of the term *direct threat* is "a significant risk to the health or safety of others that cannot be eliminated by reasonable accommodation" (Winterbauer, 1997). Employers may use the direct-threat defense only in cases where risk is significantly increased, and standards for determining how severe a risk is must be applied to all employees—both with and without disabilities (U.S. EEOC, 1992).

When the ADA employment provisions first became effective, some industries were predominantly concerned about their hiring practices and restraints against being able to ask questions about prior injuries (Setzer, 1992); other employers responded with concerns about additional facets of employment that would be affected, such as the implications of insurance benefits and compensation (Huss, 1993; Nobile, 1996; Zolkos, 1994). Now, with 6 years of experience since the employment provisions became effective, employers also have become aware of the importance of examining how they treat job incumbents with disabilities. According to statistics kept by the U.S. Equal Employment Opportunity Commission, the federal agency that oversees compliance with the ADA employment provisions, of the 90,803 charges filed from July 26, 1992, through September 30, 1997, over half (52%) related to alleged unlawful discharge. Thus, it appears that employers need assistance in navigating requirements for nondiscrimination at several points in the employment process. Informed rehabilitation professionals can be of great assistance in this process, both to these employers and to job applicants and job incumbents with disabilities.

Family Medical Leave Act

The FMLA went into effect on August 5, 1993. It establishes, for employers with 50 or more employees, a minimum labor standard with regard to leaves of absence for family or medical reasons. The law's enactment was driven by concern to protect the needs of American workforces, while attending to the productivity concerns of employers:

> In the face of an increasing number of American children and elderly who are dependent upon family members who must spend long hours at work, Congress intended that the FMLA allow employees to balance their work and family lives. . . . [It] minimizes the potential for employment discrimination on the basis of sex, while promoting equal employment opportunity for men and women. (Commerce Clearing House, 1996)

Under the FMLA, an eligible employee may take up to 12-work weeks of leave during any 12-month period for one or more of the following reasons: the birth of a child and to care for the newborn child; the placement of a child with the employee through adoption or foster care and to care for the child; to care for the employee's spouse, son, daughter, or parent with a serious health condition; and a serious health condition that makes the employee unable to perform one or more of the essential functions of his or her job.[8] An FMLA serious health condition is an illness, injury, impairment, or physical or mental condition that involves inpatient care or continuing treatment by a health care provider. During the FMLA leave, the employer must maintain the employee's existing level of coverage under a group health plan. At the end of FMLA leave, an employer must take an employee back into the same or an equivalent job. The FMLA does not require an employer to return to work an employee who is medically unable to do his job, nor does it require modification of the job or reassignment to a new position.

Some of the questions that arise in use of the FMLA that relate to the functioning of rehabilitation professionals are in the interplay of FMLA leave with accommodation and return-to-work efforts (Bell, 1995; Scott, 1996; Shalowitz, 1993). The FMLA may create difficulties for an employer attempting to get injured workers back to work and off benefits. Many employers have used "light duty" to bring an injured worker back to work within his or her medical restrictions. Light-duty jobs typically are very different from the job an employee was doing at the time of injury. Because the FMLA requires that a worker be restored to the same or an equivalent position on return from leave, an employer may not compel an injured worker to accept light duty in lieu of exercising his or her FMLA entitlement. Likewise, the Department of Labor has taken the position that an employer may not require an FMLA-eligible employee to accept reasonable accommodation instead of FMLA leave.

An employer may offer accommodation or light duty but may not compel it. On the other hand, if an employee rejects an offer of employment that is within his or her medical restrictions, an employer may contest the employee's entitlement to workers' compensation indemnity benefits. In addition, if an employee voluntarily accepts light duty, an employer may not designate time on light duty as FMLA leave, as the employee is working. However, time spent on light duty does not lessen an employee's right to be restored to the same or an equivalent position held at the time leave commenced.

Some employers raise questions about a perceived conflict between the FMLA provision allowing employers to ask for certification of a serious health condition and the ADA restrictions on disability-related inquires by employees. The EEOC issued a fact sheet to address some of these most often asked questions about the ADA and FMLA interaction.[9] This publication clarifies the point that when an employee requests leave under the FMLA for a serious health condition, employers will not violate the ADA by asking for the information specified in the FMLA certification form. The FMLA form requests only information relating to the particular serious health condition for which the person is seeking leave. An employer is entitled to know why an employee, who otherwise should be at work, is requesting time off under the FMLA. If the inquiries are strictly limited in this fashion, they would be "job-related and consistent with business necessity" under the ADA ("EEOC Answers," 1997).

Occupational Safety and Health Act

The Occupational Safety and Health Act of 1970 represents the culmination of nearly a century of Congress's growing concern for workplace safety (Rothstein, 1990). The earliest laws concerning the health and safety of employees were based at the state level and were in place in some form in 46 states by 1921. These laws were not substantially preventive, and unfortunately their existence did little to curb the actual occurrence of incidents. However, workers' compensation schemes, also at the state level, made it possible for employees to recover damages from their employers for injuries incurred on the job, as well as allow the families of victims of industrial accidents some relief for their predicaments. Throughout the 20th century, laws were passed in response to specific health issues on the job: the Esch Act of 1912 curtailed phosphorus use in match factories; the Coal Mine Safety Act of 1952 was passed after 119 miners were killed in West Frankfort, Illinois, a year earlier; the Construction Safety Act of 1969 addressed safety issues on construction sites of public works. Still, no piece of legislation covered all safety and health issues in every workplace for every employee until the passage of OSHA in 1970. Unlike some other employment regulation, OSHA is applied universally to all employers, regardless of the volume of business they conduct or the number of people in their employ (Rothstein, 1990).

At OSHA's core is the recognition that every worker has a right to a workplace that is free from recognized hazards. Therefore, when a potential hazard is identified, the OSH Administration, through the Labor Department, develops a standard against which workplace practices or conditions should be measured. Standards are issued by three procedures—one for interim standards, one for permanent standards, and one for emergency temporary standards. Investigation and evaluation of a standard-warranting situation begins when the OSH Administration becomes aware of pertinent information about that situation. With the exception of emergency hazards that require immediate precautionary treatment, a committee of no more than 15 members will be assigned to determine an appropriate standard within a 260-day period from the committee's assignment. The committee's recommendations are submitted and reviewed by all affected parties, comments are taken from interested persons, and a public hearing is held. The OSH Administration then decides to accept their recommended standard or to deny it based on stated reasons (Bureau of National Affairs, 1997).

After the implementation of a standard, the Labor Department can determine which workplaces will be inspected—either by the request of an employee in the particular workplace, or at the OSH Administration's discretion. Inspections are conducted with the permission of the employer, and according to OSHA guidelines. Violations of a standard are punishable by government ordered abatement and monetary fines, set according to the size of the business, the seriousness of the violation, the good faith of the employer and the record of prior violations.

Violations which result in the death of an employee can be punished by criminal law (Bureau of National Affairs, 1997).

Some of the issues surrounding this piece of legislation that may affect the functioning of rehabilitation professionals is the interplay with prohibitions in employment screening, medical confidentiality of records, and accommodations required under the ADA. The ADA's limitations on employee testing can be in conflict with OSHA's need for testing in furtherance of workplace safety goals.

> The ADA places significant restrictions on an employer's right to require pre-employment physicals, to make medical inquiries of employees and applicants, and to require that employees submit to physical examinations, and restrict access to such information in an effort to prevent potential discrimination. The Occupational Safety and Health Act, in contrast, affirmatively requires employers to conduct testing in a variety of situations to assure safety. For example, employees exposed to high noise levels are required to be included within an audiometric testing program which includes among other things, annual hearing tests. (Taylor, 1995, p. 24)

The ADA also requires strict confidentiality of medical records. OSHA, on the other hand, requires employers to provide employees, their representatives with signed authorizations, and OSHA personnel access to such records in the interest of exposing potential hazards and their causes. By having the employee sign an information release, the employer can better assure that the information being released stays in the appropriate hands and that the ADA confidentiality requirements are not violated.

Although OSHA requirements can often take precedence over the ADA requirements to assure that health and safety requirements are being adhered to, the reasonable accommodation element of ADA can still be applied to OSHA-mandated policies and modifications. For example, an eyewash station, which may be required by OSHA for certain positions, must be installed in such a way that a wheelchair user would have access to it.

The lines are not always so clear, however, particularly in terms of the direct threat defense to ADA claims. Take, for example, the case of an employee with epilepsy working on an assembly line. The way an employer handles the situation is largely contingent on which legislation he or she believes more likely to be invoked. Removal of the employee, satisfying the general duty clause of OSHA, may violate the ADA. The direct threat defense is so difficult to prove that employers are likely to avoid the ADA claim at all costs, often leaving themselves in violation of OSHA standards. The complications arise when OSHA doesn't explicitly call for an action such as removal of an employee who has seizures. As a general rule, OSHA standards "trump" the ADA's duty to accommodate, but employers cannot rely on using OSHA as a defense to ADA claims unless the employment action in question was specifically called for by OSHA (Skoning & McGlothlen, 1994).

National Labor Relations Act

The NLRA, also called the Wagner Act, was passed in 1935. It stands as the prevailing framework for labor relations in the United States, covering union-management relations in virtually every private firm in operation. The law protects workers from the effects of unfair labor practices by employers and requires employers to recognize and bargain collectively with a union that the workers elect to represent them (Gold, 1989).

Among the main principles of the NLRA are the idea of exclusivity of representation, the policy against direct dealing, and the duty to provide information. Seniority rights gained through collective bargaining are also among the most valued benefits of having a unionized workplace (Gold, 1989). All of these areas may yield conflict for individuals seeking to invoke protection from laws such as the ADA, FMLA, or the Rehabilitation Act. These laws rely on making exceptions to or changes in terms and conditions of employment on an individual basis. Compliance with these laws may include dealings with the employer to discuss and secure those agreements that may fall outside the scope of the union's normal interactions, the unilateral implementation of an accommodation for an employee, and often the security of medical information, which the union may feel it has the right to access under the NLRA (Evans, 1992).

Reasonable accommodations for individuals with disabilities may present an especially problematic situation for employers and unions alike. Both parties are required by law to operate in a nondiscriminatory manner: the employer must accommodate a worker so that his or her essential job functions may be performed regardless of disability and must provide terms and conditions of employment that are free of discriminatory intent. The union must represent its constituency equally and consistently, as well as allow accommodations for people with disabilities to be implemented without unreasonable opposition (President's Committee, 1994).

Whenever a modification in the terms or conditions of employment is required, a review of the collective bargaining agreement would be advisable, as well as some kind of communication between the employer and the union concerning the accommodation and the potential effects it may have on the lives of other workers (President's Committee, 1994). An effective way to approach this is the use of joint labor-management teams (Bruyère, Gomez, & Handelmann, 1996).

In a unionized workplace, the rehabilitation professional can contribute to the effective return to the workplace for an injured worker, taking into account the interests of the employee, the employer, and the union to effect a successful reintegration. Organized labor has been an important part of the history of fighting for worker rights and against job discrimination, and these social issues are very important to workers with disabilities. Yet many employment professionals have little experience with unions and little knowledge of their purpose and structure (Bruyère, 1996). Adopting a position that favors both the person with a disability *and* the union will go a long way in the service delivery process to minimize conflict and maximize union support in the accommodation process.

Workers' Compensation

Workers' compensation programs are government-sponsored and employer-financed systems for compensating employees who incur an injury or illness in connection with their employment. They are designed to ensure that employees who are injured on the job receive timely compensation for their losses without proof of fault. Workers' compensation laws allow employees or their survivors to file claims for economic losses resulting from work-related injuries or occupational diseases. Benefits provided under workers' compensation laws include medical care, disability payments, rehabilitation services, survivor benefits, and funeral expenses. Employers who participate in workers' compensation programs usually are protected against tort actions that employees might otherwise pursue to redress their losses.

State workers' compensation statutes generally provide benefits to employees for job-related injuries, whether or not the injury is permanently disabling. In addition to medical care and treatment for job-related injuries, workers' compensation statutes typically also provide benefits for temporary incapacity, scarring, and permanent impairment of specific parts of the body. Workers' compensation laws are maintained by all 50 states, the District of Columbia, American Samoa, Guam, the Virgin Islands, and Puerto Rico. In addition, the federal government administers workers' compensation programs authorized by the Federal Coal Mine Health and Safety Act, the Longshore and Harborworkers' Compensation Act, and the Federal Employers' Liability Act. Rehabilitation professionals working in private-sector rehabilitation and in the return-to-work process for persons with disabilities are interfacing with this system and its regulations regularly.

Although much emphasis early on after the passage of the ADA was on disability nondiscrimination and the hiring process, some employers were already focusing on its impact where incumbents with disabilities were concerned (Walworth, Damon, & Wilder, 1993). Now, even more attention is being paid to the ADA's impact on job retention aspects of the employment process. Of the ADA charges filed with the EEOC since the law came into effect, approximately one in five of these charges (18%) has been cited as being related to a back impairment, which is a disability or injury often seen in the workers' compensation system.

It is inevitable that the rehabilitation practitioner will deal with some persons for whom there will be an interplay of the these two pieces of legislation.

Some authors have pointed out that disability nondiscrimination legislation such as the ADA appears to rest on very different premises than the workers' compensation system (Bell, 1994). The ADA is predicated on the premise that disability does not necessarily mean inability to work and focuses on how accommodation can assist in removing barriers to employment caused by the interaction between functional limitations and the workplace. Workers' compensation legislation, however, focuses on the apparently contrasting premise that impairments are the cause of work limitations, and employees must prove loss of earning capacity because of injury.

Some areas of concern for rehabilitation professionals in this interplay of legislation relate to clarifying for individuals with disabilities and for employers some of the significant aspects of workers' compensation legislation as it relates to the protections provided by the ADA. These include such issues as the injured worker as a protected person under the ADA; queries by an employer about a worker's prior workers' compensation claims; hiring persons with a prior history of an occupational injury and application of the direct threat standard; reasonable accommodation for persons with disability-related occupational injuries; light duty issues; and exclusive remedy provisions in workers' compensation laws. In response to a need for clarification of these issues, the EEOC issued enforcement guidance concerning the interaction between Title I of the ADA and state workers' compensation laws that can greatly assist rehabilitation professionals in responding to many of these employer questions (U.S. EEOC, 1996; Welch, 1996).

IMPLICATIONS FOR REHABILITATION SERVICE DELIVERY

To prepare persons with disabilities appropriately for initial entry or reentry into the workplace and to provide effective consultation to employers on disability nondiscrimination and equal access in the workplace, rehabilitation professionals must be apprised of state and federal legislation that affects both safety and equity practices in the workplace. The issues presented here in the implementation of specific pieces of legislation and more specifically as they interrelate with disability nondiscrimination legislation, such as the ADA, point to areas where rehabilitation professionals need more knowledge and expertise and also where they can provide effective service. A listing of specific skill and knowledge areas needed by rehabilitation professionals in implementing the ADA as a consultant were identified by Pape and Tarvydas (1994) as cutting across the following three distinct areas: core rehabilitation principles, knowledge, and functions; disability concepts, functions, and knowledge; and ADA knowledge and functions. The implications of disability nondiscrimination legislation specifically for the role of psychologists were addressed by Crewe (1994), who encourages specialized pre- or postdoctoral preparation in disability and rehabilitation for psychologists who are planning to apply their clinical or counseling psychology training to services for people with disabilities. The implications of disability nondiscrimination legislation such as the ADA for preparation of rehabilitation undergraduate and graduate professionals is discussed by Stude (1994), who encourages rehabilitation educators to include this information in existing course work rather than isolating it into a specialized course.

The ADA has afforded rehabilitation professionals who contribute to employment opportunities for persons with disabilities a tool to more effectively combat discrimination in the recruitment, hiring, retention, and termination processes. Under the ADA, a significant service that vocational rehabilitation counselors might provide is to assist employers to do job analyses, write job descriptions, and help develop or design the reasonable accommodations that will make initial hiring or return to work feasible for workers with disabilities (Walker & Heffner, 1992). Employers need assistance in the development of policies and procedures that do not discriminate against people with disabilities in the recruitment, hiring, health and other employment benefits, promotion and training, and termination processes.

The workers' compensation system is one that is often cited as being difficult for both employees and employers, seemingly fanning the fires for a contentious and litigious relationship. One of the most important things rehabilitation professionals can do is to facilitate communication between the employer and the employee (Commerce Clearing House, 1997). Rehabilitation professionals can either be that bridge with employers themselves or serve as a consultant to encourage supervisors and others in the workplace to address the employee's questions and provide supportive follow-up during disability leave. Rehabilitation professionals also can play a role in bringing human resource, safety, and health professionals together within a given organization to begin a unified approach to the ADA and workers' compensation (Walker & Hefner, 1992).

In all facets of this legislation, working both with individuals with disabilities and with employers, teaching them how to communicate their respective needs effectively is imperative. Often, when coached appropriately, both employees with disabilities and their supervisors or the human resources staff in a given organization can effectively address accommodation requests and resolve any conflicts that arise in negotiating the final decision on accommodations. Problems arise when there has been a prior history of poor performance, of poor relationship between supervisor and employee, or of general discordance or conflict in a unit or workplace environment, creating a culture of mistrust in responding to employee needs.

SUMMARY

The purpose of this chapter has been to provide rehabilitation professionals with a basic overview of some of the pieces of disability and employment legislation that may affect their functioning in the rehabilitation and return-to-work process. Several pieces of this legislation, such as the NLRA and the OSHA, are designed to protect workers' rights before injury occurs and to emphasize employer responsibilities in the safety and equitable treatment of workers across terms and conditions of employment. Regulatory requirements such as the FMLA, short-term disability leave requirements as dictated by state regulations, and workers' compensation legislation are designed to deal with the rights of employees once an injury or illness has occurred. These laws protect the right to a medical leave that affords the worker the time needed for the rehabilitation process and assure the security of benefits to cover part of the medical costs and salary lost to time off due to illness or injury, as well as a job to return to. Legislation such as the Rehabilitation Act of 1973 as amended and the ADA is designed more specifically to focus on the rights of workers with disabilities. These pieces of legislation require equal access in the seeking and securing of employment, as well as retention and equitable access to other terms and conditions of employment. Regulatory requirements such as confidentiality of medical information also serve a role here, in terms of providing requirements for employers to keep confidential any medical diagnostic information on employees that they may gain access to.

Working with the individual in the rehabilitation process to assist him or her to return to productive functioning in the community and in the workplace is the core of the rehabilitation professional's job. A knowledge of the regulatory requirements that surround the workplace and have an impact on employer and employee behavior is necessary if rehabilitation professionals are to function as effectively as possible for the person with a disability when employment outcomes are part of the rehabilitation goal process. The purpose of this chapter has been to point out some of the possible areas of conflict or concern that may influence both the worker's and the employer's behaviors and to provide a basic introduction for practitioners to pursue further information, given the nature of their services and interventions for persons with disabilities.

ACKNOWLEDGMENTS

The authors' efforts in writing this material were supported by a grant from the U.S. Department of Education National Institute on Disability and Rehabilitation Research for a research demonstration project entitled "Improving Employment Practices Covered by Title I of the ADA" (Grant #H133A70005). The authors would like to acknowledge the helpful review and editing of an earlier version of this manuscript by Risa Lieberwitz, Associate Professor of Collective Bargaining, Cornell University School of Industrial and Labor Relations.

NOTES

1. A brief publication discussing these pieces of legislation, entitled *A Guide to Disability Rights Laws,* is available from the U.S. Department of Justice, Civil Rights Division, Disability Rights Section, P. O. 66738, Washington, DC 20035-6738; (800) 514-0301 (voice), (800) 514-0383 (TDD).
2. FY 1997 appropriation, as reported in the House Labor, Health and Human Services and Education Appropriations bill before the U.S. House of Representatives, August 1997.
3. For further information, contact the Council for State Administrators in Vocational Rehabilitation (CSAVR) Executive Office, P.O. Box 3776, Washington, DC 20007; phone (202) 638-4634; fax (202) 333-5881.
4. As reported in personal conversation with Roseanne Ashby, chief of the Basic State Grant Branch, Rehabilitation Services Administration, U.S. Department of Education, August 11, 1997.
5. To obtain more information or to file a complaint, employees should contact their agency's Equal Employment Opportunity Office.
6. For more information on section 503, contact Office of Federal Contract Compliance Programs, U.S. Department of Labor, 200 Constitution Ave., NW, Washington, DC 20210; (202) 219-9423 (voice/relay).
7. For information on how to file 504 complaints with the appropriate agency, contact Disability Rights Section, Civil Rights, Divisions, U.S. Department of Justice, PO Box 66738, Washington, DC 20035-6738; (800) 514-0301 (voice), (800) 514-0383 (TDD).
8. For additional information about the FMLA or to file an FMLA complaint, individuals should contact the nearest office of the Wage and Hour Division, Employment Standards Administration, U.S. Department of Labor. The Wage and Hour division is listed in most directories under U.S. Government, Department of Labor. For further information, contact the Office of Legal Counsel's Attorney of the Day at (202) 663-4691.
9. The EEOC fact sheet, the *Family and Medical Leave Act, the Americans with Disabilities Act, and Title VII of the Civil Rights Act* can be ordered by writing or calling the EEOC's Office of Communications and Legislative Affairs at 1801 L St., NW, Washington, DC 20507; telephone (202) 663-4900, TDD (202) 663-4494, or by accessing the EEOC Web site at eeoc.gov.

REFERENCES

Bell, C. (1994). The Americans with Disabilities Act and injured workers: Implications for rehabilitation professionals and the workers' compensation system. In S. Bruyère & J. O'Keeffe (Eds.), *Implications of the Americans with Disabilities Act for psychology* (pp. 137–149). New York: Springer Publishing/Washington, DC: American Psychological Association.

Bell, C. (1995). Integrating ADA and FMLA into workers' compensation and STD policies and practices. *Employee Benefits Digest*, *32*(5), 3–12.

Bruyère, S. (Ed.). (1996). *A job developer's guide to working with unions: Obtaining the support of organized labor for the hiring of employees with disabilities*. St. Augustine, FL: Training Resource Network.

Bruyère, S., Gomez, S., & Handelmann, G. (1996). The reasonable accommodation process in unionized environments. *Labor Law Journal*, *48*, 629–647.

Bureau of National Affairs. (1997). Job safety and health (No. 228). In *The Laws in Brief: OSHA*. Washington, DC: Author.

Commerce Clearing House. (1996). Family and medical leave. In *Employment practices guide* (pp. 1501–1503). Chicago: Author.

Commerce Clearing House. (1997). Communication and concern help workers return to work. In *Workers' Compensation Business Management Guide* (pp. 299–301). Chicago: Author.

Crewe, N. (1994). Implications of the Americans with Disabilities Act for the training of psychologists. *Rehabilitation Education*, *8*(1), 9–16.

EEOC answers biggest FMLA/ADA questions. (1997). *Disability Leave and Absence Reporter*, *104*, 4.

Evans, B. (1992). Will employers and unions cooperate? *HR Magazine*, *37*(11), 59–63.

Gault, R., & Kinnane, A. (1996). Navigating the maze of employment law. *Management Review*, *85*(2), 9–11.

Gold, M. (1989). *An introduction to labor law*. Ithaca, NY: Cornell University, ILR Press.

Huss, A. (1993). ADA, insurance, and employee benefits. *Journal of the American Society of CLU and ChFC*, *47*(5), 82–89.

Nobile, R. (1996). How discrimination laws affect compensation. *Compensation and Benefits Review*, *28*(4), 38–42.

O'Keeffe, J. (1994). Disability, discrimination, and the Americans with Disabilities Act. In S. Bruyère & J. O'Keeffe (Eds.), *Implications of the Americans with Disabilities Act for psychology* (pp. 1–14). New York: Springer Publishing/Washington, DC: American Psychological Association.

Pape, D., & Tarvydas, V. (1994). Responsible and responsive rehabilitation consultation on the ADA: The importance of training for psychologists. In S. Bruyère and J. O'Keeffe (Eds.), *Implications of the Americans with Disabilities Act for psychology* (pp. 169–186). New York: Springer Publishing/Washington, DC: American Psychological Association.

Pechman, L. (1995). Coping with mental disabilities in the workplace. *New York State Bar Journal*, *67*(5), 22, 24–26, 49.

President's Committee on Employment of People with Disabilities. (1994). *Seniority and collective bargaining issues and the Americans with Disabilities Act: A strategy for implementation.* Final Report of the Seniority/Collective Bargaining Agreement Work Group. Washington, DC: Author.

Rothstein, M. A. (1990). *Occupational safety and health law* (3rd ed., pp. 1–25). St. Paul, MN: West Publishing Co.

Scott, M. (1996). Compliance with ADA, FMLA, workers' compensation, and other laws requires road map. *Employee Benefit Plan Review, 50*(9), 20–30.

Setzer, S. (1992, February 24). Hiring restraints loom in disability law. *ENR News*, pp. 8–9.

Shalowitz, D. (1993, December 6). Return to work obstacle. *Business Insurance*, 2, 53.

Skoning, G., & McGlothlen, C. (1994). Other laws shape ADA policies. *Personnel Journal, 73*(4), 116.

Stude, E. (1994). Implications of the ADA for master's and bachelor's level rehabilitation counseling and rehabilitation services professionals. *Rehabilitation Education, 8*(1), 17–25.

Taylor, R. W. (1995). Medical examinations under the ADA and OSH Act: A camarinan dilemma for employers. *Employment in the Mainstream, 20*(6), 23–25.

U.S. Department of Justice. (1997). *A guide to disability rights laws*. Washington, DC: Author.

U.S. Equal Employment Opportunity Commission. (1992). *A technical assistance manual on the employment provisions (Title I) of the Americans with Disabilities Act*. Washington, DC: Author.

U.S. Equal Employment Opportunity Commission. (1996). *EEOC enforcement guidance: Workers' compensation and the ADA*. Washington, DC: Author.

U.S. Equal Employment Opportunity Commission. (1997). *EEOC enforcement guidance on the Americans with Disabilities Act and psychiatric disabilities* (No. 915.002). Washington, DC: Author.

Walker, J., & Heffner, F. (1992). The Americans with Disabilities Act and workers compensation. *CPCU Journal, 45*(3), 151–152.

Walworth, C., Damon, L., & Wilder, C. (1993). Walking a fine line: Managing the conflicting obligations of the Americans with Disabilities Act and workers' compensation laws. *Employee Relations, 19*(2), 221–232.

Welch, E. (1996). The EEOC, the ADA, and WC. *Ed Welch on Workers' Compensation, 6*(9), 178–179.

Winterbauer, S. (1997). The direct threat defense: Striking a balance between the duties to accommodate and to provide a safe workplace. *Employee Relations Law Journal, 23*(1), 5–35.

Wright, G. (1980). *Total rehabilitation*. Boston: Little, Brown.

Zolkos, R. (1994, July 18). Avoiding charges of bias. *Business Insurance*, p. 85.

Index